Endocrine and Metabolic Disorders

Endocrine and Metabolic Disorders

Edited by Dante Banks

hayle
medical

New York

Hayle Medical,
750 Third Avenue, 9th Floor,
New York, NY 10017, USA

Visit us on the World Wide Web at:
www.haylemedical.com

ISBN: 978-1-63241-596-7

Cataloging-in-Publication Data

Endocrine and metabolic disorders / edited by Dante Banks.
   p. cm.
Includes bibliographical references and index.
ISBN 978-1-63241-596-7
1. Endocrine glands--Diseases. 2. Metabolism--Disorders. 3. Endocrinology.
4. Metabolism. I. Banks, Dante.
RC648 .E53 2019
616.4--dc23

Table of Contents

Preface

The disorders of the endocrine system are known as endocrine disorders. Major endocrine glands are the pineal and the pituitary glands, the thymus, thyroid gland, adrenal gland, the pancreas and the ovary and the testes. Endocrine disorders include endocrine gland hypersecretion that leads to excessive hormone production, endocrine gland hyposecretion which leads to hormone deficit, and benign or malignant tumors of the endocrine glands. When abnormal chemical reactions occur in the body and alters the normal metabolic process of the body, it results in a metabolic disorder. It is an inherited genetic condition that creates an enzyme deficiency. The symptoms of metabolic disorders can be categorized as acute, progressive general, late-onset acute and permanent. Some common symptoms are weight loss, lethargy, seizures and jaundice. This book contains some path-breaking studies related to endocrine and metabolic disorders. It unravels the recent studies in the diagnosis, prevention and management of these disorders. For all readers who are interested in these domains, the case studies included in this book will serve as an excellent guide to develop a comprehensive understanding.

This book has been the outcome of endless efforts put in by authors and researchers on various issues and topics within the field. The book is a comprehensive collection of significant researches that are addressed in a variety of chapters. It will surely enhance the knowledge of the field among readers across the globe.

It gives us an immense pleasure to thank our researchers and authors for their efforts to submit their piece of writing before the deadlines. Finally in the end, I would like to thank my family and colleagues who have been a great source of inspiration and support.

Editor

Association of thyroid nodules with adiposity: a community-based cross-sectional study in China

Bin Song[1,2], Zhihua Zuo[1], Juan Tan[3], Jianjin Guo[4], Weiping Teng[5], Yibing Lu[1]* and Chao Liu[6]*

Abstract

Background: The association between thyroid nodules and adiposity remains controversial. We performed a cross-sectional, community-based study to examine whether thyroid nodules are associated with overweight and obesity, as defined with body mass index (BMI) and waist circumference.

Methods: The study included 1482 subjects (≥20 years of age; residing in Nanjing, China) receiving questionnaire interview, anthropometric measurements, laboratory tests and thyroid ultrasonography in 2009–2010. Overweight and obesity were defined as BMI ≥24 and ≥28 kg/m^2, respectively. Central obesity was defined as waist circumference at ≥90 cm in men and ≥80 cm in women. A sensitivity analysis was conducted using the American Diabetes Association (ADA) criteria for overweight and obesity (BMI ≥ 23 and ≥25 kg/m^2).

Results: Thyroid nodules were identified in 12.6% of the subjects. A greater proportion of the subjects with thyroid nodules had a BMI at ≥24 kg/m^2 (51.9% vs. 40.5% in those without thyroid nodules, $P = 0.003$) and central obesity (43. 3% vs. 24.2%, $P < 0.001$). After adjustment for other confounders, central obesity was still associated with significantly elevated risk of thyroid nodules (OR 1.62, 95%CI 1.14–2.28), whereas obesity/overweight based on BMI was not in both the main analysis and sensitivity analysis with the alternative criteria. In the subgroup analysis, BMI ≥24 kg/m^2 (OR 1.61, 95%CI 1.01–2.54), as well as BMI ≥25 kg/m^2 (OR 1.95, 95%CI 1.14–3.34), was significantly associated with higher risk of thyroid nodules among women. Using the ADA criteria, overweight and obesity were associated with thyroid nodules (OR 5.59, 95%CI 1.39–22.51 and 5.15, 95%CI 1.30–20.37) in thyroid-stimulating hormone (TSH) > 4.2 mIU/L subgroup. Central obesity correlated with higher risk of thyroid nodules regardless of age (< 50 years: OR 1.87, 95%CI 1.05–3.32: ≥50 years: OR 1.54, 95%CI 1.00–2.37) and in the following subgroups: men (OR 1.91, 95%CI 1.14–3.20), TSH > 4.2 mIU/L (OR 3.05, 95%CI 1.01–9.22), and urine iodine ≥200 μg/L (OR 1.79, 95%CI 1.14–2.81).

Conclusion: Waist circumference is superior to BMI for assessing risk of thyroid nodules in Chinese subjects.

Keywords: Thyroid nodules, Body mass index, Overweight, Waist circumference, Central obesity

Background

Thyroid nodules are one of the most common thyroid diseases and their incidence has been rising in recent decades worldwide. Although most thyroid nodules are benign, detecting them early is important because there is always risk that the nodules may be cancerous [1].

Several factors have been associated with the formation of thyroid nodules, including gender [2–4], age [2–9], thyroid-stimulating hormone (TSH) [9], and iodine intake [10, 11]. Numerous studies have also associated thyroid nodules with adiposity [3–5, 8, 9, 12–14], which is traditionally evaluated based on body mass index (BMI). While some studies have supported a positive correlation between BMI and risk of thyroid nodules [3, 5, 13], particularly in women, other studies have failed to detect this association [2, 6, 7], including our own work with children [15]. In addition, two case–control studies from different countries found that morbid obesity in

* Correspondence: luyibing2003@163.com; liuchao@nfmcn.com
[1]Department of Endocrinology, The Second Affiliated Hospital of Nanjing Medical University, 125 Jiangjiayuan Road, Nanjing 211166, China
[6]Endocrine and Diabetes Center, Affiliated Hospital of Integrated Traditional Chinese and Western Medicine, Nanjing University of Chinese Medicine, 8 Huadian East Road, Nanjing 210028, China
Full list of author information is available at the end of the article

women (BMI ≥40 kg/m^2) was associated with lower prevalence of thyroid nodules [12, 14]. These findings call into question whether BMI is useful as a predictor of thyroid nodule risk.

Another measure of adiposity is waist circumference. While BMI cannot distinguish between general adiposity and central (or abdominal) obesity, waist circumference reflects specifically central obesity. In several types of chronic diseases, including cardiovascular disease [16], renal disease [17] and metabolic syndrome [18], central obesity correlates more strongly with adverse health outcomes than higher BMI. Several studies have associated metabolic syndrome with increased prevalence of thyroid nodules [2, 4, 8, 9, 19], and one of these studies found waist circumference to correlate positively with thyroid nodules in men, although not in women [9].

Whether central obesity is associated with thyroid nodules is unclear. Studies from our group [4] and others [8] involving individuals showing moderate iodine intake have linked central obesity to higher prevalence of thyroid nodules, whereas another study of individuals with mild to moderate iodine deficiency failed to find this association after adjusting for insulin resistance [19]. These discrepancies may reflect differences in study design, sample size, ethnicity, gender and iodine levels.

Therefore we undertook the present study to clarify whether central obesity is significantly associated with the presence of thyroid nodules and may therefore serve as a useful indicator of thyroid nodule risk. In addition, we compared the association of thyroid nodule risk with higher waist circumference or elevated BMI in order to determine whether one of these adiposity indicators is superior to the other. Our study population came from our previous study designed to investigate thyroid diseases and iodine nutrition in a Chinese community-based population. Median urinary iodine concentration in this population was 239 μg/L, indicating more than adequate iodine intake [11].

Methods
Subjects
Participants in the present study were taken from the population analyzed in our multicenter, cross-sectional epidemiological investigation of thyroid diseases in 10 Chinese cities [11]. From among this population originally recruited in 2009–2010, we selected a community in Nanjing where most inhabitants had lived for more than 5 years. To avoid recruitment bias, we screened the residents based on their household registrations and stratified sampling by age to mirror the average age composition of Chinese urban populations, based on 2008 data from the Chinese National Bureau of Statistics. This led us to enroll 1572 individuals older than 20 years old (men: women, 1:1.2), who showed the following age distribution: 20–

29 years, 17.5%; 30–39 years, 23.2%; 40–49 years, 23.3%; 50–59 years, 17.9%; 60–69 years, 10.1%; ≥70 years, 7.9%.

Participants were excluded if they were pregnant women or women who had given birth during the preceding year; if they had adrenocortical insufficiency, renal insufficiency or other serious systemic disease; or if they were receiving any treatment that might affect thyroid function and iodine excretion, such as glucocorticoids, antiepileptic drugs, amiodarone or iodine-containing contrast agents. Details of the study design, eligibility, recruitment, survey procedures and participant characteristics were reported elsewhere [11, 20]. This study was conducted in accordance with the Declaration of Helsinki and approved by the medical ethics committee of China Medical University (serial number: IRB [2008]34) [11]. Written informed consent was obtained from all participants before any sample or data collection.

Data collection
As previously described [11], a structured questionnaire was administered by trained staff during a face-to-face interview in order to collect data on demographic characteristics, smoking status, dietary habits, type of salt used, and personal or family history of thyroid disease. Physical examination included weight (measured to nearest 0.5 kg), height (nearest 0.1 cm), waist circumference (nearest 0.1 cm) and blood pressure (nearest 1 mmHg). Height and weight were evaluated using a calibrated balance beam scale when subjects wore light clothes and were barefoot. Waist circumference was measured midway between the lowest rib and iliac crest using a tape measure while participants were standing and breathing normally. Systolic and diastolic blood pressure was measured using a standard manual mercury sphygmomanometer while the subject was seated. Pressure was measured twice at an interval of 30 s, and the readings were averaged. Overnight fasting blood and urine samples from all subjects were assayed for serum levels of TSH, thyroid peroxidase antibodies (TPOAb), thyroglobulin antibodies (TgAb) and urine iodine concentration (UIC). Normal reference ranges were 0.27–4.2 mIU/L for TSH, 0–34 IU/L for TPOAb and 0–115 IU/L for TgAb [11]. Thyroid ultrasonography was performed by professional physicians who had received centralized training using a portable instrument (LOGIQ a50, 7.5 MHz; GE Healthcare).

Definition of variables
A thyroid nodule was defined as a discrete lesion that was distinct from the surrounding thyroid parenchyma and that had a solid portion, regardless of whether a cystic portion was present [21]. Central obesity was defined as waist circumference ≥ 90 cm for men or ≥80 cm for women, based on the criteria recommended for Chinese adults by the International Diabetes Federation [22]. BMI

was calculated as weight (kg) divided by height (m) squared, and definition of overweight and obesity was BMI ≥ 24 and ≥28 kg/m^2, respectively, according to the 2016 China consensus statement on management of overweight/obesity [23]. Additionally, a sensitivity analysis was conducted using the American Diabetes Association definition for overweight (≥23 kg/m^2) and obesity (≥25 kg/m^2) for Asians [24]. Elevated TSH was defined as > 4.2 mIU/L, and the presence of antithyroid antibodies was defined as TPOAb > 34 IU/L or TgAb > 115 IU/L. UIC was classified as low if < 200 μg/L and high if ≥200 μg/L based on World Health Organization guidelines.

Statistical analysis

Continuous data are reported as mean ± standard deviation (SD) or median (interquartile range), while categorical data are reported as count and percentage. Differences in means, medians or proportions between individuals with or without thyroid nodules were assessed for significance using the Mann–Whitney U and chi-squared tests. Logistic regression was used to calculate odds ratios (ORs) and 95% confidence intervals (95%CIs) to assess the association of thyroid nodules with waist circumference or BMI. Adjusted logistic regression models took into account age, gender, education, profession, smoking status, systolic and diastolic blood pressure, TSH and UIC.

Subgroup analyses were performed by treating BMI and waist circumference as categorical variables and stratifying subjects based on four potential risk factors for thyroid nodules: gender, age (< 50 or ≥50 years), TSH (≤4.2 or > 4.2 mIU/L), and UIC (< 200 or ≥200 μg/L). Heterogeneity in the influence of BMI or waist circumference on thyroid nodules between participants with or without these factors was evaluated by adding an interaction term to the relevant adjusted model. All analyses were performed using EmpowerStats (http://www.empowerstats.com; X&Y Solutions, Boston, MA). A two-sided significance level of 0.05 was used to evaluate statistical significance.

Results

Baseline characteristics

Of the 1572 individuals recruited, 40 were excluded from the study because they did not complete the survey, resulting in a response rate of 97.4%. We excluded another 50 participants because of previous thyroid disease. In the end, 1482 subjects were included in the study (mean age, 44.5 ± 15.4 years), of whom 682 (46.0%) were males and 187 (12.6%) had thyroid nodules (Table 1). Mean BMI was 23.52 ± 3.33 kg/m^2 and mean waist circumference was 79.68 ± 9.56 cm; 41.9% of subjects had BMI ≥ 24 kg/m^2, and 26.7% had central obesity based on waist circumference. Individuals with thyroid nodules were significantly older than those without nodules (54.6 vs. 43.0 years, $P < 0.001$) and had significantly higher BMI

(24.10 vs. 23.44 kg/m^2, $P = 0.011$) and waist circumference (82.38 vs. 79.29 cm, $P = 0.030$), as well as significantly lower TSH (2.17 vs. 2.52 mIU/L, $P < 0.001$). The proportion of individuals with BMI ≥ 24 kg/m^2 was significantly higher among individuals with nodules (51.9% vs. 40.5%, $P = 0.003$), as was the proportion of individuals with central obesity (43.3% vs. 24.2%, $P < 0.001$). Individuals with or without thyroid nodules were similar in terms of gender composition, UIC, smoking status, family history of thyroid disease, iodized salt intake, seafood intake, and TPOAb or TgAb positivity.

Associations of thyroid nodules with waist circumference and BMI

Associations of BMI and waist circumference with thyroid nodules across the entire study population are shown in Table 2. BMI considered as a continuous variable (per 1 kg/m^2 increase) was associated with increased risk of thyroid nodules in the unadjusted model (OR 1.06, 95%CI 1.01–1.11), but this association was no longer significant after adjusting for age, gender, education, profession, smoking status, systolic and diastolic pressure, TSH and UIC (OR 1.02, 95%CI 0.97–1.07). BMI as a categorical variable was also associated with elevated risk of thyroid nodules: the OR for individuals with BMI ≥24 kg/m^2-relative to those with BMI < 24 kg/m^2 was 1.59 (95%CI 1.17–2.16) in the unadjusted model. Again, this association was not significant in the adjusted model (OR 1.33, 95%CI 0.95–1.86). Additionally, using the ADA definition for overweight (≥23 kg/m^2) and obesity (≥25 kg/m^2) for Asians, results are consistent and shown in Additional file 1: Table S1. In the unadjusted model, the ORs for individuals with BMI ≥23, < 25 kg/m^2 and BMI ≥25 kg/m^2 relative to those with BMI < 23 kg/m^2 were 1.62 (95%CI 1.10–2.40) and 1.70 (95%CI 1.19–2.44), respectively. Those associations were not significant in the adjusted model (OR 1.47, 95%CI 0.97–2.23 and OR 1.43, 95%CI 0.96–2.13, respectively).

Waist circumference considered as a continuous variable (per 1 cm increase) was significantly associated with increased risk of thyroid nodules in an unadjusted model (OR 1.03, 95%CI 1.02–1.05) as well as in the adjusted model (OR 1.02, 95%CI 1.00–1.04). Central obesity, defined according to a gender-specific waist circumference cut-off, was significantly associated with higher risk of thyroid nodules in the unadjusted model (OR 2.39, 95%CI 1.74–3.27) and adjusted model (OR 1.62, 95%CI 1.14–2.28).

Subgroup analyses based on gender, age, TSH and UIC

Possible relationships of thyroid nodules with BMI or waist circumference, both considered as categorical variables, were explored in different subgroups of study participants (Table 3). BMI ≥ 24 kg/m^2 was significantly associated with higher thyroid nodule risk only in

Table 1 Baseline characteristics of a community-based Chinese population with or without thyroid nodules

Characteristic	Total (n = 1482)	No nodules (n = 1295)	Nodules (n = 187)	P
Male	682 (46.0)	605 (46.7)	77 (41.2)	0.155
Age (years)	44.5 ± 15.4	43.0 ± 14.8	54.6 ± 15.3	< 0.001
BMI (kg/m^2)	23.52 ± 3.33	23.44 ± 3.35	24.10 ± 3.18	0.011
WC (cm)	79.68 ± 9.56	79.29 ± 9.53	82.38 ± 9.36	< 0.001
SBP (mmHg)	123.22 ± 16.83	122.38 ± 16.43	129.06 ± 18.38	< 0.001
DBP (mmHg)	78.42 ± 10.74	78.11 ± 10.70	80.55 ± 10.76	0.004
UIC (μg/L)	240.6 (163.6–336.5)	243.0 (165.2–338.1)	222.0 (151.6–328.6)	0.193
TSH (mIU/L)	2.48 (1.67–3.46)	2.52 (1.71–3.45)	2.17 (1.44–3.59)	0.030
Education				< 0.001
Primary school or illiterate	132 (8.9)	106 (8.2)	26 (13.9)	
Junior high school	399 (26.9)	334 (25.8)	65 (34.8)	
Senior high school	697 (47.0)	627 (48.4)	70 (37.4)	
Undergraduate or above	254 (17.1)	228 (17.6)	26 (13.9)	
Profession				< 0.001
Employed	1045 (70.5)	947 (73.1)	98 (52.4)	
Unemployed	354 (23.9)	271 (20.9)	83 (44.4)	
Not reported	83 (5.6)	77 (5.9)	6 (3.2)	
Smoking status				0.187
Never	1084 (73.1)	937 (72.4)	147 (78.6)	
Currently	386 (26.0)	347 (26.8)	39 (20.9)	
Formerly	12 (0.8)	11 (0.8)	1 (0.5)	
Family history of thyroid disease	43 (2.9)	35 (2.7)	8 (4.3)	0.241
Iodized salt	1450 (97.8)	1266 (97.8)	184 (98.4)	0.789
Seafood intake				0.851
Never	83 (5.6)	73 (5.6)	10 (5.3)	
Occasionally	1166 (78.7)	1021 (78.8)	145 (77.5)	
Frequently	233 (15.7)	201 (15.5)	32 (17.1)	
TPOAb positive	139 (9.4)	122 (9.4)	17 (9.1)	0.885
TgAb positive	163 (11.9)	141 (10.9)	22 (11.8)	0.720
BMI ≥24 kg/m^2	621 (41.9)	524 (40.5)	97 (51.9)	0.003
Central obesity	395 (26.7)	314 (24.2)	81 (43.3)	< 0.001

Continuous data are shown as the mean ± standard deviation or median (interquartile), and categorical data as n (%)

Table 2 Analysis of associations of thyroid nodules with BMI and waist circumference

Predictor	Unadjusted OR, 95%CI	P	[a]Adjusted OR, 95%CI	P
BMI (per kg/m^2)	1.06 (1.01, 1.11)	0.011	1.02 (0.97, 1.07)	0.459
BMI				
< 24 kg/m^2	Ref		Ref	
≥ 24 kg/m^2	1.59 (1.17, 2.16)	0.003	1.33 (0.95, 1.86)	0.100
Waist circumference (per cm)	1.03 (1.02, 1.05)	< 0.001	1.02 (1.00, 1.04)	0.034
Central obesity				
No	Ref		Ref	
Yes	2.39 (1.74, 3.27)	< 0.001	1.62 (1.14, 2.28)	0.007

[a]The adjusted OR controls for age, gender, education, profession, smoking status, systolic and diastolic blood pressure, TSH, and UIC

Table 3 Associations of thyroid nodules with BMI and waist circumference in subgroups of subjects stratified by gender, age, TSH or UIC

Predictor	N	BMI ≥24 kg/m²			Central obesity		
		Adjusted OR, 95%CI	P	P interaction	Adjusted OR, 95%CI	P	P interaction
Gender[a]							
Male	682	1.14 (0.68, 1.90)	0.626	0.372	1.91 (1.14, 3.20)	0.013	0.272
Female	800	1.61 (1.01, 2.54)	0.044		1.44 (0.89, 2.35)	0.142	
Age[b]							
< 50 years	958	1.61 (0.94, 2.74)	0.081	0.185	1.87 (1.05, 3.32)	0.033	0.632
≥ 50 years	524	1.14 (0.74, 1.75)	0.559		1.54 (1.00, 2.37)	0.048	
TSH[c]							
≤ 4.2 mIU/L	1259	1.17 (0.81, 1.68)	0.408	0.161	1.41 (0.97, 2.05)	0.069	0.194
> 4.2 mIU/L	223	2.52 (0.91, 6.99)	0.076		3.05 (1.01, 9.22)	0.048	
UIC[d]							
< 200 μg/L	543	1.08 (0.63, 1.85)	0.785	0.375	1.30 (0.75, 2.24)	0.351	0.373
≥ 200 μg/L	939	1.48 (0.95, 2.29)	0.082		1.79 (1.14, 2.81)	0.012	

[a]Adjusted for age, education, profession, smoking status, systolic and diastolic blood pressure, TSH, and UIC
[b]adjusted for gender, education, profession, smoking status, systolic and diastolic blood pressure, TSH, and UIC
[c]adjusted for age, gender, education, profession, smoking status, systolic and diastolic blood pressure, and UIC
[d]adjusted for age, gender, education, profession, smoking status, systolic and diastolic blood pressure, and TSH

women (OR 1.61, 95%CI 1.01–2.54), while central obesity significantly correlated with increased risk of thyroid nodules in men (OR 1.91, 95%CI 1.14–3.20), individuals younger than 50 years (OR 1.87, 95%CI 1.05–3.32), individuals at least 50 years (OR 1.54, 95%CI 1.00–2.37), individuals with TSH > 4.2 mIU/L (OR 3.05, 95%CI 1.01–9.22) and UIC ≥200 μg/L (OR 1.79, 95%CI, 1.14–2.81). Neither BMI ≥ 24 kg/m² nor central obesity interacted significantly with any of the four potential thyroid nodule risk factors of gender, age, TSH, or UIC (all P for interaction > 0.05).

Additionally, in the sensitivity analysis according to ADA definition for Asians (Additional file 2: Table S2), compared with BMI < 23 kg/m², BMI ≥ 25 kg/m² was significantly associated with higher thyroid nodule risk among women (OR 1.95, 95%CI 1.14–3.34) and individuals with TSH > 4.2 mIU/L (OR 5.15, 95%CI 1.30–20.37). Similarly, individuals with BMI ≥23, < 25 kg/m² relative to those with BMI < 23 kg/m² was 5.59 (95%CI 1.39–22.51) in TSH > 4.2 mIU/L subgroup. Interestingly, BMI based on 23 and 25 kg/m² interacted significantly with TSH (P for interaction = 0.044).

Discussion

In this cross-sectional study of a community-based population in China showing more than adequate iodine intake, we were unable to confirm a significant association between high BMI and risk of thyroid nodules, except for the subgroup of women. In contrast, we found an independent, positive correlation between waist circumference – treated as a categorical or continuous variable – and risk of thyroid nodules. Participants with

central obesity were at 1.62-fold higher risk of thyroid nodules than those with normal waist circumference, and this relationship was also observed in nearly all subgroup analyses. Our findings suggest that in Chinese individuals with more than adequate iodine intake, higher waist circumference is more strongly associated than higher BMI with elevated risk of thyroid nodules. This may mean that adipose tissue in the waist area may influence risk of thyroid nodules differently from adipose tissue elsewhere in the body.

Previous studies in different populations have reached conflicting conclusions about the association between BMI and risk of thyroid nodules. Two community-based studies in China reported that overweight and general obesity (as measured using BMI) were associated with higher risk of thyroid nodules only in women [5, 13], and we found the same result in our population when we treated BMI as a categorical variable. However, another Chinese study did not detect this association, perhaps because of insufficient sample size [2]. A previous community-based study in China found that BMI defined as a continuous variable correlated positively with risk of thyroid nodules [3], but two other studies involving healthy individuals undergoing physical exams failed to detect this association [6, 7], similar to our negative result in the present study. To make things more complicated, two studies outside Asia reported a negative relationship between BMI and risk of thyroid nodules [12, 14]. In light of the literature, we speculate that BMI may not correlate linearly with thyroid nodule risk, and so it may be unsuitable for assessing the influence of adiposity on the presence of thyroid nodules. Whether this is true only for Chinese populations or more broadly requires further study.

The poor performance of BMI as an indicator of thyroid nodules may relate to the fact that it is a quite nonspecific measure of adiposity, aggregating measures of muscle mass, peripheral and abdominal adipose tissue, and bone mass [17]. Waist circumference, in contrast, specifically reflects abdominal adipose distribution, which mainly consists of subcutaneous and visceral adipose tissue [25, 26]. This specificity may help to explain why waist circumference appears to be a better indicator of thyroid nodule risk. Central obesity has already been linked to greater likelihood of adverse metabolic health conditions [18, 27], including hyperglycemia, hypertension and dyslipidemia, which reflect a cluster of components in metabolic syndrome. Only approximately 20% of obese individuals (based on BMI) have metabolic disorders because of their smaller proportion of visceral adipose tissue [25]. In other words, larger waist circumference appears to be a stronger risk factor than BMI for metabolic syndrome [18]. Our finding of a strong correlation between waist circumference and thyroid nodule risk may therefore reflect the well-established correlation between metabolic syndrome and thyroid nodule risk [2, 4, 8, 9, 19]. Indeed, several of those previous studies have reported correlations between central obesity and thyroid nodule risk [4, 8, 9]. Central obesity lies at the core of metabolic syndrome [22], so it may not be surprising that our results show central obesity to be more closely associated with thyroid nodules than overweight and general obesity.

In our association analyses, we took into account age, gender, TSH and UIC as potential confounders. Thyroid nodules are known to be more prevalent in women [2–4] and older individuals [2–9], while waist circumference tends to larger in males and in the elderly. Thyroid nodule formation has been associated with TSH [9] and UIC [10, 11], and TSH has been associated with waist circumference [28]. Our observation that the increased risk of thyroid nodules was markedly attenuated after adjustment for these potential confounders suggests that these covariates also contribute to overall risk. Subgroup analyses showed that central obesity was significantly and independently associated with higher risk of thyroid nodules in nearly all subgroups, while BMI ≥ 24 kg/m^2 significantly correlated with increased risk of thyroid nodules only in women. This provides further evidence that, overall, central obesity is more strongly associated with risk of thyroid nodules than overweight and general obesity. The present study shows no evidence that gender, age, TSH, or UIC affects the observed relationship between risk of nodules and either BMI ≥ 24 kg/m^2 or central obesity. Certainly, according to American Diabetes Association definition for overweight (≥ 23 kg/m^2) and obesity (≥ 25 kg/m^2) for Asians [24], higher BMI was also significantly associated with higher thyroid nodule risk among individuals with TSH > 4.2 mIU/L, and TSH

played an interactive role in the association between BMI and TNs, which might deserve further researches.

We found central obesity to be significantly related to higher thyroid nodule risk in men but not in women. While further work is needed to confirm that this is not merely a sample size effect, we suggest that it may reflect sex differences in the proportion of abdominal fat components. Women tend to have larger stores of subcutaneous fat than visceral fat, while men tend to have more visceral fat than subcutaneous fat for any given waist circumference [25, 26]. This implies that increasing waist circumference represents, in men, primarily accumulation of visceral fat. Obese individuals with greater proportion of subcutaneous fat than visceral fat are at lower risk of metabolic syndrome than those with more visceral than subcutaneous fat [25]. These findings, when taken together with our present results, suggest that waist circumference-associated visceral fat may play a key role in the development of thyroid nodules.

These considerations may point to a key role of insulin resistance in formation of thyroid nodules. Visceral fat is the strongest predictor of insulin resistance [22, 25], which is a central contributor to metabolic syndrome [22]. One study in Italy found that while waist circumference was significantly associated with the presence of thyroid nodules, this association was no longer significant after adjusting for insulin resistance [19]. These results suggest that insulin resistance may be associated with thyroid nodule formation more strongly than even waist circumference. Indeed, our previous study of a large population suggested that insulin resistance is associated with the distribution, construction, and density of blood vessels in thyroid nodules [29]. Differences in such vascularization may help determine nodule growth and progression. It is possible that insulin resistance may cause changes in proliferative pathways activated directly by insulin or insulin-like growth factor-1 (IGF-1), which helps regulate thyroid gene expression and may be important in thyrocyte proliferation and differentiation [4, 30, 31]. Previous studies and the present work argue for focusing future research on the potential role of waist circumference-associated insulin resistance in the formation of thyroid nodules. The available evidence further suggests that effective diagnosis and treatment of insulin resistance may help prevent such nodules.

The present study extends previous work on associations of thyroid nodules with BMI or waist circumference to the case of a population with more than adequate iodine intake (UIC = 239 μg/L). In addition, our study was able to show that waist circumference was associated with thyroid nodules independently of TSH and UIC. These two thyroid nodule risk factors are usually ignored as potential confounders in the literature. Finally, our study systematically compared two adiposity measures, whereas most previous studies have focused on one or the other.

Nevertheless, the results of the present work should be interpreted with caution in light of several limitations. First, the cross-sectional study design does not allow us to establish causal links between obesity measures and thyroid nodules. Second, although the multivariate model adjusted for as many confounders as possible, we did not control for other components of metabolic syndrome, including hyperglycemia, hypertension and dyslipidemia. This reflects the fact that the original purpose of our study was to investigate relationships between iodine nutrition and thyroid diseases, so we did not collect information about history of hypertension, diabetes or dyslipidemia. Third, we did not examine whether the relationship of thyroid nodule risk to BMI or waist circumference depends on the specific nodule subtype.

Conclusions

In this community-based Chinese population showing more than adequate iodine intake, waist circumference was consistently and more strongly associated than BMI with higher risk of thyroid nodules. These results suggest that waist circumference may be the better indicator of thyroid nodule risk. Maintaining normal waist circumference may help prevent thyroid nodules, particularly in men.

Abbreviations

ADA: American Diabetes Association; BMI: body mass index; CI: Confidence interval; DBP: Diastolic blood pressure; IGF-1: Insulin-like growth factor-1; OR: Odds ratio; SBP: Systolic blood pressure; TgAb: Thyroglobulin antibodies; TPOAb: Thyroid peroxidase antibodies; TSH: Thyroid-stimulating hormone; UIC: Urine iodine concentration; WC: Waist circumference

Acknowledgements

Not applicable

Funding

Design and data collection were supported by the International Cooperation Foundation of the Ministry of Health of the People's Republic of China (2009); The development of the analytical methods and software used in this work was supported by the Foundation of Jiangsu Subei People's Hospital (yzucms201204), and writing the manuscript was supported in part by the Key Research and Development Project of Jiangsu Province (BE2015723)

Authors' contributions

WT developed the research questionnaire and wrote the protocol for this study. CL was responsible for the original study design and data collection together with the other authors. BS and ZZ analysed the data; BS and YL interpreted the results; BS, JT and ZZ wrote the article and the other authors revised it critically for important intellectual content. All authors agreed to take responsibility for the integrity of the data and the accuracy of the data analysis. All authors have approved the final version of the manuscript.

Competing interests

The authors declare that they have no competing interests.

Author details

[1]Department of Endocrinology, The Second Affiliated Hospital of Nanjing Medical University, 125 Jiangjiayuan Road, Nanjing 211166, China. [2]Department of Endocrinology, Clinical Medical College, Yangzhou University, 98 Nantong West Road, Yangzhou 225001, China. [3]Department of Gerontology, Huai'an First People's Hospital, Nanjing Medical University, 6 Beijing West Road, Huai'an 223300, China. [4]Department of Endocrinology, Second Hospital of Shanxi Medical University, 382 Wuyi Road, Taiyuan 030001, China. [5]Department of Endocrinology and Metabolism, The First Hospital of China Medical University, 155 Nanjing Road, Shenyang 110001, China. [6]Endocrine and Diabetes Center, Affiliated Hospital of Integrated Traditional Chinese and Western Medicine, Nanjing University of Chinese Medicine, 8 Huadian East Road, Nanjing 210028, China.

References

1. Burman KD, Wartofsky L. CLINICAL PRACTICE. Thyroid nodules. N Engl J Med. 2015;373(24):2347–56.
2. Guo H, Sun M, He W, Chen H, Li W, Tang J, Tang W, Lu J, Bi Y, Ning G, et al. The prevalence of thyroid nodules and its relationship with metabolic parameters in a Chinese community-based population aged over 40 years. Endocrine. 2014;45(2):230–5.
3. Jiang H, Tian Y, Yan W, Kong Y, Wang H, Wang A, Dou J, Liang P, Mu Y. The prevalence of thyroid nodules and an analysis of related lifestyle factors in Beijing communities. Int J Environ Res Public Health. 2016;13(4):442.
4. Feng S, Zhang Z, Xu S, Mao X, Feng Y, Zhu Y, Liu C. The prevalence of thyroid nodules and their association with metabolic syndrome risk factors in a moderate iodine intake area. Metab Syndr Relat Disord. 2017;15(2):93–7.
5. Xu W, Chen Z, Li N, Liu H, Huo L, Huang Y, Jin X, Deng J, Zhu S, Zhang S, et al. Relationship of anthropometric measurements to thyroid nodules in a Chinese population. BMJ Open. 2015;5(12):e008452.
6. Kim JY, Jung EJ, Park ST, Jeong SH, Jeong CY, Ju YT, Lee YJ, Hong SC, Choi SK, Ha WS. Body size and thyroid nodules in healthy Korean population. J Korean Surg Soc. 2012;82(1):13–7.
7. Sharen G, Zhang B, Zhao R, Sun J, Gai X, Lou H. Retrospective Epidemiological study of thyroid nodules by ultrasound in asymptomatic subjects. Chin Med J. 2014;127(9):1661–5.
8. Yin J, Wang C, Shao Q, Qu D, Song Z, Shan P, Zhang T, Xu J, Liang Q, Zhang S, et al. Relationship between the prevalence of thyroid nodules and metabolic syndrome in the iodine-adequate area of Hangzhou, China: a cross-sectional and cohort study. Int J Endocrinol. 2014;2014:675796.
9. Shin J, Kim MH, Yoon KH, Kang MI, Cha BY, Lim DJ. Relationship between metabolic syndrome and thyroid nodules in healthy Koreans. Korean J Intern Med. 2016;31(1):98–105.
10. Chen Z, Xu W, Huang Y, Jin X, Deng J, Zhu S, Liu H, Zhang S, Yu Y. Associations of noniodized salt and thyroid nodule among the Chinese population: a large cross-sectional study. Am J Clin Nutr. 2013;98(3):684–92.
11. Shan Z, Chen L, Lian X, Liu C, Shi B, Shi L, Tong N, Wang S, Weng J, Zhao J, et al. Iodine status and prevalence of thyroid disorders after introduction of mandatory universal salt iodization for 16 years in China: a cross-sectional study in 10 cities. Thyroid. 2016;26(8):1125–30.
12. Cappelli C, Pirola I, Mittempergher F, De Martino E, Casella C, Agosti B, Nascimbeni R, Formenti A, Rosei EA, Castellano M. Morbid obesity in women is associated to a lower prevalence of thyroid nodules. Obes Surg. 2012;22(3):460–4.
13. Zheng L, Yan W, Kong Y, Liang P, Mu Y. An epidemiological study of risk factors of thyroid nodule and goiter in Chinese women. Int J Environ Res Public Health. 2015;12(9):11608–20.
14. Sousa PA, Vaisman M, Carneiro JR, Guimarães L, Freitas H, Pinheiro MF,

Liechocki S, Monteiro CM, Teixeira PF. Prevalence of goiter and thyroid nodular disease in patients with class III obesity. Arq Bras Endocrinol Metabol. 2013;57(2):120–5.

15. Chen H, Zhang H, Tang W, Xi Q, Liu X, Duan Y, Liu C. Thyroid function and morphology in overweight and obese children and adolescents in a Chinese population. J Pediatr Endocrinol Metab. 2013;26(5–6):489–96.

16. Lo K, Wong M, Khalechelvam P, Tam W. Waist-to-height ratio, body mass index and waist circumference for screening paediatric cardio-metabolic risk factors: a meta-analysis. Obes Rev. 2016;17(12):1258–75.

17. Kramer H, Gutiérrez OM, Judd SE, Muntner P, Warnock DG, Tanner RM, Panwar B, Shoham DA, McClellan W. Waist circumference, body mass index, and ESRD in the REGARDS (reasons for geographic and racial differences in stroke) study. Am J Kidney Dis. 2016;67(1):62–9.

18. Zhang P, Wang R, Gao C, Jiang L, Lv X, Song Y, Li B. Prevalence of central obesity among adults with normal BMI and its association with metabolic diseases in Northeast China. PLoS One. 2016;11(7):e0160402.

19. Ayturk S, Gursoy A, Kut A, Anil C, Nar A, Tutuncu NB. Metabolic syndrome and its components are associated with increased thyroid volume and nodule prevalence in a mild-to-moderate iodine-deficient area. Eur J Endocrinol. 2009;161(4):599–605.

20. Yan YR, Liu Y, Huang H, Lv QG, Gao XL, Jiang J, Tong NW. Iodine nutrition and thyroid diseases in Chengdu, China: an epidemiological study. QJM. 2015;108(5):379–85.

21. Cooper DS, Doherty GM, Haugen BR, Hauger BR, Kloos RT, Lee SL, Mandel SJ, Mazzaferri EL, McIver B, Pacini F, et al. Revised American Thyroid Association management guidelines for patients with thyroid nodules and differentiated thyroid cancer. Thyroid. 2009;19(11):1167–214.

22. Alberti KG, Zimmet P, Shaw J. The metabolic syndrome–a new worldwide definition. Lancet. 2005;366(9491):1059–62.

23. Chen W. Consensus statement of the Chinese medical and nutritional experts on management for overweight/obesity in China (2016). Chin J Diabetes Mellitus. 2016;8(9):525–40.

24. American Diabetes Association. Standards of medical Care in Diabetes-2017 abridged for primary care providers. Clin Diabetes. 2017;35(1):5–26.

25. Power ML, Schulkin J. Sex differences in fat storage, fat metabolism, and the health risks from obesity: possible evolutionary origins. Br J Nutr. 2008;99(5):931–40.

26. Lemieux S, Prud'homme D, Bouchard C, Tremblay A, Després JP. Sex differences in the relation of visceral adipose tissue accumulation to total body fatness. Am J Clin Nutr. 1993;58(4):463–7.

27. Janssen I, Katzmarzyk PT, Ross R. Waist circumference and not body mass index explains obesity-related health risk. Am J Clin Nutr. 2004;79(3):379–84.

28. Mamtani M, Kulkarni H, Dyer TD, Almasy L, Mahaney MC, Duggirala R, Comuzzie AG, Samollow PB, Blangero J, Curran JE. Increased waist circumference is independently associated with hypothyroidism in Mexican Americans: replicative evidence from two large, population-based studies. BMC Endocr Disord. 2014;14:46.

29. Wang K, Yang Y, Wu Y, Chen J, Zhang D, Mao X, Wu X, Long X, Liu C. The association between insulin resistance and vascularization of thyroid nodules. J Clin Endocrinol Metab. 2015;100(1):184–92.

30. Marcello MA, Cunha LL, Batista FA, Ward LS. Obesity and thyroid cancer. Endocr Relat Cancer. 2014;21(5):T255–71.

31. Pappa T, Alevizaki M. Obesity and thyroid cancer: a clinical update. Thyroid. 2014;24(2):190–9.

2

Distinct metabolic profile according to the shape of the oral glucose tolerance test curve is related to whole glucose excursion: a cross-sectional study

Leonardo de Andrade Mesquita[1]* iD, Luciana Pavan Antoniolli[1], Giordano Fabricio Cittolin-Santos[1] and Fernando Gerchman[1,2]

Abstract

Background: The shapes of the plasma glucose concentration curve during the oral glucose tolerance test are related to different metabolic risk profiles and future risk of type 2 DM. We sought to further analyze the relationship between the specific shapes and hyperglycemic states, the metabolic syndrome and hormones involved in carbohydrate and lipid metabolism, and to isolate the effect of the shape by adjusting for the area under the glucose curve.

Methods: One hundred twenty one adult participants underwent a 2-h oral glucose tolerance test and were assigned to either the monophasic ($n = 97$) or the biphasic ($n = 24$) group based upon the rise and fall of their plasma glucose concentration. We evaluated anthropometric measures, blood pressure, lipid profile, high-sensitivity C-reactive protein, glycated hemoglobin, insulin sensitivity, beta-cell function, C-peptide, glucagon, adiponectin and pancreatic polypeptide.

Results: Subjects with monophasic curves had higher fasting and 2-h plasma glucose levels, while presenting lower insulin sensitivity, beta-cell function, HDL cholesterol, adiponectin and pancreatic polypeptide levels. Prediabetes and metabolic syndrome had a higher prevalence in this group. Glycated hemoglobin, total cholesterol, triglycerides, high-sensitivity C-reactive protein and glucagon were not significantly different between groups. After adjusting for the area under the glucose curve, only the differences in the 1-h and 2-h plasma glucose concentrations and HDL cholesterol levels between the monophasic and biphasic groups remained statistically significant.

Conclusions: Rates and intensity of metabolic dysfunction are higher in subjects with monophasic curves, who have lower insulin sensitivity and beta-cell function and a higher prevalence of prediabetes and metabolic syndrome. These differences, however, seem to be dependent on the area under the glucose curve.

Keywords: Shape of the glucose curve, Area under the glucose curve, Metabolic syndrome, Insulin resistance, Diabetes mellitus

* Correspondence: leonardodeamesquita@gmail.com
[1]Faculdade de Medicina da Universidade Federal do Rio Grande do Sul,
Ramiro Barcelos, 2400, Porto Alegre 90035-003, Brazil
Full list of author information is available at the end of the article

Background

Criteria for the diagnosis of diabetes mellitus (DM) and at-risk categories of glucose tolerance were established using the oral glucose tolerance test (OGTT) [1]. For this purpose, we currently use only plasma glucose measurements at fasting and 2 h after ingestion of 75 g of dextrose. Interestingly, insights into the natural history of glucose tolerance and DM have been derived from data such as the 1-h plasma glucose (1hPG) concentration [2–5], the relationship between the fasting and 2-h plasma glucose levels [6] and the shape of the glucose concentration curve.

Cross-sectional studies in diverse populations, including Latinos and obese youths [7–14], have assessed the shape of the glucose curve during the 2-h 75 g OGTT and demonstrated patterns associated with insulin resistance and beta-cell dysfunction. Two cohort studies [15, 16] showed a different future risk of impaired glucose metabolism and type 2 DM in individuals with distinct shapes of the OGTT glucose curve. Another cohort study [17] found a distinct risk of progression to type 1 DM according to the shape of the glucose curve in subjects with positivity for autoantibodies who were relatives of people with type 1 DM. On the other hand, a cross-sectional study [18] did not find different odds of prediabetes (PDM). Recent research in obese young subjects with distinct shapes of the glucose curve [19] demonstrated differences in free fatty acid response, plasma incretin levels and insulin sensitivity and insulin secretion, which were directly measured using the euglycemic hyperinsulinemic and hyperglycemic clamp techniques, respectively.

In the current study, we examined how the shape of the plasma glucose concentration curve during the OGTT relates to hyperglycemic states, the metabolic syndrome (MetS) and its components, and hormones involved in the carbohydrate and lipid metabolism. We also investigated whether any differences found were dependent only on the shape of the glucose curve.

Methods

Study design and setting

We performed a secondary analysis on data obtained between 2008 and 2015 from patients without a previous diagnosis of metabolic syndrome referred for outpatient care to the Metabolism Unit of Hospital de Clínicas de Porto Alegre, a tertiary hospital linked to Universidade Federal do Rio Grande do Sul, a public university in southern Brazil. These patients were enrolled in a cross-sectional study designed to examine the mechanisms and risk factors related to the development of type 2 diabetes and the metabolic syndrome. Additional information regarding the study protocol may be accessed elsewhere [20]. The study protocol was approved by the Institutional Review Board of Hospital de Clínicas de Porto Alegre.

Subjects

We included in the analysis adult individuals who had a complete, 2-h OGTT with five equally spaced measurements of plasma glucose and insulin concentration. Exclusion criteria included insulin treatment, autoimmune diseases, uncompensated hypo or hyperthyroidism, malignant disease that could affect 5-year survival, stage IV-V chronic kidney disease, HIV infection, pregnancy or lactation, dementia, cirrhosis, hepatitis, glucocorticoid treatment and malnutrition. Application of the criteria above resulted in the exclusion of 41 subjects from an initial population of 228. Of the remaining 187 individuals, 31 were excluded from the analysis due to presenting glucose curve shapes that did not fit criteria for any group. We excluded 35 subjects with DM from the main analysis, because of the possible distortion of the results when including extremes of insulin resistance. The final sample size consisted of 121 individuals (156 for the alternative analysis including subjects with DM).

All subjects provided written informed consent.

Measurements

We weighed subjects wearing light clothing without shoes. We used a stadiometer to measure height. We calculated body mass index (BMI) dividing the weight in kilograms by the height squared in meters. We measured waist circumference at the midpoint between the lower costal margin and the iliac crest, rounding values to the lowest 0.5 cm. We performed blood pressure (BP) measurements 1 week after the withdrawal of all antihypertensive medications. We measured office BP with an oscillometric monitor device (OMRON H-003D) with the appropriate cuff placed on the right arm of the patient, who had to be sitting for at least 5 min. We used the mean of the last two measurements to estimate systolic and diastolic BP.

Blood samples were taken after a 12-h overnight fast for analysis of plasma lipids (triglycerides, HDL and total cholesterol), glycated hemoglobin (HbA1c), high-sensitivity C-reactive protein (hs-CRP), adiponectin, glucagon, C-Peptide and pancreatic polypeptide (PP). Lipids were determined by an enzymatic method (Siemens ADVIA 1800 Chemistry System), HbA1c by high performance liquid chromatography (Tosoh Plus) and hs-CRP by turbidimetry (Siemens ADVIA 1800 Chemistry System). C-peptide was measured by chemiluminescent microparticle immunoassay (Abbott ARCHITECT; intra-assay coefficient of variation [CV] 2.7–3.2% and inter-assay CV < 10%). The enzyme-linked immunosorbent assay technique was used to determine glucagon (Yanaihara Institute; intra-assay CV < 5.1% and inter-assay CV < 18.9%), adiponectin (Invitrogen; intra-assay CV < 3.84% and inter-assay CV < 5.50%) and PP (Uscn Life Science; intra-assay CV < 10% and inter-assay CV < 12%).

After a 12-h overnight fast, subjects underwent a 75 g OGTT, with plasma glucose and serum insulin measured at baseline and 30, 60, 90 and 120 min. Plasma glucose was determined by an enzymatic method (Roche Cobas c501) and serum insulin by electrochemiluminescence (Centaur XP; inter-assay CV < 7.0%).

Calculations

We estimated insulin sensitivity with data obtained from the OGTT, using the Gutt insulin sensitivity index [21]:

$$\text{Gutt index} = \{[(75,000 \text{ mg} + (\text{FPG–2hPG}) \times 0.19 \times \text{body weight}) \div 120 \text{ min}] \div \text{mean plasma glucose}\} \div \log(\text{mean serum insulin}).$$

(FPG: fasting plasma glucose, 2hPG: 2-h plasma glucose; weight should be entered in kilograms, plasma glucose concentration in mg/dL and serum insulin levels in μU/mL)

This index was the most accurate in determining the presence of metabolic syndrome in our sample [22].

We calculated the insulinogenic index as the ratio between the changes in plasma insulin and glucose concentrations from baseline to 30 min after the oral glucose challenge, using the same units as in the Gutt index. We used the disposition index, obtained from the multiplication of the Gutt index and the insulinogenic index, to estimate beta-cell function.

Classification of glucose curves

We classified glucose curves according to previous studies [8, 12–14]. The "monophasic" (M) curve is defined by a rise in plasma glucose until a peak is reached, followed by a continuous fall. In subjects with a "biphasic" (B) curve, plasma glucose rises until a peak at 30′ or 60′, decreases and increases again from 90′ to 120′. In "triphasic" curves, plasma glucose increases from 0′ to 30′, decreases from 30′ to 60′, rises again from 60′ to 90′ and falls from 90′ to 120′. In this study, we included triphasic individuals ($n = 10$) in the biphasic group. We deemed a glucose curve shape "unclassifiable" if the difference in plasma glucose between 90′ and 120′ was lower than 0.25 mmol/L (except for triphasic curves, in which we applied this threshold to the change in plasma glucose between 60′ and 90′ instead). We also excluded subjects with a steady rise in plasma glucose concentration not followed by a fall, who did not fit into the previous groups. Models of each shape are shown in Fig. 1.

Definition of glucose tolerance statuses and metabolic syndrome

We used the American Diabetes Association criteria (based on FPG and 2hPG) [1] not considering HbA1c to categorize subjects as having normal glucose tolerance (FPG < 5.6 mmol/L and 2hPG < 7.8 mmol/L),

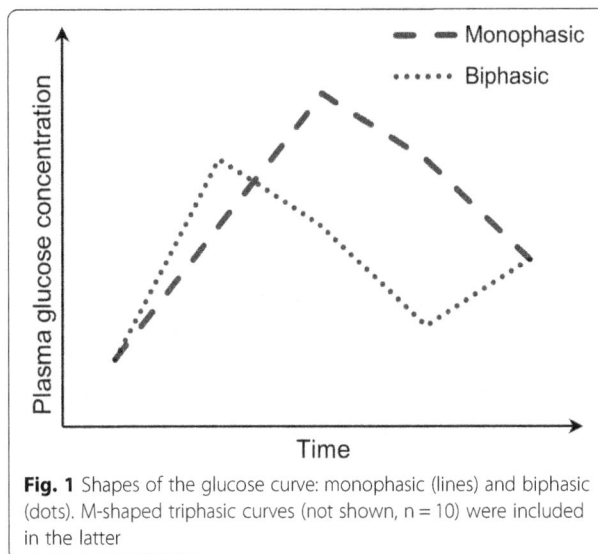

Fig. 1 Shapes of the glucose curve: monophasic (lines) and biphasic (dots). M-shaped triphasic curves (not shown, n = 10) were included in the latter

impaired fasting glucose (FPG 5.6–6.9 mmol/L, 2hPG < 7.8 mmol/L), impaired glucose tolerance (FPG < 5.6 mmol/L, 2hPG 7.8–11.0 mmol/L) or diabetes (FPG ≥ 7.0 mmol/L and/or 2hPG ≥ 11.1 mmol/L or use of medication for the control of DM). Subjects with either impaired fasting glucose or impaired glucose tolerance were considered to have prediabetes.

We defined the presence or absence of MetS according to the harmonization of metabolic syndrome criteria from the International Diabetes Federation, the American Heart Association and the National Heart, Lung and Blood Institute, among other organizations [23]. The chosen cut-off points for waist circumference were those of the previous International Diabetes Federation definition. We considered that a subject had MetS if he or she presented at least three of the following: waist circumference ≥ 94 cm for men or ≥ 80 cm for women; plasma triglyceride concentration ≥ 1.7 mmol/L or receiving drug treatment for this abnormality; HDL cholesterol < 1.0 mmol/L in males or < 1.3 mmol/L in females or receiving drug treatment for this abnormality; systolic BP ≥ 130 mmHg or diastolic BP ≥ 85 mmHg or receiving treatment for previously diagnosed hypertension; FPG ≥ 5.6 mmol/L or previous diagnosis of type 2 DM.

Statistical analysis

All data are reported in SI units (except for HbA1c, the Gutt, insulinogenic and disposition indices, adiponectin, glucagon and pancreatic polypeptide) and expressed as absolute number (%), mean ± standard deviation, or median [P25-P75]. For continuous variables, we assessed the normality of distribution using the Kolgomorov-Smirnov and Shapiro-Wilk tests. We compared demographic characteristics and clinical and laboratory data between groups using the chi-squared test, the Student's t-test or the

Mann-Whitney U test as appropriate. We adjusted for confounding variables by means of ANCOVA for continuous dependent variables (after log or reciprocal transformation of variables with non-normal distributions) and multiple logistic regression analysis for categorical dependent variables. In these analyses, the shape of the glucose curve was included as categorical independent variable (or factor) and each suspected confounding variable as the covariate in separate models. A p-value < 0.05 was considered statistically significant. Statistical analyses were performed in PASW Statistics 18 (IBM Corporation, Armonk, NY, USA). We used G-Power 3.1 (Heinrich Heine Universität Düsseldorf, Düsseldorf, Germany) to conduct a *post-hoc* power analysis, in which we determined the β error probability of this study and the sample size required to achieve a power of 80% to detect, in the multiple logistic regression analysis adjusted for glucose AUC, a difference in the prevalence of the metabolic syndrome according to the shape of the glucose curve similar to the one we found in the unadjusted comparison, setting the alpha error rate to 0.05. We would need a total sample size of 231 subjects in order to reach such power in this analysis.

Results

Data related to the OGTT and lipid profile were available for all subjects. For some subjects, data was missing as follows: waist circumference (1 female for B), blood pressure (2 for M, 1 for B), HbA1c (9 for M, 5 for B), hs-CRP (13 for M, 3 for B), adiponectin (13 for M, 3 for B), PP (28 for M, 10 for B), C-peptide (21 for M, 5 for B) and glucagon (39 for M, 13 for B).

97 subjects had glucose curves classified as monophasic and 24 as biphasic. The two groups had similar age,

sex and ethnic composition. The monophasic group showed a trend toward obesity when compared to the biphasic group, with higher BMI and waist circumference (in both males and females), though these differences did not achieve statistical significance. Details on demographic and anthropometric characteristics are shown in Table 1.

The monophasic group had higher plasma glucose levels at all timepoints and a greater area under the glucose curve (glucose AUC). While fasting and 2-h serum insulin levels and plasma C-peptide concentration were also higher in this group, insulin sensitivity, disposition index, HDL cholesterol, adiponectin and PP levels were lower, and we found no statistically significant difference between groups in hs-CRP, total cholesterol, triglycerides or glucagon levels. The same group also presented a higher prevalence of prediabetes and metabolic syndrome. Data regarding laboratory characteristics are displayed in Table 2 and the prevalence of PDM and MetS is depicted in Fig. 2.

In order to account for the potential confounding effect of the higher waist circumference in the monophasic group, we performed ANCOVA and logistic regression analyses. After adjustment, the differences in 30-min (30minPG), 1-h and 90-min (90minPG) plasma glucose concentration, glucose AUC, Gutt, insulinogenic and disposition indices, and HDL cholesterol levels remained statistically significant, and, while a trend for the monophasic group to have higher 2-h plasma glucose and serum insulin concentrations persisted, the differences did not reach statistical significance. Also, although not statistically significant, we observed a trend for the monophasic curve to predict the presence of the metabolic syndrome (odds ratio = 2.512 [95% CI: 0.959–6.585]).

Table 1 Demographic and clinical characteristics according to the shape of the plasma glucose curve

		Shape of the glucose curve		p-value
		Monophasic	Biphasic	
N		97	24	–
Age – years		51.96 ± 12.49	51.58 ± 10.73	0.893
Female sex – n (%)		73 (75.3)	20 (83.3)	0.401
White ethnicity – n (%)		82 (87.2)	18 (75.0)	0.137
BMI – kg/m²		31.36 ± 6.34	29.56 ± 4.48	0.192
Nutritional status – n (%)[a]	Lean	15 (15.5)	3 (12.5)	0.140
	Overweight	28 (28.9)	12 (50.0)	
	Obese	54 (55.7)	9 (37.5)	
Waist circumference – cm	Male	109.02 ± 14.98	94.00 ± 9.06	0.065
	Female	101.04 ± 14.42	96.71 ± 7.37	0.075
Blood pressure – mmHg	Systolic	136.93 ± 23.32	134.24 ± 18.93	0.608
	Diastolic	84.05 ± 13.00	86.63 ± 11.76	0.387

[a]Lean: BMI < 25 kg/m²; Overweight: BMI ≥ 25 kg/m² and < 30 kg/m²; Obese: BMI ≥ 30 kg/m²

Table 2 Laboratory characteristics according to the shape of the glucose curve

	Shape of the glucose curve		p-value
	Monophasic	Biphasic	
N	97	24	–
FPG – mmol/L	5.38 ± 0.63	5.15 ± 0.44	0.044[ab]
30minPG – mmol/L	9.22 [8.19–10.53]	7.83 [6.76–9.04]	0.001[ab]
1hPG – mmol/L	9.83 [8.36–11.64]	6.03 [5.33–8.71]	< 0.001[ab]
90minPG – mmol/L	9.16 ± 2.40	6.60 ± 1.87	< 0.001[ab]
2hPG – mmol/L	8.11 [5.92–9.39]	6.33 [5.07–8.49]	0.028[ab]
Glucose AUC – mmol/L.h	17.55 ± 3.49	13.79 ± 2.99	< 0.001[a]
HbA1c - %	5.81 ± 0.63	5.74 ± 0.51	0.630
Fasting serum insulin – pmol/L	66.18 [45.15–100.47]	44.07 [32.10–67.65]	0.016[ab]
2-h serum insulin – pmol/L	476.70 [284.07–1017.51]	301.50 [148.98–470.16]	0.012[ab]
Gutt index	3.22 [2.43–4.12]	3.95 [3.06–5.29]	0.006[ab]
Insulinogenic index	0.91 [0.53–1.48]	1.48 [0.70–2.95]	0.017[ab]
Disposition index	2.99 [1.76–5.82]	6.42 [3.16–11.55]	0.002[ab]
C-Peptide – nmol/L	0.76 [0.43–0.96]	0.43 [0.38–0.70]	0.027[ab]
Glucagon – ng/L	332.50 [200.00–640.00]	600.00 [220.00–780.00]	0.115
Total cholesterol – mmol/L	5.41 ± 1.14	5.41 ± 1.10	0.990
HDL cholesterol – mmol/L	1.22 [1.01–1.37]	1.53 [1.23–1.76]	< 0.001[ab]
Triglycerides – mmol/L	1.54 [1.04–2.14]	1.29 [0.80–1.67]	0.106
hs-CRP – nmol/L	25.67 [11.90–67.83]	25.71 [13.48–63.29]	0.930
Adiponectin – μg/mL	11.93 [9.06–15.74]	15.42 [11.24–21.20]	0.018[ab]
PP – pg/mL	194.20 [103.65–392.15]	464.45 [204.90–808.15]	0.049[ab]

[a]After adjustment for waist circumference: 0.254 for FPG, 0.004 for 30minPG, < 0.001 for 1hPG, < 0.001 for 90minPG, 0.075 for 2hPG, < 0.001 for glucose AUC, 0.311 for fasting serum insulin, 0.050 for 2-h serum insulin, 0.024 for Gutt index, 0.011 for insulinogenic index, 0.012 for disposition index, 0.291 for C-peptide, 0.003 for HDL cholesterol, 0.094 for adiponectin and 0.096 for PP.

[b]After adjustment for glucose AUC: 0.273 for FPG, 0.583 for 30minPG, < 0.001 for 1hPG, 0.348 for 90minPG, 0.049 for 2hPG, 0.379 for fasting serum insulin, 0.436 for 2-h serum insulin, 0.767 for Gutt index, 0.464 for insulinogenic index, 0.819 for disposition index, 0.697 for C-peptide, 0.005 for HDL cholesterol, 0.420 for adiponectin and 0.205 for PP

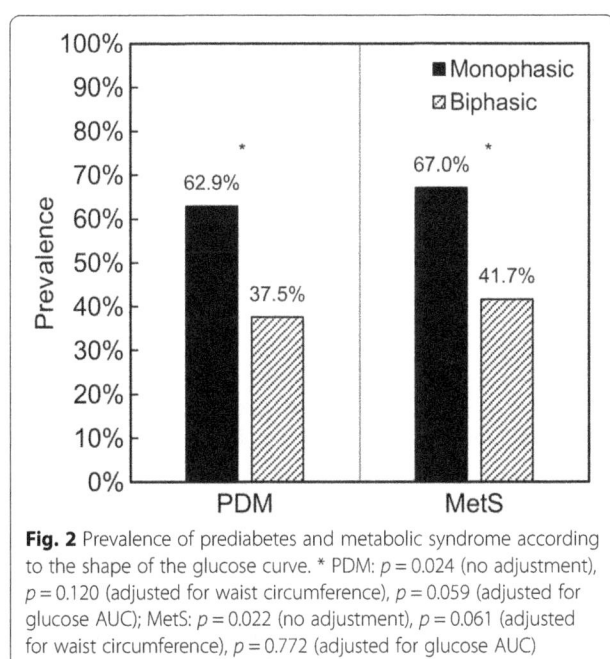

Fig. 2 Prevalence of prediabetes and metabolic syndrome according to the shape of the glucose curve. * PDM: $p = 0.024$ (no adjustment), $p = 0.120$ (adjusted for waist circumference), $p = 0.059$ (adjusted for glucose AUC); MetS: $p = 0.022$ (no adjustment), $p = 0.061$ (adjusted for waist circumference), $p = 0.772$ (adjusted for glucose AUC)

We used the same approach to check whether the findings were related purely to the shape of the glucose curve or dependent on the whole glucose excursion, represented by the glucose AUC. In other words, we would like to know whether two subjects with the same glucose load, i.e. the same glucose AUC in the OGTT, but with different shapes of the glucose curve, would still present a diverse phenotype. Only the differences in 1hPG, 2hPG and HDL cholesterol levels achieved statistical significance after this adjustment. In the model, the monophasic curve showed a trend to have a negative effect on the probability of prediabetes (odds ratio = 0.186 [95% CI: 0.032–1.066]).

Considering data on the OGTT, clinical and laboratory characteristics were available for 35 subjects with DM, whom we did not include in the main analysis because of the possibility of distortion of the results due to their condition as a metabolic extreme, we performed an alternative analysis including those individuals (Additional file 1: Table S1). In this expanded sample of 128 monophasic and 28 biphasic individuals, the comparisons yielded mostly similar results to the main analysis. However, the difference in C-peptide levels between the groups did not achieve statistical significance, while the waist circumference (in males) was higher and glucagon levels were lower in the monophasic group before adjustment. Also, we observed statistically significant differences in PP and glucagon, after adjusting for waist circumference, and in waist circumference (in males), FPG, 90minPG, 2-h serum insulin, glucagon, PP and the prevalence of impaired glucose metabolism, after adjusting for glucose AUC. On the other hand, the Gutt index was not significantly different after adjustment for waist circumference and 2hPG was not significantly different after adjustment for glucose AUC.

Discussion

This study demonstrates that subjects with monophasic glucose curves in the OGTT, compared with individuals with biphasic curves, have higher fasting plasma glucose and insulin concentrations at all time points. This group has, also, lower insulin sensitivity, insulin secretion, beta-cell function, HDL cholesterol, adiponectin and PP levels. The prevalence of impaired glucose metabolism and metabolic syndrome is also higher in the monophasic group. However, except for 1hPG, 2hPG and HDL cholesterol levels, these differences are not significant after adjusting for glucose AUC, a variable which reflects the whole glucose excursion these individuals are submitted to during the OGTT.

This relationship between the shape of the glucose curve and distinct metabolic profiles found in our study, with the monophasic group being at higher risk for metabolic dysfunction, corroborates the results of previous studies [8, 9, 11–14, 16, 18, 19]. Also, the finding that most differences were not significant after adjustment for glucose AUC is in agreement with the study by Tschritter et al. [8], which, to our knowledge, is the only one to have published results adjusted for glucose AUC, showing that most linear correlations between clinical/laboratory characteristics and the shape index (a quantitative measure for the shape of the glucose curve) were not significant. This added evidence brings up the hypothesis that the glucose AUC may be a better parameter for predicting metabolic dysfunction.

Surprisingly, even though the monophasic group has a higher prevalence of prediabetes in the unadjusted analysis, we found a trend for the monophasic curve to be associated with a lower probability of impaired glucose metabolism after adjustment for glucose AUC. We believe this may happen due to the diagnosis of prediabetes and diabetes being based on the fasting and 2-h plasma glucose values only [1]. Hence, if we consider subjects with the same glucose AUC, those who have an elevation at 120 min (biphasic) may be more prone to be diagnosed with impaired glucose metabolism. Nevertheless, since it did not reach statistical significance in the main analysis, this finding needs to be checked in high-powered studies.

In our study, in agreement with previous ones, subjects with biphasic curves displayed a better early-phase insulin secretion (as the insulinogenic index) [8, 9, 12–15]. This finding, along with the greater insulin sensitivity, may explain in part the biphasic curve, as plasma glucose concentration would fall in the early timepoints, followed by a rebound increase in the late OGTT [8, 9, 13, 14]. The exact reason for the existence of different shapes of the glucose curve, however, has not been elucidated yet. It may also involve differences in incretin levels and gastrointestinal physiology, requiring specific studies to explore the physiological intricacies behind the different shapes.

The main limitations of our study are the following. First, it has a limited sample size, with which we may not have been able to detect subtler differences between groups, especially in variables with a more significant proportion of missing data, such as the polypeptide hormones. HbA1c and hs-CRP also had a substantial amount of missing data, yet this had not affected the major outcome. As for the main analysis, we found that our study had a power of 53% and that we would need a total sample of 231 subjects to achieve a power of 80%. Hence, there is a need for studies with a higher sample size to analyze whether the null hypothesis of no difference in most metabolic parameters after controlling for glucose AUC holds true, since we expected to find the same differences despite the adjustment. Second, the cross-sectional design restrains the evaluation of the risk of developing impaired glucose metabolism and metabolic syndrome. Third, we performed a single execution of the OGTT, which does not allow us to make inferences on reproducibility of the shape of the glucose curve in this sample, something other studies [16, 24] have pointed out as relatively poor, and even describing that the combination of shapes of glucose curve from two OGTTs defines groups with different clinical and laboratory characteristics. Also, we estimated insulin sensitivity and beta-cell function with the Gutt and oral disposition indices respectively, instead of directly measuring them through the euglycemic-hyperinsulinemic and hyperglycemic clamp techniques. Nevertheless, previous studies have validated these surrogate measures against the gold standard clamp studies and demonstrated their relationship with clinical outcomes such as the presence of metabolic syndrome and future risk of diabetes [21, 22, 25]. Lastly, our classification of the shapes of the glucose curve - merging the biphasic and triphasic patterns and excluding individuals with a continuously rising plasma glucose concentration - is not based on solid scientific evidence, but is akin to the classification used in previous studies on the subject [8, 13, 18, 19].

Our study does not evaluate the use of the shape of the glucose curve as a tool in clinical practice. Our search did not return any article about the applicability of this parameter in the clinical setting (e.g. as criteria for differential testing or treatment). While the low reproducibility of this parameter and the neutralization of its impact after adjustment for the glucose AUC may limit its usefulness, specific studies are needed to give a definitive answer.

Conclusions

The monophasic curve is associated with a greater prevalence of prediabetes and metabolic syndrome, as well as with higher plasma glucose and insulin levels, and lower insulin sensitivity and beta-cell function, but most of the differences found between the groups are driven by the area under the glucose curve. Future studies are necessary to examine the reasons behind the existence of distinct behaviors of the glucose curve and why they are associated with different metabolic and clinical phenotypes.

Abbreviations

1hPG: 1-h plasma glucose; 2hPG: 2-h plasma glucose; 30minPG: 30-min plasma glucose; 90minPG: 90-min plasma glucose; B: Biphasic; BMI: Body mass index; BP: Blood pressure; CV: Coefficient of variation; DM: Diabetes mellitus; FPG: Fasting plasma glucose; glucose AUC: Area under the glucose curve; HbA1c: Glycated hemoglobin; hs-CRP: High-sensitivity C-reactive protein; M: Monophasic; MetS: Metabolic syndrome; OGTT: Oral glucose tolerance test; PDM: Prediabetes mellitus; PP: Pancreatic polypeptide

Acknowledgements

We would like to thank Dr. Ralph A. DeFronzo for reviewing the preliminary manuscript and making valuable comments. We would also like to recognize the work of the following persons, who integrate (or integrated) our research group and helped in the execution of the study: Anize D. von Frankenberg, Bárbara L. Nedel, Carina de Araújo, Giovana F. Piccoli, Letícia M. T. Silva, Lucas E. Gatelli, Mayara A. Beer, Monique de M. Machado, Raquel C. Fitz, Rodrigo S. de S. Marques, Tássia C. Pazinato and Vanessa Piccoli.

Funding

This work was supported by the Research Support Foundation of the State of Rio Grande do Sul (Fundação de Amparo à Pesquisa do Estado do Rio Grande do Sul – FAPERGS; grant number: 5989.284.18921.12062013), the Brazilian National Council for Scientific and Technologic Development (Conselho Nacional de Desenvolvimento Científico e Tecnológico – CNPq; grant number: 486802/2013–2) and the Hospital de Clínicas de Porto Alegre Research and Events Incentive Funds (Fundo de Incentivo à Pesquisa e Eventos – FIPE-HCPA). The funding sources had no role in the design of the study, collection, analysis and interpretation of data, nor in the drafting of the manuscript.

Authors' contributions

LdAM designed the analysis, interpreted the data and was a major contributor in writing the manuscript. LPA participated in the acquisition, sorting and analysis of data. GFCS contributed in drafting the manuscript. FG designed the original study and contributed in every stage of the present analysis. All authors read and approved the final manuscript.

Competing interests

The authors declare that they have no competing interests.

Author details

[1]Faculdade de Medicina da Universidade Federal do Rio Grande do Sul, Ramiro Barcelos, 2400, Porto Alegre 90035-003, Brazil. [2]Serviço de Endocrinologia do Hospital de Clínicas de Porto Alegre, Ramiro Barcelos, 2350, Porto Alegre 90035-903, Brazil.

References

1. Classification and diagnosis of diabetes. Diabetes Care [Internet]. 2017;40: S11–24. Available from: http://care.diabetesjournals.org/lookup/doi/10.2337/dc17-S005
2. Abdul-Ghani MA, Abdul-Ghani T, Ali N, Defronzo RA. One-hour plasma glucose concentration and the metabolic syndrome identify subjects at high risk for future type 2 diabetes. Diabetes Care. 2008;31:1650–5. [Internet] Available from: http://www.ncbi.nlm.nih.gov/pubmed/18487478%5Cnhttp://www.pubmedcentral.nih.gov/articlerender.fcgi?artid=PMC2494641
3. Bergman M, Chetrit A, Roth J, Dankner R. One-hour post-load plasma glucose level during the OGTT predicts mortality: observations from the Israel Study of Glucose Intolerance, Obesity and Hypertension. Diabet Med. 2016;33:1060–6. [Internet] [cited 2018 Jan 22] Available from: http://doi.wiley.com/10.1111/dme.13116
4. Bergman M, Chetrit A, Roth J, Jagannathan R, Sevick M, Dankner R. One-hour post-load plasma glucose level during the OGTT predicts dysglycemia: observations from the 25 year follow-up of the Israel study of glucose intolerance, obesity and hypertension. Diabetes Res Clin Pract. 2016;120:221–8. [Internet]. Elsevier. Available from: https://doi.org/10.1016/j.diabres.2016.08.013
5. Pareek M, Bhatt DL, Nielsen ML, Jagannathan R, Eriksson K-F, Nilsson PM, et al. Enhanced predictive capability of a 1-hour oral glucose tolerance test: A prospective population-based cohort study. Diabetes Care. 2018;41:171 LP–177. [Internet]. Available from: http://care.diabetesjournals.org/content/41/1/171.abstract
6. Abdul-Ghani MA, Williams K, DeFronzo R, Stern M. Risk of progression to type 2 diabetes based on relationship between postload plasma glucose and fasting plasma glucose. Diabetes Care. 2006;29:1613–8. [Internet] [cited 2017 May 2]. Available from: http://care.diabetesjournals.org/cgi/doi/10.2337/dc05-1711
7. Fuchigami M, Nakano H, Oba K, Metori S. Oral glucose tolerance test using a continuous blood sampling technique for analysis of the blood glucose curve (article in Japanese). Japanese J Geriatr. 1994;31:518–24.
8. Tschritter O, Fritsche A, Shirkavand F, Machicao F, Häring H, Stumvoll M. Assessing the shape of the glucose curve during an oral glucose tolerance test. Diabetes Care. 2003;26:1026–33.
9. Kanauchi M, Kimura K, Kanauchi K, Saito Y. Beta-cell function and insulin sensitivity contribute to the shape of plasma glucose curve during an oral glucose tolerance test in non-diabetic individuals. Int J Clin Pract. 2005;59: 427–32. [Internet] [cited 2017 Feb 13]. Available from: https://onlinelibrary.wiley.com/doi/abs/10.1111/j.1368-5031.2005.00422.x
10. Zhou W, Gu Y, Li H, Luo M. Assessing 1-h plasma glucose and shape of the glucose curve during oral glucose tolerance test. Eur J Endocrinol [Internet]. 2006;155:191–7. Available from: http://www.eje-online.org/content/155/1/191.abstract
11. Tura A, Morbiducci U, Sbrignadello S, Winhofer Y, Pacini G, Kautzky-Willer A. Shape of glucose, insulin, C-peptide curves during a 3-h oral glucose tolerance test: any relationship with the degree of glucose tolerance? AJP Regul Integr Comp Physiol [Internet]. 2011;300:R941–8. Available from: http://ajpregu.physiology.org/cgi/doi/10.1152/ajpregu.00650.2010
12. Nolfe G, Spreghini MR, Sforza RW, Morino G, Manco M. Beyond the morphology of the glucose curve following an oral glucose tolerance test in obese youth. Eur J Endocrinol [Internet]. 2012;166:107–14. Available from: http://www.eje-online.org/content/166/1/107.abstract

13. Kim JY, Coletta DK, Mandarino LJ, Shaibi GQ. Glucose response curve and type 2 diabetes risk in Latino adolescents. Diabetes Care [Internet]. 2012;35: 1925–30. Available from: http://care.diabetesjournals.org/cgi/doi/10.2337/dc11-2476

14. Bervoets L, Mewis A, Massa G. The shape of the plasma glucose curve during an oral glucose tolerance test as an indicator of beta cell function and insulin sensitivity in end-pubertal obese girls. Horm Metab Res. 2015;47: 445–51. [Internet]. Germany. Available from: http://www.thieme-connect.de/DOI/DOI?10.1055/s-0034-1395551

15. Abdul-Ghani MA, Lyssenko V, Tuomi T, DeFronzo RA, Groop L. The shape of plasma glucose concentration curve during OGTT predicts future risk of type 2 diabetes. Diabetes Metab Res Rev. 2010;26:280–6. [Internet] [cited 2017 Feb 13]. Available from: https://onlinelibrary.wiley.com/doi/abs/10.1002/dmrr.1084

16. Manco M, Nolfe G, Pataky Z, Monti L, Porcellati F, Gabriel R, et al. Shape of the OGTT glucose curve and risk of impaired glucose metabolism in the EGIR-RISC cohort. Metabolism. 2017;70:42–50. [Internet] . Elsevier. Available from: http://dx.doi.org/10.1016/j.metabol.2017.02.007

17. Ismail HM, Xu P, Libman IM, Becker DJ, Marks JB, Skyler JS, et al. The shape of the glucose concentration curve during an oral glucose tolerance test predicts risk for type 1 diabetes. Diabetologia. 2018;61:84-92. [Internet]. Springer Berlin Heidelberg. [cited 2017 Oct 29]. Available from: http://link.springer.com/10.1007/s00125-017-4453-6

18. Chung ST, Ha J, Onuzuruike AU, Kasturi K, Galvan-De La Cruz M, Bingham BA, et al. Time to glucose peak during an oral glucose tolerance test identifies prediabetes risk. Clin Endocrinol (Oxf). 2017;87:484–91. [Internet] . Available from: http://doi.wiley.com/10.1111/cen.13416

19. Kim JY, Michaliszyn SF, Nasr A, Lee SJ, Tfayli H, Hannon T, et al. The shape of the glucose response curve during an oral glucose tolerance test heralds biomarkers of type 2 diabetes risk in obese youth. Diabetes Care [Internet]. 2016;39:1431–9. Available from: http://care.diabetesjournals.org/content/39/8/1431.abstract

20. von Frankenberg AD, do Nascimento FV, Gatelli L, Nedel BL, Garcia SP, de Oliveira CS, et al. Major components of metabolic syndrome and adiponectin levels: a cross-sectional study. Diabetol Metab Syndr [Internet]. 2014;6:26. Available from: http://dmsjournal.biomedcentral.com/articles/10.1186/1758-5996-6-26

21. Gutt M, Davis CL, Spitzer SB, Llabre MM, Kumar M, Czarnecki EM, et al. Validation of the insulin sensitivity index (ISI0,120): Comparison with other measures. Diabetes Res Clin Pract. 2000;47:177–84. [Internet]. Elsevier. [cited 2017 Feb 13]. Available from: http://www.diabetesresearchclinicalpractice.com/article/S0168822799001163/fulltext

22. Antoniolli LP, Piccoli V, Beer MA, Nedel BL, Pazinato TC, Gatelli LE, et al. Accuracy of insulin resistance indices for metabolic syndrome in a population with different degrees of glucose tolerance. Diabetol Metab Syndr. 2015;7:51. [Internet]. BioMed Central. Available from: http://www.embase.com/search/results?subaction=viewrecord&from=export&id=L615888373%5Cnhttp://sfx.library.uu.nl/utrecht?sid=EMBASE&issn=17585996&id=doi:&atitle=Accuracy+of+insulin+resistance+indices+for+metabolic+syndrome+in+a+population+with+different+de

23. KGMM A, Eckel RH, Grundy SM, Zimmet PZ, Cleeman JI, Donato KA, et al. Harmonizing the metabolic syndrome: A joint interim statement of the international diabetes federation task force on epidemiology and prevention; National heart, lung, and blood institute; American heart association; World heart federation; International. Circulation [Internet]. 2009; 120:1640–5. Available from: http://circ.ahajournals.org/content/120/16/1640.abstract%5Cnhttp://circ.ahajournals.org/content/120/16/1640.full.pdf

24. Kramer CK, Vuksan V, Choi H, Zinman B, Retnakaran R. Emerging parameters of the insulin and glucose response on the oral glucose tolerance test: Reproducibility and implications for glucose homeostasis in individuals with and without diabetes. Diabetes Res Clin Pract. 2014;105:88–95. [Internet].

Elsevier. [cited 2017 Feb 14]. Available from: http://www.diabetesresearchclinicalpractice.com/article/S016882271400206X/fulltext

25. Utzschneider KM, Prigeon RL, Faulenbach MV, Tong J, Carr DB, Boyko EJ, et al. Oral Disposition Index Predicts the Development of Future Diabetes Above and Beyond Fasting and 2-h Glucose Levels. Diabetes Care [Internet]. 2009;32:335 LP–341. Available from: http://care.diabetesjournals.org/content/32/2/335.abstract

3

Postoperative tight glycemic control significantly reduces postoperative infection rates in patients undergoing surgery: a meta-analysis

Yuan-yuan Wang[1], Shuang-fei Hu[2], Hui-min Ying[1], Long Chen[2], Hui-li Li[1], Fang Tian[1] and Zhen-feng Zhou[2]* ⓘ

Abstract

Background: The benefit results of postoperative tight glycemic control (TGC) were controversial and there was a lack of well-powered studies that support current guideline recommendations.

Methods: The EMBASE, MEDLINE, and the Cochrane Library databases were searched utilizing the key words "Blood Glucose", "insulin" and "Postoperative Period" to retrieve all randomized controlled trials evaluating the benefits of postoperative TGC as compared to conventional glycemic control (CGC) in patients undergoing surgery.

Results: Fifteen studies involving 5053 patients were identified. As compared to CGC group, there were lower risks of total postoperative infection (9.4% vs. 15.8%; RR 0.586, 95% CI 0.504 to 0.680, $p < 0.001$) and wound infection (4.6% vs. 7.2%; RR 0.620, 95% CI 0.422 to 0.910, $p = 0.015$) in TGC group. TGC also showed a lower risk of postoperative short-term mortality (3.8% vs. 5.4%; RR 0.692, 95% CI 0.527 to 0.909, $p = 0.008$), but sensitivity analyses showed that the result was mainly influenced by one study. The patients in the TGC group experienced a significant higher rate of postoperative hypoglycemia (22.3% vs. 11.0%; RR 3.145, 95% CI 1.928 to 5.131, $p < 0.001$) and severe hypoglycemia (2.8% vs. 0.7%; RR 3.821, 95% CI 1.796 to 8.127, $p < 0.001$) as compared to CGC group. TGC showed less length of ICU stay (SMD, − 0.428 days; 95% CI, − 0.833 to − 0.022 days; $p = 0.039$). However, TGC showed a neutral effect on neurological dysfunction (1.1% vs. 2.4%; RR 0.499, 95% CI 0.219 to 1.137, $p = 0.098$), acute renal failure (3.3% vs. 5.4%, RR 0.610, 95% CI 0.359 to 1.038, $p = 0.068$), duration of mechanical ventilation ($p = 0.201$) and length of hospitalization ($p = 0.082$).

Conclusions: TGC immediately after surgery significantly reduces total postoperative infection rates and short-term mortality. However, it might limit conclusion regarding the efficacy of TGC for short-term mortality in sensitivity analyses. The patients in the TGC group experienced a significant higher rate of postoperative hypoglycemia. This study may suggest that TGC should be administrated under close glucose monitoring in patients undergoing surgery, especially in those with high postoperative infection risk.

Keywords: Tight glycemic control, Postoperative, Infection

* Correspondence: zhenfeng9853@163.com
[2]Department of Anesthesiology, Zhejiang Provincial People's Hospital
(People's Hospital of Hangzhou Medicine College), Hangzhou 315000, China
Full list of author information is available at the end of the article

Background

Tight glycemic control (TGC) was found to decrease the mortality and morbidity in critically ill patients [1] and it has therefore been recommended as the standard treatment for the duration of the perioperative intensive care unit (ICU) throughout the world. However, subsequent trials have failed to confirm the benefits of this recommendation [2, 3].

Perioperative hyperglycemia is reported in approximately 20–40% of patients after general surgery [4] and almost 80% of patients undergoing cardiac surgery [5]. Several studies in cardiac surgery and general surgery have shown a clear association between perioperative hyperglycemia and adverse clinical outcomes including delayed wound healing, surgical site infections, and prolonged hospital stay [4, 6]. However, the optimal glucose target during the post-operative period is widely controversial. No significant difference was found between TGC and conventional glycemic control (CGC) when evaluating the variety of complications [5, 7, 8]. However, another study. [9] including cardiac surgery patients reported a reduction of postoperative complications in TGC group.

Given the conflicting results and the lack of well-powered studies that support current guideline recommendations, the present study employed meta-analysis to evaluate the current evidence and analyze the association between the strategies of postoperative glycemic control and outcomes in patients undergoing elective surgery.

Methods

This meta-analysis was performed according to meta-analyses (PRISMA) format guidelines [10].

Search strategy

EMBASE, MEDLINE, and the Cochrane Library were searched electronically by two investigators (Long CHEN and Fang TIAN) for relevant studies, and the following key words were used: "Blood Glucose" "insulin" and "Postoperative Period". The searches were last updated in 16th April 2018. Search strategies are available in Additional file 1. Two investigators (Long CHEN and Fang TIAN) independently screened the titles and abstracts to exclude irrelevant articles. Then, they reviewed the full-text articles to ensure all relevant articles had been included. A third author resolved any controversies.

Study selection and data extraction

We only included randomized controlled trials (RCTs) with surgery patients who had received postoperative TGC. Specific eligibility criteria were as follows: (a) published in English; (b) treatment with postoperative TGC; and (c) the study documented any endpoints including

infection or mortality. Two authors (Long CHEN and Fang TIAN) evaluated all records according to the above eligibility criteria (Table 1). We abstracted the year of publication, sample size, type of surgery, population type (adult or infant), patient age, gender, history of diabetes, baseline BG (blood glucose level), time of TGC intervention (only during the post-operative or intra-operative plus post-operative), target BG and trigger BG for intervention, any insulin infusion protocol, and reported clinical outcomes.

Outcomes definition and quality assessment

The primary endpoint for the current review was any postoperative infection including wound infection, pneumonia, urinary tract infection and sepsis. Secondary efficacy outcomes were the duration of mechanical ventilation, length of ICU stay, length of hospital stay (LOS) and other adverse events included the following: (1) short-term mortality (30-day mortality or hospital mortality). Any postoperative mortality including the following outcomes: 30-day mortality, hospital mortality, 6-month mortality and 1-year mortality; (2) neurological dysfunction including delirium, seizures and stroke; (3) acute renal failure that required postoperative CRRT (continuous renal replacement therapy); and (4) hypoglycemia, which was defined as a BG < 70 mg/dL, and the reported severe hypoglycemia (BG < 40 mg/dL).

Quality of the included studies

The quality assessment of studies was independently performed by two investigators (Long CHEN and Fang TIAN) and the Jadad scale was used to assess the methodological quality of individual studies [11]. These evaluative criteria included the generation of allocation sequence (2 points), allocation concealment (2 points), investigator blindness (2 points), description of withdrawals and drop-outs (1 points), and the efficacy of randomization (2 points) (Additional file 2). The discrepancies were resolved by a third author.

Data synthesis and analysis

The statistical analysis was performed using STATA (Version 12.0). Dichotomous data were expressed as the risk ratio (relative risk [RR]) with 95% confidence interval (CI). Data were pooled using a random-effects model (M-H heterogeneity). Statistical heterogeneity was tested by the I^2 statistic and the $\chi 2$ test and heterogeneity was considered to be significant when values $I^2 > 50\%$ and $p \leq 0.05$. Subgroup analyses and meta-regression analyses were applied to detect the potential sources of heterogeneity. Sensitivity analysis was performed to assess the stability of the results. Publication bias was evaluated by Egger's and Begg's test, but it was not performed as the number of included studies was less than 10 [12]. All reported p values were two-tailed

Table 1 Main characteristics of the included trials

First author	Type of surgery	Patient type	Sample	Time of intervention	Insulin infusion protocol	Mean age (mean ± SD, year)		Male (%)		BMI(mean ± SD)	
			TGC/CGC			TGC	CGC	TGC	CGC	TGC	CGC
Van Den et al. (2001)	various surgeries	adult	1548(765/783)	postoperative	Yes	63.4 ± 13.6	62.2 ± 13.9	71	71	26.2 ± 4.4	25.8 ± 4.7
Salah M et al. (2013)	cardiac surgery	adult	100(50/50)	Intra + post operative	Yes	46.0 ± 9.0	49.0 ± 8.0	60	70	28.0 ± 0.8	26.0 ± 2.0
Konstantinos et al. (2013)	cardiac surgery	adult	212(105/107)	postoperative	Yes	64.9 ± 11.5	66.9 ± 11.1	66	68	27.8 ± 4.4	28.0 ± 3.9
Amisha et al. (2017)	liver transplantation	adult	164(82/82)	postoperative	Yes	58.1 ± 8.0	56.9 ± 7.6	65	65	30.3 ± 6.0	30.0 ± 6.6
Rehong Zheng et al. (2010)	cardiac surgery	adult	100(50/50)	Intra + post operative	Yes	43.3 ± 11.7	44.0 ± 11.5	48	46		
Raquel Pei Chen Chan et al. (2009)	cardiac surgery	adult	108(54/55)	Intra + post operative	Yes	57.0 ± 12.0	58 ± 12	43	56	24.0 ± 3.4	26.0 ± 4.9
Shou-gen Cao et al. (2011)	elective radical gastrectomy with D2 lymphadenectomy	adult	248(125/123)	postoperative	Yes	58.5 ± 8.1	59.9 ± 7.6	67	64	20.8 ± 2.1	21.2 ± 2.1
Shou-gen Cao et al. (2011)	elective radical gastrectomy with D2 lymphadenectomy	adult	179(92/87)	postoperative	Yes	58.2 ± 6.3	59.4 ± 7.3	30	34	21.1 ± 2.0	22.2 ± 2.6
Takehiro Okabayashi et al. (2014)	hepatectomy or pancreatectomy	adult	447(222/225)	Intra + post operative	No	66.7 ± 10.1	66.4 ± 10.4	64	67	23.3 ± 3.6	23.1 ± 3.4
Ehab A. Wahby et al. (2016)	cardiac surgery	adult	135(67/68)	Intra + post operative	No	54.99 ± 6.49	56.40 ± 7.79	73	68		
Federico Bilotta et al. (2009)	Neurosurgical	adult	483(241/242)	postoperative	Yes	57.3 ± 11.9	56.9 ± 12.7	63	52		
Shalin P. Desai et al. (2012)	cardiac surgery	adult	189(91/98)	postoperative	Yes	62.5 ± 10.2	62.8 ± 9.5	89	80		
Federico Bilotta et al. (2007)	Intracranial Aneurysm Clipping	adult	78(40/38)	Intra + post operative	Yes	53.0 ± 16.0	52.0 ± 15.0	30	32		
Michael SD Agus et al. (2012)	cardiac surgery	birth to 36 months	980(490/490)	postoperative	Yes	4.3(1.8–9.7) months	4.9(2.3–10.8) months	51	56		
Harold L et al. (2011)	cardiac surgery	adult	82(40/42)	Intra + post operative	Yes	63 ± 9	65 ± 9	65	76		
First author	History of diabetes (%)	Baseline blood glucose (mean ± SD, mg/dL)	Target blood glucose(mean ± SD, mg/dL)	Trigger blood glucose(mean/ mg/dL)	Postoperatively maintain blood glucose(mean ± SD, mg/dL)	Glucocorti-coids used		postoperative follow-up		Jadad Score	

Table 1 Main characteristics of the included trials *(Continued)*

First author	Type of surgery TGC	Type of surgery CGC	Patient type TGC	Sample CGC	Time of intervention TGC	Time of intervention CGC	Insulin infusion protocol TGC	Mean age (mean ± SD, year) CGC	Male (%) TGC	Male (%) CGC	BMI (mean ± SD)		
Van Den et al. (2001)	13	13			80–110	180–200	110	215	103 ± 19	153 ± 33	No	in-hospital	6
Salah M et al. (2013)	100	100			80–110	110–180	110	180			No	6 months	2
Konstantinos et al. (2013)	26	31			120–160	161–200	160	200	153.9 ± 13.9	173.9 ± 17.4	No	30 days or in-hospital	1
Amisha et al. (2017)	28	32					140	180	146.4 ± 16.4	178.8 ± 24.0	Yes	1 year	4
Rehong Zheng et al. (2010)	0	0	78.4 ± 3.8	77.5 ± 2.6	70–110		110				No		2
Raquel Pei Chen Chan et al. (2009)	0	0	113.4 ± 42.5	138 ± 75	80–130	160–200	130	200	126.7 ± 10.8	168.2 ± 28.3	No	30 days	3
Shou-gen Cao et al. (2011)	0	0	99.0 ± 14.4	95 ± 13	80–110	< 200	110	200	94.5 ± 15.3	184.0 ± 16.7	No	28 days	2
Shou-gen Cao et al. (2011)	100	100	122.4 ± 10.8	126 ± 13	80–110	180–215	110	215	99 ± 14.4	178.2 ± 18	No	28 days	1
Takehiro et al. (2014)	24	26			80–110	140–180	110	180			No	1 day	2
Ehab A. Wahby et al. (2016)	100	100	164.1 ± 12.1	167 ± 17	110–149	150–180					No	weaned from mechanical ventilation	2
Federico Bilotta et al. (2009)	10	10	179 ± 32	181 ± 29	80–110	180–215	110	215	92.3 ± 2.5	143.3 ± 20.3	Yes	6 months	6
Shalin P. Desai et al. (2012)	41	45			90–120	121–180					No	30 days	1
Federico Bilotta et al. (2007)	10	11			80–120	80–220					Yes	6 months	5
Michael SD Agus et al. (2012)	0	0			80–110		110		112(104–120)	121(109–136)	Yes	30 days	6
Harold L et al. (2011)	100	100	161 ± 50	151 ± 35	80–120	120–180	120	180	103 ± 17	135 ± 12	No	30 days	1

TGC tight glycemic control, CGC conventional glycemic control

and values of less than 0.05 were considered to be statistically significant.

Sample size calculation and power analysis

Previous study showed a significant benefit for an intensive compared with a conventional glucose control protocol in reducing post-operative infection (OR 0·43, 0·29 to 0·64), but no significant benefit of death was found (OR 0·74, 0·45 to 1·23) [13]. A two-tailed power analysis with 0.80 power and an α of 0.05 was used. The post-operative infection and short-term mortality in CGC group was 15.8 and 5.4% respectively, with an estimated standard deviation of 249 patients were needed for post-operative infection and 4020 patients were needed for short-term mortality per study group. About 2233 patients per group were included in the study so the analysis was underpowered to identify an effect of TGC on mortality. Analysis was computed using GPower 3.1.9.2 Software.

Results

Study selection and characteristics

Our search strategy identified 4191 articles. After screening the titles and abstracts, 4119 articles were excluded. The remaining 72 articles underwent a full-text review, although the study by van den Berghe et al. included adults receiving mechanical ventilation who were admitted to intensive care unit (which included mainly surgical patients (about 92%) and 62.5% had undergone cardiac surgery), because of the importance of this study, we still included it in our meta-analysis. Finally a total of 15 articles that had enrolled 5053 patients were finally included in this meta-analysis [1, 14–27] (Fig. 1). The detailed characteristics of these studies are presented in Table 1. About 1056 (20.9%) patients had diabetes, nine articles of included 15 articles mainly reported cardiac surgery including 3455 patients (68.4%). Among the included 15 articles, eight articles define tight glycemic control and trigger blood glucose as blood glucose ≤110 mg/dL, three articles were ≤ 120 mg/dL, the last four articles were ≤ 130 mg/dL, ≤140 mg/dL, ≤150 mg/dL and ≤ 160 mg/dL respectively. Eight articles only tight control the blood glucose postoperatively, the other seven articles were during intra and post operative period. The average Jadad Score of the studies included in the meta-analyses was 2.9, only five studies have exceeded 4.

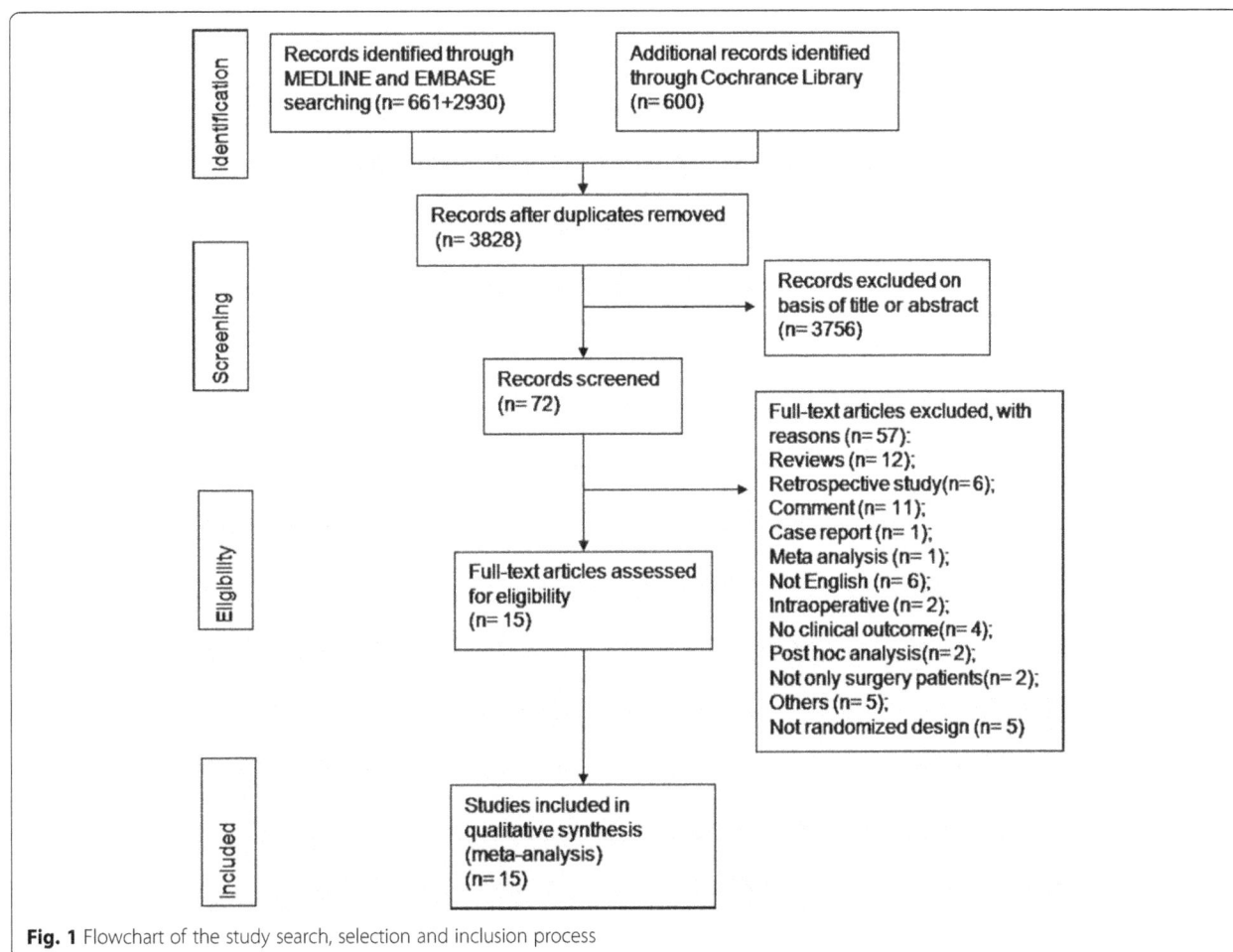

Fig. 1 Flowchart of the study search, selection and inclusion process

Primary outcomes

Risk of postoperative infection

Fourteen studies ($n = 4952$) compared the effectiveness of TGC versus CGC with respect to postoperative infection. These studies revealed that the risk of total postoperative infection (9.4% vs. 15.8%; RR 0.586, 95% CI 0.504 to 0.680, $p < 0.001$; Fig. 2) and sepsis (2.7% vs. 4.7%; RR 0.594, 95% CI 0.418 to 0.842, $p = 0.003$) were significantly lower in the TGC group than in the CGC group. The most frequent type of infection in the TGC group and CGC group was wound infection (4.6% vs. 7.2%; RR 0.620, 95% CI 0.422 to 1.910, $p = 0.015$). However, no difference was found in pneumonia (2.0% vs. 2.9%; RR 0.692, 95% CI 0.400 to 1.196, $p = 0.187$) and urinary tract infection (3.6% vs. 4.4%; RR 0.843, 95% CI 0.548 to 1.297, $p = 0.437$). In addition, there was no significant heterogeneity between articles ($I^2 < 50\%$, $p > 0.05$; Table 2).

Sensitivity analysis and publication Bias

The results of sensitivity analyses showed consistency in the results with the omission of a single article per replication (Additional file 3: Table S1). A funnel plot of the risk of postoperative infection identified all studies in the 95% confidence limits (Additional file 4: Figure S1).

Risk of postoperative short-term mortality

Of the 15 studies included, 13 studies ($n = 4492$) compared the effectiveness of TGC versus CGC to assess the risk of postoperative short-term mortality. TGC showed a lower risk of postoperative short-term mortality (3.8% vs. 5.4%; RR 0.692, 95% CI 0.527 to 0.909, $p = 0.008$; Fig. 3) and any postoperative mortality (6.3% vs. 8.0%; RR 0.792, 95% CI 0.653 to 0.960, $p = 0.018$; Additional file 5: Figure S2) without evidence of heterogeneity between articles ($I^2 < 0.001\%$, $p > 0.05$; Table 2).

Sensitivity analysis and publication Bias

Sensitivity analyses showed that the result was mainly influenced by the study of van den Berghe when eliminating one single study per replication (Additional file 6: Table S2). A funnel plot of the risk of postoperative short-term mortality revealed that no included studies exceeded the 95% confidence limits (Additional file 7: Figure S3). Begg's ($p = 0.533$ for short-term mortality and $p = 0.951$ for any postoperative mortality; Additional

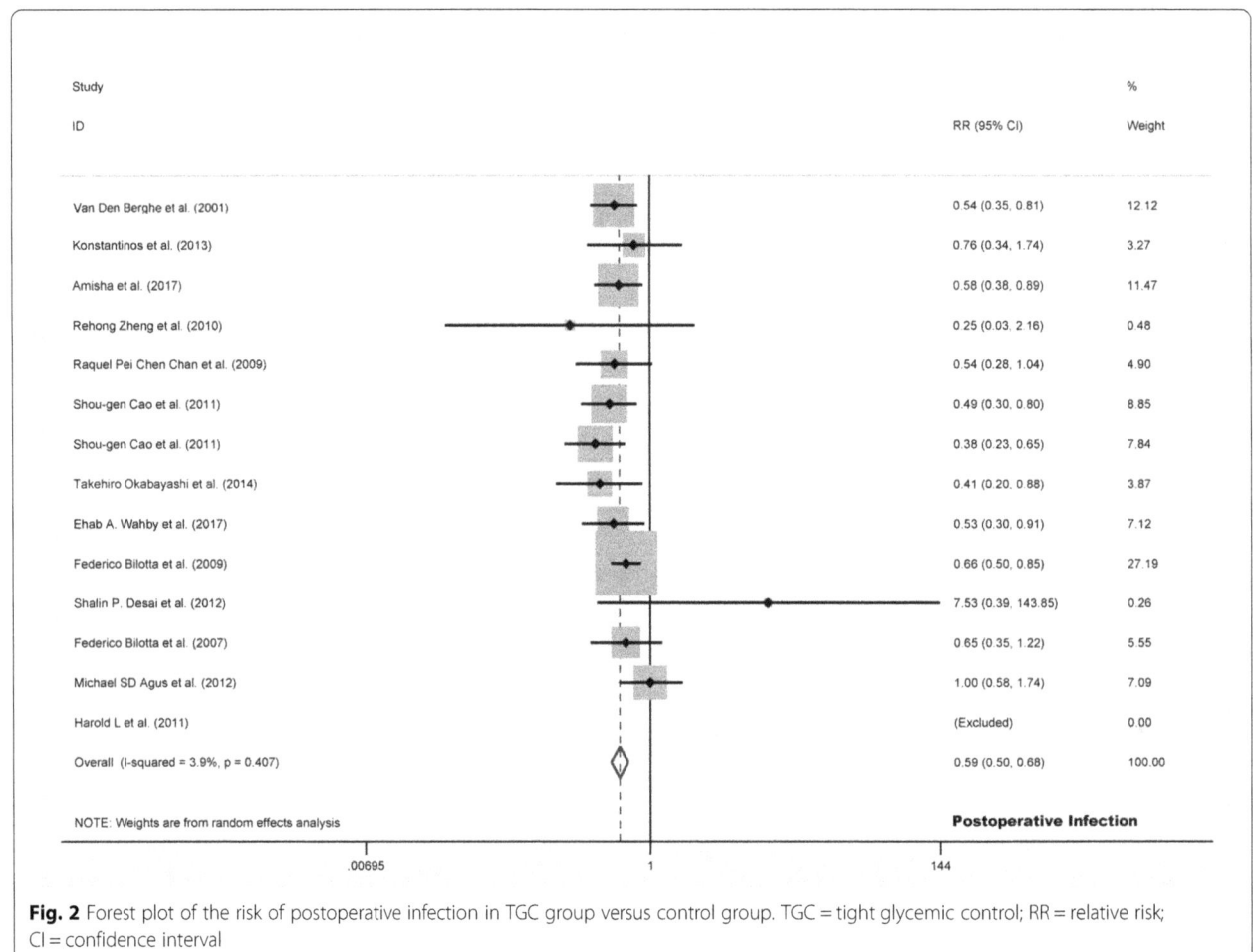

Fig. 2 Forest plot of the risk of postoperative infection in TGC group versus control group. TGC = tight glycemic control; RR = relative risk; CI = confidence interval

Table 2 Postoperative adverse events and other outcomes

Events	Studies	TGC		CGC		Overall event rates (%)	M-H pooled RR		Heterogeneity	
		N+(%)	Total	N+(%)	Total		RR/ SMD (95%CI)	p	I^2 (%)	p
Infection	[1, 15–27]	231(9.4%)	2464	392(15.8%)	2488	12.6%	0.586(0.504, 0.680)	< 0.001	3.9	0.407
Sepsis	[1, 19, 20, 23, 25, 26]	48(2.7%)	1753	82(4.7%)	1763	3.7%	0.594(0.418, 0.842)	0.003	< 0.001	0.945
Pneumonia	[19, 20, 23–26]	22(2.0%)	1079	31(2.9%)	1078	2.5%	0.692(0.400, 1.196)	0.187	< 0.001	0.511
Urinary tract infection	[19, 20, 23, 25, 30]	36(3.6%)	988	43(4.4%)	980	4.0%	0.843(0.548, 1.297)	0.437	< 0.001	0.682
Wound infection	[19, 20, 22–27]	54(4.6%)	1186	86(7.2%)	1188	6.1%	0.620(0.422, 0.910)	0.015	18.8	0.287
Short-term mortality	[1, 14–22, 24, 27]	85(3.8%)	2233	122(5.4%)	2259	4.6%	0.692(0.527, 0.909)	0.008	< 0.001	0.769
Any mortality	[1, 14–27]	159(6.3%)	2514	204(8.0%)	2539	7.2%	0.792(0.653, 0.960)	0.018	< 0.001	0.738
Neurological dysfunction	[14, 18, 22, 24, 26]	8(1.1%)	752	18(2.4%)	761	1.7%	0.499(0.219, 1.137)	0.098	< 0.001	0.651
Acute renal failure	[1, 22, 24, 26]	46(3.3%)	1413	78(5.4%)	1439	4.3%	0.610(0.359, 1.038)	0.068	16.0	0.312
Hypoglycemia	[1, 16–20, 22–24, 27]	467(22.3%)	2097	233(11.0%)	2118	16.6%	3.145(1.928, 5.131)	< 0.001	81.4	< 0.001
Severe hypoglycemia	[15, 16, 19–21, 24, 26]	34(2.8%)	1207	8(0.7%)	1210	1.7%	3.821(1.796, 8.127)	< 0.001	< 0.001	0.894
ICU stay	[1, 15, 16, 18, 23, 26, 27]						−0.428(−0.833, −0.022)	0.039	96.6	< 0.001
Mechanical ventilation	[1, 15, 16, 18, 23, 26, 27]						−0.275(−0.695,0.146)	0.201	96.9	< 0.001
LOS	[15, 16, 18–20, 26, 27]						−0.233(−0.496,0.030)	0.082	85.4	< 0.001

N^+ the number of patient with adverse event, *Total* the number of the total patients, *RR* relative risk, *SMD* standardised mean difference, *LOS* length of hospital stay

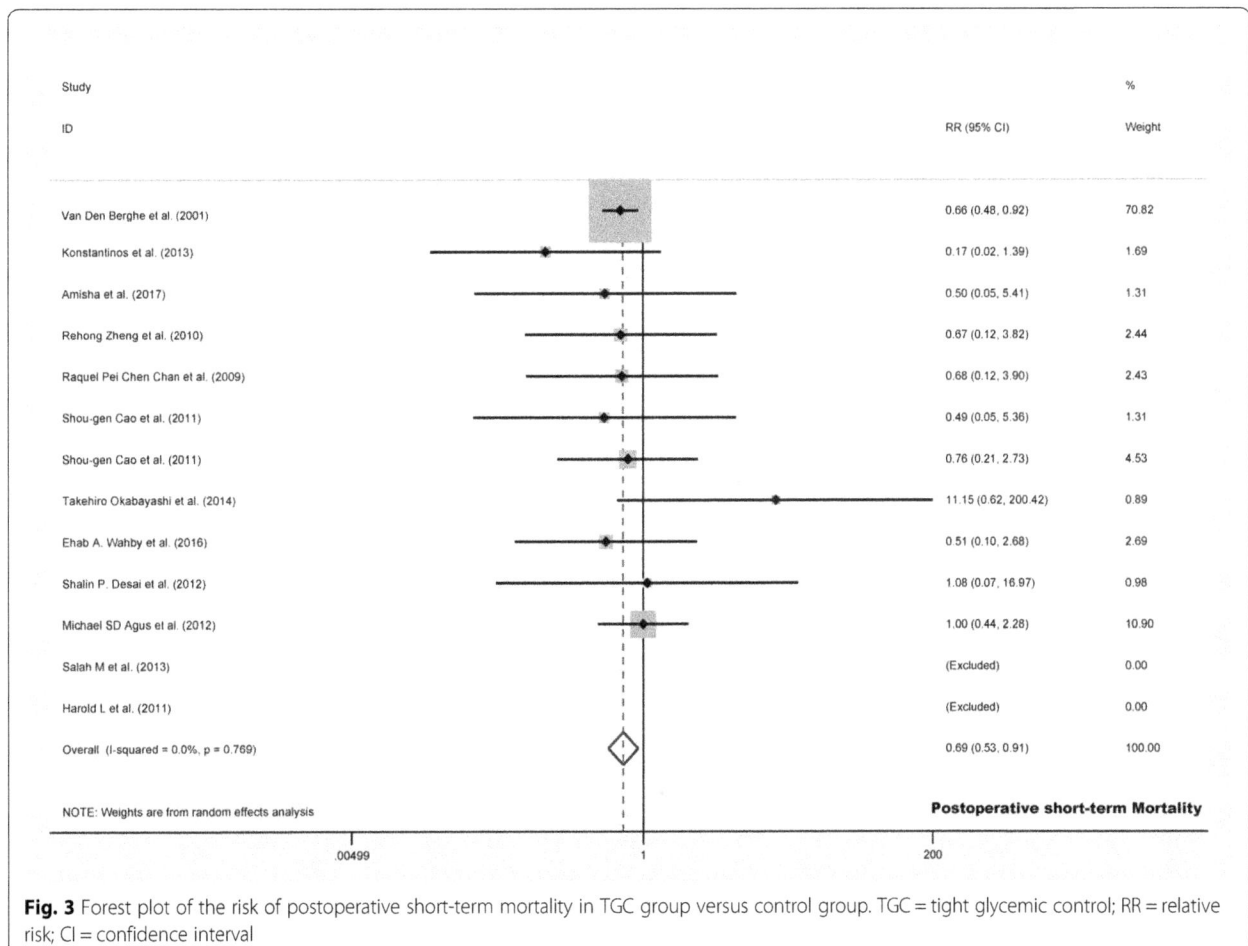

Fig. 3 Forest plot of the risk of postoperative short-term mortality in TGC group versus control group. TGC = tight glycemic control; RR = relative risk; CI = confidence interval

file 8: Figure S4A) and Egger's test ($p = 0.741$ for short-term mortality and $p = 0.814$ for any postoperative mortality; Additional file 8: Figure S4B) did not identify significant publication bias.

Risk of postoperative neurological dysfunction and acute renal failure

Only five ($n = 1513$) and four ($n = 2852$) articles reported postoperative neurological dysfunction and postoperative acute renal failure respectively. No significant difference was observed in postoperative neurological dysfunction (1.1% vs. 2.4%; RR 0.499, 95% CI 0.219 to 1.137, $p = 0.098$) and postoperative acute renal failure (3.3% vs. 5.4%; RR 0.610, 95% CI 0.359 to 1.038, $p = 0.068$), and no significant heterogeneity was observed between articles ($I^2 < 50\%$, $p > 0.05$; Table 2). In addition, sensitivity analyses revealed a consistency of the results based on the omission of a single article at a time for acute renal failure, but not for neurological dysfunction (Additional file 9: Table S3, Additional file 10: Table S4). Publication bias analysis was not performed as the number of included studies was less than 10 [12].

Risk of postoperative hypoglycemia

Eleven ($n = 4215$) studies compared the safety of TGC versus CGC to assess the risk of postoperative hypoglycemia. We observed more patients experiencing postoperative hypoglycemia (22.3% vs. 11.0%; RR 3.145, 95% CI 1.928 to 5.131, $p < 0.001$; Fig. 4) and severe hypoglycemia (2.8% vs. 0.7%; RR 3.821, 95% CI 1.796 to 8.127, $p < 0.001$; Additional file 11: Figure S5) in the TGC group as compared to the CGC group. No significant heterogeneity was observed respect to severe hypoglycemia ($I^2 < 0.001\%$, $p = 0.894$), however, there was significant heterogeneity between articles with a corresponding I^2 of 81.4% ($p < 0.001$) with respect to postoperative hypoglycemia (Table 2).

Sensitivity analysis and publication Bias

Sensitivity analyses revealed that there was no significant heterogeneity of postoperative hypoglycemia ($I^2 = 33.9\%$, $p = 0.137$ Additional file 12: Table S5) when we omitted Federico Bilotta's study of neurosurgical patients. The result was consisted with a significant higher rate of postoperative hypoglycemia in the TGC groups (13.0% vs. 4.3%; RR 3.361, 95% CI 2.311 to 4.890, $p < 0.001$;

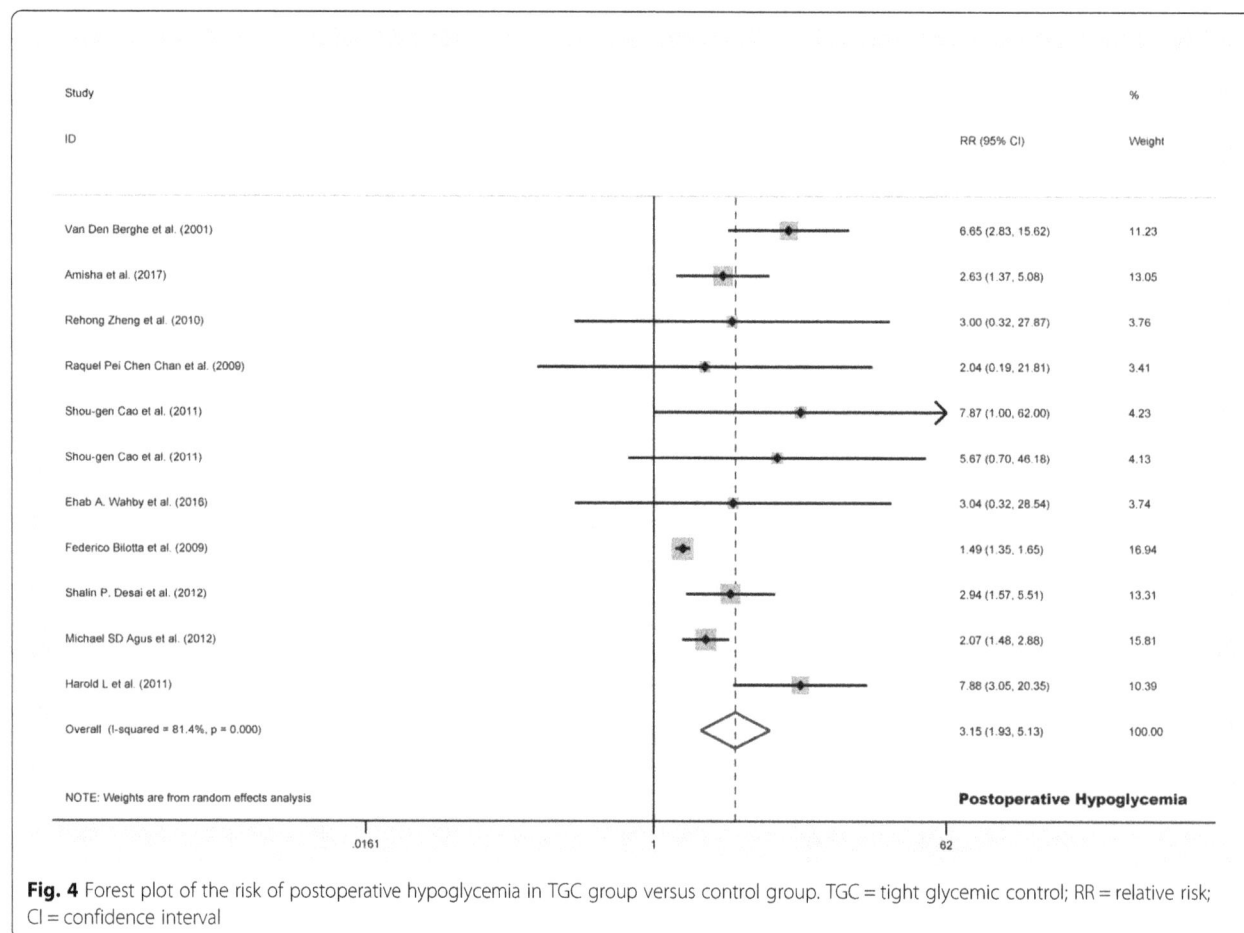

Study ID	RR (95% CI)	% Weight
Van Den Berghe et al. (2001)	6.65 (2.83, 15.62)	11.23
Amisha et al. (2017)	2.63 (1.37, 5.08)	13.05
Rehong Zheng et al. (2010)	3.00 (0.32, 27.87)	3.76
Raquel Pei Chen Chan et al. (2009)	2.04 (0.19, 21.81)	3.41
Shou-gen Cao et al. (2011)	7.87 (1.00, 62.00)	4.23
Shou-gen Cao et al. (2011)	5.67 (0.70, 46.18)	4.13
Ehab A. Wahby et al. (2016)	3.04 (0.32, 28.54)	3.74
Federico Bilotta et al. (2009)	1.49 (1.35, 1.65)	16.94
Shalin P. Desai et al. (2012)	2.94 (1.57, 5.51)	13.31
Michael SD Agus et al. (2012)	2.07 (1.48, 2.88)	15.81
Harold L et al. (2011)	7.88 (3.05, 20.35)	10.39
Overall (I-squared = 81.4%, p = 0.000)	3.15 (1.93, 5.13)	100.00

NOTE: Weights are from random effects analysis

Postoperative Hypoglycemia

.0161   1   62

Fig. 4 Forest plot of the risk of postoperative hypoglycemia in TGC group versus control group. TGC = tight glycemic control; RR = relative risk; CI = confidence interval

Additional file 12: Table S5). A funnel plot of the risk of postoperative hypoglycemia identified two studies beyond the 95% confidence limits (Additional file 13: Figure S6).

Sensitivity analyses showed consistency in the results of severe hypoglycemia with the omission of a single article per replication (Additional file 14: Table S6).

Subgroup analysis and meta-regression of postoperative hypoglycemia

Then, subgroup analyses and meta-regression were further applied to examine the sources of the heterogeneity. In the subgroup analyses, we found that the type of surgery, but not preoperative diabetes, the type of patient, the time of intervention, the trigger of blood glucose level, and the use of glucocorticoids in the hospital, could explain the heterogeneity (Additional file 15: Table S7).

However, the result of meta-regression could not identify that the type of surgery was the source of the heterogeneity. The use of glucocorticoids in the hospital was seem to be the source of the observed heterogeneity, but factors such as preoperative diabetes, the type of patient, the time of intervention, trigger of blood glucose level, the mean age, the sample size and the quality of the study did not seem to be the source of the observed heterogeneity (Additional file 16: Table S8).

Length of ICU stay and hospitalization

About half of the included studies reported duration of mechanical ventilation, length of ICU stay and hospitalization. TGC showed less length of ICU stay (SMD, – 0.428 days; 95% CI, – 0.833 to – 0.022 days; p = 0.039, Additional file 17: Figure S7), but TGC showed neutral effect on postoperative duration of mechanical ventilation (SMD, – 0.275 h; 95% CI, – 0.695 to 0.146 h; p = 0.201, Additional file 18: Figure S8) and length of hospitalization (SMD, – 0.233 days; 95% CI, – 0.496 to 0.030 days; p = 0.082, Additional file 19: Figure S9) (Table 2). In the sensitivity analysis, we found significant heterogeneity between the studies (Additional file 20: Table S9, Additional file 21: Table S10, Additional file 22: Table S11).

Subgroup analysis and meta-regression of ICU stay and hospitalization

The results of the subgroup analyses and meta-regression analyses revealed that the type of surgery, preoperative diabetes, type of patient, time of intervention, trigger of blood glucose level and use of glucocorticoids in hospital, the year of publication, the mean age, the sample size, and the quality of the study could not identify the heterogeneity; thus, heterogeneity persisted between the included articles (Additional file 23: Table S12, Additional file 24:

Table S13, Additional file 25: Table S14, Additional file 26: Table S15, Additional file 27: Table S16, Additional file 28: Table S17).

Discussion

In the current meta-analysis of randomized trials, we found that when compared to CGC, TGC immediately after surgery significantly reduces total postoperative infection rates and short-term mortality. However, it might limit conclusion regarding the efficacy of TGC for short-term mortality in sensitivity analyses. The patients in the TGC group experienced a significant higher rate of postoperative hypoglycemia. TGC had a neutral effect on the risk of postoperative neurological dysfunction and acute renal failure in patients undergoing surgery. Although there was significant heterogeneity of hypoglycemia between studies, which was primarily caused by the study of Federico Bilotta et al., the pooled RR still derived the same results after omitting this study.

There was still some controversy on the positive effects of TGC in reducing postoperative infection. Some meta-analysis found that intra-operative TGC [28] or using a TGC strategy in the perioperative period (< 150 mg/dl) [13] decreased the infection rate when compared to the conventional therapy; however, other meta-analyses have reported negative effects [29, 30]. Furthermore, most of those studies just focused on cardiac surgery. A recent retrospective analysis [31] found that the basal + premeal insulin regimen was associated with a reduced rate of postoperative infective complications than the premeal insulin alone therapy, without increasing the number of severe hypoglycemic events. These results suggest that type of treatments more than levels of glycemic controls might have on beneficial effect these outcomes. This meta-analysis has shown that TGC significantly reduced total postoperative infection, wound infection and sepsis regardless of whether TGC was commenced during or after surgery, but no difference was found in pneumonia and urinary tract infection. This study may suggest that TGC should be administrated especially in those with high postoperative infection risk.

Our meta-analysis further supported the study of van den Berghe [1] that perioperative TGC reduce the rates of postoperative short-term mortality, but sensitivity analyses showed a negative result when eliminating the study of van den Berghe. It might limit conclusion regarding the efficacy of TGC for mortality. Another meta-analysis [32] also found that moderate perioperative glycemic control (BG 150–200 mg/dL) was associated with lower postoperative mortality and stroke in patients with diabetes, whereas no additional benefit was found in a stricter glycemic control group (BG < 150 mg/dL). We should also note that this meta-analysis not only includes randomized studies, but also retrospective studies. A recent retrospective study analyzed a large database of patients in critical care units [33] and found that TGC (80–110 mg/dL) was associated with the lowest mortality. However, previous meta-analysis found that perioperative TGC did not reduce the rates of short-term mortality in ICU settings [29] or in various hospital settings [28, 34] when compared to the conventional therapy. In the NICE-SUGAR trial (Normoglycemia in Intensive Care Evaluation-Survival Using Glucose Algorithm Regulation trial), 6104 critically ill patients in intensive care units (ICUs) were randomized to an intensive blood glucose control (81–108 mg/dL) or conventional glucose control (< 180 mg/dL) group. It showed that TGC actually increased 90-day mortality and hypoglycemia compared to a more liberal glucose target in the ICU setting [2, 3]. Recently, in the GLUCO-CABG trial [5], CABG patients were randomized to TGC (100 to 140 mg/dL) and CGC (141 to 180 mg/dL) groups just in the ICU. The two groups had no significant difference in complications rates of mortality, wound infection, acute kidney injury, or other outcomes, and in the incidence of hypoglycemia or length of hospital stay.

Most studies [8, 9] and meta-analysis [29, 32] found a neutral effect of TGC on other clinical outcomes including neurological dysfunction, acute renal failure and length of hospital stay; our result further supported those findings. Our finding was not consistent with the clinical practice guideline from the American College of Physicians [30] that they found TGC was not associated with a reduction of ICU stay in the mixed medical intensive care unit/surgical intensive care unit environment. Another recent study [9] found that only nondiabetic cardiac surgery patients, but not patients with diabetes, could gain significant benefit of postoperative complications from intraoperative TGC.

The major harm of TGC was that it might increase hypoglycemia, especially in critically ill patients [2, 35, 36]. The study by Finfer S et al. found that intensive glucose control leads to moderate and severe hypoglycemia in critically ill patients [2]. Our finding was also consistent with many studies [13] and other meta-analysis [29, 34], which have also noted that using a TGC protocol in the perioperative period increased the risk of hypoglycemia, but without a significant increase in serious adverse events in various hospital settings. However, a recent meta-analysis [28] that found intraoperative insulin therapy may not increase the rate of hypoglycemia. The consequences of hypoglycemia in hospitalized patients remain unclear as few studies report clinical adverse effects and explain how hypoglycemia harms patients in the long-term consequences. The study of Finfer S [2] has confirmed that both of moderate and severe hypoglycemia was associated with

an increased risk of death in critically ill patients, however, others argued [37] that hyperglycemia was more similar to a signal of illness severity rather than the cause of clinical adverse outcomes. Indeed, the hyperglycemia level was related to the activation of the stress response.

The conflict of the results between the present meta-analysis and others can be explained by different inclusion criteria, patient characteristics, time of TGC, type of treatments, hospital setting, and the definition of hypoglycemia. Furthermore, the markedly variation in blood glucose target levels, the protocols of glucose monitoring and managing among studies may also influence the results.

There are some strengths of this study. For the first time, the present meta-analysis was conducted to evaluate the association between postoperative glycemic control and outcomes in patients undergoing elective surgery. Second, we have included the most rigorous analysis of TGC studies to date and conducted a comprehensive meta-analysis to elevate the effect of postoperative TGC on outcomes. However, high-quality evidence to support the routine use of postoperative TGC is still lacking.

Limitations

There are some limitations in this meta-analysis. First, the source data were extracted from diverse types of surgery and glycemic targets. In addition, there were variations in the timing of the intervention (postoperative versus intra-operative plus post-operative). Finally, the number of eligible studies was small; thus the results were likely biased. This may underestimate the benefit of TGC. Despite these differences, no significant heterogeneity was observed between studies with respect to the primary endpoint and most other outcomes and our results were consistent in the sensitivity analyses.

Conclusions

The results of this study show that TGC immediately after surgery significantly reduces total postoperative infection rates and short-term mortality. However, it might limit conclusion regarding the efficacy of TGC for short-term mortality in sensitivity analyses. The patients in the TGC group experienced a significant higher rate of postoperative hypoglycemia. TGC had a neutral effect on the risk of postoperative neurological dysfunction and acute renal failure as compared to CGC. This study may suggest that TGC should be administrated under close glucose monitoring in patients undergoing surgery, especially in those with high postoperative infection risk. In addition, large, prospective, randomized and high quality trials on the efficacy and safety of TGC in the postoperative period are needed to investigate the ideal

BG target to optimize clinical outcomes and minimize adverse events in patients undergoing surgery.

Additional files

Additional file 1: Search strategies for this study. (DOC 38 kb)

Additional file 2: The Jadad scale for assessing the methodological quality of clinical trials. (DOC 27 kb)

Additional file 3: Table S1. Sensitivity analysis for the outcome of the risk of postoperative infection. (DOC 49 kb)

Additional file 4: Figure S1. A funnel plot of the risk of postoperative infection. (TIF 301 kb)

Additional file 5: Figure S2. Forest plot of the risk of any postoperative mortality in TGC group versus control group. TGC = tight glycemic control; RR = relative risk; CI = confidence interval. (TIF 445 kb)

Additional file 6: Table S2. Sensitivity analysis for the outcome of the risk of postoperative short-term mortality. (DOC 48 kb)

Additional file 7: Figure S3. A funnel plot of the risk of postoperative short-term mortality. (TIF 299 kb)

Additional file 8: Figure S4. A: Begg's test for short-term mortality; B: Egger's test for short-term mortality. (TIF 365 kb)

Additional file 9: Table S3. Sensitivity analysis for the outcome of the risk of postoperative neurological dysfunction. (DOC 38 kb)

Additional file 10: Table S4. Sensitivity analysis for the outcome of the risk of postoperative acute renal failure. (DOC 35 kb)

Additional file 11: Figure S5. Forest plot of the risk of postoperative servese hypoglycemia in TGC group versus control group. TGC = tight glycemic control; RR = relative risk; CI = confidence interval. (TIF 300 kb)

Additional file 12: Table S5. Sensitivity analysis for the outcome of the risk of postoperative hypoglycemia. (DOC 47 kb)

Additional file 13: Figure S6. A funnel plot of the risk of postoperative hypoglycemia. (TIF 293 kb)

Additional file 14: Table S6. Sensitivity analysis for the outcome of the risk of postoperative servese hypoglycemia. (DOC 40 kb)

Additional file 15: Table S7. Subgroup analyses for the outcome of the risk of postoperative hypoglycemia. (DOC 68 kb)

Additional file 16: Table S8. Meta-regression for the outcome of the risk of postoperative hypoglycemia. (DOC 44 kb)

Additional file 17: Figure S7. Forest plot of the risk of postoperative ICU stay in TGC group versus control group. TGC = tight glycemic control; SMD = standardised mean difference; CI = confidence interval . (TIF 296 kb)

Additional file 18: Figure S8. Forest plot of the risk of postoperative duration of mechanical ventilation in TGC group versus control group. TGC = tight glycemic control; SMD = standardised mean difference; CI = confidence interval. (TIF 300 kb)

Additional file 19: Figure S9. Forest plot of the risk of postoperative LOS in TGC group versus control group. TGC = tight glycemic control; SMD = standardised mean difference; CI = confidence interval; LOS = length of hospitalization. (TIF 297 kb)

Additional file 20: Table S9. Sensitivity analysis for the outcome of the risk of postoperative ICU stay. (DOC 40 kb)

Additional file 21: Table S10. Sensitivity analysis for the outcome of the risk of postoperative duration of mechanical ventilation. (DOC 40 kb)

Additional file 22: Table S11. Sensitivity analysis for the outcome of the risk of postoperative length of hospitalization. (DOC 41 kb)

Additional file 23: Table S12. Subgroup analyses for the outcome of the risk of postoperative ICU stay. (DOC 55 kb)

Additional file 24: Table S13. Meta-regression for the outcome of the risk of postoperative ICU stay. (DOC 45 kb)

Additional file 25: Table S14. Subgroup analyses for the outcome of the risk of postoperative duration of mechanical ventilation. (DOC 55 kb)

Additional file 26: Table S15. Meta-regression for the outcome of the risk of postoperative duration of mechanical ventilation. (DOC 44 kb)

Additional file 27: Table S16. Subgroup analyses for the outcome of the risk of postoperative length of hospitalization. (DOC 60 kb)

Additional file 28: Table S17. Meta-regression for the outcome of the risk of postoperative length of hospitalization. (DOC 45 kb)

Abbreviations

BG: Blood glucose level; CGC: Conventional glycemic control; CI: Confidence interval; CRRT: Continuous renal replacement therapy; ICU: Intensive care unit; LOS: Length of hospital stay; RR: Relative risk; SMD: Standardised mean difference; TGC: Tight glycemic control

Acknowledgements

The authors sincerely thank Yun-xian YU (Department of Epidemiology and Health Statistics, School of Public Health, Zhejiang University) for the help of data analyzed in this study.

Authors' contributions

YYW, SFH and ZFZ designed the study. SFH, HMY, LC and HLL did the work of data collecting, and data was analyzed by LC and FT. YYW and ZFZ wrote the paper. HMY and HLL revised the paper. Any controversies of the paper were discussed and resolved by all authors. All authors have read and approved the manuscript.

Competing interests

The authors declare that they have no competing interests.

Author details

[1]Department of Endocrinology, Xixi Hospital of Hangzhou, Hangzhou, Hangzhou 315000, Zhejiang Province, China. [2]Department of Anesthesiology, Zhejiang Provincial People's Hospital (People's Hospital of Hangzhou Medicine College), Hangzhou 315000, China.

References

1. van den Berghe G, Wouters P, Weekers F, et al. Intensive insulin therapy in critically ill patients. N Engl J Med. 2001;345(19):1359–67.
2. Finfer S, Liu B, Chittock DR, et al. Hypoglycemia and risk of death in critically ill patients. N Engl J Med. 2012;367(12):1108–18.
3. Finfer S, Chittock DR, Su SY, et al. Intensive versus conventional glucose control in critically ill patients. N Engl J Med. 2009;360(13):1283–97.
4. Kwon S, Thompson R, Dellinger P, Yanez D, Farrohki E, Flum D. Importance of perioperative glycemic control in general surgery: a report from the surgical care and outcomes assessment program. Ann Surg. 2013;257(1):8–14.
5. Umpierrez G, Cardona S, Pasquel F, et al. Randomized controlled trial of intensive versus conservative glucose control in patients undergoing coronary artery bypass graft surgery: GLUCO-CABG trial. Diabetes Care. 2015; 38(9):1665–72.
6. Kotagal M, Symons RG, Hirsch IB, et al. Perioperative hyperglycemia and risk of adverse events among patients with and without diabetes. Ann Surg. 2015;261(1):97–103.
7. Agus MS, Wypij D, Hirshberg EL, et al. Tight Glycemic Control in Critically Ill Children. N Engl J Med. 2017;376(8):729–41.
8. Pezzella AT, Holmes SD, Pritchard G, Speir AM, Ad N. Impact of perioperative glycemic control strategy on patient survival after coronary bypass surgery. Ann Thorac Surg. 2014;98(4):1281–5.

9. Bláha J, Mráz M, Kopecký P, et al. Perioperative tight glucose control reduces postoperative adverse events in nondiabetic cardiac surgery patients. J Clin Endocrinol Metab. 2015;100(8):3081–9.

10. Moher D, Liberati A, Tetzlaff J, Altman DG. Preferred reporting items for systematic reviews and meta-analyses: the PRISMA statement. Int J Surg. 2010;8(5):336–41.

11. Bañares R, Albillos A, Rincón D, et al. Endoscopic treatment versus endoscopic plus pharmacologic treatment for acute variceal bleeding: a meta-analysis. Hepatology. 2002;35(3):609–15.

12. Sterne JA, Sutton AJ, Ioannidis JP, et al. Recommendations for examining and interpreting funnel plot asymmetry in meta-analyses of randomised controlled trials. BMJ. 2011;343:d4002.

13. de Vries FE, Gans SL, Solomkin JS, et al. Meta-analysis of lower perioperative blood glucose target levels for reduction of surgical-site infection. Br J Surg. 2017;104(2):e95–e105.

14. Asida SM, Atalla MMM, Gad GS, Eisa KM, Mohamed HS. Effect of perioperative control of blood glucose level on patient's outcome after anesthesia for cardiac surgery. Egyptian Journal of Anaesthesia Egypt. 2013; 29(1):71–6.

15. Giakoumidakis K, Eltheni R, Patelarou E, et al. Effects of intensive glycemic control on outcomes of cardiac surgery. Heart and lung: journal of acute and critical CareHeart lung J. Acute Crit Care. 2013;42(2):146–51.

16. Wallia A, Schmidt K, Oakes DJ, et al. Glycemic control reduces infections in post-liver transplant patients: results of a prospective, randomized study. Journal of clinical endocrinology and MetabolismJ. Clin Endocrinol Metab. 2017;102(2):451–9.

17. Zheng R, Gu C, Wang Y, et al. Impacts of intensive insulin therapy in patients undergoing heart valve replacement. Heart Surgery Forum Heart Surg Forum. 2010;13(5):E292–8.

18. Chan RP, Galas FR, Hajjar LA, Bello CN, Piccioni MA, Auler JO Jr. Intensive perioperative glucose control does not improve outcomes of patients submitted to open-heart surgery: a randomized controlled trial. Clinics (Sao Paulo). 2009;64(1):51–60.

19. Cao S, Zhou Y, Chen D, et al. Intensive versus conventional insulin therapy in nondiabetic patients receiving parenteral nutrition after D2 gastrectomy for gastric cancer: a randomized controlled trial. J Gastrointest Surg. 2011; 15(11):1961–8.

20. Cao SG, Ren JA, Shen B, Chen D, Zhou YB, Li JS. Intensive versus conventional insulin therapy in type 2 diabetes patients undergoing D2 gastrectomy for gastric cancer: a randomized controlled trial. World J Surg. 2011;35(1):85–92.

21. Okabayashi TYTATTTMMK. Intensive versus intermediate glucose control in surgical intensive care unit patients. Diabetes Care. 2014;37(6):1516–24.

22. Wahby EEMMSM. Perioperative glycemic control in diabetic patients undergoing coronary artery bypass graft surgery. Journal of the egyptian society of cardio-thoracic surgery. 2017;24(2):143–9.

23. Bilotta F, Caramia R, Paoloni FP, Delfini R, Rosa G. Safety and efficacy of intensive insulin therapy in critical neurosurgical patients. Anesthesiology. 2009;110(3):611–9.

24. Desai SLSSCSN. Strict versus liberal target range for perioperative glucose in patients undergoing coronary artery bypass grafting: a prospective randomized controlled trial. J Thorac Cardiovasc Surg. 2012;143(2):318–25.

25. Bilotta F, Spinelli A, Giovannini F, Doronzio A, Delfini R, Rosa G. The effect of intensive insulin therapy on infection rate, vasospasm, neurologic outcome, and mortality in neurointensive care unit after intracranial aneurysm clipping in patients with acute subarachnoid hemorrhage: a randomized prospective pilot trial. J Neurosurg Anesthesiol. 2007;19(3):156–60.

26. Agus MS, Steil GM, Wypij D, et al. Tight glycemic control versus standard care after pediatric cardiac surgery. N Engl J Med. 2012;367(13):1208–19.

27. Lazar HL, McDonnell MM, Chipkin S, Fitzgerald C, Bliss C, Cabral H. Effects of aggressive versus moderate glycemic control on clinical outcomes in diabetic coronary artery bypass graft patients. Ann Surg. 2011;254(3):458–63. discussion 463-4

28. Hua J, Chen G, Li H, et al. Intensive intraoperative insulin therapy versus conventional insulin therapy during cardiac surgery: a meta-analysis. J Cardiothorac Vasc Anesth. 2012;26(5):829–34.

29. Marik PE, Preiser JC. Toward understanding tight glycemic control in the ICU: a systematic review and metaanalysis. Chest. 2010;137(3):544–51.

30. Qaseem A, Humphrey LL, Chou R, Snow V, Shekelle P. Use of intensive insulin therapy for the management of glycemic control in hospitalized patients: a clinical practice guideline from the American College of Physicians. Ann Intern Med. 2011;154(4):260–7.

31. Piatti PM, Cioni M, Magistro A, et al. Basal insulin therapy is associated with beneficial effects on postoperative infective complications, independently from circulating glucose levels in patients admitted for cardiac surgery. J Clin Transl Endocrinol. 2017;7:47–53.

32. Sathya B, Davis R, Taveira T, Whitlatch H, Wu WC. Intensity of peri-operative glycemic control and postoperative outcomes in patients with diabetes: a meta-analysis. Diabetes Res Clin Pract. 2013;102(1):8–15.

33. Badawi O, Waite MD, Fuhrman SA, Zuckerman IH. Association between intensive care unit-acquired dysglycemia and in-hospital mortality. Crit Care Med. 2012;40(12):3180–8.

34. Kansagara D, Fu R, Freeman M, Wolf F, Helfand M. Intensive insulin therapy in hospitalized patients: a systematic review. Ann Intern Med. 2011;154(4): 268–82.

35. Krinsley J. Glycemic control in critically ill patients: Leuven and beyond. Chest. 2007;132(1):1–2.

36. Vriesendorp TM, van Santen S, DeVries JH, et al. Predisposing factors for hypoglycemia in the intensive care unit. Crit Care Med. 2006;34(1):96–101.

37. Marik PE, Bellomo R. Stress hyperglycemia: an essential survival response. Crit Care. 2013;17(2):305.

4

Factors associated with type 2 diabetes in patients with vascular dementia: a population-based cross-sectional study

Chun-Lin Liu[1,2], Ming-Yen Lin[3,4*†], Shang-Jyh Hwang[1,3,4,6], Ching-Kuan Liu[1,7], Huei-Lan Lee[4]
and Ming-Tsang Wu[1,5,8,9*†]

Abstract

Background: Incidence of dementia is growing rapidly and affects many people worldwide. Type 2 diabetes mellitus (DM) might link cognitive decline and dementia, but the reasons for this association remain unclear. Our study explored the factors associated with type 2 DM in patients with dementia.

Methods: Patients ($n = 40,404$) with vascular dementia were identified in Taiwan's 1997 to 2008 National Health Insurance Research Database and divided into a DM group and non-DM group. Eleven comorbidities were identified and categorized into four groups: cardiovascular and cerebrovascular diseases, digestive system diseases, renal and metabolic system diseases, and cancer. The associations of these factors with type 2 DM were explored through multivaraible logistic regression.

Results: Of the patients with dementia, 22.5% had DM. Associated with a higher likelihood of DM in this population were female sex (adjusted odds ratio [OR]: 1.44, 95% confidence interval [CI]: 1.36–1.52), young age (range of adjusted OR: 0.55–1.13), low income (range of adjusted OR: 1.09–1.18), and renal and metabolic system diseases (OR: 2.81, 95% CI: 2.64–2.98).

Conclusions: The findings of this study suggest that clinicians should encourage patients with dementia to receive regular glucose impairment screening if they are female, have low socioeconomic status, or have renal or metabolic diseases.

Keywords: Type 2 diabetes, Comorbidity, Dementia, Socioeconomic status

Background

Dementia, including Alzheimer's disease and vascular dementia (VaD), is a progressive neurodegenerative disease affecting more than 35 million people worldwide [1]. It can shorten human life, reduce patient and caregiver quality of life, and cause substantial economic burden [2–4]. As the number of patients with dementia increases, understanding the natural course of dementia is crucial for identifying vulnerable populations and appropriate interventions.

Type 2 diabetes mellitus (DM), which is found in 13–20% of patients with dementia [5], is a major disease linked with cognitive decline and dementia [6]. However, the reasons for this close association remain unclear. Through poorly controlled blood sugar, DM may damage blood vessels and produce long-term complications such as cerebrovascular disease, cardiovascular disease, or hypertension, all of which further accelerate progression toward cognitive impairment [7]. Following the interrelationships between DM, rare complications, and dementia may be possible by tracing large DM populations over a long period. Until then, the prevalences of DM related comorbidities in the dementia population should be determined to help identify patients at high risk, and cognitive impairment screening is required to help physicians prevent or treat DM-related complications that can lead

* Correspondence: 1030475@kmuh.org.tw; 960021@kmuh.org.tw
†Ming-Yen Lin and Ming-Tsang Wu contributed equally to this work.
[3]Department of Renal Care, College of Medicine, Kaohsiung Medical University, No. 100, Shih-Chuan 1st Road, Kaohsiung 80708, Taiwan
[1]Graduate Institute of Medicine, College of Medicine, Kaohsiung Medical University, No. 100, Shih-Chuan 1st Road, Kaohsiung 80708, Taiwan
Full list of author information is available at the end of the article

to dementia. To begin this line of research, we conducted a population-based cross-sectional study to estimate the prevalence of type 2 DM in patients with dementia and explored factors associated with the development of DM in the study population.

Methods
Data source
The Department of Health in Taiwan implemented the National Health Insurance (NHI) program in 1995. By the end of 1996, approximately 96% of all residents in Taiwan had enrolled [8]. The coverage rate increased steadily from 96.1 to 98.6% from 2000 to 2007. All hospitals and clinics contracted with the NHI program are required to submit patient claims to receive reimbursements from the program. To verify the accuracy of claims data, the Bureau of NHI Management performs quarterly expert reviews on a random sample of inpatient claims at each hospital and clinic. Severe penalties are issued for false reports. We linked data from Taiwan's Registry for Catastrophic Illness Database and related outpatient and inpatient claims datasets from 1997 to 2008.

Study design and population
For this population-based cross-sectional study, we included all patients in Taiwan with dementia who were newly registered to receive the catastrophic illness certification for senile dementia according to the International Classification of Diseases, Ninth Revision, Clinical Modification (ICD-9-CM; code 290.X) from 1997 to 2008. These designations are based on rigid diagnostic criteria evaluated by a neurologist or psychiatrist. The registry date found on the catastrophic illness certification was considered the index date for this study. All patients were defined as having comorbid diabetes if diagnostic ICD-9-CM code 250.XX appeared on at least two ambulatory care claims records or at least one inpatient care claims record within 1 year leading up to dementia diagnosis.

Assessment of associated factors
Several factors were considered to assess their potential associations with type 2 DM, namely demographic factors (age, sex, area of residence, urbanization level, and insurance amount), comorbidities (myocardial infarction, congestive heart failure, peripheral vascular disease, cerebrovascular disease, chronic pulmonary disease, peptic ulcer disease, mild liver disease, renal disease, cancer, hypertension, and hyperlipidemia), and disease severity. Area of residence was classified into four regions of Taiwan (north central, south, and east); urbanization level was divided into urban and rural; and insurance amount was divided into dependent, < NT$20,000 per month, and ≥ NT$20,000 per month. Patients were defined as "low income" when their insurance amount was

dependent, "medium income" when their insurance amount was < NT$20,000 per month, and "high income" when their insurance amount was ≥ NT$20,000 per month. Comorbidities were defined based on ICD-9-CM codes (Additional file 1: Table S1) listed on two or more ambulatory care claims records or one or more inpatient care claims records during the year prior to dementia diagnosis. To further evaluate the associations of various systematic diseases with diabetes, we grouped these comorbidities into four main categories based on similar manageable risk factors. These categories were (1) cardiovascular and cerebrovascular diseases (myocardial infarction, congestive heart failure, peripheral vascular disease, cerebrovascular disease, chronic pulmonary disease, and hypertension), (2) digestive system diseases (peptic ulcer disease and mild liver disease), (3) renal and metabolic system diseases (renal disease and hyperlipidemia), and (4) cancer. Disease severity was defined based on Charlson comorbidity index scores, which are listed in a previous report [9], calculated based on diseases.

Statistical analysis
Participant characteristics were analyzed as follows. Distributions of continuous variables were expressed as mean ± standard deviation (SD) or median (interquartile range), and those of categorical variables were expressed as numbers and percentages. The differences in the distributions of count variables between DM and non-DM were analyzed through Mann–Whitney U testing, and those of categorical variables were analyzed through the chi-squared (χ^2) testing. Multivariable logistic regressions adjusted for all demographic factors, and comorbidities or various systematic diseases were tested to identify independent factors associated with DM. In addition, we investigated associations among various systematic disease groups, the number of each systematic disease, and DM by using multivariable logistic regression adjusted for patient characteristics. Data were represented as odds ratios (ORs) and 95% confidence intervals (CIs). To further explore the effects of income and comorbidities on the prevalence of DM, the proportion of DM and high income by number of comorbidities, and the proportions of various systematic diseases by DM and income were also investigated. To validate our main findings, we conducted sensitivity analysis after redefining the DM group as ICD-9-CM code 250.XX appearing on at least three ambulatory care claims records or at least one inpatient care claims record within 1 year leading up to dementia diagnosis. All statistical operations were performed in SAS (version 9.4, SAS Institute, Cary, NC, USA). A p value of < 0.05 was considered significant.

Results

Patient characteristics

In the study cohort, 22.5% patients with dementia also had diabetes. Table 1 provides a summary of patient characteristics. Compared with patients without diabetes, those with diabetes were significantly more likely to be female, young, and living in south and rural areas (Table 1). They were also more likely to have low incomes, more comorbidities (myocardial infarction, congestive heart failure, peripheral vascular disease, cerebrovascular disease, chronic pulmonary disease, peptic ulcer disease, mild liver disease, renal disease, cancer), and a greater number of severe diseases. The top three largest differences in the distributions of comorbidities between the DM and non-DM groups were

Table 1 Patient Characteristics

	DM		Non-DM		P-value
	N	%	N	%	
Gender					
Male	3261	35.9	13,830	44.2	< 0.001
Female	5816	64.1	17,484	55.8	
Age (mean ± SD), yr	75.7 ± 8.1		77.1 ± 9.4		< 0.001
< 65	843	9.3	2878	9.2	< 0.001
65–74	3088	34.0	8165	26.1	
75–84	4149	45.7	14,584	46.5	
≥ 85	997	11.0	5687	18.2	
Area of residence					
North	3237	35.7	12,357	39.4	< 0.001
Central	2192	24.1	7310	23.3	
South	3269	36.0	10,287	32.9	
East	379	4.2	1360	4.4	
Urbanization level					
Urban	2837	31.2	10,419	33.3	< 0.001
Rural	6240	68.8	2,0895	66.7	
Insurance amount, NT$/month					
Dependent	4522	49.8	13,554	43.3	< 0.001
< 20,000	3013	33.2	12,043	38.4	
≥ 20,000	1542	17.0	5717	18.3	
Charlson comorbidity index					
Mean ± SD	3.9 ± 1.9		1.7 ± 1.5		< 0.01
Median (Interquartile range)	4.0 (2.0–5.0)		1.0 (1.0–2.0)		< 0.01
Selective comorbidities					
Myocardial infarction	176	1.9	359	1.2	< 0.01
Congestive heart Failure	1071	11.8	2219	7.1	< 0.01
Peripheral vascular disease	317	3.5	671	2.1	< 0.01
Cerebrovascular disease	4499	49.6	9608	30.7	< 0.01
Chronic pulmonary disease	1969	21.7	5593	17.9	< 0.01
Peptic ulcer disease	1800	19.8	3981	12.7	< 0.01
Mild liver disease	790	8.7	1601	5.1	< 0.01
Renal disease	855	9.42	1166	3.7	< 0.01
Cancer	499	5.5	1250	4.1	< 0.01
Hypertension	6537	72.0	12,669	40.5	< 0.01
Hyperlipidemia	1854	20.4	1791	5.72	< 0.01

DM, diabetes mellitus, *DM; NT$*, New Taiwan dollar
Differences in characteristics between the DM and non-DM groups were tested through the Mann–Whitney U test or χ^2 test; $p < 0.05$ was considered significant

Table 2 Associations of baseline characteristics and comorbidities with type 2 diabetes mellitus

Parameters	Multivariable-adjusted model	
	Odds ratio	95%CI
Gender		
Male	1.00 [Reference]	
Female	1.44	1.36–1.52
Age, yr		
< 65	1.00 [Reference]	
65–74	1.13	1.02–1.24
75–84	0.86	0.78–0.95
≥ 85	0.55	0.49–0.62
Area of residence		
North	1.00 [Reference]	
Central	1.14	1.06–1.22
South	1.12	1.06–1.19
East	1.17	1.05–1.19
Urbanization level		
Urban	1.00 [Reference]	
Rural	1.12	1.06–1.19
Insurance amount, NT$/month		
≥ 20,000	1.00 [Reference]	
< 20,000	1.09	1.09–1.27
Dependent	1.18	1.01–1.17
Selected comorbidities		
Myocardial infarction	1.01	0.83–1.23
Congestive heart failure	1.12	1.06–1.26
Peripheral vascular disease	1.12	0.99–1.34
Cerebrovascular disease	1.56	1.48–1.64
Chronic pulmonary disease	1.03	0.97–1.09
Peptic ulcer disease	1.25	1.17–1.34
Mild liver disease	1.42	1.28–1.56
Renal disease	2.00	1.81–2.21
Cancer	1.27	1.13–1.42
Hypertension	2.79	2.65–2.95
Hyperlipidemia	2.93	2.72–3.15

CI, confidence interval; *NT$*, New Taiwan dollar
Multivariable logistic regressions adjusted for sex, age, income, area of residence, urbanization level, and comorbidities were run to identify independent factors associated with type 2 diabetes mellitus; $p < 0.05$ was considered significant

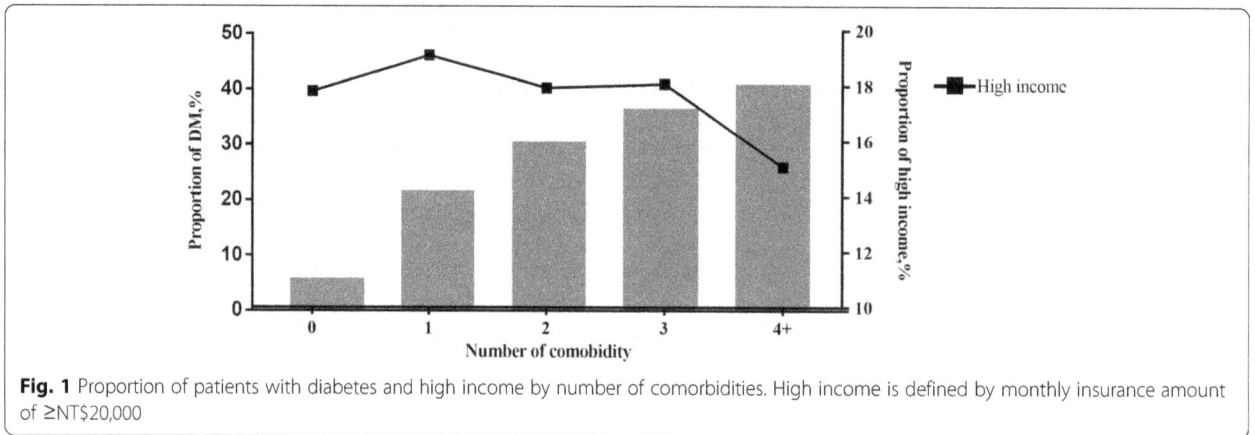

Fig. 1 Proportion of patients with diabetes and high income by number of comorbidities. High income is defined by monthly insurance amount of ≥NT$20,000

cerebrovascular disease (percentage difference: 18.9), peptic ulcer disease (percentage difference: 7.1), and renal disease (percentage difference: 5.7).

Factors related to DM prevalence

Table 2 shows the associations of baseline characteristics and comorbidities with DM. Age, sex, area of residence, urbanization level, insurance amount, congestive heart failure, cerebrovascular disease, peptic ulcer disease, mild liver disease, renal disease, hypertension, and hyperlipidemia were significantly and independently associated with DM in patients with dementia (Table 2). Notably, patients with DM were more likely to be female (adjusted OR: 1.44, 95% CI: 1.36–1.52) and young (range of adjusted OR: 0.55–1.13). Those with DM were significantly more likely to have more comorbidities, have lower incomes, and live in rural areas. We analyzed the associations of DM with income, number of comorbidities, and systematic diseases (Figs. 1 and 2). As can be seen in Fig. 1, which shows the results of our analysis regarding the prevalence of DM,

number of comorbidities, income, the prevalence of DM was higher in patients with four or more comorbidities and lower in those with high incomes (Fig. 1). Figure 2 depicts the results of our analysis regarding the proportion of comorbidity-related diseases based on diabetes status and insurance amount. Patients with DM had substantially more comorbidities than did those without DM. Those with DM and those in the lower income group had the highest proportion of renal and metabolic system diseases (Fig. 2). The sensitivity analysis strongly supported these model findings (Additional file 1: Table S2).

Systematic diseases and DM prevalence

Table 3 shows the results of our study regarding association between systematic comorbidities and DM in patients with dementia. Prevalence of DM was significantly associated with the following systematic comorbidities: cardiovascular diseases (adjusted OR: 3.93, 95% CI: 3.68–4.19); digestive system diseases (adjusted OR: 1.34, 95% CI: 1.26–1.42); renal and metabolic system diseases

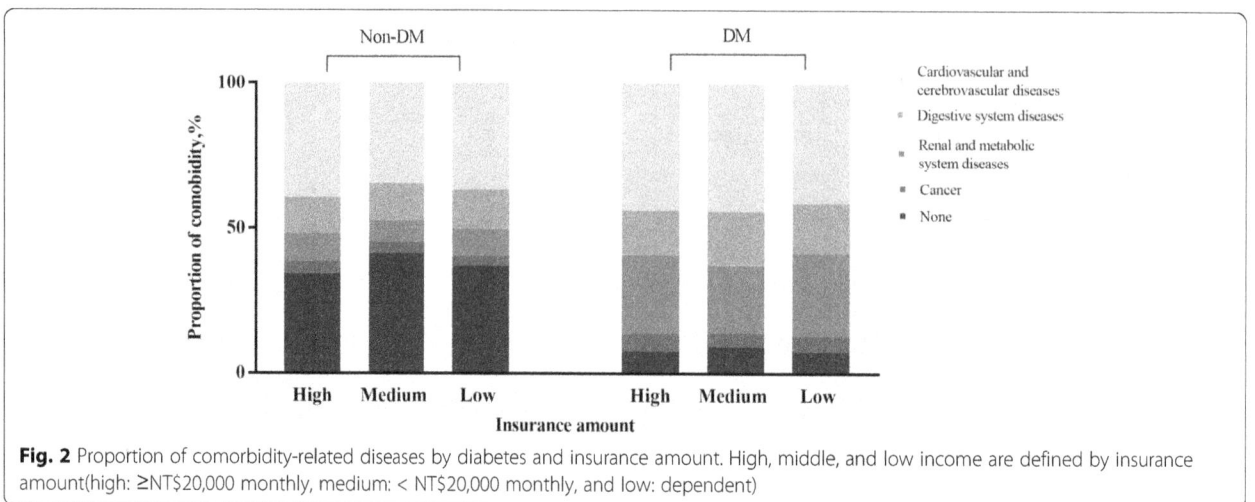

Fig. 2 Proportion of comorbidity-related diseases by diabetes and insurance amount. High, middle, and low income are defined by insurance amount(high: ≥NT$20,000 monthly, medium: < NT$20,000 monthly, and low: dependent)

Table 3 Associations of systemic comorbidities with type 2 diabetes mellitus

Parameters	Univariable model		Multivariable-adjusted model[d]	
	OR	95%CI	OR	95%CI
Cardiovascular and cerebrovascular diseases[a]				
No	1.00 [Reference]		1.00 [Reference]	
Yes	4.67	4.38–4.98	3.93	3.68–4.19
Number				
0	1.00 [Reference]		1.00 [Reference]	
1–3	2.57	2.45–2.69	2.28	2.17–2.41
4–6	2.81	2.39–3.29	2.34	1.97–2.76
Digestive system diseases[b]				
No	1.00 [Reference]		1.00 [Reference]	
Yes	1.79	1.69–.189	1.34	1.26–1.42
Number				
0	1.00 [Reference]		1.00 [Reference]	
1	1.78	1.67–1.88	1.43	1.35–1.53
2	1.93	1.66–2.25	1.55	1.32–1.82
Renal and metabolic system diseases[c]				
No	1.00 [Reference]		1.00 [Reference]	
Yes	3.85	3.63–4.09	2.81	2.64–2.98
Number				
0	1.00 [Reference]		1.00 [Reference]	
1	3.72	3.49–3.95	3.05	2.86–3.25
2	7.07	5.60–8.93	5.32	4.18–6.78
Cancer				
No	1.00 [Reference]	1.00 [Reference]		
Yes	1.39	1.26–1.56	1.23	1.09–1.38

OR, odds ratio; *CI*, confidence interval

[a]Cardiovascular and cerebrovascular diseases comprised myocardial infarction, congestive heart failure, peripheral vascular disease, cerebrovascular disease, chronic pulmonary disease, and hypertension

[b]Digestive system diseases comprised peptic ulcer disease and mild liver disease

[c]Renal and metabolic system diseases comprised renal disease and hyperlipidemia

[d]Multivariable logistic regressions adjusted for sex, age, income, area of residence, and urbanization, and various systematic comorbidities were run to identify independent factors associated with type 2 diabetes mellitus; $p < 0.05$ was considered significant

(adjusted OR: 2.81, 95% CI: 2.64–2.98); and cancer (adjusted OR: 1.23, 95% CI: 1.09–1.38) (Table 3). The likelihood of DM was clearly higher in patients with one or two renal or metabolic system diseases than in those without (adjusted OR: 3.05, 95% CI: 2.86–3.25 and adjusted OR: 5.32, 95% CI: 4.18–56.78, respectively). Similar results from the sensitivity analysis are shown in Additional file 1: Table S3.

Discussion

Although epidemiology studies have reported that type 2 DM is associated with an increased risk of Alzheimer's disease and VaD [10], few studies have focused on the prevalence of type 2 DM in patients with dementia. The present population-based cross-sectional study found several factors independently associated with high prevalence of diabetes in patients with dementia. We found that likelihood of DM was higher in female, young, and low-income patients as well as those with one or more comorbidities and those with both hyperlipidemia and renal disease.

More than one-fifth of the patients with dementia had type 2 DM, suggesting that improved glucose management is required during the predementia phase. Previous studies have suggested that in the population with DM, long-term poor DM management and repeated serious glycemic episodes result in cognitive impairment in older adults [11, 12]. Consistent with one previous report [13], in the present study, female sex was associated with an increased likelihood of having DM with dementia. We also found that the patients with dementia who had DM were nearly 2 years younger on average than those without DM. This finding is similar to a prior observation in an Australian population [14] and might suggest a need for more targeted blood glucose management for women, considering other targeting criteria.

Previous studies have found high prevalences of comorbid medical conditions and related complications in patients with dementia. In a recent review of 54 primary studies, Bunn et al. concluded that DM and stroke were the most prevalent comorbid conditions in patients with dementia (13–20% and 16–29%, respectively) [15]. Another study identified 12 chronic commodities associated with dementia, most of which have similar pathophysiologies [5]. These chronic diseases may share similar risk factors or etiologies. Although anthropometric, dietary, and lifestyle factors were associated with type 2 DM in the general population [16], measurements of these risk factors were not easily obtained from patients with cognitive disorders. Identification of disease factors associated with type 2 DM may be more intuitive and more efficient than that of traditional type 2 DM risk factors for physicians providing optimal DM care for patients with dementia. The current study found that comorbidities with similar manageable risk factors, including cerebrovascular disease, renal disease, hypertension, and hyperlipidemia, were more likely to be grouped with DM in our study population, thereby emphasizing the need for comanagement of related metabolic system diseases to prevent DM-related complications in dementia.

This study found that lower income was associated with a higher prevalence of DM; the mechanisms underlying this association may be complex. A plausible explanation is that low-income patients tend to exert poor control over their glycemic levels, putting themselves at excessive risk of cardiovascular disease and accelerating progress toward cognitive dysfunction [17]. Alongside income differences may come differences in lifestyle factors, including education, occupation, and leisure activities, which have been increasingly recognized as factors that may affect the development of dementia [18–20]. Although having a privileged socioeconomic background might be associated with protection of brain function after damage, which reduces the risk of senile dementia [21], its potential moderation of the relationship between DM and dementia requires further study.

Several limitations of this study should be declared. It is unlikely, but possible, that the observed associations between diseases and DM resulted from more effective treatments and higher disease awareness among physicians and patients in the DM group compared with those in the non-DM group. Because of the long development from cognition impairment to dementia, we were unable to obtain the time of dementia onset. We were also unable to accurately differentiate types of dementia based on only diagnosis codes. Given that the study population was old and had high prevalence of chronic conditions, most of our patients likely had VaD. Finally, we were unable to control various potential confounders associated with DM and dementia, including educational status, life habits, and clinical laboratory data, that may have contributed to our findings. These factors may be helpful for clarifying the interrelationships between type 2 DM, comorbidities, and dementia in further research.

Conclusions

This study found significant associations of gender, socioeconomic status, and comorbidities with DM in patients with dementia. Based on our findings, patients with dementia who are female, have low income, and have comorbid renal or metabolic disease should undergo routine glucose impairment examinations to facilitate the management of blood glucose and prevention of adverse glycemic events.

Abbreviations
CI: Confidence Interval; DM: Diabetes Mellitus; ICD-9-CM: International Classification of Disease, Ninth Revision, Clinical Modification; NHI: National Health Insurance; NT$: New Taiwan Dollar; OR: Odds Ratio; VaD: Vascular Dementia

Acknowledgements
We thank the Statistical Analysis Laboratory of the Department of Internal Medicine of Kaohsiung Medical University Hospital for providing access to the NHI database (registration number 99324). We also thank James Steed and Wallace Academic Editing for editing this manuscript.

Funding
This study was partially supported by grants from the Ministry of Science and Technology (grant number: NSC102–2314-B-037-012-MY3), Ministry of Health and Welfare (grant numbers: MOHW103-TD-B-111-05, MOHW104-TDU-B-212-124-003, and MOHW105-TDU-B-212-134007; health and welfare surcharge of tobacco products), and Research Center for Environmental Medicine, Kaohsiung Medical University, Kaohsiung (SH000183), Taiwan.

Authors' contributions
CLL conducted the literature review and composed the initial draft. MYL designed the study, interpreted the results, and rewrote the manuscript. HLL performed the analyses and prepared the results. SJH acquired the data and provided critical input on earlier versions of the manuscript. MTW and CKL reviewed the manuscript critically for intellectual content. All authors read and approved the final manuscript.

Competing interests
The authors declare that they have no competing interests.

Author details
[1]Graduate Institute of Medicine, College of Medicine, Kaohsiung Medical University, No. 100, Shih-Chuan 1st Road, Kaohsiung 80708, Taiwan. [2]Calo Psychiatric Center, No.12-200, Jinhua Rd., Xinpi Township, Pingtung County 925, Taiwan. [3]Department of Renal Care, College of Medicine, Kaohsiung Medical University, No. 100, Shih-Chuan 1st Road, Kaohsiung 80708, Taiwan. [4]Division of Nephrology, Department of Internal Medicine, Kaohsiung Medical University Hospital, Kaohsiung Medical University, No. 100, Shih-Chuan 1st Road, Kaohsiung 80708, Taiwan. [5]Research Center for Environmental Medicine, Kaohsiung Medical University, No. 100, Shih-Chuan 1st Road, Kaohsiung 80708, Taiwan. [6]Institute of Population Health Sciences, National Health Research Institutes, No. 35 Keyan Road, Zhunan, Miaoli 35053, Taiwan. [7]Department of Neurology, Kaohsiung Medical University Hospital, Kaohsiung Medical University, No. 100, Shih-Chuan 1st Road, Kaohsiung 80708, Taiwan. [8]Department of Public Health, Kaohsiung Medical University, No. 100, Shih-Chuan 1st Road, Kaohsiung 80708, Taiwan. [9]Graduate Institute of Clinical Medicine, Kaohsiung Medical University, No. 100, Shih-Chuan 1st Road, Kaohsiung 80708, Taiwan.

References
1. Prince M, Bryce R, Albanese E, Wimo A, Ribeiro W, Ferri CP. The global prevalence of dementia: a systematic review and metaanalysis. Alzheimers Dement. 2013;9(1):63–75. e62
2. Van De Vorst IE, Vaartjes I, Geerlings MI, Bots ML, Koek HL. Prognosis of patients with dementia: results from a prospective nationwide registry linkage study in the Netherlands. BMJ Open. 2015;5(10):e008897.
3. Barca ML, Engedal K, Laks J, Selbæk G. Quality of life among elderly patients with dementia in institutions. Dement Geriatr Cogn Disord. 2011;31(6):435–42.
4. Wimo A, Jönsson L, Bond J, Prince M, Winblad B, International AD. The worldwide economic impact of dementia 2010. Alzheimers Dement. 2013;9(1):1–11. e13.
5. Poblador-Plou B, Calderón-Larrañaga A, Marta-Moreno J, Hancco-Saavedra J, Sicras-Mainar A, Soljak M, Prados-Torres A. Comorbidity of dementia: a cross-sectional study of primary care older patients. BMC psychiatry. 2014;14(1):84.
6. Xu W, Qiu C, Gatz M, Pedersen NL, Johansson B, Fratiglioni L. Mid-and late-life diabetes in relation to the risk of dementia. Diabetes. 2009;58(1):71–7.
7. Ninomiya T. Diabetes mellitus and dementia. Current Diabetes Reports. 2014;14(5):1.
8. J-FR L, Hsiao WC. Does universal health insurance make health care unaffordable? Lessons from Taiwan. Health Aff. 2003;22(3):77–88.
9. Deyo RA, Cherkin DC, Ciol MA. Adapting a clinical comorbidity index for use with ICD-9-CM administrative databases. J Clin Epidemiol. 1992;45(6):613–9.
10. Pasquier F, Boulogne A, Leys D, Fontaine P. Diabetes mellitus and dementia. Diabetes & metabolism. 2006;32(5):403–14.
11. Yaffe K, Falvey C, Hamilton N, Schwartz AV, Simonsick EM, Satterfield S, Cauley JA, Rosano C, Launer LJ, Strotmeyer ES. Diabetes, glucose control, and 9-year cognitive decline among older adults without dementia. Arch Neurol. 2012;69(9):1170–5.
12. Whitmer RA, Karter AJ, Yaffe K, Quesenberry CP, Selby JV. Hypoglycemic episodes and risk of dementia in older patients with type 2 diabetes mellitus. Jama. 2009;301(15):1565–72.
13. Kuo S-C, Lai S-W, Hung H-C, Muo C-H, Hung S-C, Liu L-L, Chang C-W, Hwu Y-J, Chen S-L, Sung F-C. Association between comorbidities and dementia

in diabetes mellitus patients: population-based retrospective cohort study. J Diabetes Complicat. 2015;29(8):1071–6.

14. Zilkens R, Davis W, Spilsbury K, Semmens J, Bruce D. Earlier age of dementia onset and shorter survival times in dementia patients with diabetes. Am J Epidemiol. 2013;177(11):1246–54.

15. Bunn F, Burn A-M, Goodman C, Rait G, Norton S, Robinson L, Schoeman J, Brayne C. Comorbidity and dementia: a scoping review of the literature. BMC Med. 2014;12(1):192.

16. Kengne AP, Beulens JWJ, Peelen LM, Moons KGM, van der Schouw YT, Schulze MB, Spijkerman AMW, Griffin SJ, Grobbee DE, Palla L, et al. Non-invasive risk scores for prediction of type 2 diabetes (EPIC-InterAct): a validation of existing models. Lancet Diabetes Endocrinology. 2014;2(1):19–29.

17. Seligman HK, Jacobs EA, López A, Tschann J, Fernandez A. Food insecurity and glycemic control among low-income patients with type 2 diabetes. Diabetes Care. 2012;35(2):233–8.

18. Scazufca M, Menezes PR, Vallada HP, Crepaldi AL, Pastor-Valero M, Coutinho LM, Di Rienzo VD, Almeida OP. High prevalence of dementia among older adults from poor socioeconomic backgrounds in Sao Paulo, Brazil. *Int Psychogeriatrics*. 2008;20(2):394–405.

19. Nitrini R, Caramelli P, Herrera E Jr, Bahia V, Caixeta L, Radanovic M, Anghinah R, Charchat-Fichman H, Porto C, Carthery M. Incidence of dementia in a community-dwelling Brazilian population. Alzheimer Dis Assoc Disord. 2004;18(4):241–6.

20. Keskinoglu P, Giray H, Pıcakcıefe M, Bilgic N, Ucku R. The prevalence and risk factors of dementia in the elderly population in a low socio-economic region of Izmir, Turkey. Arch Gerontol Geriatr. 2006;43(1):93–100.

21. Valenzuela MJ, Sachdev P. Brain reserve and dementia: a systematic review. Psychol Med. 2006;36(4):441–54.

5

Socioeconomic status and time in glucose target range in people with type 2 diabetes: a baseline analysis of the GP-OSMOTIC study

Mei Lyn Tan[1], Jo-Anne Manski-Nankervis[1*] (iD), Sharmala Thuraisingam[1], Alicia Jenkins[2], David O'Neal[3] and John Furler[1]

Abstract

Background: Optimal glycaemia, reflected by glycated haemoglobin (HbA1c) levels, is key in reducing type 2 diabetes (T2D) complications. However, most people with T2D have suboptimal recall and understanding of HbA1c. Continuous glucose monitoring (CGM) measures glucose levels every 5 to 15-min over days and may be more readily understood. Given that T2D is more common in lower socioeconomic settings, we aim to study relationships between socioeconomic status (SES) and percentage time in glucose target range (TIR) which is a key metric calculated from CGM.

Methods: Analysis of baseline data from the General Practice Optimising Structured MOnitoring To Improve Clinical outcomes (GP-OSMOTIC) randomised controlled trial (October 2016 – November 2017) of 300 people with T2D from 25 Victorian General Practices. *FreeStyle Libre Pro®* sensor patch was used for this study. SES was defined by the Index of Relative Socio-economic Disadvantage (IRSD) and educational attainment. Univariable and multivariable mixed-effects linear regression analyses controlling for age, BMI, diet, exercise and study arm were performed.

Results: One hundred and sixty-seven (60.1%) participants were male, the mean (SD) participant age was 61.0 (9.7) years, and the mean (SD) duration of CGM use was 12.3 (2.5) days. The 10th IRSD decile (least disadvantaged) was associated with a 15% higher TIR vs. the 1st decile (most disadvantaged) (95% CI 5, 25; $p = 0.003$) and a 0.6% lower HbA1c (95% CI 0.1, 1; $p = 0.03$). There was no evidence of an association between educational attainment and TIR/HbA1c.

Conclusion: Higher SES measured at an area level is associated with better achievement of glycaemic target using complementary measures of HbA1c and TIR in the GP-OSMOTIC cohort. Given that TIR may be more easily used in patient education and self-management support compared to HbA1c values, the social gradient identified in TIR provides an opportunity for clinicians and policy makers to address health inequities in T2D.

Keywords: Type 2 diabetes mellitus, Primary care, Continuous glucose monitors, Time in glucose target range, Socioeconomic status

* Correspondence: jomn@unimelb.edu.au
[1]Department of General Practice, University of Melbourne, Level 1, 200
Berkeley St, Carlton, VIC 3010, Australia
Full list of author information is available at the end of the article

Background

Approximately 1.2 million (5%) Australians are currently living with type 2 diabetes (T2D), increasing from 840,000 people (3.8%) in 2011–2012 [1, 2]. Strategies aimed at optimising blood glucose levels are a fundamental premise for the prevention and progression of complication in people with T2D. Current Australian guidelines set targets for glycated haemoglobin (HbA1c), an index of average blood glucose level over three months to assess glycaemia and as a measure of risk for the development of diabetes-related vascular and neurological complications [3]. Self-management (adherence to medications, managing diet and exercise) is an important way for people with T2D to achieve and maintain glycaemic targets.

Significant inequities exist with prevalence, mortality and hospitalisations all twice as common in people with T2D from low socioeconomic backgrounds compared to people from high socioeconomic backgrounds [1, 4]. Increasing levels of socioeconomic disadvantage are also associated with higher likelihood of out of target (high) HbA1c [5].

Research has shown that patients with diabetes have suboptimal levels of recall and understanding of HbA1c (only around 25% report a good understanding), which in turn impacts significantly on patients' diabetes self-care behaviours [6–8]. This is particularly important in the setting of socioeconomic disadvantage which is associated with low levels of health literacy and education [9–11].

Continuous glucose monitoring (CGM) technology provides a level of detail when assessing glucose control not provided by HbA1c measurements. CGM measures interstitial glucose levels nearly continuously allowing insights into short and medium-term fluctuations in glucose levels. Several parameters can be derived from CGM data including a measurement of percentage of time in glucose target range (TIR), a measure of the amount of time an individual spends within a specified glucose target range. Previous studies have identified a correlation between TIR and HbA1c. Having 50% of self-monitored glucose levels within 3.9–10 mmol/l (70.2–180 mg/dL) is correlated with an HbA1c of around 7% [12–15]. TIR, dependent on fluctuations in diet and physical activity, medication and adherence, is known to be an independent predictor of diabetes complications and mortality [13, 16].

Understanding the association between TIR and socioeconomic status (SES) may provide important insights in addition to those of HbA1c when evaluating the socioeconomic disparity seen in T2D prevalence and the development of complications. Importantly, TIR may also be a measurement that is easier for people with T2D to interpret and comprehend, empowering them to optimise their self-care behaviours. This is because TIR directly relates to measurements that are being made (i.e. blood glucose levels and a range), whereas HbA1c is one remove from that as it indirectly references blood glucose levels, therefore possibly making this harder conceptually for people to understand.

The General Practice Optimising Structured MOnitoring To Improve Clinical outcome (GP-OSMOTIC) randomised controlled trial is a study on the impact of a retrospective CGM device (*Abbott FreeStyle Libre Pro® Flash Glucose Monitoring System*) used in the clinical care of people with T2D in General Practice in Australia [17]. We report here on the relationship found between SES and TIR based on analysis of baseline data from the GP-OSMOTIC randomised controlled trial.

Methods

Design and study participants

This is an analysis of baseline data obtained from the GP-OSMOTIC trial (ACTRN12616001372471) that recruited a total of 300 patients from 25 General Practices in Victoria, Australia, between October 2016 and November 2017.

GP-OSMOTIC trial inclusion criteria are ages 18–80 years old, patients diagnosed with T2D, patients with the most recent (in the previous 3 months) HbA1c level 0.5% above their individualised target, patients prescribed at least 2 non-insulin anti-hyperglycaemic agents and/or insulin, and patients who have had stable anti-hyperglycaemic therapy for the last four months. Individualised target refers to an HbA1c target based on the participant's clinical characteristics and risk profile.

GP-OSMOTIC trial exclusion criteria are patients with debilitating medical conditions (e.g. unstable CVD, severe mental illness, end-stage cancer), eGFR < 30 ml/min/1.73m^2, proliferative retinopathy, patients who are pregnant/lactating/planning pregnancy, patients unable to speak English/give consent, patients unwilling to use CGM device or follow the GP-OSMOTIC study protocol, a history of allergy to plaster/tape and any condition that makes monitoring diabetes using the HbA1c unreliable (e.g. haemoglobinopathies).

Baseline data

Baseline survey, anthropometric measures and pathology collection were undertaken by clinically-trained research assistants at each participant's general practice. The survey included questions on educational attainment, employment and occupation, ethnicity and smoking status. Participant's medications, co-morbidities and diabetes-related complications were retrieved from clinical medical electronic health records. Chronic kidney disease was present if participants had evidence of microalbuminuria/macroalbuminuria and/or eGFR of < 60 mL/min/1.73 m^2 from urine and blood samples performed up to 30 days prior to baseline. eGFR was calculated by pathology labs using the Chronic Kidney Disease Epidemiology Collaboration (CKD-EPI) formula as per the Australasian Creatinine Consensus Working Group's position statements [18]. Similarly, HbA1c measures performed up to 30 days prior to the baseline visit were accepted, otherwise research assistants performed blood collection during the baseline visit. All HbA1c measurements were reported in both International Federation of Clinical Chemistry and Laboratory Medicine (IFCC) units (mmol/mol) and National Glycohaemoglobin Standardisation Programme (NGSP) units (%). These pathology measurements were undertaken at different laboratories based on General Practice clinic preferences. Masked CGM data was collected at baseline, prior to any therapeutic intervention, using a *FreeStyle Libre Pro* sensor patch. This was applied by study staff to the underside of the participant's upper arm to measure individual glucose levels in 15-min intervals for 2-weeks. After 2-weeks, the sensor was removed, and data were uploaded to a secure computer onto Microsoft Office Excel 2007 (Microsoft Corp., Seattle, WA, USA). Survey and clinical data were entered into REDCap© (REsearch Data CAPture software), a secure, web-based application designed to support research data capture [19].

Measures

TIR, defined in this study as 3.9-10 mmol/l (70.2 – 180 mg/dL), is calculated using the CGM data. TIR was calculated using Microsoft Office Excel 2007 (Microsoft Corp., Seattle, WA, USA). The range of CGM data for inclusion in this study was 5 to 14 days, consistent with manufacturer's recommendations [20].

We used the Socio-Economic Indexes For Areas (SEIFA) Index of Relative Socioeconomic Disadvantage (IRSD) as one measure of SES in our analysis. The SEIFA IRSD scores for each postcode are calculated by summarising attributes of the population collected through Australia's national household census, such as income, educational attainment, employment and occupation. These scores are grouped into deciles where decile 1 represents the most disadvantaged and decile 10 represents the least disadvantaged [21].

The second measure of SES we used was the level of educational attainment. Educational levels were categorised into never attended, primary level, secondary level, Trade/Vocational training course (TAFE) and University diploma/degree.

Information on diet and exercise were obtained through a baseline questionnaire. Participants were asked to write down the number of days in the last week in which carbohydrates were evenly spaced, and the numbers of days in the last week in which ≥30 min of physical activity was undertaken.

Data analysis

Normally distributed continuous variables are expressed as mean ± standard deviation, non-normally distributed continuous variables as median (IQ range) and categorical variables as frequency (percentage). Mixed-effects linear regression analysis was used to examine the four associations: TIR and IRSD, HbA1c and IRSD, TIR and educational attainment, and HbA1c and educational attainment. Never attended, primary education and secondary education were grouped into one category and used as a baseline to compare with other categories of education in our analysis. Univariable and multivariable analyses controlling for age, BMI, diet, exercise and study arm were performed to examine each association. Adjustment for study arm was performed as randomisation occurred after the CGM sensor was attached and before it was removed. Robust standard errors were specified to allow for clustering at the clinic level. As baseline HbA1c and IRSD deciles were non-normally distributed, log and square transformations of these variables were considered. Residual graphs were plotted for both transformed and untransformed data. Following review of the residual graphs, data transformation was not applied in our data analysis for all models of analyses. This is because the transformation did not significantly improve the random spread of the residuals, which results in limited benefit of the added complexity transformation would add to the interpretation. All statistical analyses were performed using STATA version 13.0 software (StataCorp, College Station, TX, USA).

Ethics

The GP-OSMOTIC trial, incorporating this study, was approved by The University of Melbourne Human Research Ethics Committee (ID 1647151.3).

Results
Patient characteristics

Data from 278 of the 300 participants in the GP-OSMOTIC trial were included in this study. Ten participants were excluded from data analysis as their CGM data duration were < 5 days, thus limiting the accuracy of glucose profile output obtained from insufficient number of data points [20]. Three participants were excluded from this study's analysis due to absent Socio-Economic Indexes for Areas (SEIFA) data based on the provided postcodes, and a further nine participants were excluded due to missing CGM data.

There was no difference in essential characteristics between included and excluded participants. Of the 22 participants excluded from this study, 10 (45.5%) were males, mean (SD) age was 57.4 (11.2) years, mean (SD) duration of T2D was 14.9 (4.6) years and mean (SD) BMI was 33.0 (4.6) kg/m^2. Information obtained on diet and exercise were also similar with a median (IQR) of 4 (1,5) days and 5 (2, 6.75) days respectively.

The baseline characteristics of participants are summarised in Table 1.

Association between TIR and IRSD

Table 2 shows the association between TIR and IRSD using unadjusted and adjusted models. There is evidence of a positive correlation between TIR and IRSD following adjustment for confounding variables. As the mean difference in TIR between one decile change of IRSD is 1.5% (95% CI 0.5, 2.5), thus on average, TIR was 15% higher for those least disadvantaged (IRSD = 10th decile) compared to those most disadvantaged (IRSD = 1st decile) (95% CI 5, 25).

Association between baseline HbA1c and IRSD

Multivariable mixed effects linear regression identified an inverse correlation between HbA1c and IRSD. As the mean difference in HbA1c between one decile change of IRSD is 0.06% (95% CI 0.01, 0.1), thus on average, HbA1c was 0.6% lower for those least disadvantaged (IRSD = 10th decile) compared to those most disadvantaged (IRSD = 1st decile) (95% CI 0.1, 1).

Association between TIR/HbA1c and education

Table 2 shows results of the association between TIR and educational attainment, as well as HbA1c and educational attainment following univariable and multivariable mixed effects linear regression. Educational attainment was not shown to be associated with either TIR or baseline HbA1c.

Discussion

Our analysis of CGM data obtained over a 2-week period from participants with T2D and sub-optimal HbA1c in primary care as part of the GP-OSMOTIC trial provides novel insight into glycaemia in this population. Least disadvantaged IRSD deciles, a composite area level measure of socioeconomic disadvantage, were correlated with better glycaemic control (both TIR and HbA1c). Our results support that an increase of 5 deciles in IRSD was associated with bringing the mean TIR in this population to almost 50%. As having 50% of self-monitored glucose levels within 3.9-10 mmol/l(70.2 – 180 mg/dL) is correlated with an HbA1c of around 7% [12], this would be associated with significantly improved health outcomes and reduced risk of diabetes-related complications. However, we found no association between educational attainment, a single, individual level measure of SES, and glycaemic control (either TIR or HbA1c).

Our finding that educational attainment was not shown to be associated with achieving glycaemic targets

despite the strong association seen for IRSD highlights the complexity of studying the concept of SES and its relationship with chronic disease parameters. Our finding is in contrast to international studies suggesting that socioeconomic advantage measured at the individual level such as higher educational attainment [22–25], higher income [26, 27] and higher residential stability [28], were associated with a greater likelihood of achieving HbA1c targets. However, there are many different measures and ways of defining SES, a concept that is made up of individual characteristics (e.g. educational attainment, income level, occupation), as well as contextual levels where the individual is situated within a physical and social location with characteristics relating to the built environment, social networks and social and supportive relationships. There is no single best indicator of SES suitable for all study aims and applicable at all stages in life. Rather there are many different possible measures, each with its own implications as well as strengths and limitations [29, 30]. It is thus important for policy, practice and research to be aware of this complexity, to use relevant SES measures and concepts that are suitable for their objectives and to interpret findings in relation to SES appropriately.

Individual and environmental factors likely interact with each other to affect glycaemia. People from more advantaged socio-economic backgrounds may have higher health literacy, with improved capacity to obtain, process, understand and act upon health information to support self-management of their condition [24]. However, our findings suggest that area level disadvantage is associated with glycaemia. Environmental and neighbourhood characteristics that we know are associated with more socio-economically advantaged areas such as greater accessibility to greenspace to engage in physical activities, a lower density of unhealthy food options such as fast food outlets, community norms and emphasis on healthy living and more opportunities to access health care services may all contribute to the social gradient in TIR and HbA1c that we identified [31].

It is important to acknowledge study limitations. The SEIFA IRSD represents an average of all people living in an area and does not represent individual situations. This is especially so in larger areas where there is more likely to be greater diversity [21]. The association between SES as measured by the IRSD and TIR is thus a generalised way of studying the link between neighbourhood level disadvantage with achievement of glycaemic targets. Other limitations of our study also include reliance on participants' recall for certain information, such as duration of diabetes and the likelihood that T2D may have existed for months or even years before formal diagnosis. Information regarding participant medications, medical history and diabetes-related

Table 1 Demographic characteristics of 278 participants with T2D

Characteristics	n (%) (unless otherwise stated)	Missing data, n (%)
Male	167 (60.1)	–
Age in years[a]	61.0 ± 9.7	–
Country of birth		14 (5.0)
Australia	186 (70.5)	
Others[b]	78 (29.5)	
Healthcare Card Holder[c]	132 (49.4)	11 (4.0)
Private Health Insurance Owner	111 (41.6)	11 (4.0)
IRSD Decile[d]	4 (1, 6)	–
Education level		11 (4.0)
Never attended	1 (0.4)	
Primary	18 (6.7)	
Secondary	128 (47.9)	
Trade/TAFE	51 (19.1)	
University diploma/degree	69 (25.8)	
Employed	113 (42.3)	11 (4.0)
Smoking Status		12 (4.3)
Current Smoker	40 (15.0)	
BMI (kg/m^2)[a]	34.0 ± 9.1	2 (0.7)
Diet[d,e]	3 (1, 5)	2 (0.7)
Exercise[d,f]	5 (3, 7)	2 (0.7)
Number of hypoglycaemic agents used		1 (0.4)
One agent	5 (1.8)	
Two agents	110 (39.7)	
Three agents	113 (40.8)	
Four or more agents	49 (17.7)	
Number of co-morbidities[d]	3 (2, 4)	–
Years of Diabetes[a]	14.3 ± 7.8	11 (4.0)
Diabetes-related Complications		
Micro-vascular	161 (57.9)	–
≥ 1 microvascular complication		
Macro-vascular	52 (18.7)	–
≥ 1 macrovascular complication		
Both micro- and macro-vascular complications	38 (13.7)	–
Duration of CGM use (days)[a]	12.3 ± 2.5	–
TIR(%)[a]	41.6 ± 25.4	
HbA1c[d]		
%	8.6 (8.0, 9.7)	1 (0.4)
mmol/mol	70.5 (64.0, 82.5)	1 (0.4)
Intervention study arm	144 (51.8)	–

[a]Represents mean ± standard deviation
[b]Comprises Philippines, India, China, Singapore, Sri Lanka, East Timor, Afghanistan, Sudan, Timor, Indonesia, New Zealand, USA, Fiji and South Africa, UK, Poland, Former Yugoslavia, Malta, Northern Ireland, Italy, Poland and Netherlands
[c]Healthcare card holders are people in Australia who have a concession card provided by the Australian Government to enable them to get cheaper medicines and some healthcare cost discounts
[d]Represents median (IQ range)
[e]Represents number of days in the last week in which carbohydrates were evenly spaced
[f]Represents numbers of days in the last week in which ≥30 min of physical activity was undertaken
IRSD Index of Relative Socioeconomic Disadvantage, *BMI* Body Mass Index, *CGM* Continuous Glucose Monitor, *TIR* Percentage Time in Range, *HbA1c* Glycated Haemoglobin

Table 2 Association between TIR/HbA1c and IRSD/Education using unadjusted and adjusted models

Variable	Unadjusted	Adjusted[a]
TIR		
	Mean difference in TIR (95% Confidence Interval)	Mean difference in TIR (95% Confidence Interval)
IRSD Decile	1.7% (0.7, 2.6)	1.5% (0.5, 2.5)
Educational attainment		
Trade/TAFE	−5.7% (−16.2, 4.8)	−4.9% (−15.0, 5.3)
University/diploma	1.6% (−5.4, 8.7)	1.4% (− 5.5, 8.2)
HbA1c		
	Mean difference in HbA1c (95% Confidence Interval)	Mean difference in HbA1c (95% Confidence Interval)
IRSD Decile	−0.06% (− 0.1, − 0.01)	−0.06% (− 0.1, − 0.01)
Educational attainment		
Trade/TAFE	0.3% (− 0.06, 0.6)	0.2% (− 0.1, 0.6)
University/diploma	− 0.07% (− 0.3, 0.2)	−0.08% (− 0.4, 0.2)

[a]Multivariable analysis was adjusted for age, BMI, diet, exercise and study arm

complications were retrieved from clinic medical electronic health records that may not be up to date. Our data were also sourced from only Victorian general practices and cannot be generalised to the whole Australian population. Lastly, heterogeneity in laboratory measurements (e.g. creatinine, albumin:creatinine ratio, HbA1c) which were performed in a variety of pathology laboratories may have weakened the correlation, though all laboratories would have been accredited and participate in a national quality control programme.

No studies have used TIR to look at the association with SES. As TIR may be a measure of glycaemic control that is easier for patients to understand, utilising TIR in clinical care particularly for patients from lower socio-economic backgrounds may aid in increasing patient engagement, which in turn could assist in optimising self-care behaviours, improving health outcomes, and could contribute to reducing health inequities seen in T2D. Our findings, in conjunction with previous international [22–28] and Australian [5] studies, also have significant implications for resource allocation of community-based health services to reduce the health inequity gap in patients with T2D. It also aids in highlighting the importance for GPs to consider and understand patient context when engaging and supporting patients with their diabetes self-management. Further studies involving larger patient sample sizes over a longer period throughout Australia to investigate this association are warranted, as well as further studies investigating patient and practitioner perceptions of TIR as a measure of glycaemic control. Further studies of the relative effectiveness and cost of CGMs in this population would also be useful and will be conducted as part of the GP-OSMOTIC trial at a later stage.

Conclusion

Our study showed a clinically and statistically significant association between an area-based measure of SES and glycaemic targets with more socio-economically disadvantaged people less likely to achieve glycaemic targets. Lower socioeconomic groups and areas may require prioritisation in resource allocation of primary health care services as well as policies aimed at ensuring equitable access to healthy environments to reduce health inequity. Our study highlights the importance of considering patient context during GP consultations and introduces a novel measure of glycaemia that may help with patient engagement to improve diabetes outcomes.

Abbreviations
CGM: Continuous glucose monitor; GP-OSMOTIC: General Practice Optimising Structured MOnitoring To Improve Clinical outcomes (GP-OSMOTIC); HbA1c: Glycated Haemoglobin; IRSD: Index of Relative Socioeconomic Disadvantage; SEIFA: Socio-Economic Indexes For Areas; SES: Socioeconomic Status; T2D: Type 2 Diabetes; TIR: Percentage Time in Range

Acknowledgements
We gratefully acknowledge the GP-OSMOTIC study team, especially research coordinators Katie De La Rue and Rebecca Hannam, for their hard work in patient and clinic recruitment, and collection of baseline study measures. We thank participating patients and general practice clinics for their support.

Funding
The GP-OSMOTIC study is supported by the National Health and Medical Research Council Project Grant (ID APP1104241). Additional funding has been provided by Sanofi-aventis Australia pty ltd. In-kind support has been provided by Abbott Diabetes Care who has provided Libre Pro reader devices, patient sensors and Libre Pro software. This research project is supported by the Royal Australian College of General Practitioners with funding from the Australian Government under the Australian General Practice Training programme.
The funding bodies and industry partners have no say in the design of the study and have no role in the collection, analysis, and interpretation of data or in writing the manuscript describing the outcomes of the study.

Authors' contributions

MLT collected data, performed data analysis, data interpretation and drafting of the manuscript. JAMN performed data analysis and interpretation, and was a major contributor in writing the manuscript. ST performed data analysis and interpretation. AJ and DO designed this study and interpreted study results. JF interpreted study results and was a major contributor in writing the manuscript. All authors read and approved the final manuscript.

Competing interests

JF has received unrestricted educational grants for research support from Roche, Sanofi and Medtronic.
DO is on the advisory boards to Abbott Diabetes Care, and Novo-Nordisk. DO and JAMN have had various financial relationships with pharmaceutical industries outside the submitted work including consultancies, grants, lectures, educational activities and travel. AJ is on an advisory board to Abbott Diabetes care and has had research grants and educational activities supported by various pharmaceutical industries outside the submitted work. The authors declare that they have no competing interests.

Author details

[1]Department of General Practice, University of Melbourne, Level 1, 200 Berkeley St, Carlton, VIC 3010, Australia. [2]NHMRC Clinical Trials Centre, University of Sydney, Levels 4-6 Medical Foundation Building, 92-94 Parramatta Rd, Camperdown, NSW 2050, Australia. [3]Department of Medicine, St Vincent's Hospital, The University of Melbourne, Level 4, Clinical Sciences Building, 29 Regent St, Fitzroy, VIC 3065, Australia.

References

1. National Health Survey First Results, Cat. No. 4363.0.55.001. Australian bureau of Statistics; 2015.
2. Diabetes Map. http://www.diabetesmap.com.au/#/. Accessed 24 Aug 2017.
3. General Practice Management of Type 2 Diabetes: 2016-2018. Royal Australian College of General Practitioners; 2016.
4. Diabetes: Australian facts 2008. In Diabetes series no8 Cat no CVD 40 Australian Institute of Health and Welfare; 2008.
5. Cross R, Bonney A, Mayne DJ, Weston KM. Cross-sectional study of area-level disadvantage and glycaemic-related risk in community health service users in the Southern.IML research (SIMLR) cohort. Aust Health Rev. 2017;
6. Beard E, Clark M, Hurel S, Cooke D. Do people with diabetes understand their clinical marker of long-term glycemic control (HbA1c levels) and does this predict diabetes self-care behaviours and HbA1c? Patient Educ Couns. 2010;80:227–32.
7. Heisler M, Piette JD, Spencer M, Kieffer E, Vijan S. The relationship between knowledge of recent HbA1c values and diabetes care understanding and self-management. Diabetes Care. 2005;28:816–22.
8. Harwell TS, Dettori N, McDowall JM, Quesenberry K, Priest L, Butcher MK, Flook BN, Helgerson SD, Gohdes D. Do persons with diabetes know their (AIC) number? The Diabetes Educator. 2002;28:99–105.
9. Perspectives on Education and Training: Social Inclusion, 2009. http://abs. gov.au/ausstats/abs@.nsf/Latestproducts/4250.0.55.001Main%20Features 12009?opendocument&tabname=Summary&prodno=4250.0.55.001&issue= 2009&num=&view=. Accessed 11 Oct 2017.
10. Ayotte BJ, Allaire JC, Bosworth H. The associations of patient demographic characteristics and health information recall: the mediating role of health literacy. Neuropsychol Dev Cogn B Aging Neuropsychol Cogn. 2009;16:419–32.
11. Scott TL, Gazmararian JA, Williams MV, Baker DW. Health literacy and preventive health care use among Medicare enrollees in a managed care organization. Med Care. 2002;40:395–404.
12. Brewer KW, Chase HP, Owen S, Garg SK. Slicing the pie. Correlating HbA--values with average blood glucose values in a pie chart form. Diabetes Care. 1998;21:209–12.
13. The Diabetes Control Complications Trial Research Group. The Effect of Intensive Treatment of Diabetes on the Development and Progression of Long-Term Complications in Insulin-Dependent Diabetes Mellitus. N Engl J Med. 1993;329:977–86.
14. Effect of intensive blood-glucose control with metformin on complications in overweight patients with type 2 diabetes (UKPDS 34). UK prospective diabetes study (UKPDS) group. Lancet. 1998;352:854–65.
15. National Evidence Based Guideline for Blood Glucose Control in Type 2 Diabetes. The Boden Institue of obesity, nutrition and exercise. The University of Sydney; 2009.
16. Ohkubo Y, Kishikawa H, Araki E, Miyata T, Isami S, Motoyoshi S, Kojima Y, Furuyoshi N, Shichiri M. Intensive insulin therapy prevents the progression of diabetic microvascular complications in Japanese patients with non-insulin-dependent diabetes mellitus: a randomized prospective 6-year study. Diabetes Res Clin Pract. 1995;28:103–17.
17. GP-OSMOTIC Study. http://medicine.unimelb.edu.au/mms/gp/gp-osmotic-study. Accessed 12 Dec 2017.
18. Johnson DW, Jones GRD, Mathew TH, Ludlow MJ, Doogue MP, Jose MD, Langham RG, Lawton PD, McTaggart SJ, Peake MJ, et al. Chronic kidney disease and automatic reporting of estimated glomerular filtration rate: new developments and revised recommendations. Med J Aust. 2012;197:224–5.
19. Harris PA, Taylor R, Thielke R, Payne J, Gonzalez N, Conde JG. Research electronic data capture (REDCap) - a metadata-driven methodology and workflow process for providing translational research informatics support. J Biomed Inform. 2009;42:377–81.
20. Freestyle Libre Flash Glucose Monitoring System User's Manual. https:// freestyleserver.com/Payloads/IFU/2017_oct/ART28697-409_rev-A_Web.pdf. Accessed 12 Dec 2017.
21. Pink B: Technical paper: socio-economic indexes for areas (SEIFA). 2013.
22. Emoto N, Okajima F, Goto R. A socioeconomic and behavioral survey of patients with difficult-to-control type 2 diabetes mellitus reveals an association between diabetic retinopathy and educational attainment. Patient Preference & Adherence. 2016;10:2151–62.
23. Xiaoming T, Jihu L, Xiaolin Z, Bin Z, Jiao S, Linong J, Dayi H, Changyu P, Yuxin H, Suyuan J, et al. Association between socioeconomic status and metabolic control and diabetes complications: a cross-sectional nationwide study in Chinese adults with type 2 diabetes mellitus. Cardiovasc Diabetol. 2016;15:1–10.
24. Schillinger D, Barton LR, Karter AJ, Wang F, Adler N. Does literacy mediate the relationship between education and health outcomes? A study of a low-income population with diabetes. Public Health Rep. 2006;121:245–54.
25. Goudswaard AN, Stolk RP, Zuithoff P, Rutten GE. Patient characteristics do not predict poor glycaemic control in type 2 diabetes patients treated in primary care. Eur J Epidemiol. 2004;19:541–5.
26. Saydah SH, Imperatore G, Beckles GL. Socioeconomic status and mortality: contribution of health care access and psychological distress among U.S. adults with diagnosed diabetes. Diabetes Care. 2013;36:49–55.
27. Bachmann MO, Eachus J, Hopper CD, Davey Smith G, Propper C, Pearson NJ, Williams S, Tallon D, Frankel S. Socio-economic inequalities in diabetes complications, control, attitudes and health service use: a cross-sectional study. Diabet Med. 2003;20:921–9.
28. Laraia BA, Karter AJ, Warton EM, Schillinger D, Moffet HH, Adler N. Place matters: neighborhood deprivation and cardiometabolic risk factors in the diabetes study of northern California (DISTANCE). Soc Sci Med. 2012;74: 1082–90.
29. Morgan M. Measuring social inequality: occupational classifications and their alternatives. Community Med. 1983;5:116–24.
30. Dutton TT, Gavid; Oldenburg, Brian: Measuring socioeconomic position in population health monitoring and health research. 2005.
31. de Vries McClintock HF, Wiebe DJ, Odonnell AJ, Morales KH, Small DS, Bogner HR, O'Donnell AJ. Neighborhood social environment and patterns of adherence to oral hypoglycemic agents among patients with type 2 diabetes mellitus. Family & Community Health. 2015;38:169–79.

6

Effect of hypothyroidism on the hypothalamic–pituitary–ovarian axis and reproductive function of pregnant rats

Jianran Sun[1†], Cancan Hui[1†], Tongjia Xia[1†], Min Xu[1], Datong Deng[1*] ⓘ, Faming Pan[2] and Youmin Wang[1]

Abstract

Background: This study aimed to detect changes in hormone levels in the hypothalamic–pituitary–ovarian axis in Sprague-Dawley (SD) rats with hypothyroidism, and identify differences in the pregnancy and abortion rates of female adult rats. The potential role of gonadotropin releasing hormone (GnRH) as the link between the hypothalamic–pituitary–ovarian axis and reproductive function regulated by thyroid hormones was also investigated.

Methods: Female SD rats ($n = 136$) were causally classified into two groups: the normal-drinking-water group ($n = 60$) and the 0.05% propylthiouracil-drinking-water group (PTU 2 mg/kg/day, $n = 76$) to establish an adult rat model of hypothyroidism (6 weeks). Female and male rats at a ratio of 1:2 were used to establish a hypothyroidism pregnancy model. GnRH mRNA and GnRH receptor (GnRHR) expression in rats was detected using real time quantitative PCR(qRT-PCR) and immunohistochemistry, respectively.

Results: The abortion rate differed significantly between the hypothyroidism pregnancy group and the normal pregnancy group ($P < 0.05$). No significant differences were found in the distribution of the GnRHR among the five nuclei (hypothalamic arcuate nucleus, hypothalamic ventromedial nucleus, hypothalamic anterior nucleus, paraventricular nucleus of the hypothalamus, and ventral premammillary nucleus) of the hypothalamus and ovary ($P > 0.05$). Hypothyroidism had no significant effect on GnRH mRNA expression in the hypothalamic–pituitary–ovarian axis in the four groups (normal control group, normal pregnancy group, hypothyroidism pregnancy group, and hypothyroidism group) ($P > 0.05$).

Conclusions: Hypothyroidism had an adverse impact on pregnancy in rats and may affect the distribution of pituitary GnRHR, whereas it did not obviously affect the distribution of GnRHR in the nuclei of the hypothalamus and ovary. Hypothyroidism had no effect on GnRH mRNA expression.

Keywords: Hypothyroidism, Hypothalamic–pituitary–ovarian axis, GnRH, GnRHR

Background

The regulation of reproductive function is mainly accomplished by the hypothalamic–pituitary–ovarian axis. The amount of thyroid hormone (TH) contributes to maintaining the stability of the pituitary ovarian axis [1]. Metabolic disorders caused by abnormal thyroid function further increase the risk of infertility [2]. Gonadotropin

releasing hormone (GnRH) plays an important role in the cascade mediating the release of reproductive hormones in the hypothalamic–pituitary–ovarian axis [3]. Clinical findings identified bidirectional communication between thyroxine and the hypothalamic–pituitary–ovarian axis; however, the underlying mechanism remains unclear [4]. In the present study, we sought to determine whether GnRH is the central link between the hypothalamic–pituitary–ovarian axis and reproductive function regulated by TH.

In primates, puberty is initiated by a surge of pulsatile GnRH that begins a prolonged phase of juvenile

* Correspondence: dengdayong@ahmu.edu.cn
†Equal contributors
[1]Department of Endocrinology, Institute of Endocrinology and Metabolism, The First Affiliated Hospital of Anhui Medical University, 218 Jixi Road, Hefei 230022, Anhui, China
Full list of author information is available at the end of the article

development in which the hypothalamic network regulates the release of GnRH, which is held in check by mechanisms that are poorly understood [5]. At the initial stage of infancy and prior to GnRH release, circulating gonadotropin levels are elevated and, in infantile female primates, are associated with blood estradiol levels in the adult range [6]. Therefore, primate adolescence is thought to be dominated by two primary postnatal switches [7]. During infancy, the first switch is activated and inhibits GnRH pulsation discharge, which leads to a hypogonadotropic condition that secures gonadal silencing before puberty. At the end of adolescent growth, the second switch is invoked, which leads to the recurrence of puberty in the discharge of pulsatile GnRH and the formation of the hypothalamic–pituitary–ovarian axis (gonadarche), the major physiological process underlying primate puberty [8].

The release of GnRH from approximately 1000 neurons within the hypothalamus in a pulsatile manner, which is characteristic of postnatal development in primates, is largely independent of the gonad [9]. Although the switch of pulsatile GnRH discharge leading to the recurrence of puberty has been researched widely, few studies have explored the causes of the inhibition of the GnRH pulse generators at the start of youth. In any case, the potential neurobiology is difficult to comprehend [10]. Under both conditions, one can assume that significant developmental variations in GnRH pulsation are associated with structural remolding of the GnRH pulse generator and/or with molecular variations in the hypothalamus.

Pulsed GnRH discharge during pubertal relapse depends on the allowable action of TH in this developmental phase. The action of TH during infancy is not related to the constraint that affects pulsatile GnRH release during infancy-youth switching or during pubertal reactivation of the pulse generators of GnRH [11]. TH deficiency during infancy also fails to have an effect on the timing of the pubertal resurgence of gonadotropin secretion [12].

Methods
Materials
Propylthiouracil (PTU) was purchased from Sigma-Aldrich (St. Louis, MO, USA). Distilled water with 3% H_2O_2 and mouse monoclonal antibody against human GnRH receptor (GnRHR) (clone F1G4) were purchased from Beijing ZhongShan Golden Bridge Biological Technology, Co., Ltd. (Beijing, China). Phosphate-buffered saline (2 mg/mL, pH: 7.4), bovine serum albumin, SYBR Premix Ex Taq II (Tli RNaseH Plus), ROX Reference Dye, and ROX Reference Dye II were purchased from Takara Bio Dalian Co., Ltd. (Dalian, China). Rat tri-iodothyronine (T_3) enzyme-linked immunosorbent assay (ELISA) kit, rat thyroxine (T_4) ELISA

kit, and rat thyroid-stimulating hormone (TSH) ELISA kit were purchased from Shanghai Yuan Ye Biotechnology Co., Ltd. (Shanghai, China).

Protocols and experimental design
All animal experiments were performed in accordance with the principles approved by the Animal Ethics Committee of Anhui Medical University. A total of 280 SD rats (7 days old, 55–70 g) were obtained from the Experimental Animal Center of Anhui Medical University. Food and tap water were continuously available in the cage top. Lights in the colony were on from 04:00 to 20:00 h and temperatures were maintained between 21 °C and 25 °C. All conditions and treatments were in accordance with the recommended humane conditions. The rats were randomly mated in polycarbonate cages (40 × 30 × 26 cm) with grid floors from 18:00 to 18:30 h each day, and the female-to-male sex ratio of the SD rats was 1:2. The period of mating was 3 days and the frequency was three times per day. Cages were checked daily, and the day in which an avaginal plug was secreted and detected was considered to be day 1 of gestation (G-1). Stainless steel wire lids and wood shavings were used as bedding material, and parturition occurred between G-21 and G-2. Pregnant rats were housed individually in polycarbonate cages (38 × 30 × 27 cm).

Infertile female SD rats
The SD rats that were mated three times but did not secrete a vaginal plug were considered infertile.

Establishment of a hypothyroid pregnant rat model
A total of 136 female SD rats were included and randomly divided into two groups, a normal-drinking-water group ($n = 60$) and a 0.05% PTU-drinking-water group (2 mg/kg/day, $n = 76$) to establish an adult rat model of hypothyroidism (6 weeks). Five rats were randomly selected from each group to measure the level of TH and determine whether the model of hypothyroidism was successfully established. Twenty-five SD rats from the normal-drinking-water group were randomly selected as the normal control group ($n = 25$). The remaining 30 SD rats in the normal-drinking-water group were subdivided into the normal caged-group ($n = 30$), and the remaining 71 rats in the PTU-drinking-water group were established as the hypothyroidism caged-group ($n = 71$). Thirty-two SD rats from the hypothyroidism caged-group were randomly picked as the hypothyroidism group ($n = 32$). The female and normal male rats at a respective ratio of 1:2 were mated to establish a pregnancy model, and the pregnant rats were further divided into the normal pregnancy group ($n = 24$) and the hypothyroidism pregnancy group ($n = 28$). One day after G-21, 11 rats that were not pregnant from the hypothyroidism pregnancy group and

six rats that were not pregnant from the normal pregnancy group were humanely killed by cervical dislocation under anesthesia. Finally, there were 25, 24, 28, and 32 rats in the normal control group, normal pregnancy group, hypothyroidism pregnancy group, and hypothyroidism group, respectively. The establishment of the hypothyroid pregnant rat model is described in Fig. 1.

Specimen preparation

After 12 h of fasting, the rats were anesthetized by intraperitoneal injection of 10% chloral hydrate (0.3 mL/100 g). Blood was collected from the abdominal aorta, and samples of brain tissues, pituitary tissues, and ovarian tissues were harvested. Portions of the samples were placed in 10% formaldehyde fixative, followed by gradient alcohol dehydration, xylene dewaxing, and serial sectioning.

Immunohistochemistry staining detection

The tissue blocks were cut into 3–4 μm thick sections for histological analysis, dehydrated in an ascending series of ethanol, and dewaxed in xylene. For increased specificity and sensitivity, tissues were microwaved for 10 min for antigen retrieval, followed by cooling and rinsing in distilled water. Endogenous peroxidase activity was blocked with 3% H_2O_2 for 30 min at room temperature, followed by a serum-free protein block for 1 h at room temperature. Sections were incubated with antibodies against GnRHR (20 mg/mL) overnight at 4 °C. The streptavidin–peroxidase method was used to detect the antigen–antibody complexes, and diaminobenzidine was used as the chromogen substrate. The optical density values of stained tissues photographed with a Nikon Eclipse 80i fluorescence microscope (Tokyo, Japan) were quantified using Image Pro Plus 6.0 software (Maryland, USA).

ELISA for determination of serum T_3, T_4, and TSH levels

Serum levels of T_3, T_4, and TSH were detected using ELISA following the kit protocol (Shanghai Yuanye Biological Technology Co., Ltd.). The activity of these hormones was used as a measure of thyroid function.

qRT-PCR

RNA was isolated from tissues of the arcuate nucleus (ARC) of the hypothalamus of SD rats using the TRIzol

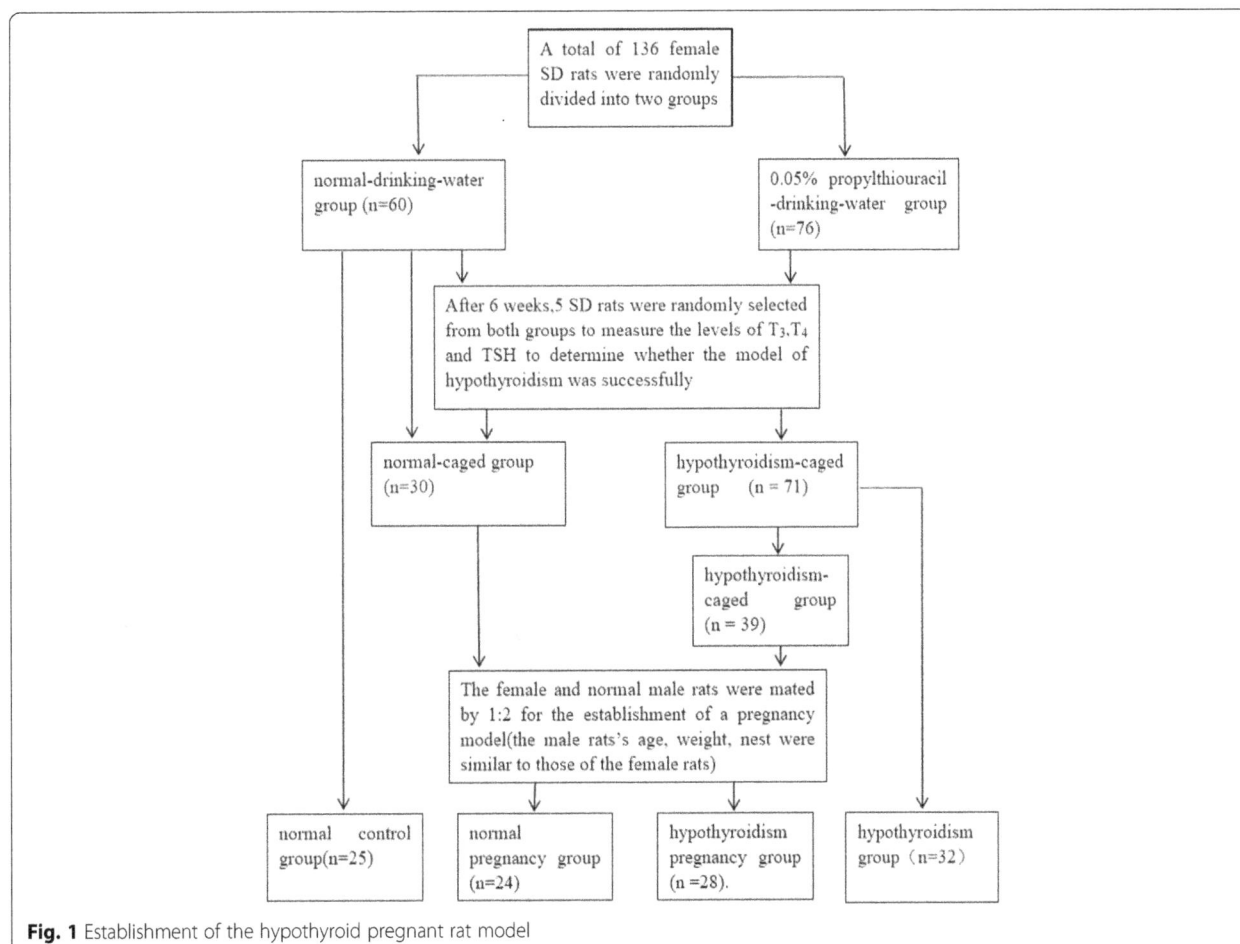

Fig. 1 Establishment of the hypothyroid pregnant rat model

reagent (Sigma–Aldrich, St Louis, MO, USA) according to the manufacturer's instructions. mRNA levels were quantified using qRT-PCR. In brief, RNA preparations were used to synthesize cDNA in all qRT-PCRs, with a reaction volume of 20 μL, including primers (forward and reverse; details in Table 1), SYBR MIX, ddH$_2$O, and 2 μL of RNA. The cycling conditions were as follows: denaturation for 0.5 min at 95 °C, followed by 40 cycles of amplification for 0.5 min at 60 °C and 5 s at 95 °C, and a final elongation step for 10 min at 72 °C. Every sample of cDNA (2 μL) was individually amplified using β-actin-specific primers to assess the RNA integrity and components of the reaction. qRT-PCR analyses were performed in duplicate with at least three individual RNA samples from each group during the period of development. The melting curves for every reaction were recorded to confirm the purity of the amplified product. The comparative cycle threshold (Ct) method was used to calculate the relative expression levels, and β-actin expression was used to normalize mRNA expression. The expression value of 7-day-old rat ARC was considered as the reference sample (Reference Value 1) for every period of development for comparisons with other groups. Every mean Ct value of β-actin was subtracted from the corresponding target-based Ct (GnRH) to obtain the ΔCt. The ΔCt of the 7-day-old rat was subtracted from each ΔCt of the period group to determine the ΔΔCt. Thus, the formula $2^{-\Delta\Delta CT}$ was used to calculate the fold expression to compare the experimental groups with the 7-day-old rat samples. The relative quantity (RQ = $2^{\wedge(-\Delta\Delta Ct)}$) value was the output by qRT-PCR, which is the comparison of the Ct value, transformed by mathematical formulas.

Statistical analysis

Statistical analysis was performed using IBM SPSS 16.0 (Armonk, NY, USA). The data of the normal distribution were represented as $\bar{x} \pm s$, and the data of the skewed distribution were represented as M (P_{25}, P_{75}). Differences between the two sets were compared using the Chi-square test for qualitative data. Differences between the two sets were compared by the paired t-test for normal distributions, and comparisons among groups were performed with one-way analysis of variance (one-way ANOVA). Differences between sets were also compared using the SNK-Q test [13, 14]. For non-normal distributions, differences between sets were compared with the

Kruskal–Wallis test. Nemenyi test is a post hoc test that can be used after a Kruskal-Wallis test to indicate significant differences between the different groups. The P-value calibration method was used to compare the differences between the two sets with Fisher's exact test using crosstabs of $n < 40$ and theoretical frequency [T ij = (n$_i$ * m$_j$)/n(n: total numbers of cases; n$_i$: total numbers of the i row; m$_j$: total numbers of the j column)] < 1. Differences with $P < 0.05$ were considered statistically significant.

Results

Establishment of a hypothyroid pregnant rat model

At the end of the 6-month period of drinking 0.05% PTU water, the female SD rats moved slowly. Their shins and hair became brownish yellow. Thyroid function was measured in blood samples collected from the angular vein. The results of paired t tests showed statistically significant differences in T$_3$ ($t = 13.749$, $P < 0.001$), T$_4$ ($t = 9.644$, $P < 0.001$, and TSH ($t = 7.009$, $P < 0.001$) between the normal-drinking-water group and the 0.05% PTU-drinking-water group. Serum T$_3$ and T$_4$ levels were lower and serum TSH levels were higher in the 0.05% PTU-drinking-water group than in the normal-drinking-water group ($P < 0.05$, both). The establishment of the hypothyroid rat model is described in Table 2.

Comparison of the pregnancy and miscarriage rates of SD rats

There were significant differences in the conception rates between the normal pregnancy group and the hypothyroidism pregnancy group *(P < 0.05)* according to the results of the Chi-square test. The abortion rate differed significantly between the normal pregnancy group and the hypothyroidism pregnancy group as determined by Fisher's exact test ($P < 0.05$). The results showed that the miscarriage rate increased and the pregnancy rate decreased in the hypothyroid pregnant SD rats. The pregnancy rate and miscarriage rate results are shown in Table 3.

Immunohistochemical analysis of the expression of GnRHR in the hypothalamus, pituitary gland, and ovary in the four groups

The immunohistochemistry results are shown in Figs. 2, 3, 4 and 5. The data of integral optical density values of pituitary GnRHR are consistent with skewed distribution. M (P_{25}, P_{75}) for figures used in the calculations are presented in a box plot. Similarly, the data of integral optical density values of ovarian GnRHR were consistent with normal distribution. $\bar{x} \pm s$ for figures used in the calculations are presented in a histogram. In the present study, we aimed to investigate the expression of GnRHR in the target gland, such as the pituitary gland, and ovary.

Table 1 Sequences of PCR primers

Gene	Primer	Sequence(5'-3')	Accession no.
GnRH	GnRH-F	TCCAGCCAGCACTGGGTCCTA	NM_012767.2
	GnRH-R	GGGTTCTGCCATTTGATCCTC	
β-actin	β-actin-F	GGAGATTACTGCCCTGGCTCCTA	NM_017008.4
	β-actin-R	GACTCATCGTACTCCTGCTTGCTG	

PCR Polymerase chain reaction

Table 2 Establishment of hypothyroidism($\bar{x} \pm s$)

Items	normal-drinking- water group($n = 5$)	0.05%PTU-drinking-water group($n = 5$)	t value	P value
T_3(ng/mL)	128.52 ± 6.57	66.27 ± 7.70[**]	13.749	< 0.001
T_4(ug/dL)	232.76 ± 9.41	174.45 ± 9.67[**]	9.644	< 0.001
TSH(ulU/L)	1111.02 ± 84.83	1476.56 ± 79.75[**]	7.009	< 0.001

[**] $P < 0.01$,compared to normal-drinking- water group

Therefore, GnRHR distribution in the hypothalamus was used as a negative control. The histogram or box plot was added as a Supplementary file, without including the integral optical density values of the hypothalamus. The relative integral optical density values of pituitary and ovarian GnRHR in the four groups are shown in Additional file 1: Figure S1 and Additional file 2: Figure S2, respectively.

3.1 The integral optical density values of hypothalamus GnRHR in the four groups are shown in Table 4

(1) In the normal control group, there were no statistically significant differences in the expression of GnRHR in the hypothalamus between the five nuclei by one-way ANOVA ($F = 0.810$, $P = 0.531$).

(2) In the hypothyroidism group, there were no statistically significant differences between the five nuclei by one-way ANOVA ($F = 0.717$, $P = 0.949$).

(3) In the normal pregnancy group, there were no statistically significant differences between the five nuclei by one-way ANOVA ($F = 0.432$, $P = 0.782$).

(4) In the hypothyroidism pregnancy group, there were no statistically significant differences between the five nuclei by one-way ANOVA ($F = 0.440$, $P = 0.779$).

(5) There were no statistically significant differences in the hypothalamic arcuate (ar) nucleus between the four groups by one-way ANOVA ($F = 0.373$, $P = 0.774$).

(6) There were no statistically significant differences in the hypothalamic ventromedial (vmh) nucleus between the four groups by one-way ANOVA ($F = 1.346$, $P = 0.291$).

(7) There were no statistically significant differences in the hypothalamic anterior (ah) nucleus between the four groups by one-way ANOVA ($F = 2.486$, $P = 0.478$).

(8) There were no statistically significant differences in the paraventricular (pa) nucleus of hypothalamus between the four groups by one-way ANOVA ($F = 0.591$, $P = 0.670$).

(9) There were no statistically significant differences in the ventral premammillary (pmv) nucleus between the four groups by one-way ANOVA ($F = 0.517$, $P = 0.676$).

No differences in the distribution of GnRHR were identified between the five nuclei (ar, vmh, ah, pa, and pmv) of the hypothalamus.

3.2 The integral optical density values of pituitary GnRHR in the four groups

(1) The Kruskal–Wallis test showed that there were statistically significant differences in the expression of the GnRHR in the pituitary between the four groups ($P = 0.037$).

(2) There were no statistically significant differences between the hypothyroidism pregnancy group and the hypothyroidism group according to the Nemenyi test (standard $\chi^2 = 0.089$, $P = 0.929$).

(3) There were no statistically significant differences between the hypothyroidism pregnancy group and normal control group (standard $\chi^2 = 1.809$, $P = 0.071$).

(4) Statistically significant differences were also found between the hypothyroidism pregnancy group and normal pregnancy group (standard $\chi^2 = 2.345$, $P = 0.019$).

(5) No statistically significant differences were observed between the hypothyroidism group and normal control group (standard $\chi^2 = 1.720$, $P = 0.086$).

(6) There were statistically significant differences between the hypothyroidism group and normal pregnancy group (standard $\chi^2 = 2.268$, $P = 0.023$).

(7) No statistically significant differences were detected between the normal control group and normal pregnancy group (standard $\chi^2 = 0.779$, $P = 0.436$).

To summarize, differences in the expression of the GnRHR in the pituitary were observed.

Table 3 Pregnancy and miscarriage rates

Items	hypothyroidism pregnancy group ($n = 39$)	normal pregnancy group ($n = 30$)	χ^2 value	P value
numbers of pregnancy	28	24		
numbers of miscarriage	10	0		
pregnancy rate(%)	71.4	80.0	0.002	0.096
miscarriage rate(%)	25.6[*]	0		0.036

In the cross table, n < 40 and T < 1; therefore, Fisher's exact test is used ($P = 0.036$) and there is no χ^2 value

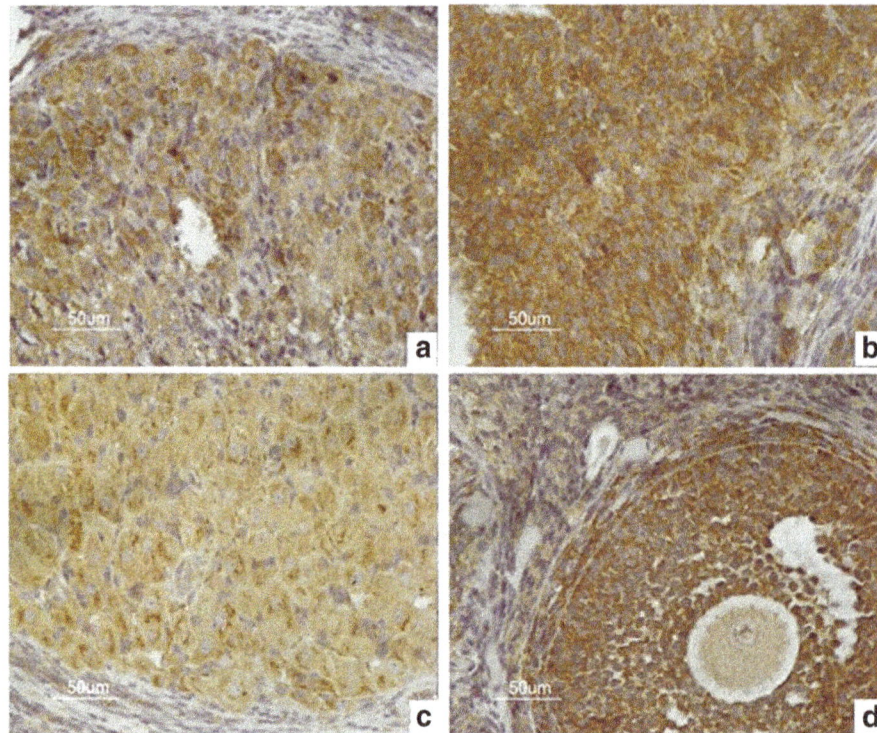

Fig. 2 Immunohistochemical analysis of GnRHR expression in the hypothalamus in four groups. **a** hypothyroidism group. **b** normal control group. **c** normal pregnant group. **d** hypothyroidism pregnant group

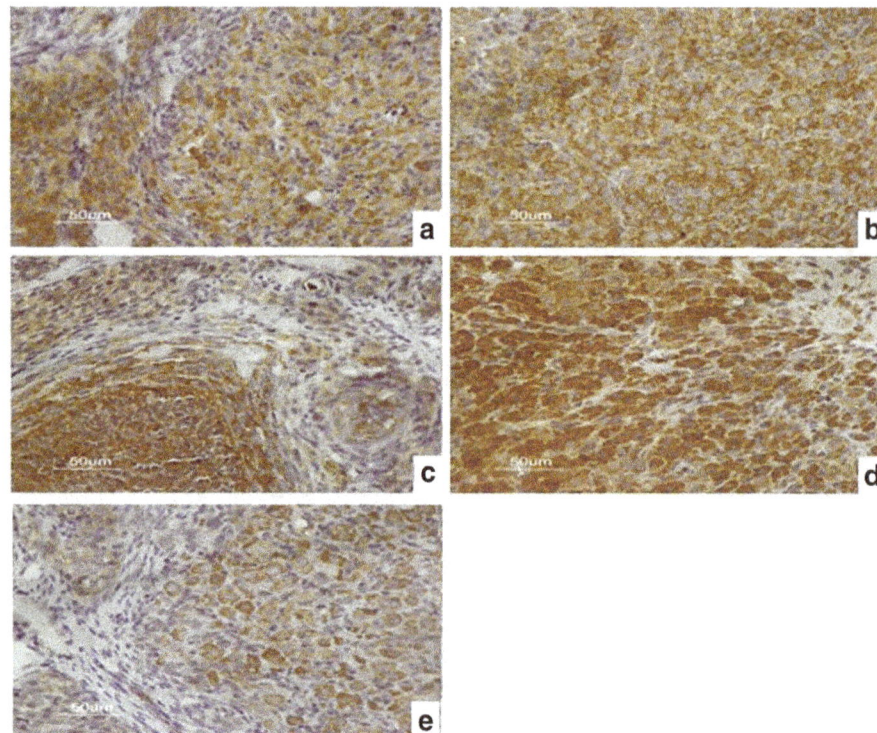

Fig. 3 Hypothalamic nuclei. **a** hypothalamic arcuate nucleus. **b** hypothalamic ventromedial nucleus. **c** hypothalamic anterior nucleus. **d** paraventricular nucleus of hypothalamus. **e** ventral premammillary nucleus

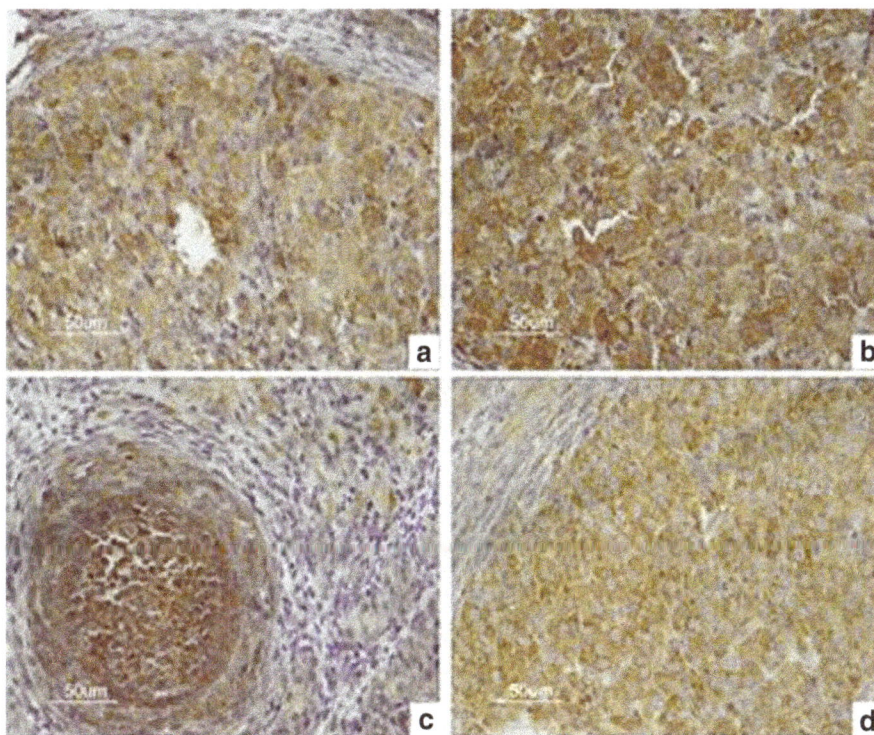

Fig. 4 Immunohistochemical analysis of GnRHR expression in the pituitary in four groups. **a** hypothyroidism group. **b** normal control group. **c** normal pregnant group. **d** hypothyroidism pregnant group

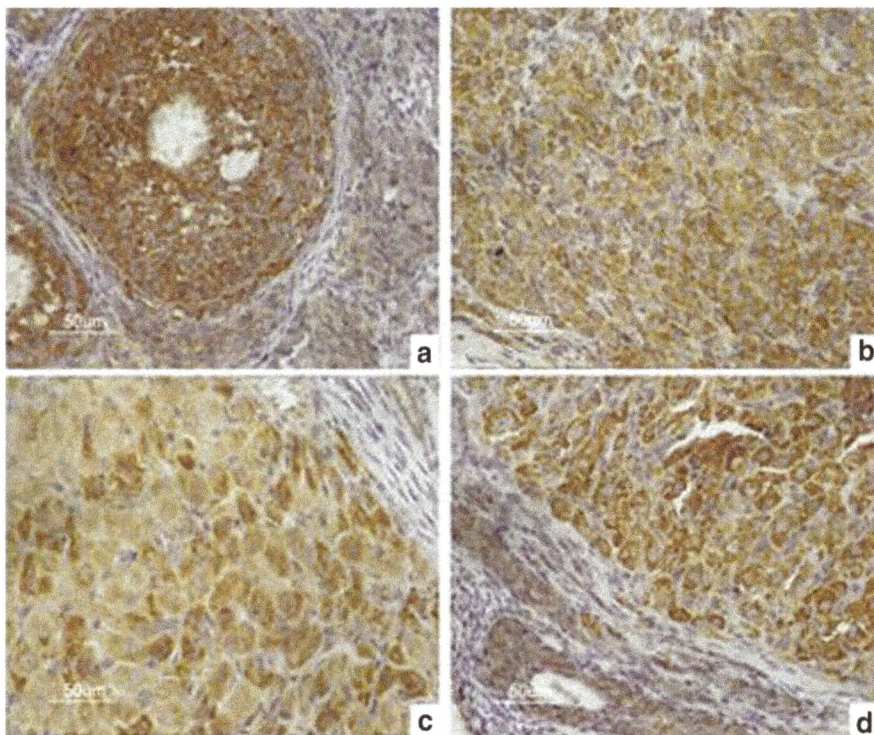

Fig. 5 Immunohistochemical results of GnRHR expression in the ovary in four groups. **a** hypothyroidism group. **b** normal control group. **c** normal pregnant group. **d** hypothyroidism pregnant group

Table 4 Comparison of integral optical density values of hypothalamus GnRHR between four groups

Groups	hypothyroidism pregnancy group	hypothyroidism group	normal control group	normal pregnancy group	F value	P value
Numbers	28	32	25	24		
arc	(61.14 ± 42.84)	(46.47 ± 18.77)	(63.12 ± 42.14)	(48.87 ± 7.24)	0.373	0.774
vmh	(65.05 ± 36.71)	(48.31 ± 14.94)	(75.97 ± 29.75)	(70.22 ± 4.00)	1.346	0.291
ah	(64.94 ± 49.85)	(48.94 ± 5.84)	(73.75 ± 43.93)	(59.33 ± 23.37)	2.486	0.478
pa	(57.62 ± 30.70)	(42.85 ± 13.95)	(50.08 ± 17.37)	(67.07 ± 43.77)	0.591	0.670
pmv	(40.76 ± 17.26)	(46.22 ± 13.09)	(62.99 ± 32.10)	(46.95 ± 1.30)	0.517	0.676
F value	0.440	0.717	0.810	0.432		
P value	0.779	0.949	0.531	0.782		

arc:arcuate hypothalamic nucleus; vmh:ventromedial hypothalamic nucleus;
ah:anterior hypothalamic nucleus; pa:paraventricular nucleus of hypothalamus; pmv:ventral premammillary nucleus

3.3 The integral optical density values of ovarian GnRHR in the four groups

No statistically significant differences in the expression of the GnRHR in the ovary were observed between the four groups by one-way ANOVA ($F = 0.544$, $P = 0.655$).

Effect of hypothyroidism on GnRH mRNA expression

The amplification curve of GnRH mRNA and β-actin mRNA showed an inverted S type. The amplification curves of GnRH mRNA ran parallel with those of β-actin mRNA, which indicated that qRT-PCR could detect β-actin in a broad range with high efficiency and in a short time. The solubility curve had a single peak, which indicated that primer specificity was high. This indicated that a single qRT-PCR product was used, and that the data obtained were reliable. The relative mRNA levels of pituitary and ovarian GnRH in the four groups are shown in Fig. 6 and Fig. 7, respectively.

Comparison of the RQ values of hypothalamus GnRH mRNA between the four groups

There was no statistically significant difference by one-way ANOVA ($F = 1.412$, $P = 0.296$) ($P > 0.05$, details in Table 5).

Comparison of the RQ values of pituitary GnRH mRNA between the four groups

There was no statistically significant difference by one-way ANOVA ($F = 1.153$, $P = 0.368$) ($P > 0.05$, details in Table 6).

Comparison of the RQ values of ovarian GnRH mRNA between the four groups

There were no statistically significant differences by Kruskal–Wallis test ($\chi^2 = 1.276$, $P = 0.077$) ($P > 0.05$, Table 7).

GnRH mRNA RQ values of the hypothalamus, pituitary gland, and ovary in the normal control group

There was a statistically significant difference between these groups ($\chi^2 = 7.372$, $P = 0.025$). The results of group-wise comparisons were as follows:

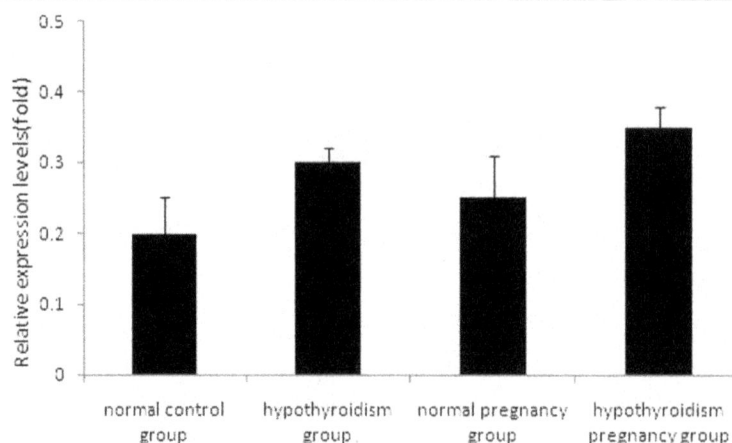

Fig. 6 Relative mRNA levels of pituitary GnRH in the four groups determined using qRT-PCR, $P > 0.05$

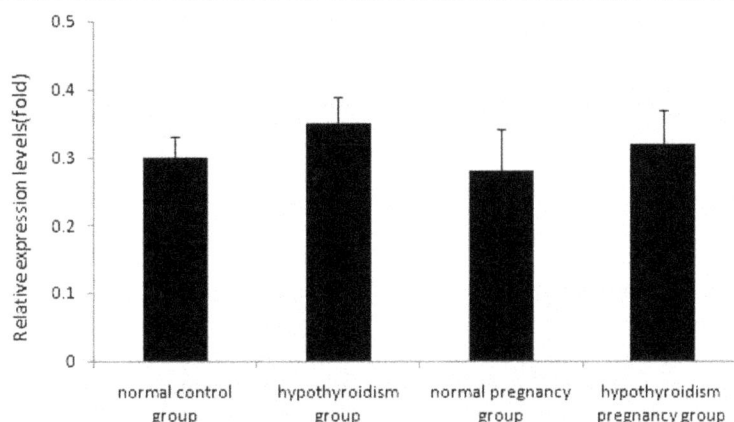

Fig. 7 Relative mRNA levels of ovarian GnRH in the four groups determined using qRT-PCR, $P > 0.05$

(1) There was no statistically significant difference in the value of GnRH mRNA RQ between the ovary and pituitary gland ($Z = 0.889$, $P = 0.374$)

(2) There was a statistically significant difference in the value of GnRH mRNA RQ between the ovary and hypothalamus ($Z = 2.666$, $P = 0.008$)

(3) There was no statistically significant difference in the value of GnRH mRNA RQ between the hypothalamus and pituitary ($Z = 1.778$, $P = 0.075$)

Comparison of GnRH mRNA RQ values of the hypothalamus, pituitary gland, and ovary in the hypothyroidism group

There was a statistically significant difference between these groups (standard $\chi^2 = 8.769$, $P = 0.012$). Group-wise comparisons were as follows:

(1) There was no statistically significant difference in the value of GnRH mRNA RQ between the ovary and pituitary gland ($Z = 1.177$, $P = 0.239$)

(2) There was a statistically significant difference in the value of GnRH mRNA RQ between the ovary and hypothalamus ($Z = 2.942$, $P = 0.003$)

(3) There was no statistically significant difference in the value of GnRH mRNA RQ between the hypothalamus and the pituitary gland ($Z = 1.765$, $P = 0.078$)

Comparison of GnRH mRNA RQ values of the hypothalamus, pituitary gland, and ovary in the normal pregnancy group

The difference was statistically significant (standard $\chi^2 = 6.144$, $P = 0.046$). Group-wise comparisons were as follows:

(1) There was a statistically significant difference in the value of GnRH mRNA RQ values between the ovary and pituitary gland ($Z = 2.204$, $P = 0.028$)

(2) There was a statistically significant difference in the value of GnRH mRNA RQ between the ovary and hypothalamus ($Z = 2.205$, $P = 0.043$)

(3) There was no statistically significant difference in the value of GnRH mRNA RQ between the hypothalamus and pituitary gland ($Z = 0.329$, $P = 0.742$)

Comparison of GnRH mRNA RQ values of the hypothalamus, pituitary gland, and ovary in the hypothyroidism pregnancy group

The differences between these groups were statistically significant (standard $\chi^2 = 8.909$, $P = 0.012$). Group-wise comparisons were as follows:

(1) There was no statistically significant difference in the value of GnRH mRNA RQ between the ovary and pituitary gland ($Z = 1.706$, $P = 0.088$)

Table 5 Comparison of RQ values of hypothalamus GnRH mRNA between four groups

Items	Hypothyroidism pregnancy group	Hypothyroidism group	normal control group	norma pregnancy group	F value	P value
C_T	(21.42,29.96)	(21.96,23.83)	(20.02,24.27)	(21.56,24.69)	–	–
$\triangle C_T$	(5.72,15.29)	(5.60,8.30)	(3.90,7.19)	(6.45,10.00)	–	–
$\triangle \triangle C_T$	(−4.27,5.29)	(−4.39,-1.70)	(−6.09,-2.81)	(−3.55,0.00)	–	–
RQ	(8.56 ± 9.85)	(16.79 ± 5.97)	(29.04 ± 27.71)	(7.62 ± 4.68)	1.412	0.296

Table 6 Comparison of RQ values of pituitary GnRH mRNA between four groups

Items	hypothyroidism pregnancy group	hypothyroidism group	normal control group	norma pregnancy group	Fvalue	P value
C_T	(30.03,31.98)	(31.79,33.24)	(31.56,32.93)	(32.60,32.73)	–	–
$\triangle C_T$	(11.82,12.18)	(11.76,33.24)	(12.53,13.32)	(13.35,14.19)	–	–
$\triangle\triangle C_T$	(0.94,1.11)	(0.69,1.38)	(1.46,2.25)	(2.28,3.11)	–	–
RQ	(0.16 ± 0.07)	(0.78 ± 0.79)	(0.49 ± 0.31)	(0.42 ± 0.40)	1.153	0.368

(2) There was a statistically significant difference in the value of GnRH mRNA RQ between the ovary and hypothalamus ($Z = 2.961$, $P = 0.003$)

(3) There was no statistically significant difference in the value of GnRH mRNA RQ between the hypothalamus and pituitary gland ($Z = 1.382$, $P = 0.167$)

Discussion

The mutual effects of the gonadal axis and the thyroid play a critical role in maintaining normal reproduction. Thyroid dysfunction can cause unnatural menstrual patterns, infertility problems, and ovulation disorders [15]. The high incidence of thyroid disease among women in sterile couples is well recorded in the literature [16].

In the present study, we demonstrated that hypothyroidism exerted an adverse effect on pregnancy in rats. Additionally, the results suggested that hypothyroidism in pregnant SD rats was associated with an increased miscarriage rate and a decreasing pregnancy rate. Hypothyroidism is associated with various conditions, such as placental abruption, pre-eclampsia, and intra-uterine fetal death [17]. Subclinical hypothyroidism is defined as a serum TSH level above the normal range despite normal serum free thyroxine levels. In addition, the side effects of subclinical hypothyroidism (SCH) include higher rates of premature delivery, abortion, and pregnancy-induced hypertension [18, 19]. Maraka et al. assessed (a) the effect of SCH during pregnancy on maternal and neonatal outcomes and (b) the impact of levothyroxine replacement therapy in these patients [20]. They found that compared with euthyroid pregnant women, pregnant women with SCH are at a higher risk of pregnancy loss [risk ratio (RR): 2.01, confidence interval (CI): 1.66–2.44], placental abruption (RR: 2.14, CI: 1.23–3.70), premature rupture of membranes (RR: 1.43, CI: 1.04–1.95), and neonatal death (RR: 2.58, CI: 1.41–4.73). The authors concluded that SCH during pregnancy is related to multiple adverse maternal and neonatal outcomes. The value of levothyroxine therapy in preventing these adverse outcomes remains uncertain.

The present results suggested that hypothyroidism affects the distribution of the pituitary GnRHR; however, we observed no evident effect on the distribution of the GnRHR of the ovary and hypothalamus. The GnRH neuronal system plays a regulatory role in the pituitary–gonadal axis hierarchy by regulating the secretion of pituitary luteinizing hormone and follicle-stimulating hormone. Variations of GnRH neurons are critical for regulating pubertas and the oestrous cycle. It is noteworthy that a "GnRH surge" triggers ovulation, and GnRH pulse secretion is not under seasonal control [21].

Although studies clearly show how hormones and other factors affect propagation, the brain remains a "black box" in that model. GnRH neurons serve as the ultimate pathway for controlling propagation; however, identification of the GnRH neurons involved in pulsatile secretion and how steroids and other factors modulate their activity remain unresolved issues, as indicated by the latest surveys among researchers. In the next sections, some key tests are reviewed. Because thyroid hormones (THs) are critical mediators, new evidence supporting this role is needed as well as evidence showing that THs directly affect GnRH neurons and may affect their developmental destiny and functionality in the brains of adults [22].

Unlike other neuroendocrine systems, GnRH neurons are scattered in various forebrain areas from the olfactory bulb to the hypothalamus, rather than in discrete nuclei or areas [23]. Since several GnRH cells form synaptic connections with other neurons and are distributed widely, it makes sense to question whether any GnRH neurons are neuroendocrine area-specific, that is, projected to median uplift, the location of release of the peptide into the pituitary portal system, which may indicate the export of neurons to different remote regions [24]. In the classic theory,

Table 7 Comparison of RQ values of ovarian GnRHmRNA between four groups

Items	hypothyroidism pregnancy group	hypothyroidism group	normal control group	norma pregnancy group	χ^2value	P value
C_T	(31.72,31.93)	(31.46,34.40)	(30.94,35.30)	(31.51,32.09)	–	–
$\triangle C_T$	(8.82,9.81)	(5.71,7.86)	(3.39,10.17)	(9.46,10.24)	–	–
$\triangle\triangle C_T$	(6.43,7.42)	(3.32,5.47)	(0.99,7.78)	(7.07,7.85)	–	–
RQ	(0.01,0.02)	(0.02,0.10)	(0.04,0.50)	(0.04,0.07)	1.276	0.077

GnRH itself is released from hypothalamic nuclei. However, three different forms of GnRH have been reported: hypothalamic GnRH or GnRH-I, mid brain GnRH or GnRH-II, and GnRH-III, which are present in various species of protochordates and vertebrates [25]. Although the hypothalamus and pituitary are the principal sources and target sites for GnRH, several recent reports suggested the presence of extra-hypothalamic GnRH and GnRH receptors in various reproductive tissues such as ovaries, placenta, endometrium, oviducts, testes, prostate, and mammary glands [26, 27]. GnRH in non-hypothalamic reproductive tissues may have interfered with our experimental results; therefore, we were unable to determine the effect of hypothyroidism on GnRH mRNA expression.

Lehman [28] and others who studied ewes as models performed most of the work in this area. Thyroidectomized ewes are different from intact animals because they do not exhibit a reduction in GnRH secretion in the pituitary portal vein. Nevertheless, thyroxine substitution reverses this effect and converts thyroid-removed ewes from anestrus to the nursery stage. The underlying participation of the thyroid is interesting, because THs are necessary for the standard mature morphology of the central nervous system.

THs act through particular receptors (THRs) that belong to the transcriptional active nuclear receptor superfamily [29]. Two THR isoforms (α and β) have been identified, and each has known subtypes (α1, α2 and β1, β2). Although THRs are located in various tissues, in the brain, there are fewer phenotypic records of specific neuronal populations that bind to THs. Surprisingly, GnRH secretion and GnRHR mRNA levels seem to be affected by the thyroid state [30]. The hypothesis that GnRH neurons include THRs has been partially sustained. In a study of double-tagging immunocytochemistry, Lehman et al. demonstrated the existence of a THR in models of GnRH neurons in hamsters (28%) and sheep (46%) [28]. Preliminary results indicate that a β2 isoform exists in GnRH neurons of sheep. It is interesting that GnRH neurons involve nuclear THR, and that nuclear THR seems to exist in the relevant glial cell nuclei. These findings indicate that THs have a direct effect on the level of GnRH neurons. A possible interpretation is that THs affect GnRH neurons by facilitating gene expression, which is required for the pulsatile release of GnRH [31].

We hypothesized that GnRH neurons may be susceptible to TH development because they express THRs [32]. To test this, rat pups were induced to develop hypothyroidism through feeding (0.4% PTU water) and drinking of 0.1% PTU water from birth until 25 days of age. At 25 days, the pups were ablactated and no further PTU therapy was performed. At 150 days, the animals were immolated, and paired tests were performed to record body weight and brain weight. In addition, the brain was immunocytochemically stained for GnRH. In the hypothyroid group, the quantity of GnRH neurons was almost double that of the saline treated control in the anterior and lateral hypothalamus. There were no differences in other areas (tendon, medial septum/diagonal band, anterior visual area, and medial basal hypothalamus) between the hypothyroid and the control pups. It is conceivable that the increase in GnRH neurons was due to the disturbance of the standard development-associated GnRH cell loss or loss of phenotype in those regions [28]. Therefore, THs may affect GnRH system development because of their presence in other brain areas [32]. Our studies in SD rats indicated that hypothyroidism may affect the allocation of the pituitary GnRHR; however, whether THs play a role in the ovaries and hypothalamus and the nature of their involvement remains unclear, and there are few relevant reports in the literature.

Conclusions

The present study showed that the GnRHR is expressed in tissues of the hypothalamic–pituitary–ovarian axis in pregnant SD rats. The expression of the GnRHR in the pituitary gland is related to the GnRH-induced synthesis and release of gonadotropins. The presence of the GnRHR in the ovary points to either direct effects of hypothalamic GnRH on ovarian function or paracrine/autocrine effects of ovarian GnRH. Because THs may act as potential mediators of GnRH neurons, hypothyroidism may affect the distribution of the pituitary GnRHR [21]. A limitation of this study was the inability to detect the frequency and amplitude of GnRH release. We were therefore unable to determine whether hypothyroidism affects the distribution of GnRHR in the nuclei of the ovary. The negative results may indicate the lack of sensitivity of the staining for measuring GnRHR expression. In addition, immunohistochemistry is only semi-quantitative at best.

Recent research in SD rats yielded new insights into which GnRH neurons mediate pulsatile secretion, the circuitry by which steroids may regulate reproductive transitions, and the potential for plasticity in that circuitry [33]. A number of important questions remain to be answered. From a long-term perspective, elucidating the mechanisms underlying the effect of THs on GnRH secretion may provide the basis for the development of new approaches to regulate fertility in animals and humans [34].

Abbreviations

Ah nucleus: hypothalamic anterior nucleus; Ar nucleus: hypothalamic arcuate nucleus; ELISA: enzyme-linked immunosorbent assay; FT_4: free thyroxine; GnRH: gonadotropin releasing hormone; GnRHR: GnRH receptor; Pa nucleus: paraventricular nucleus of hypothalamus; Pmv nucleus: ventral premammillary nucleus; PTU: propylthiouracil; qRT-PCR: real time quantitative PCR; SD rats: Sprague-Dawley rats; T_3: tri-iodothyronine; T_4: thyroxine; TH: thyroid hormone; THRs: thyroid hormone receptors; THs: thyroid hormones; TSH: thyroid-stimulating hormone; Vmh nucleus: hypothalamic ventromedial nucleus

Acknowledgements

We thank the Department of Endocrinology, Institute of Endocrinology and Metabolism, The First Affiliated Hospital of Anhui Medical University.

Funding

This work was supported by research grants from the Fund of Anhui Natural Science Foundation of China (1608085MH207).

Authors' contributions

JS, CC, and TX were involved in the concept and design of the paper. DD conceived the study and helped to draft the paper. JS, CC, TX, MX, DD, FP, YW read and approved the final paper. MX and YW contributed to the study design and performed experiments. FP takes responsibility for the integrity of the data and the accuracy of data analysis.

Competing interests

The authors declare that they have no competing interests.

Author details

[1]Department of Endocrinology, Institute of Endocrinology and Metabolism, The First Affiliated Hospital of Anhui Medical University, 218 Jixi Road, Hefei 230022, Anhui, China. [2]Department of Epidemiology and Biostatistics,School of Public Health, Anhui Medical University,81Meishan Road, Hefei 230032, Anhui, China.

References

1. Curto L, Trimarchi F. Hypopituitarism in the elderly: a narrative review on clinical management of hypothalamic-pituitary-gonadal, hypothalamic-pituitary-thyroid and hypothalamic-pituitary-adrenal axes dysfunction. J Endocrinol Investig. 2016;39:1115–24.
2. Flood DE, Fernandino JI, Langlois VS. Thyroid hormones in male reproductive development: evidence for direct crosstalk between the androgen and thyroid hormone axes. Gen Comp Endocrinol. 2013;192:2–14.
3. Park CW, Choi MH, Yang KM, et al. Pregnancy rate in women with adenomyosis undergoing fresh or frozen embryo transfer cycles following gonadotropin-releasing hormone agonist treatment. Clinical and experimental reproductive medicine. 2016;43:169–73.
4. Cortes C, Langlois DC, VS Fernandino JI. Cross over of the hypothalamic pituitary-adrenal/interrenal,-thyroid, and-gonadal axes in testicular development. Front Endocrinol. 2014;5:139.
5. Miccoli A, Olivotto I, De Felice A, et al. Characterization and transcriptional profiles of Engraulis encrasicolus' GnRH forms. Reproduction. 2016;152:727–39.
6. Duan JR, Fang DA, Zhang MY, et al. Changes of gonadotropin-releasing hormone receptor 2 during the anadromous spawning migration in Coilia nasus. BMC Dev Biol. 2016;16:42.
7. Durand A, Bashamboo A, Mcelreavey K, et al. Familial early puberty: presentation and inheritance pattern in 139 families. BMC Endocr Disord. 2016;16:50.
8. Jadhao AG, Pinelli CD. Aniello B, et al. gonadotropin-inhibitory hormone (GnRH) in the amphibian brain and its relationship with the gonadotropin

9. Ciechanowska M, Lapot M, Mateusiak K, et al. The central effect of beta-endorphin and naloxone on the biosynthesis of GnRH and GnRH receptor (GnRHR) in the hypothalamic-pituitary unit of follicular-phase ewes. Reprod Domest Anim. 2016;51:555–61.
10. Cimino I, Casoni F, Liu X, et al. Novel role for anti-Mullerian hormone in the regulation of GnRH neuron excitability and hormone secretion. Nat Commun. 2016;7:10055.
11. Kumar A, Shekhar S, Dhole B. Thyroid and male reproduction. Indian journal of. endocrinology and metabolism. 2014;18:23–31.
12. Mann DR, Plant TM. The role and potential sites of action of thyroid hormone in timing the onset of puberty in male primates. Brain Res. 2010; 1364:175–85.
13. Shaffer JP. Controlling the false discovery rate with constraints: the Newman-Keuls test revisited. Biom J. 2007;49(1):136–43.
14. De Muth JE. Basic Statistics and Pharmaceutical Statistical Applications. 2nd ed. Boca Raton, FL: Chapman and Hall/CRC; 2006. p. 229–59.
15. Yang J, Zhou X, Zhang X, et al. Analysis of the correlation between lipotoxicity and pituitary-thyroid axis hormone levels in men and male rats. Oncotarget. 2016;7:39332–44.
16. Coelho Neto MAMWP, Melo AS, et al. Subclinical hypothyroidism and intracytoplasmic sperm injection outcomes. Rev Bras Ginecol Obstet. 2016; 38:552–8.
17. Andersen SL, Olsen J. Early pregnancy thyroid function test abnormalities in biobanksera from women clinically diagnosed before or after the pregnancy. Thyroid. 2017;27:451–9.
18. Ajmani SN, Aggarwal D, Bhatia P, et al. Prevalence of overt and subclinical thyroid dysfunction among pregnant women and its effect on maternal and fetal outcome. J Obstet Gynaecol India. 2014;64:105–10.
19. Casey B, De Veciana M. Thyroid screening in pregnancy. American journal of obstetrics and gynecology. 2014;211:351–3. e1
20. Maraka S, Ospina NM, O'keeffe DT, et al. Subclinical hypothyroidism in pregnancy: a systematic review and meta-analysis. Thyroid: official journal of the American Thyroid Association. 2016;26:580–90.
21. No authors listed. Pulsatile control of reproduction. Lancet. 1984;2:382–23.
22. Vastagh C, Rodolosse A, Solymosi N, et al. Altered expression of genes encoding neurotransmitter receptors in GnRH neurons of proestrous mice. Front Cell Neurosci. 2016;10:230.
23. Kim SM, Lee M, Lee SY, et al. Discovery of an orally bioavailable gonadotropin-releasing hormone receptor antagonist. J Med Chem. 2016; 59:9150–72.
24. Piet R, Dunckley H, Lee K, et al. Vasoactive intestinal peptide excites GnRH neurons in male and female mice. Endocrinology. 2016;157:3621–30.
25. Larco DO, Semsarzadeh NN, Cho-Clark M, et al. The novel actions of the metabolite GnRH-(1-5) are mediated by a G protein-coupled receptor. Front Endocrinol. 2013;4:83.
26. Bianco SD, Kaiser UB. Molecular biology of the kisspeptin receptor: signaling, function, and mutations. Adv Exp Med Biol. 2013;784:133–58.
27. Ramakrishnappa N, Rajamahendran R, Lin YM, et al. GnRH in non-hypothalamic reproductive tissues. Anim Reprod Sci. 2005;88:95–113.
28. Lehman MN, Goodman RL, Karsch FJ, et al. The GnRH system of seasonal breeders: anatomy and plasticity. Brain Res Bull. 1997;44:445–57.
29. Singh BK, Yen PM. A clinician's guide to understanding resistance to thyroid hormone due to receptor mutations in the TRalpha and TRbeta isoforms. Clinical diabetes and endocrinology. 2017;3:8.
30. Populo H, Nunes B, Sampaio C, et al. Inhibitory effects of antagonists of growth hormone-releasing hormone (GHRH) in thyroid Cancer. Hormones & cancer. 2017;8(5–6):314–24.
31. Yoshimura T. Thyroid hormone and seasonal regulation of reproduction. Front Neuroendocrinol. 2013;34(3):157–66.
32. Liu J, Guo M, Hu X, et al. Effects of Thyroid Dysfunction on Reproductive Hormones in Female Rats. Chin J Physiol. 2018;61. [Epub ahead of print].
33. Ikegami K, Yoshimura T. Comparative analysis reveals the underlying mechanism of vertebrate seasonal reproduction. Gen Comp Endocrinol. 2016;227:64–8.
34. Nakayama T, Yoshimura T. Seasonal rhythms: the role of thyrotropin and thyroid hormones. Thyroid: official journal of the American Thyroid Association. 2018;28(1):4–10.

releasing hormone (GnRH) system: an overview. Gen Comp Endocrinol. 2016;240:69–76.

7

A proof-of-concept study to evaluate the efficacy and safety of BTI320 on post-prandial hyperglycaemia in Chinese subjects with pre-diabetes

Andrea O. Y. Luk[1,2,6*] (iD), Benny C. Y. Zee[3], Marc Chong[3], Risa Ozaki[1,2], Carl W. Rausch[4], Michael H. M. Chan[5], Ronald C. W. Ma[1,2], Alice P. S. Kong[1,2], Francis C. C. Chow[1,2] and Juliana C. N. Chan[1,2]

Abstract

Background: Galactomannan(s) are plant-derived fiber shown to reduce post-prandial blood glucose by delaying intestinal absorption of carbohydrates and slowing down gastric emptying. We examined glucose-lowering effects of BTI320, a propriety fractionated mannan(s) administered as a chewable tablet before meal in a proof-of-concept study in Chinese subjects with prediabetes.

Methods: Sixty Chinese adults aged 18–70 years with either impaired fasting glucose, impaired glucose tolerance, or glycated haemoglobin 5.7–6.4% (39-46 mmol/mol), were randomly assigned in 2:2:1 ratio to either BTI320 8 g (high dose), BTI320 4 g (low dose) or matching-placebo three times daily before meal for 16 weeks. The primary endpoint was change in fructosamine in subjects treated with BTI320 compared with placebo from baseline to week 4. Indices of glycaemic variability based on continuous glucose monitoring (CGM) and standard meal tolerance test were explored in secondary analyses.

Results: Of 60 subjects randomized, 3 subjects discontinued study treatment prematurely. In intention-to-treat analysis, no significant differences in change in serum fructosamine between low or high dose BTI320 and placebo were observed. Using random effect models, adjusted for variability by meals, treatment with low dose BTI320 was associated with reduction in 1-h ($p < 0.01$), 2-h ($p = 0.01$) and 3-h ($p = 0.02$) post-prandial incremental glucose area-under-curve and post-meal maximum glucose ($p = 0.03$) compared with placebo. Subjects receiving low dose BTI320 had greater body weight reduction than placebo group.

Conclusions: BTI320 did not change fructosamine levels compared with placebo. BTI320 reduced glycaemic variability based on CGM indices.

Keywords: Galactomannans, Prediabetes, Fructosamine

* Correspondence: andrealuk@cuhk.edu.hk
[1]Department of Medicine and Therapeutics, The Chinese University of Hong Kong, Shatin, Hong Kong
[2]Li Ka Shing Institute of Health Science, The Chinese University of Hong Kong, Prince of Wales Hospital, Shatin, Hong Kong
Full list of author information is available at the end of the article

Background

One in ten Chinese adults have diabetes and recent estimates from the International Diabetes Federation indicates that there are 11 million people living with diabetes in China [1, 2]. Individuals with impaired glucose tolerance (IGT) or impaired fasting glucose (IFG) are at increased risks of developing diabetes at estimated annual conversion rates of 3–10% depending on the presence of other risk factors [3]. Diabetes may be prevented or delayed through intensive lifestyle intervention and pharmacological treatment agents [4–7]. The Diabetes Prevention Program demonstrated that lifestyle modification reduced progression to diabetes by 58% and metformin by 31% in people with pre-diabetes during the 2.8-year in-trial period, and that the benefits persisted at up to 15 years post-intervention albeit attenuated [4, 8]. Similarly, the 3.3-year STOP-NIDDM trial reported 25% relative risk reduction of incident diabetes with acarbose compared to placebo in people with IGT [7]. Despite the best clinical evidence and international guidelines, the effects of diabetes prevention programs are often limited and not sustained in real world setting due to poor uptake and persistence as well as the safety concern of systemic drug product exposure. As such, the rising burden of type 2 diabetes and its associated morbidity and mortality remain a global health problem of enormous proportion [2].

A simple, non-systemic pharmacological approach to disease management is a universal healthcare ideal, and extracts of natural materials represent an explored opportunity. Specifically, galactomannan(s) are the active ingredient in natural gum and are used extensively in food industry as a thickener of free water [9]. Through its action in increasing viscosity of gastrointestinal content, carbohydrates are slow to interact with digestive enzymes, glucose absorption is delayed, and this results in diminution of post-prandial blood glucose excursion [10]. Galactomannan(s) have been previously examined in humans for its beneficial effects on blood glucose, blood cholesterol and body weight, although most of these studies were of small sample sizes with notable heterogeneity in doses and preparation of the plant-derived gum tested [11–17].

BTI320 is a proprietary combination of fractionated mannans derived from guar gum and other plant sources and is administered in the form of a chewable tablet. In an earlier open-label study of 24 patients with type 2 diabetes, BTI320 8 g and 16 g taken before a test meal reduced 3-h post-prandial glucose area-under-curve (AUC) in 75% of patients [18]. The main adverse events reported in that study were increased flatulence and bloating. Here, we examined the glycaemic efficacy, tolerability and safety of 16 weeks' intervention with BTI320 compared with placebo in Chinese adults with prediabetes. In the present proof-of-concept study, we utilized a continuous glucose monitor (CGM) device to monitor glucose levels at 3 multi-day periods throughout the 16 weeks' study to explore the effects of BTI320 on post-prandial glucose excursion and variability.

Methods

Study design and subjects

We undertook a randomized, double-blind, placebo-controlled, parallel arm study with the first subject enrolled on 30 March 2015 and the last subject completed the study on 19 February 2016. The study was conducted in the Diabetes and Endocrine Research Centre of the Chinese University of Hong Kong (CUHK) at the Prince of Wales Hospital, Hong Kong Special Administrative Region. Subjects were identified from non-specialist general medical or family medicine clinics at the hospital. We recruited Chinese subjects aged between 18 and 70 years inclusive, fulfilling at least two of the following three criteria: 1) fasting plasma glucose 5.6–5.9 mmol/L (IFG) and/or 2-h plasma glucose 7.8–11.0 mmol/L (IGT) during a standard 75 g oral glucose tolerance test (OGTT); 2) glycated haemoglobin (HbA1c) 5.7–6.4% (39–46 mmol/mol); and 3) at least one of the following risk factors of a) history of gestational diabetes, b) history of diabetes in first degree relatives, and c) two or more of metabolic syndrome components of triglyceride ≥1.7 mmol/L, high density-lipoprotein (HDL) cholesterol < 1.3 mmol/L in women or < 1.1 mmol/L in men, waist circumference ≥ 80 cm in women or ≥ 90 cm in men, or blood pressure (BP) ≥130/80 mmHg. Exclusion criteria included current use of dietary supplements known to affect glucose or galactose metabolism, use of anti-diabetic medications in the previous 6 weeks, cardiovascular disease in the recent 12 months, renal impairment with estimated glomerular filtration rate < 60 mL/min/1.73m^2, history of eating disorder, and known lactose or galactose intolerance. The study was registered at www.clinicaltrials.gov, reference number NCT02358668.

Randomisation

The randomization process involved the use of computer-generated random numbers. Treatment group assignment of each sequentially randomised subject were contained in individually sealed, opaque and consecutively numbered envelops, which were opened by a non-study personnel.

Intervention

Subjects meeting eligibility criteria were randomly assigned to receive BTI320 4 g ($n = 24$), BTI320 8 g ($n = 24$) or matching placebo ($n = 12$) orally three times daily, 10 min before each main meal for 16 weeks. Each 4-g tablet of BTI320, administered as a chewable tablet, contained 2.0 g of the key ingredient mannan polysaccharides.

Other ingredients included food grade sorbitol, magnesium stearate, malic acid, natural flavors and colors. Subjects were instructed to maintain their usual dietary pattern and physical exercise levels. Subjects were reviewed every 4 weeks for assessment of adverse events and drug compliance, the latter was established by counting the returned tablets.

Clinical measurements

Serum fructosamine was measured at baseline and 4-weekly interval until completion of treatment at 16 weeks, HbA1c at baseline and 16 weeks, and OGTT at screening and 30-day post-treatment visit. Meal tolerance test (MTT) using a standardized meal of 500 kcal was conducted at baseline, 4 weeks and 16 weeks measuring plasma glucose, insulin, C-peptide and glucagon-like peptide (GLP)-1 at 0, 15, 30, 60, 90 and 120 min. The standard meal consisted of two pieces of pineapple short cakes and one carton of soymilk with nutritional breakdown as follows: carbohydrates 75.7 g (57.1% of total energy intake), fat 21.2 g (35.9% of total energy intake) and protein 9.3 g (7.0% of total energy intake). Seventy-two-hour CGM using the Medtronic iPro®2 CGM and Enlite sensor was performed at baseline, 4 weeks and 16 weeks. Other metabolic parameters (body weight, waist circumference, BP, lipid [total cholesterol, HDL-cholesterol, triglyceride, low density-lipoprotein cholesterol], high-sensitivity C-reactive protein [hs-CRP]) and safety parameters (renal function, liver function and complete blood count) were measured at regular intervals.

Fructosamine was measured using colorimetric test by reaction with nitroblue tetrazolium. The measuring range of the fructosamine assay was 14–1000 μmol/L, intra-assay coefficient of variations (CVs) were 0.8% and 0.5% at concentration of 275 μmol/L and 515 μmol/L, respectively, and inter-assay CVs were 1.5% and 1.2% at concentrations of 262 μmol/L and 489 μmol/L, respectively. Glycated haemoglobin was measured using immunoassay traceable to the National Glycohaemoglobin Standardisation Program and the International Federation of Clinical Chemistry standards. The measuring range of HbA1c assay was 0.3–3.4 g/dL, inter-assay CVs were 1.2% and 0.7% at concentrations of 5.3% Hb and 9.6% Hb, respectively, and inter-assay CVs were 2.2% and 1.9% at concentrations of 5.0% and 10.4% Hb, respectively. Insulin was measured by immunoassay which had a measuring range of 2–300 mIU/L with intra-assay CVs of 3.6% and 2.9% at concentrations of 11.7 mIU/L and 51.2 mIU/L, respectively, and inter-assay CVs of 6.7% and 5.3% at concentrations of 11.2 mIU/L and 47.4 mIU/L, respectively. C-peptide was measured using immunoassay which had measuring range of 0.1–20 μg/L with intra-assay CV of 2.8% and 1.7% at concentrations of 0.7 μg/L and 6.2 μg/L, respectively, and inter-assay CVs of 3.5% and 6.3% at

concentrations of 0.8 μg/L and 6.3 μg/L, respectively. Glucagon-like peptide 1 was measured by enzyme-linked immunosorbent assay (Immuno-Biological Laboratories Co. Ltd., Japan). The measuring range of GLP-1 was 1.25–80 pmol/L, intra-assay CVs were 9.8% and 2.2% at concentrations of 5.0 pmol/L and 7.8 pmol/L, respectively, and inter-assay CVs were 10.3% and 5.7% at concentrations of 6.1 pmol/L and 11.0 pmol/L, respectively. Glucose, total cholesterol, HDL-cholesterol and triglyceride were measured using the enzymatic colorimetric method. Insulin and C-peptide were analysed by the Siemens IMMULITE® 2000 XPi Immunoassay System, HbA1c was measured on the Roche Cobas Integra 800 System (Roche Diagnostic GmbH, Mannheim, Germany), GLP-1 was measured manually, and the rest of the assays were measured on the Roche Cobas c8000 Analytical System (Roche Diagnostic GmbH, Mannheim, Germany). All laboratory tests were performed in the Department of Chemical Pathology, the CUHK, the Prince of Wales Hospital, which was accredited by the National Association of Testing Authorities, Australia and the Royal College of Pathologists of Australasia for medical testing.

All subjects completed Food Frequency Questionnaire, Hill and Blundell questionnaire on appetite, International Physical Activity Questionnaire, and World Health Organisation Quality of Life questionnaire at baseline, 4 weeks and 16 weeks.

Efficacy endpoints

The primary endpoint was change in serum fructosamine in subjects treated with low dose and high dose BTI320 compared with placebo from baseline to 4 weeks. The main secondary endpoints were changes in calculated indices of glycaemic variability (mean post-prandial incremental AUC [AUCpp] at 1 h, 2 h and 3 h, mean post-meal maximum glucose [MPMG], AUC-180, mean amplitude of glucose excursion [MAGE], standard deviation [SD], and percent CV) based on CGM data in subjects treated with low dose and high dose BTI320 compared with placebo during the study. The AUCpp is the area above pre-prandial glucose starting from the beginning of each main meal to 1 h, 2 h and 3 h after the meal, obtained using the trapezoidal rule. The MPMG is the mean maximal glucose value within 3 h after each main meal. The AUC-180 is the AUC for glucose level above 180 mg/dL (10 mmol/L). The MAGE is the mean difference in glucose values between consecutive peaks and nadirs, only considering changes above and below mean glucose of more than 1 SD [19]. The percent CV is SD divided by mean glucose values. Other secondary endpoints included changes in HbA1c, 2-h AUC of plasma glucose, insulin, C-peptide and GLP-1 post-MTT, body weight, BPs, lipids, hs-CRP, as well as changes in self-reported dietary intake and satiety from baseline to end of treatment in subjects treated with low dose and high dose BTI320 compared with placebo.

Safety endpoints

Laboratory safety variables analyzed were renal function, liver function and complete blood counts. Self-reported adverse events including hypoglycaemic events were captured and analyzed.

Statistical analysis

In our estimation of sample size, we assumed a mean serum fructosamine level of 273 µmol/L with SD of 22.5 µmol/L in the placebo arm, and a change of 10% in fructosamine level would be detected using a two-sided 5% level test with 80% power if there were 11 subjects per arm.

Efficacy analyses were performed in the intention-to-treat population which consisted of all randomized subjects who have received at least one dose of the assigned treatment. A *per protocol* analysis was also performed in subjects who have taken at least 70% of the treatment. Analysis of covariance (ANCOVA) was used to measure the changes in serum fructosamine, and changes in other glycaemic and metabolic indices from baseline to week 4 and week 16 between intervention arms, adjusted for age, gender and baseline measurements. The effects of low or high dose BTI320 compared with placebo on CGM glycaemic variability indices were further explored using random effect models with repeated measurements adjusted for intra-individual between-meal and between meal-day variability, age and gender. Linear mixed effect is a common statistical method to address repeated measurements [20, 21]. Post-hoc subgroup analysis was conducted on significant CGM glycaemic variability indices by dividing the population into 1) Low and high body mass index (BMI) stratified by the population BMI median; 2) Younger and older age groups by population age median; and 3) With IFG and/or IGT at baseline and without IGF and IGT at baseline. Analysis was performed using Statistical Analysis Software Version 9.4.

Results

Subject disposition and baseline clinical characteristics

A total of 77 subjects were screened and 60 subjects met eligibility for randomisation (Additional file 1: Figure S1). Twenty-four subjects were assigned to treatment with low dose BTI320, 24 subjects to high dose BTI320, and 12 subjects to placebo. Two subjects receiving low dose BTI320 withdrew from the study due to adverse events (one withdrew due to serious adverse event of osteosarcoma, and another due to abdominal pain), and 1 subject receiving high dose BTI320 withdrew consent for non-medical reasons. Overall 55 subjects have taken more

than 70% of the study treatment and were included in the *per protocol* analysis.

The mean age of the cohort was 56.4 ± 9.1 years and 46.7% were male. At baseline, 4 subjects (6.7%) had IFG only, 23 subjects (38.3%) had IGT only, 15 (25.0%) had both IFG and IGT, and 18 (30.0%) had normal fasting glucose and glucose tolerance but HbA1c between 5.7–6.4% (39–46 mmol/mol). Mean serum fructosamine and HbA1c were 272.1 ± 19.9 µmol/L and 6.0 ± 0.3% (42 ± 2.1 mmol/mol), respectively. Glycaemic indices were comparable among the three intervention arms at baseline (Table 1).

Primary endpoint

In the intention-to-treat analysis, changes in serum fructosamine levels from baseline to 4 weeks were − 5.2, − 9.4 and − 8.8 µmol/L in subjects receiving low dose BTI320, high dose BTI320 and placebo, respectively (Fig. 1). The estimated mean differences in the change in serum fructosamine levels from baseline to 4 weeks were not significant for the comparison between low dose BTI and placebo (mean difference 2.5 [95% confidence interval {CI} -6.3, 11.2] µmol/L, $p = 0.57$) and between high dose BTI and placebo (mean difference − 1.6 [95% CI -10.3, 7.1] µmol/L, $p = 0.72$), adjusted for gender, age, and baseline fructosamine (Table 2, Fig. 1). Analysis of the *per protocol* population yielded similar results.

Secondary endpoints

Parameters of post-prandial glucose excursion and glycaemic variability were calculated for each subject based on data from CGM. Using ANCOVA with adjustment for gender, age and baseline values, we did not detect significant differences in CGM glycaemic parameters between treatment with low dose or high dose BTI320 and placebo. Using random effect models adjusted for variability by meals, treatment with low dose BTI320 was associated with reduction in 1-h, 2- h and 3-h AUCpp and MPMG compared with placebo by 16 weeks (Table 3). The SDs at 1-h, 2-h and 3-h post-meal were lower in the low dose BTI320 group although the differences just missed statistical significance. Treatment with high dose BTI320 did not differ from placebo with respect to CGM parameters in random effect models.

At 16 weeks, serum fructosamine levels were reduced by 5.0 and 6.8 µmol/L in subjects receiving low dose and high dose BTI320, respectively but the changes did not differ from placebo. Similarly, there were no differences in changes in HbA1c from baseline to 16 weeks between intervention with BTI320 and placebo (Table 2). The AUC of glucose, C-peptide, insulin and GLP-1 over 2 h post-MTT were similar in the 3 groups at 4 weeks and 16 weeks (Table 2). At 30 days following treatment completion, 0% of subjects on low dose BTI320, 4.3% of

Table 1 Baseline clinical characteristics of subjects in low dose BTI320, high dose BTI320 and placebo groups

	Placebo	Low Dose BTI320	High Dose BTI320
Number	12	24	24
Demographics			
Age, years	57.1 ± 10.9	54.1 ± 8.6	58.5 ± 8.5
Male, % (n)	25.0 (3)	54.2 (13)	50.0 (12)
Metabolic Parameters			
Body weight, kg	63.9 ± 20.0	74.2 ± 16.9	71.0 ± 16.2
Body mass index, kg/m^2	25.1 ± 4.3	28.0 ± 5.8	26.9 ± 4.4
Waist, cm	88.0 ± 15.7	95.0 ± 15.6	90.6 ± 9.1
Systolic BP, mmHg	127.8 ± 8.7	121.7 ± 13.2	125.4 ± 16.2
Diastolic BP, mmHg	80.4 ± 7.3	78.4 ± 6.8	78.7 ± 7.2
Total cholesterol, mmol/L	5.3 ± 0.8	4.9 ± 1.1	4.9 ± 1.0
LDL-cholesterol, mmol/L	3.3 ± 0.6	2.9 ± 0.9	2.9 ± 0.8
Triglyceride, mmol/L	1.4 ± 0.6	1.2 ± 0.4	1.4 ± 0.8
HDL-cholesterol, mmol/L	1.5 ± 0.3	1.5 ± 0.3	1.4 ± 0.4
Fructosamine, μmol/L	278.9 ± 22.0	268.5 ± 18.3	272.2 ± 20.2
HbA1c, % (mmol/mol)	6.1 ± 0.3 (43 ± 2.2)	6.0 ± 0.3 (42 ± 2.1)	6.0 ± 0.30 (42 ± 2.1)
Hypertension, % (n)	58.3 (7)	45.8 (11)	54.2 (13)
Dyslipidemia, % (n)	33.3 (4)	25.0 (6)	41.7 (10)
Obesity, % (n)	25.0 (3)	16.7 (4)	20.8 (5)
Glycemic Status			
IFG, % (n)	0.0 (0)	12.5 (3)	4.2 (1)
IGT, % (n)	41.7 (5)	41.7 (10)	33.3 (8)
Both IFG/IGT, % (n)	33.3 (4)	16.7 (4)	29.2 (7)
NGT and HbA1c 5.7–6.4% (39–46 mmol/mol) only, % (n)	25.0 (3)	29.2 (7)	33.3 (8)
CGM Parameters			
1-h AUCpp, mmol/L×hour	6.33 ± 0.64	5.91 ± 0.53	6.22 ± 0.72
2-h AUCpp, mmol/L×hour	13.49 ± 1.43	12.68 ± 1.21	13.64 ± 1.87
3-h AUCpp, mmol/L×hour	20.20 ± 2.20	18.90 ± 1.69	20.20 ± 2.59
72-h AUC-180, mmol/L×hour	2.73 ± 7.64	0.40 ± 1.85	1.71 ± 3.35
MBG, mmol/L	6.45 ± 0.54	6.01 ± 0.45	6.20 ± 0.63
MPMG, mmol/L	8.07 ± 1.00	7.45 ± 0.78	8.20 ± 1.31
MAGE, mmol/L	3.21 ± 3.16	2.06 ± 0.69	2.68 ± 1.01
CV, %	18.00 ± 7.60	15.49 ± 4.43	19.07 ± 6.61
SD, mmol/L	1.18 ± 0.59	0.93 ± 0.28	1.19 ± 0.44

Expressed as mean ± standard deviation, or percentage (number) as appropriate
AUC area-under-curve, *AUCpp* post-prandial incremental area-under-curve, *BP* blood pressure, *CGM* Continuous Glucose monitoring, *CV* coefficient of variation, *HbA1c* glycated haemoglobin, *HDL* high density-lipoprotein, *IFG* impaired fasting glucose, *IGT* impaired glucose tolerance, *LDL* low density-lipoprotein, *MAGE* mean amplitude of glucose excursion, *MBG* mean blood glucose, *MPMG* mean post-meal maximum glucose, *NGT* normal glucose tolerance, *SD* standard deviation

those on high dose BTI320, 0% of those on placebo had normal glucose tolerance and HbA1c < 5.7% (39 mmol/mol).

Body weight was significantly reduced in the low dose but not the high dose BTI320 group. At 16 weeks, the mean change in body weight relative to placebo was − 1.7 (95% CI -3.2, − 0.1) kg in subjects receiving low dose BTI320 ($p = 0.03$) and − 0.1 (95% CI -1.7, 1.4) kg in those receiving high dose BTI320 ($p = 0.86$) (Table 2). There were no differences in changes in total cholesterol, LDL-cholesterol, triglyceride, HDL-cholesterol, urate, hs-CRP, systolic and diastolic BPs between treatment with either doses of BTI320 and placebo. Caloric intake as estimated using food frequency questionnaire as well

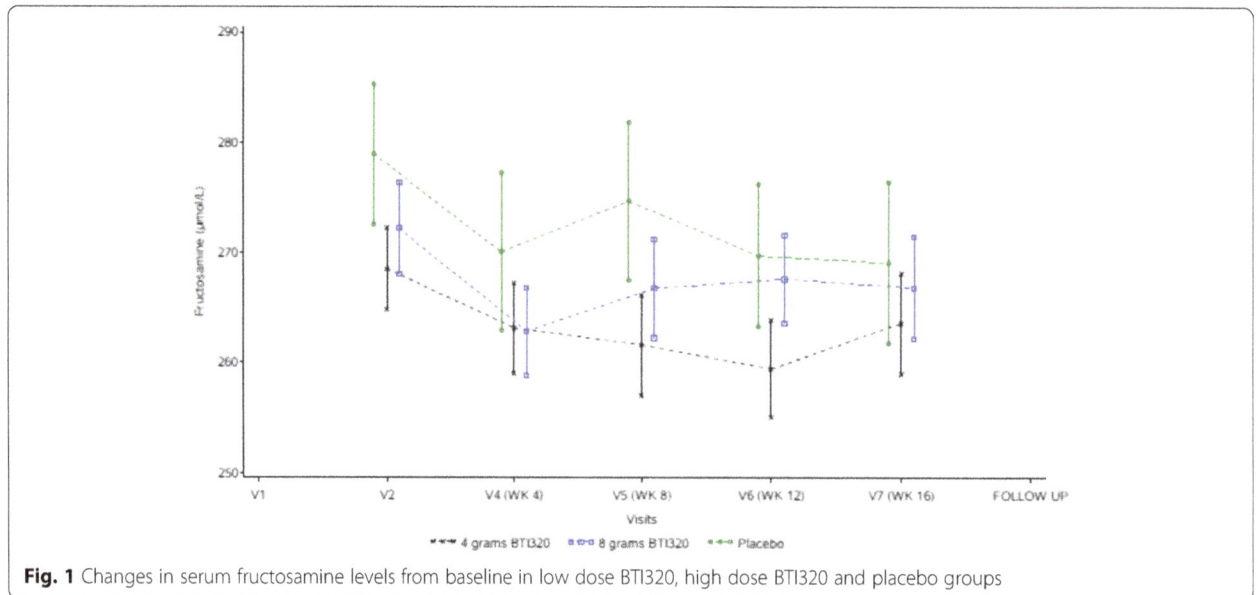

Fig. 1 Changes in serum fructosamine levels from baseline in low dose BTI320, high dose BTI320 and placebo groups

as self-reported satiety did not differ between the 3 groups.

Subgroup analysis
Post-hoc subgroup analysis was conducted to test the effects of low dose and high dose BTI320 on changes in 1-h, 2- h and 3-h AUCpp from baseline. Firstly, treatment effects were examined in subjects of high (BMI $\geq$26 kg/m^2) and low (BMI < 26 kg/m^2) BMI (Additional file 2: Table

S1). In the high BMI group, BTI320 in both low and high doses reduced AUCpp compared with placebo, whereas in the low BMI group, AUCpp was decreased with low but not high dose BTI320. Next, we examined treatment effects by IFG and IGT status (Additional file 2: Table S2). In the group with IFG and/or IGT, low dose and not high dose BTI320 reduced AUCpp, consistent with results from the main analysis. In contrast, in the group without IFG and IGT, treatment effects were not demonstrated with

Table 2 Changes in glycemic and metabolic indices from baseline between low dose or high dose BTI320 and placebo in the intention-to-treat analysis

Clinical Variable	Low Dose BTI320				High Dose BTI320			
	Week 4		Week 16		Week 4		Week 16	
	Mean Difference (95% CI)	p^*	Mean Difference (95% CI)	p^*	Mean Difference (95% CI)	p^*	Mean Difference (95% CI)	p^*
Serum fructosamine, μmol/L	2.46 (−6.28, 11.20)	0.57	1.14 (−9.17, 11.45)	0.83	−1.57 (− 10.3, 7.11)	0.72	− 0.92 (− 11.1, 9.27)	0.86
HbA1c, %	–	–	− 0.01 (− 0.13, 0.10)	0.83	–	–	− 0.04 (− 0.16, 0.08)	0.48
2-h glucose AUC post-MTT, mmol/L×min	65.0 (− 14.4, 144.5)	0.11	−13.6 (− 99.6, 72.3)	0.75	68.9 (− 9.9, 147.7)	0.09	40.0 (−43.9, 123.9)	0.34
2-h insulin AUC post-MTT, mIU/L×min	1219.2 (− 1129.0, 3567.7)	0.30	−980.0 (− 2604.0, 643.8)	0.23	1111.2 (− 1211.0, 3433.2)	0.34	323.9 (− 1269.0, 1916.6)	0.68
2-h C-peptide AUC post-MTT, μg/L×min	128.4 (−22.4, 279.2)	0.09	15.0 (− 99.6, 129.6)	0.79	101.8 (− 47.3, 250.9)	0.18	60.1 (− 52.5, 172.6)	0.29
2-h GLP-1 AUC post-MTT, pmol/L×min	42.8 (− 144.8, 230.3)	0.65	− 120.2 (− 385.3, 144.9)	0.37	32.2 (− 149.7, 214.1)	0.72	49.0 (− 198.1, 296.2)	0.69
Systolic BP, mmHg	−6.4 (− 15.3, 2.5)	0.16	−2.2 (− 9.8, 5.5)	0.57	− 2.4 (− 11.2, 6.4)	0.58	1.0 (− 6.6, 8.6)	0.79
Body weight, kg	0.0 (−1.2, 1.3)	0.95	−1.7 (−3.2, − 0.1)	0.03	0.7 (− 0.5, 1.9)	0.26	− 0.1 (− 1.7, 1.4)	0.86
Total cholesterol, mmol/L	0.06 (− 0.31, 0.43)	0.75	0.03 (− 0.39, 0.44)	0.90	− 0.21 (− 0.58, 0.16)	0.26	− 0.22 (− 0.63, 0.20)	0.30
LDL-cholesterol, mmol/L	0.07 (− 0.28, 0.41)	0.69	0.10 (− 0.28, 0.48)	0.59	− 0.26 (− 0.60, 0.09)	0.14	− 0.18 (− 0.56, 0.20)	0.35
hs-CRP, mg/L	0.77 (−0.79, 2.33)	0.33	0.62 (− 1.32, 2.57)	0.52	0.15 (− 1.39, 1.70)	0.84	1.13 (−0.78, 3.05)	0.24

*The *p*-values of treatment effects were obtained by ANCOVA analysis adjusted for age, gender and baseline measurements
AUC area under curve, *BP* blood pressure, *CI* confidence interval, *CRP* C-reactive protein, *GLP-1* glucagon-like peptide-1, *HbA1c* glycated haemoglobin, *hs-CRP* high-sensitivity C-reactive protein, *LDL* low density-lipoprotein, *MTT* meal tolerance test

Table 3 Changes in CGM glycaemic indices from baseline between low dose or high dose BTI320 and placebo using random effect models with repeated measurements adjusted for intra-individual between-meal and between meal-day variability

CGM Parameter	Low Dose BTI320		High Dose BTI320	
	Mean Difference (95% CI)	p	Mean Difference (95% CI)	p
AUCpp at 1 h	−0.30 (− 0.48, − 0.11)	< 0.01	−0.14 (− 0.32, 0.04)	0.13
AUCpp at 2 h	−0.59 (− 1.01, − 0.18)	0.01	−0.17 (− 0.57, 0.24)	0.42
AUCpp at 3 h	−0.74 (− 1.35, − 0.14)	0.02	−0.17 (− 0.75, 0.42)	0.57
MPMG	−0.42 (− 0.81, − 0.03)	0.03	−0.09 (− 0.48, 0.29)	0.63
SD at 1 h	−0.05 (− 0.13, 0.02)	0.18	0.01 (− 0.06, 0.09)	0.73
SD at 2 h	−0.07 (− 0.15, 0.00)	0.06	0.03 (− 0.05, 0.10)	0.46
SD at 3 h	−0.07 (− 0.15, 0.00)	0.06	0.03 (− 0.05, 0.10)	0.46
% CV at 1 h	−0.48 (− 1.46, 0.50)	0.34	0.22 (− 0.73, 1.18)	0.64
% CV at 2 h	−0.62 (− 1.50, 0.26)	0.17	0.39 (− 0.46, 1.24)	0.37
% CV at 3 h	−0.65 (− 1.62, 0.31)	0.18	0.42 (− 0.51, 1.36)	0.37

AUCpp post-prandial incremental area-under-curve, *CGM* Continuous Glucose monitoring, *CI* Confidence interval, *CV* coefficient of variation, *MPMG* mean post-meal maximum glucose, *SD* standard deviation

BTI320 of either doses, although subject number was small in this group ($n = 18$). Lastly, in subgroup analysis conducted in younger (< 59 years) and older (≥59 years) age groups, we detected reduction in AUCpp with high dose but not low dose BTI320 among younger subjects whilst reduction was observed with low dose but not high dose BTI320 in older subjects (Additional file 2: Table S3).

Safety endpoints

Treatment with BTI320 for 16 weeks had no effects on pre-specified safety parameters of renal function, liver function and blood counts. Significantly more subjects receiving either low or high dose BTI320 reported abdominal distension and increased flatulence (Additional file 2: Table S4). There was no difference in the frequency of gastrointestinal symptoms between the low dose and high dose groups. One subject randomized to low dose BTI320 was diagnosed to have osteosarcoma of the left femur during the study and later required chemotherapy and amputation of the affected leg. The serious adverse event was deemed unrelated to BTI320 as the subject reported history of leg pain at screening prior to commencement of study intervention. Hypoglycaemia was not reported in any of the subjects throughout the treatment period.

Discussion

In this proof-of-concept study of Chinese subjects with prediabetes, treatment with BTI320 at either low or high doses was not associated with significant changes in serum fructosamine levels compared with placebo at 4 weeks. Despite absence of significant reduction in

serum fructosamine, subjects assigned BTI320 experienced less glycaemic variability as evidenced by diminished post-prandial glucose AUC and MPMG during CGM. Post-prandial glucose control is difficult to achieve in individuals with type 2 diabetes and results from the present study suggest that therapeutic action of BTI320 may be extended to this disease population.

Glycaemic action of BTI320

The glucose-lowering effect of galactomannan in the form of guar gum in patients with type 2 diabetes has been examined in previous studies. In an early double-blind cross-over study of 11 patients with non-insulin treated diabetes, Aro and colleagues observed reduction in fasting and post-prandial glucose following 3 months of dietary supplementation with 21 g of guar gum per day in divided doses [12]. Fuessel and colleagues evaluated the effects of guar gum administered in the form of granules sprinkled over meals at a dose of 5 g per meal in 18 patients with type 2 diabetes and similarly found a diminution of post-prandial glucose AUC when guar gum was consumed prior to standard meal tolerance test [14]. In a single arm study by Groop and colleagues of 15 patients with diet-controlled diabetes, 15 g of guar gum granules per day taken with water or added to food resulted in significant lowering of HbA1c and fructosamine but not fasting plasma glucose over a 48-week intervention period [22]. Dall'alba and colleagues confirmed modest reduction in HbA1c and not fasting glycaemia following 6 weeks' treatment with 10 g per day of partially hydrolyzed guar gum in a recent study of 44 patients with metabolic syndrome and type 2 diabetes [17]. Although these studies were of small number sample sizes and many were not placebo-controlled, the predominant effect of guar gum supplementation on post-prandial over fasting glucose was consistently observed, in keeping with the proposed interfering action of galactomannan on absorption of carbohydrates in the gastrointestinal tract [10].

In the present study, we detected significant attenuation in several CGM glycaemic variability parameters among subjects with prediabetes receiving low dose BTI320. Accordingly, treatment with low dose BTI320 reduced 1-h, 2-h and 3-h incremental post-prandial glucose AUC by 0.30, 0.59 and 0.74 mmol/L×hour, respectively, compared with placebo. The maximum blood glucose within 3 h post-meal was lowered by 0.42 mmol/L in subjects receiving low dose BTI320 compared with placebo. Reductions were also observed in the high dose group albeit not reaching statistical significance. Contrary to effects on glycaemic variability, there were no significant changes in serum fructosamine or HbA1c at up to 16 weeks of intervention when compared with placebo. The predominant action of BTI320 in suppressing post-prandial glucose excursion might not be of sufficient magnitude to translate into discernable changes in serum fructosamine and HbA1c which comprise both fasting and post-prandial periods of glycaemia. It is also noteworthy that mannans-containing compounds such as BTI320 theoretically blunts post-prandial hyperglycaemia by slowing down the rate of glucose absorption more so than reducing the absolute amount absorbed, which in part explains the absence of reduction in overall glycaemia as measured using conventional glycaemic markers. As we have conducted our study in subjects with prediabetes who have less pronounced glucose fluctuation, this might have limited the study power to demonstrate significant glycaemic effects compared with testing in population with overt diabetes.

In previous investigations of healthy individuals and in patients with type 2 diabetes, addition of guar gum to a standard oral glucose load or test meal dampened post-prandial rise in plasma insulin and gastric inhibitory polypeptide [23, 24]. In our study, the reduction in post-prandial glucose was not accompanied by changes in 2-h AUC of insulin, C-peptide and GLP-1 during MTT, although there were non-significant trends of lower insulin and GLP-1 levels in the low dose BTI320 group compared with placebo.

Mechanisms of action of galactomannan

The mechanisms of blood glucose lowering and metabolic effects of guar gum have been extensively studied in the last two decades. For instance, galactomannan has been shown to increase viscosity of gastrointestinal content which in turn resists the movement of carbohydrates to the absorptive surface of the intestine, thus reducing accessibility of digestive enzymes to their substrates resulting in delayed glucose absorption [25]. Other evidence suggested that galactomannan may directly bind to and inhibit digestive enzymes such as alpha-amylase [26]. More recently, colonic fermentation of ingested guar gum has been demonstrated to alter short-chain fatty acid composition in the colon and modulate colonic microbiota [27, 28]. For example, consumption of guar gum promotes the production of propionic acid which has been reported to have favorable action on cholesterol and glucose metabolism [29]. Given our increasing knowledge regarding the roles of incretin biology [30] and microbiome [31] on intermediary metabolism as well as the proven effects of alpha-glucosidase inhibitor, a compound sharing similar actions as guar gum, in preventing diabetes in subjects with IGT [7], long-term use of galactomannan has the potential to stall progression to diabetes in at-risk individuals.

Weight effects of BTI320

Rodents being fed guar gum consistently exhibited reduced food intake and less weight gain [32]. In a small study of 21 obese subjects, administration of 10 g of guar gum twice daily for 8 weeks lowered body weight and was associated with fall in hunger rating [33]. The viscous nature of the food bolus mixed with guar gum slows down gastric emptying which augments satiety and facilitates portion control [34]. In the present study, we also observed modest decrease in body weight in the low dose BTI320 group, although we did not detect differences in caloric intake and in measures of satiety between subjects exposed and those not exposed to BTI320.

Tolerance

BTI320 was relatively well tolerated. Between 17 and 25% of participants assigned BTI320 developed abdominal distension and 29–33% reported increased flatulence but only 3 subjects had to stop study drug prematurely because of adverse effects. These gastrointestinal symptoms were likely due to increased bacterial digestion of complex carbohydrates in the colon producing gas. Hypoglycaemic symptoms were not reported in any of the subjects. In the STOP-NIDDM study, about one third of participants discontinued acarbose prematurely [7]. Advantages of BTI320 over acarbose which shares similar action mechanisms are the improved tolerability and ease of administration.

Study limitations

We acknowledge the following limitations of our study. Firstly, as our ultimate goal was to explore the clinical utility of this drug derived from natural compounds in prevention of diabetes, we have only included subjects with prediabetes. As such, our results cannot be extrapolated to people with diabetes. Secondly, fructosamine was used as a measure of short term glycaemia and there are limitations associated with this test. Fructosamine does not fully capture post-prandial hyperglycaemia which may be better reflected using other markers such as 1,5-anhydroglucitol, which were not measured in the present study. Thirdly, only subjects of Chinese ethnicity were tested and our results may not be generalised to people of other ethnic or cultural groups who have different dietary pattern. Fourly, we did not demonstrate a dose-related response and only low dose BTI320 showed statistical efficacy in the reduction of both blood glucose and body weight. The small sample size might have limited the study power to conclusively examine glucose-lowering action of BTI320. Inter-individual variability with respect to meal content, meal size and post-prandial glucose absorption might challenge the strength of the study to assess dose response, particularly if subjects in the three intervention groups might not have been balanced in this respect due to small numbers. Importantly, differences in age, BMI and IFG / IGT status between the three groups at baseline might also have contributed to the unexpected absence of treatment effects with the higher dose in the main analysis. In this regard, post-hoc subgroup analysis was conducted to explore whether treatment effects differ by these parameters. Here, we observed reductions in AUCpp with high dose as well as low dose BTI320 among obese subjects, whilst changes were not seen with high dose BTI320 in the non-obese group, suggesting that baseline BMI is one of the explanatory variables for the lack of treatment effects in the high dose group when the cohort was analysed in its entirety. We speculate that obese subjects, who are likely to have different eating habits to non-obese individuals, derive greater weight and hence glucose benefits than lean subjects.

Conclusions

In this proof-of-concept study of subjects with prediabetes, low dose BTI320 (4 g three times daily) did not reduce fructosamine levels at 4 weeks as specified in the primary endpoint but attenuated post-prandial rise in blood glucose based on CGM with modest weight loss. Future research will be required to test and confirm the glycaemic and weight effects of BTI320 in a larger sample.

Additional files

Additional file 1: Figure S1. Subject disposition. (DOCX 37 kb)

Additional file 2: Table S1. Subgroup analysis (high and low BMI groups) on the changes in post-prandial incremental area-under-curve from baseline between low dose or high dose BTI320 and placebo using random effect models with repeated measurements adjusted for intra-individual between-meal and between meal-day variability. **Table S2.** Subgroup analysis (patients with IFG and IGT, and without with IFG and IGT) on the changes in post-prandial incremental area-under-curve from baseline between low dose or high dose BTI320 and placebo using random effect models with repeated measurements adjusted for intra-individual between-meal and between meal-day variability. **Table S3.** Subgroup analysis (younger and elder groups) on the changes in post-prandial incremental area-under-curve from baseline between low dose or high dose BTI320 and placebo using random effect models with repeated measurements adjusted for intra-individual between-meal and between meal-day variability. **Table S4.** Frequencies of gastrointestinal adverse events among subjects in low dose BTI320, high dose BTI320 and placebo groups. (DOCX 18 kb)

Abbreviations

ANCOVA: Analysis of Covariance; AUC: Area-under-curve; BP: Blood pressures; CGM: Continuous glucose monitoring; CI: Confidence interval; CUHK: Chinese University of Hong Kong; CV: Coefficient of variations; GLP: Glucagon-like peptide; HbA1c: Glycated haemoglobin; HDL: High density-lipoprotein; hs-CRP: high-sensitivity-C reactive protein; IFG: Impaired fasting glucose; IGT: Impaired glucose tolerance; LDL: Low density-lipoprotein; MAGE: Mean amplitude of glucose excursion; MPMG: Mean post-meal maximum glucose; MTT: Meal tolerance test; OGTT: Oral glucose tolerance test; SD: Standard deviation

Acknowledgements
We thank the nursing and research staff at the Diabetes and Endocrine Research Centre, the Prince of Wales Hospital, for their tremendous efforts in recruiting and managing study subjects.

Funding
The study was sponsored by Sugardown Company Limited, Hong Kong. The Sponsor was involved in study design but had no role in data collection, analysis and data interpretation.

Authors' contributions
AOYL contributed to conception of the study, acquisition of data, interpretation of results, drafted the manuscript, and approved the final version. BCYZ and MC contributed to statistical analysis, conception of the study, and approved the final version. RO, MHMC, RCWM, APSK, FCCC, and JCNC contributed to conception of the study, acquisition of data, and approved the final version. CWR contributed to conception of the study and approved the final version. AOYL is the guarantor of this work and has full access to all the data in the study and takes responsibility for the integrity of the data and the accuracy of the analysis.

Competing interests
Andrea O.Y, Luk is a member of advisory boards for Astra Zeneca and Amgen, and has previously received research grants from Sanofi, Boehringer Ingelheim and Merck. Juliana C.N. Chan is a member of advisory boards, speaker bureaus and steering committees of multinational studies sponsored by companies including Bayer, Merck, Pfizer, Sanofi, Astra Zeneca, Lilly and Novo-Nordisk with consultancy fees which have been donated to the Chinese University of Hong Kong for supporting education and research in diabetes. Carl W. Rausch is the Chairman and Chief Executive Officer of Boston Therapeutics Inc., and Boston Therapeutics Inc. is involved in the development of BTI320. The remaining authors have no competing interests to declare.

Author details
¹Department of Medicine and Therapeutics, The Chinese University of Hong Kong, Shatin, Hong Kong. ²Li Ka Shing Institute of Health Science, The Chinese University of Hong Kong, Prince of Wales Hospital, Shatin, Hong Kong. ³School of Public Health and Primary Care, The Chinese University of Hong Kong, Prince of wales Hospital, Shatin, Hong Kong. ⁴Boston Therapeutics Inc., 354 Merrimack Street #4, Lawrence, MA 01843, USA. ⁵Department of Chemical Pathology, The Chinese University of Hong Kong, Prince of Wales Hospital, Shatin, Hong Kong. ⁶Diabetes and Endocrine Research Centre, The Prince of Wales Hospital, Shatin, New Territories, Hong Kong.

References
1. Wang L, Gao P, Zhang M, et al. Prevalence and ethnic pattern of diabetes and prediabetes in China in 2013. JAMA. 2017;317:2515–23.
2. International Diabetes Federation. IDF Diabetes Atlas. 8th ed. Brussels, Belgium: International Diabetes Federation; 2017.
3. Inzucchi SE, Sherwin RS. The prevention of type 2 diabetes mellitus. Endocrinol Metab Clin N Am. 2005;34:199–219.
4. Knowler WC, Barette-Conner E, Fowler SE, et al. Diabetes prevention program research group. Reduction in the incidence of type 2 diabetes with lifestyle intervention or metformin. N Engl J Med. 2002;346:393–403.
5. Tuomilehto J, Lindstrom J, Eriksson JG, et al. Finnish diabetes prevention study group. Prevention of type 2 diabetes mellitus by changes in lifestyle among subjects with impaired glucose tolerance. N Engl J Med. 2001;344:1343–50.
6. Gerstein HC, Yusuf S, Bosch J, et al. DREAM (diabetes reduction assessment with Ramipril and rosiglitazone medication) trial investigators. Effect of rosiglitazone on the frequency of diabetes in patients with impaired glucose tolerance or impaired fasting glucose: a randomized controlled trial. Lancet. 2006;368:1096–105.
7. Chiasson JL, Josse RG, Gomis R, et al. STOP-NIDDM trial research group. Acarbose for prevention of type 2 diabetes mellitus: the STOP-NIDDM randomized trial. Lancet. 2002;359:2072–7.
8. Diabetes Prevention Program Research Group. Long-term effects of lifestyle intervention or metformin on diabetes development and microvascular

complications over 15-year follow-up: the diabetes prevention program outcomes study. Lancet Diabetes Endocrinol. 2015;3:866–75.

9. Butt MS, Shahzadi N, Sharif MK, et al. Guar gum: a miracle therapy for hypercholesterolemia, hyperglycemia and obesity. Crit Rev Food Sci Nutr. 2007;47:389–96.

10. Papathanasopoulos A, Camilleri M. Dietary fiber supplements: effects in obesity and metabolic syndrome and relationship to gastrointestinal functions. Gastroenterology. 2010;138:65–72.

11. Jenkins DJ. Diabetic glucose control, lipids and trace elements on long-term guar. Br Med J. 1980;1:1353.

12. Aro A, Uusitupa M, Voutilainen E, et al. Improved diabetic control and hypocholesterolaemic effect induced by long-term dietary supplementation with guar gum in type 2 (insulin-independent) diabetes. Diabetologia. 1981;21:29–33.

13. Vaaler S, Hanssen KF, Dahl-Jorgensen K, et al. Diabetic control is improved by guar gum and wheat bran supplementation. Diabet Med. 1986;3:230–3.

14. Fuessl HS, Williams G, Adrian TE, et al. Guar sprinkled on food: effect on glycaemic control, plasma lipids and gut hormones in non-insulin dependent diabetic patients. Diabet Med. 1987;4:463–8.

15. Uusitupa M, Siitonen O, Savolainen K, et al. Metabolic and nutritional effects of long-term use of guar gum in the treatment of non-insulin dependent diabetes of poor metabolic control. Am J Clin Nutr. 1989;49:345–51.

16. Morgan LM, Tredger JA, Wright J, et al. The effect of soluble and insoluble-fibre supplementation on post-prandial glucose tolerance, insulin and gastric inhibitory polypeptide secretion in healthy subjects. Br J Nutr. 1990; 64:103–10.

17. Dall'alba V, Silva FM, Antonio JP, et al. Improvement of the metabolic syndrome profile by soluble fibre – guar gum – in patients with type 2 diabetes, a randomized clinical trial. Br J Nutr. 2013;110:1601–10.

18. Trask LE, Kasid N, Homa K, et al. Safety and efficacy of the nonsystemic chewable complex carbohydrate dietary supplement paz320 on postprandial glycemia when added to oral agents or insulin in patients with type 2 diabetes mellitus. Endocr Pract. 2013;19:627–32.

19. Service FJ, Molnar GD, Rosevear JW, et al. Mean amplitude of glycemic excursions, a measure of diabetic instability. Diabetes. 1970;19:644–55.

20. McCulloch CE, Neuhaus JM. Generalized linear mixed models. John Wiley & Sons, Ltd 2001.

21. Laird NM, Ware JH. Random-effects models for longitudinal data. Biometrics. 1982;38:963–74.

22. Groop PH, Aro A, Stenman S, et al. Long-term effects of guar gum in subjects with non-insulin-dependent diabetes mellitus. Am J Clin Nutr. 1993;58:513–8.

23. Braaten JT, Wood PJ, Scott FW, et al. Oat gum lowers glucose and insulin after an oral glucose load. Am J Clin Nutr. 1991;53:1425–30.

24. Morgan LM, Tredger JA, Wright J, et al. The effect of soluble and insoluble-fibre supplementation on post-prandial glucose tolerance, insulin and gastric inhibitory polypeptide secretion in health subjects. Br J Nutr. 1990;64:103–10.

25. Edwards CA, Johnson IT, Read NW. Do viscous polysaccharides slow absorption by inhibiting diffusion or convection? Eur J Clin Nutr. 1988; 42:307–12.

26. Slaughter SL, Ellis PR, Jackson EC, et al. The effect of guar galactomannan and water availability during hydrothermal processing on the hydrolysis of starch catalyzed by pancreatic alpha-amylase. Biochim Biophys Acta. 2002; 1571:55–63.

27. Topping DL, Clifton PM. Short-chain fatty acids and human colonic function: roles of resistant starch and nonstarch polysaccharides. Physiol Rev. 2001;81:1031–64.

28. Den Besten G, Bleeker A, Gerding A, et al. Short-chain fatty acids protect against high-fat diet-induced obesity via a PPARγ-dependent switch from lipogenesis to fat oxidation. Diabetes. 2015;64:2398–408.

29. Berggren AM, Nyman EM, Lundquist I, et al. Influence of orally and rectally administered propionate on cholesterol and glucose metabolism in obese rats. Br J Nutr. 1996;76:287–94.

30. Nauck MA, Baller B, Meier JJ. Gastric inhibitory polypeptide and glucagon-like peptide-1 in the pathogenesis of type 2 diabetes. Diabetes. 2004; 53(Suppl 3):S190–6.

31. Karlsson F, Tremaroli V, Nielsen J, Backhed F. Assessing the human gut microbiota in metabolic diseases. Diabetes. 2013;62:3341–9.

32. Frias ACD, Sgarbieri VC. Guar gum effects on food intake, blood serum lipids and glucose levels of Wistar rats. Plants Foods Human Nutr. 1999;53:15–28.

33. Krotkiewski M. Effect of guar gum on body-weight, hunger ratings and metabolism in obese subjects. Br J Nutr. 1984;52:97–105.

34. Jenkins DJ, Wolever TM, Leeds AR, et al. Dietary fibres, fibre analogues, and glucose tolerance: importance of viscosity. Br Med J. 1978;1:1392–4.

8

Variability of the Ki-67 proliferation index in gastroenteropancreatic neuroendocrine neoplasms - a single-center retrospective study

Huiying Shi[1] (iD), Qin Zhang[2], Chaoqun Han[1], Ding Zhen[1] and Rong Lin[1*]

Abstract

Background: The Ki-67 index in gastroenteropancreatic neuroendocrine neoplasms (GEP-NENs) may change throughout the disease course. However, the definitive effect of Ki-67 variability on GEP-NENs remains unknown. The aims of this study were to evaluate changes in Ki-67 levels throughout the disease course and investigate the role of Ki-67 index variability in GEP-NENs.

Methods: Specimens with multiple pathologies were evaluated from 30 patients who were selected from 514 patients with GEP-NENs, being treated at Wuhan Union Hospital from July 2009 to February 2018. The Ki-67 index was evaluated among multiple specimens over the disease course. Univariable and multivariable Cox proportional hazards regression analyses were performed to assess the prognostic significance of various clinical and histopathologic features.

Results: Among the 514 patients with GEP-NENs, metastases were seen in 182 (35.41%). Among the 30 patients from whom specimens with multiple pathologies were obtained, 24 were both primary and metastatic specimens and six were specimens collected over the course of the disease. Changes in Ki-67 levels were detected in 53.3% of the patients, of whom 40% had up-regulated Ki-67 levels, and 13.3% had down-regulated Ki-67 levels. Kaplan–Meier survival analysis showed that the group with Ki-67 variability had a shorter overall survival ($p = 0.0297$). The Cox regression analysis indicated that Ki-67 variability ($p = 0.038$) was the only independent prognostic factor for overall survival.

Conclusions: Our data suggest that patients with GEP-NENs and Ki-67 variability had a poorer prognosis. The re-assessment of Ki-67 at sites of metastasis or during the disease course might play a role in predicting the prognosis of patients with GEP-NENs. This finding could have implications for how GEP-NENs are monitored and treated.

Keywords: Gastroenteropancreatic neuroendocrine neoplasms, Ki-67, Metastases, Variability, Prognostic factors

Background

The Ki-67 protein, a cell proliferation-associated nuclear marker, has become a useful tool in assessing the malignant potential of neuroendocrine neoplasms (NENs) [1–3]. With respect to gastroenteropancreatic neuroendocrine neoplasms (GEP-NENs), the Ki-67 labeling index had already become an integral part of the World Health Organization (WHO) classification, from as early as the 2004 edition [4]. Subsequently, in the WHO-2010 classification schemes, GEP-NENs were further subdivided into three grades by the Ki-67 index as follows: grade 1 (G1) tumors with a Ki-67 index ≤2%; (grade 2) G2 tumors with an index of 3–20%; and (grade 3) G3 tumors, > 20% [5]. For NENs, a higher Ki-67 labeling index is associated with a poorer prognosis [2, 6, 7]. Accordingly, the grading system based on Ki-67 facilitates identification of the aggressive subset of NENs and provides a standardized

* Correspondence: selinalin35@hotmail.com
[1]Department of Gastroenterology, Union Hospital, Tongji Medical College, Huazhong University of Science and Technology, Wuhan 430022, China
Full list of author information is available at the end of the article

diagnostic pathway that is appropriate for effective decision-making in the management of NENs.

The GEP-NENs, one kind of heterogeneous tumors, frequently present with metastatic deposits at initial diagnosis; distant metastases have been suggested to be one of the strongest predictors of survival in GEP-NENs [1, 8–10]. In recent years, several publications have noted that the Ki-67 index varies from the site of the primary tumor to those of metastases, and even throughout the disease course [1, 2, 11]. In addition, researchers have also advocated that a sufficient evaluation of the Ki-67 index in metastatic tumors could have prognostic value and might be necessary to optimize clinical decision-making.

Despite the fact that discordant expression of Ki-67 exists at the primary and metastatic tumor sites, little is known about the manner in which Ki-67 variability changes throughout the disease, and thus affects prognosis. This is partly due to low prevalence and a lack of large sample data on GEP-NENs. We reviewed 514 patients with GEP-NENs and assessed the Ki-67 levels in the subgroup whose specimens bore multiple pathologies. Our aims were to explore the relationship between Ki-67 variability and prognosis in patients with GEP-NENs and provide the basis for more accurate decision-making in GEP-NENs.

Methods

We conducted a single-center retrospective study. The present study retrospectively reviewed patients diagnosed with GEP-NENs at Wuhan Union Hospital from July 2009 to February 2018. A total of 514 patients were included in the study, among which, 30 had multiple specimens taken from the primary tumor and a metastatic focus, or during the course of the disease. The diagnosis of NENs was performed through conventional histological and immunohistochemical analysis of specimens from the primary tumor and/or metastatic lesions. All specimens obtained by surgical resection, fine needle aspiration, and/or core biopsy were made available for all enrolled patients. The medical records were retrospectively reviewed to collect the following data: age, sex, primary and metastatic tumor sites, and Ki-67 labeling index.

The study was approved by the Ethics Committee of Tongji Medical College, Huazhong University of Science and Technology (IORG No: IORG0003571), and performed in accordance with the Declaration of Helsinki. As it was a retrospective study, all data were collected from a medical records system. Therefore, the study was exempt from the requirement to obtain individual informed consent, based on the Ethical Guidelines of the Ethics Committee of Tongji Medical College, Huazhong University of Science and Technology.

Immunohistochemistry

The specimens were fixed in 4% paraformaldehyde and embedded in paraffin wax. To evaluate the Ki-67 proliferation index of tumors, the paraffin-embedded tissue blocks were cut into 4 μm thick sections, and tissue sections were then assessed by immunohistochemistry with a Ki-67 antibody (MIB-1, DAKO), using the Ventana Discovery staining system (Ventana Medical Systems). The Ki-67 index was determined by calculating the percentage of tumor cells with positive staining, among up to 2000 tumor cells in the densest field of each slide. All results were verified by two pathologists (QZ and the pathologist responsible for the original pathology report).

Statistical analysis

Clinical and pathologic characteristics of patients were expressed as median and range, or percentage. Overall survival was defined as that time from the date of diagnosis to the date of death, or last follow-up. Survival curves were drawn according to the Kaplan–Meier analysis, and differences between groups were assessed using the log-rank test. Cox proportional hazards regression analysis was used to assess prognostic factors for survival. Statistical calculations and data manipulation were performed using the SPSS software v21.0 (IBM, USA), and $p < 0.05$ was considered statistically significant.

Results

Patient characteristics

Among the 514 patients with a GEP-NENS diagnosis, 302 (58.75%) were men and 212 were (41.25%) women. The median age at the time of diagnosis was 55 years (range: 12–85 years). Of the 514 GEP-NENs patients, 196 (38.13%) cases were of low grade G1; 102 (19.84%) of intermediate grade G2; and 216 (42.02%) of high grade G3. Metastases were observed in 35.41% (182/514) of all cases, and in 9.18% (18/196) of G1 tumors, 39.22% (40/102) of G2 tumors, and 57.41% (124/216) of G3 tumors. The clinical characteristics of these patients and tumors are shown in Table 1. The subset of 30 patients with specimens showing multiple pathologies were analyzed, to evaluate the heterogeneity of the Ki-67 index throughout the disease course (Table 2).

Variability of Ki-67 throughout the disease course of NENs

Among the 30 patients, 10 (33.3%) were G1; 7 (23.3%) G2; and 13 (43.3%) G3. Assessment of the Ki-67 index in those 30 cases with specimens showing multiple pathologies revealed discrepancies in 53.3% cases, among which, 40% and 13.3% patients had up-regulated and down-regulated Ki-67 levels, respectively. The up-regulation of the Ki-67 index from primary to metastatic specimens, or during the disease course was as follows: G1 to G2, 25.0% (4/16); G2 to

Table 1 Clinical characteristics in 514 patients with GEP-NENs

Variables	Total $n = 514$ (%)
Sex	
Male	302 (58.75)
Female	212 (41.25)
Grade (Ki-67)	
G1	196 (38.13)
G2	102 (19.84)
G3	216 (42.02)
Primary tumor site	
Pancreas	149 (28.99)
Large colon	148 (28.79)
Stomach	100 (19.46)
Esophagus	22 (4.28)
Duodenum	16 (3.11)
Other sites	79 (15.37)
Metastasis	182 (35.41)
Age at diagnosis (years)	55 (12–85)

G3, 6.25% (1/16); G2 to G2, 6.25% (1/16); G3 to G3, 37.5% (6/16).

Some Ki-67 variability was observed in 41.18% (7/17) of the patients with primary tumors categorized as G1/G2; 35.29% (6/17) showed up-regulation of Ki-67 and 5.88% (1/17) showed down-regulation of Ki-67 (Fig. 1a). For primary tumors categorized as G3 (as confirmed by both Ki-67 and mitotic count), the Ki-67 variability was 57.1% (9/13), including 46.15% (6/13) showing up-regulation, and 23.08% (3/13) showing down-regulation (Fig. 1a).

The rectum was the most variable of the primary sites, whereas grade 3 (G3) tumors had the most variable intervals. Among the 11 patients with primary tumors in the rectum, Ki-67 variability was present in 72.72% (8/11) of all cases; 54.54% (6/11) showed up-regulation, and 18.18% (2/11) showed down-regulation (Fig. 1b). About 28.6% of the patients with primary tumors in the pancreas had up-regulated Ki-67 levels in metastatic loci and were upstaged to a higher WHO class (from G2 to G3) (Table 2, Fig. 1b). For ten patients with primary tumors in the stomach, 60% (6/10) showed Ki-67 variability, with 40% (4/10) showing up-regulation, and 20% (2/10) showing down-regulation of Ki-67 levels (Fig. 1b).

Survival analysis
Kaplan–Meier survival analysis showed a significant discrepancy in mortality between Ki-67 variable and non-variable groups; the group with Ki-67 variability had a poorer prognosis than the group without Ki-67 variability ($p = 0.0297$) (Fig. 2). Cox regression analysis included age, sex, primary and metastatic tumor sites, Ki-67 level, and Ki-67 variability,

and showed that Ki-67 variability ($p = 0.038$) was the only prognostic factor for survival in patients with metastatic GEP-NENs (Table 3).

Discussion
In this study, we explored the relationship between the Ki-67 variability and the prognosis of patients with GEP-NENs. Our data support the fact that the Ki-67 index in GEP-NENs can change throughout the disease course, often with progression to increased malignancy and greater aggressiveness after metastasis. Moreover, this study further demonstrates that patients with Ki-67 variability have a poorer prognosis. Thus, re-assessment of Ki-67 at the sites of metastases, or during the disease course may prove to be a significant step in determining the prognosis of patients with GEP-NENs.

The GEP-NENs represent a heterogeneous family with variable biological and clinical characteristics [7, 12, 13]. Over the last few decades, neuroendocrine tumors (NETs) have been commonly considered rare tumors. However, the real incidence and prevalence of NETs, that has increased 6.4-fold from 1973 (1.09 per 100,000) to 2012 (6.98 per 100,000), according to Surveillance, Epidemiology, and End Results (SEER) data, may be underestimated [14].

Although the role of the Ki-67 index in GEP-NENs has been widely recognized since 2004, some recent studies have found that the Ki-67 index might change throughout the disease course or between primary and metastatic sites [1, 2, 11, 15]. One UK study showed that Ki-67 variability existed in 41.2% GEP-NEN cases from the primary tumor to metastatic sites [1]. Singh et al. (2014) proposed that Ki-67 might vary during the disease course, from primary stage to metastasis, and these changes throughout the course of the disease might have a significant impact on the monitoring and management of NETs [2]. Along with those observations, we also found that variability of the Ki-67 index between primary and metastatic specimens, or during the disease course was identified in about 53.3% of the patients in the present study.

We further analyzed the cases with Ki-67 index variability. Among 30 patients, the Ki-67 levels were found to be up- and down-regulated in 40% and 13.3% of the cases, respectively from the primary site to the metastatic site or during the disease course. The up-regulation of Ki-67 levels was as follows: G1 to G2, 25.0%; G2 to G3, 6.25%; G3 to G3, 37.5%. Shifting to a higher grade was mainly observed between G1 and G2, and as both G1 and G2 tumors received the same treatment, the clinical management based on the current criteria was not affected [16, 17]. In about 6.25% of the patients showing Ki-67 index variability, the tumor grades were upstaged from G2 to G3. However, without re-assessments of the metastasis or during the disease

Table 2 Ki-67 index variability and WHO class change in patients with multiple pathology specimens

Patient #	Primary tumor site Site1#	Metastatic/Re-biopsy tumor site Site2#	Ki-67 index (%)		Survival time	WHO class change
			Site1#	Site2#		
1	pancreas	peritoneum	70	70	12	–
2	pancreas	lymph node	10	30	15	G2 → G3
3	pancreas	peritoneum	5	20	6	G2 → G2
4	pancreas	liver	5	5	11	–
5	pancreas	liver	2	2	12	–
6	pancreas	pancreas	1	1	24	–
7	pancreas	liver	1	1	38	–
8	rectum	lymph node	70	70	12	–
9	rectum	liver	50	80	16	G3 → G3
10	rectum	liver	2	5	13	G1 → G2
11	rectum	liver	2	1	5	G1 → G1
12	rectum	liver	2	5	3	G1 → G2
13	rectum	lymph node	70	90	8	G3 → G3
14	rectum	lymph node	2	5	7	G1 → G2
15	rectum	liver	2	2	14	–
16	rectum	liver	10	10	–	–
17	rectum	rectum	80	60	12	G3 → G3
18	rectum	lymph node	60	80	–	G3 → G3
19	stomach	lymph node	2	5	12	G1 → G2
20	stomach	lymph node	60	80	14	G3 → G3
21	stomach	liver	1	1	24	–
22	stomach	lymph node	60	40	22	G3 → G3
23	stomach	lymph node	5	5	27	–
24	stomach	stomach	50	80	–	G3 → G3
25	stomach	stomach	70	30	33	G3 → G3
26	stomach	stomach	30	40	21	G3 → G3
27	stomach	pancreas	70	70	8	–
28	stomach	stomach	5	5	60	–
29	ileocecal junction	lymph node	70	70	16	–
30	duodenum	liver	5	5	12	–

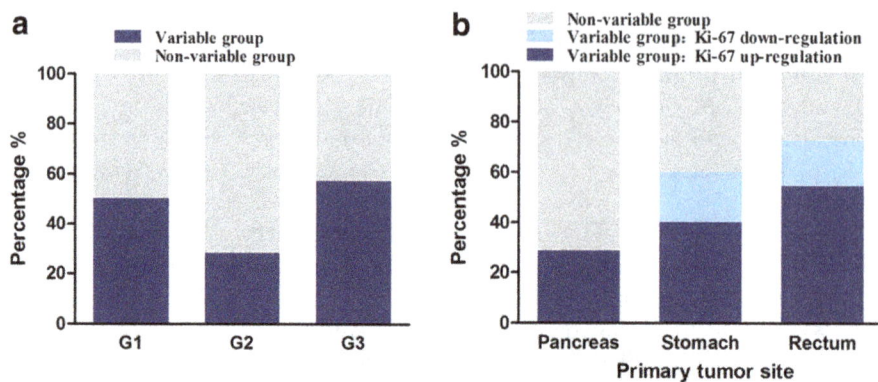

Fig. 1 Distribution of variable cases according to GEP-NENs grade (**a**) and primary tumor site (**b**)

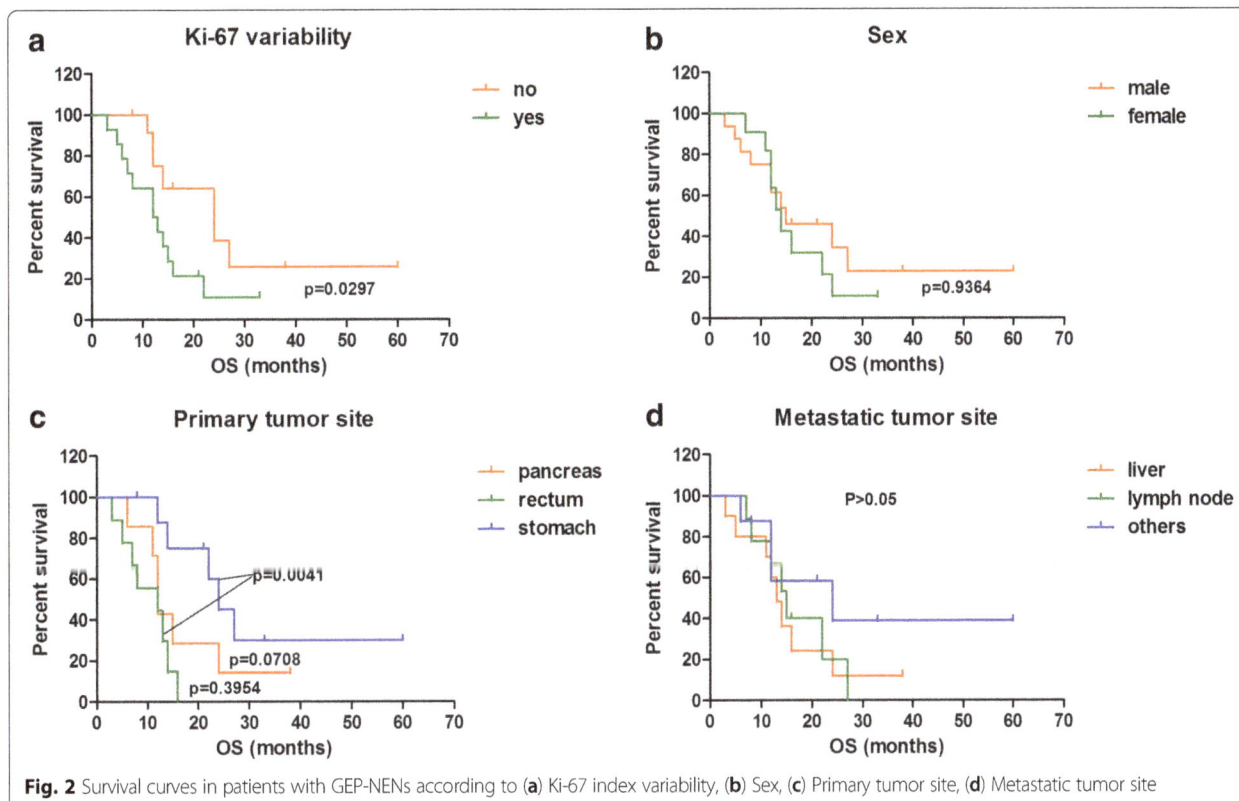

Fig. 2 Survival curves in patients with GEP-NENs according to (**a**) Ki-67 index variability, (**b**) Sex, (**c**) Primary tumor site, (**d**) Metastatic tumor site

course, those G1/G2 NENs might not have been recognized as potential candidates for chemotherapy. Therefore, our results suggest that identification of the upstaged subset of G1/G2 was significantly useful to clinical doctors in determining appropriate treatment options and evaluating prognosis.

Although previous papers [1, 2, 11] have advocated re-assessment of the Ki-67 index throughout the disease course, or the progression from primary to metastatic sites, reports on whether variability in Ki-67 levels affects the prognosis of GEP-NENs are lacking. Kaplan–Meier survival analysis of the patients of the present study showed that the group with Ki-67 variability had a significantly

shorter overall survival. Furthermore, results of the Cox regression analysis further confirmed that Ki-67 variability was the only independent prognostic factor for survival in those patients. These results emphasize the need for biopsies from metastatic lesions, or over the course of the disease. Moreover, the assessment of Ki-67 levels at all sites could significantly improve patient management.

To date, the reasons for Ki-67 index variability in GEP-NENs remain unclear. Miller et al. [1] hypothesized that variation of Ki-67 expression within a tumor is due to genetic intramural heterogeneity of NENs, as had been shown in other solid cancers [18–20]. However, Singh et al. [2] supposed that Ki-67 index changes during

Table 3 Cox regression analysis on prognostic baseline factors for survival in patients with multiple pathology specimens

Characteristics	Univariate analysis		Multivariate Cox regression analysis	
	HR (95%CI)	P value	HR (95%CI)	P value
Age	0.994 (0.954–1.037)	0.789		
Sex, female vs. Male	1.312 (0.530–3.248)	0.559		
Primary tumor site		0.068		0.310
Pancreas vs. Stomach	2.379 (0.720–7.852)	0.155	2.031 (0.564–7.311)	0.278
Rectum vs. Stomach	5.468 (1.570–19.041)	0.008	3.320 (0.956–11.523)	0.059
Metastasis, Yes vs. No	6.142 (0.810–46.551)	0.079	6.963 (0.814–59.588)	0.076
Ki-67 index	0.995 (0.979–1.011)	0.565		
Ki-67 Variability, Yes vs. No	2.612 (0.999–6.834)	0.045	3.487 (1.069–11.380)	0.038

the disease course could be due to treatment effects and therapy resistance. Although the present study showed that the Ki-67 index varies from primary to metastatic sites, or during the disease course, we were not able to draw solid conclusions about the reasons behind the Ki-67 variability observed because of the relatively small sample size. The underlying mechanisms need to be explored in further studies with larger sample sizes.

Conclusions

In summary, our study confirms that discordant expressions of Ki-67 in primary tumors and metastases are common in GEP-NENs. Furthermore, we also presented strong evidence that patients with Ki-67 variability have a poorer prognosis in GEP-NENs, and there is need for increased vigilance with this subgroup. Therefore, we recommend as a matter of great importance, a re-biopsy and re-estimation of the Ki-67 index at metastatic sites, or during the disease course. Although both intra-tumor heterogeneity and therapy resistance are speculated to be the underlying mechanisms of Ki-67 variability, the manner in which they affect patient prognosis requires further study.

Abbreviations
GEP-NENs: Gastroenteropancreatic Neuroendocrine Neoplasms; NETs: Neuroendocrine tumors; OS: Overall survival; SEER: Surveillance, Epidemiology, and End Results program; WHO: World Health Organization

Acknowledgements
The authors wish to acknowledge all participants in this study and everybody involved in the set-up and implementation of the study.

Funding
This study was supported by the National Natural Science Foundation of China (Nos. 81572428 and 81770539).

Authors' contributions
RL and HYS designed/performed most of the investigation, data analysis and wrote the manuscript; QZ provided pathological assistance; CQH and ZD contributed to interpretation of the data and analyses. All of the authors have read and approved the manuscript.

Competing interests
The authors declare that they have no competing interests.

Author details
[1]Department of Gastroenterology, Union Hospital, Tongji Medical College, Huazhong University of Science and Technology, Wuhan 430022, China. [2]Department of Pathology, Union Hospital, Tongji Medical College, Huazhong University of Science and Technology, Wuhan 430022, China.

References
1.   Miller HC, Drymousis P, Flora R, Goldin R, Spalding D, Frilling A. Role of Ki-67 proliferation index in the assessment of patients with neuroendocrine neoplasias regarding the stage of disease. World J Surg. 2014;38(6):1353–61.
2.   Singh S, Hallet J, Rowsell C, Law CH. Variability of Ki67 labeling index in multiple neuroendocrine tumors specimens over the course of the disease. European journal of surgical oncology : the journal of the European Society of Surgical Oncology and the British Association of Surgical Oncology. 2014; 40(11):1517–22.
3.   Foltyn W, Zajecki W, Marek B, Kajdaniuk D, Sieminska L, Zemczak A, Kos-Kudla B. The value of the Ki-67 proliferation marker as a prognostic factor in gastroenteropancreatic neuroendocrine tumours. Endokrynologia Polska. 2012;63(5):362–6.
4.   Kleihues PSL. World Health Organization classification of Tumours. Pathology and genetics of endocrine organs. In: Lyon: IARC press; 2004.
5.   Bosman FT CF, Hruban RH et al: WHO Classification of Tumours of the Digestive System, 4th edition. Geneva, Switzerland: WHO Press 2010, ISBN978–92–832–2432–7.
6.   Khan MS, Luong TV, Watkins J, Toumpanakis C, Caplin ME, Meyer T. A comparison of Ki-67 and mitotic count as prognostic markers for metastatic pancreatic and midgut neuroendocrine neoplasms. Br J Cancer. 2013;108(9): 1838–45.
7.   Adsay V. Ki67 labeling index in neuroendocrine tumors of the gastrointestinal and pancreatobiliary tract: to count or not to count is not the question, but rather how to count. Am J Surg Pathol. 2012;36(12):1743–6.
8.   Yao JC, Hassan M, Phan A, Dagohoy C, Leary C, Mares JE, Abdalla EK, Fleming JB, Vauthey JN, Rashid A, et al. One hundred years after "carcinoid": epidemiology of and prognostic factors for neuroendocrine tumors in 35,825 cases in the United States. Journal of clinical oncology : official journal of the American Society of Clinical Oncology. 2008;26(18):3063–72.
9.   Lewkowicz E, Trofimiuk-Muldner M, Wysocka K, Pach D, Kieltyka A, Stefanska A, Sowa-Staszczak A, Tomaszewska R, Hubalewska-Dydejczyk A. Gastroenteropancreatic neuroendocrine neoplasms: a 10-year experience of a single center. Polskie Archiwum Medycyny Wewnetrznej. 2015;125(5):337–46.
10. Scarpa A, Mantovani W, Capelli P, Beghelli S, Boninsegna L, Bettini R, Panzuto F, Pederzoli P. Delle Fave G, Falconi M. pancreatic endocrine tumors: improved TNM staging and histopathological grading permit a clinically efficient prognostic stratification of patients. Modern pathology: an official journal of the United States and Canadian Academy of Pathology, Inc. 2010;23(6):824–33.
11. Grillo F, Albertelli M, Brisigotti MP, Borra T, Boschetti M, Fiocca R, Ferone D, Mastracci L. Grade increases in Gastroenteropancreatic neuroendocrine tumor metastases compared to the primary tumor. Neuroendocrinology. 2016;103(5):452–9.
12. Yang Z, Tang LH, Klimstra DS. Gastroenteropancreatic neuroendocrine neoplasms: historical context and current issues. Semin Diagn Pathol. 2013; 30(3):186–96.
13. Cives M, Soares HP, Strosberg J. Will clinical heterogeneity of neuroendocrine tumors impact their management in the future? Lessons from recent trials. Curr Opin Oncol. 2016;28(4):359–66.
14. Dasari A, Shen C, Halperin D, Zhao B, Zhou S, Xu Y, Shih T, Yao JC. Trends in the incidence, prevalence, and survival outcomes in patients with neuroendocrine tumors in the United States. JAMA oncology. 2017;3(10):1335–42.
15. Dhall D, Mertens R, Bresee C, Parakh R, Wang HL, Li M, Dhall G, Colquhoun SD, Ines D, Chung F, et al. Ki-67 proliferative index predicts progression-free survival of patients with well-differentiated ileal neuroendocrine tumors. Hum Pathol. 2012;43(4):489–95.
16. Modlin IM, Oberg K, Chung DC, Jensen RT, de Herder WW, Thakker RV, Caplin M, Delle Fave G, Kaltsas GA, Krenning EP, et al. Gastroenteropancreatic neuroendocrine tumours. The Lancet Oncology. 2008;9(1):61–72.
17. Pape UF, Perren A, Niederle B, Gross D, Gress T, Costa F, Arnold R, Denecke T, Plockinger U, Salazar R, et al. ENETS consensus guidelines for the management of patients with neuroendocrine neoplasms from the jejuno-ileum and the appendix including goblet cell carcinomas. Neuroendocrinology. 2012;95(2): 135–56.
18. Kumler I, Balslev E, Knop AS, Brunner N, Klausen TW, Jespersen SS, Nielsen SL, Nielsen DL. Expression patterns of biomarkers in primary tumors and corresponding metastases in breast Cancer. In: Applied immunohistochemistry & molecular morphology : AIMM; 2016.

9

Estrogen receptor 1 gene polymorphisms are associated with metabolic syndrome in postmenopausal women in China

Lingxia Zhao[1,2], Xuemei Fan[1,2], Lin Zuo[3], Qiang Guo[4], Xiaole Su[5], Guangxia Xi[2], Ziyan Zhang[1], Jianlin Zhang[1] and Guoping Zheng[1,6*]

Abstract

Background: Metabolic syndrome (MetS) includes obesity, diabetes, dyslipidemia and hypertension. Its incidence is rapidly increasing worldwide, particularly in postmenopausal women. Estrogens regulate glucose homeostasis and lipid metabolism via estrogen receptors 1 (ESR1) and 2 (ESR2). The current study aimed to elucidate associations of MetS with ESR1 and ESR2 gene polymorphisms in postmenopausal Chinese women.

Methods: This case-control study included 304 postmenopausal women (154 and 150 control and MetS patients, respectively). Clinical indicators related to MetS were assessed. Two ESR1 (Pvull and Xbal) and two ESR2 (Rsal and Alul) polymorphisms were evaluated by polymerase chain reaction (PCR)-restriction fragment length polymorphism analysis.

Results: ESR1 polymorphisms were significantly different between MetS patients and healthy controls. G allele frequency for the Xbal polymorphism was significantly higher in patients than in control patients ($p = 0.004$, OR = 1. 610, 95%CI 1.169–2.18). The haplotypes A–T ($p = 0.015$) and G–C ($p = 0.024$) showed significant differences. The minor alleles of the Xbal and Pvull gene polymorphisms in both homozygous and heterozygous forms showed associations with elevated waist circumference, fasting serum insulin and HOMA-IR. The minor G allele in homozygous and heterozygous forms of the Rsal and Alul gene polymorphisms showed associations with elevated total cholesterol and LDL-C.

Conclusions: In postmenopausal Chinese women, ESR1 polymorphism and the haplotypes A–T and G–C of Xbal–Pvull are associated with MetS, unlike ESR2 polymorphisms. Patients harboring the G allele of Xbal have elevated BMI, waist circumference, systolic and diastolic BP, FBG, HOMA-IR, total cholesterol, TG, LDL-C and NAFLD (%), and reduced HDL-C.

Keywords: Metabolic syndrome, Postmenopausal women, Estrogen receptors 1 and 2, Gene polymorphisms

Background

Metabolic syndrome (MetS) constitutes a threat to human health, with estimated prevalence rates of 17–40 and 16.3% in the Middle East and North Africa, respectively [1]. Its prevalence has also increased from 23.8% between 2000 and 2005, to 27% between 2010 and 2015 in China

[2]. MetS increases the risk of coronary artery disease, stroke, fatty liver disease, diabetes mellitus (DM), insomnia, and several cancers [3, 4]. Adult Treatment Panel III (ATP III) proposed that MetS encompasses at least three of the following ailments: abdominal obesity, high triglyceride (TG) levels, low high-density lipoprotein cholesterol (HDL-C) amounts, high blood pressure (BP), and high fasting blood glucose (FBG) [5]. All MetS variations increase the risk of cardiovascular disease (CVD). CVD incidence and mortality are significantly reduced in premenopausal women compared with men, but this difference

* Correspondence: zhengguoping2@126.com
[1]Department of Biochemistry and Molecular Biology, Shanxi Medical University, Taiyuan, No.56, Xinjian South Road, Taiyuan, Shanxi 030001, People's Republic of China
[6]Centre for Transplantation and Renal Research, University of Sydney at Westmead Millennium Institute, Sydney, NSW 2145, Australia
Full list of author information is available at the end of the article

gradually diminishes after menopause [6], with a corresponding increase in MetS incidence [7].

Hormones have critical functions in MetS pathogenesis and progression. Estrogen is associated with many aspects of MetS [8] such as glucose tolerance, fat metabolism, and BP [9]. Estrogen exerts its physiological functions in combination with estrogen receptors (ERs). ERs are nuclear hormone receptors (transcription factors) found in macrophages, adipose cells, vascular smooth muscle cells, and vascular endothelial cells [10, 11]. Estrogen receptor-α (ESR1) and β (ESR2) represent two known estrogen receptors that have been assessed using transgenic ERa (ERa-/-) and/or ERb (ERb-/-) knockout mice [12, 13].

The subtypes of ER, ESR1, and ESR2 are distinct in structure and function (likely in carbohydrate and lipid metabolism) [14]. ESR1 and ESR2 are found on chromosomes 6q25.1 and 14q23.2, respectively [15]. Single nucleotide polymorphisms (SNPs) in ESR1, such as PvuII (rs2234693) and XbaI (rs9340799), are involved in MetS [16]. As for ESR2, the risk of MetS is determined by the RsaI (1082A > G) (rs1256049) and AluI (1730A > G) (rs4986938) polymorphisms [17]. ESR1 and ESR2 SNPs are associated with metabolic factors in Western populations [18]. Here we assessed associations of four representative ESR1 and ESR2 polymorphisms with MetS and related phenotypes in postmenopausal Han Chinese women.

Methods
Study population and laboratory measurements
This case control study was performed between January and November 2016 at the medical center of Shanxi Dayi Hospital (Taiyuan, China). Three hundred and four postmenopausal women aged 46–71 years were enrolled. Inclusion criteria were: ≥60 years old; permanent menstrual period discontinuation because of natural menopause.

At baseline, the subjects were assigned to 2 groups, including the control (154 healthy individuals; mean age of 63.0 ± 4.1 years) and MetS (150 MetS patients; mean age of 62.9 ± 4.8 years) groups. All subjects were Han Chinese and of the same ethnic group. All cases were diagnosed according to the Chinese type 2 diabetes Prevention Guide (2013) diagnostic guidelines [19]. MetS was reflected by ≥3 of the following parameters: waist circumference ≥ 85 cm; FBG ≥6.1 mM or 2 h post glucose–load blood glucose ≥7.8 mM or known diabetes; serum TG ≥1.70 mM; HDL-C < 1.04 mM; and BP ≥130/85 mmHg or treated hypertension. Non-alcoholic fatty liver disease (NAFLD) diagnosis was performed by abdominal ultrasonography, as described previously [20]. Exclusion criteria were: severe psychological ailments, physical disability, any type of malignancy, or history of smoking, heart failure, myocardial infarction (MI), type I diabetes, kidney failure, and

chronic liver disease. The subjects were not undergoing hormone replacement.

Data collection
The main measurements and clinical data of the participants, including age, height, weight, body mass index (BMI), waist circumference, and systolic and diastolic BPs, were measured and recorded by specifically trained individuals. Waist circumference measurement was carried out in the horizontal plane at the midpoint between the lower border of ribs and the iliac crest. Systolic and diastolic BPs were obtained in right upper arm twice following a 15 min-rest with the patient sitting. Measurements were performed at 5 min intervals and averaged.

FBG, hemoglobin A1C (HbA1C), TG, total cholesterol (TC), HDL-C, low density lipoprotein (LDL-C; direct measurement), estradiol (E2), and fasting serum insulin levels in all participants were measured from fasting blood samples on an AutoAnalyzer (AU5400, Olympus, Tokyo, Japan), with reagents and calibrators provided by the manufacturer. Abdominal ultrasonography was conducted by specialized radiologists based on unified NAFLD diagnostic criteria. Insulin resistance (homeostasis model assessment of insulin resistance, HOMA-IR) was determined for each subject.

This study followed the Declaration of Helsinki, as well as institutional regulations regarding human subjects. Written informed consent was provided by all participants. The study protocol had approval from the ethics committee of the Shanxi Da Yi Hospital Institute for Biological Sciences, Chinese Academy of Sciences.

Genomic DNA extraction and genotyping
Venous blood (2 ml) specimens were obtained in EDTA anticoagulation tubes and used for DNA extraction. Genomic DNA extraction from 200 μL whole blood was carried out with the TIANamp Blood DNA Kit (Tiangen Biotech, China), as instructed by the manufacturer.

The PvuII (c454-397 T > C) and XbaI (c454-351A > G) polymorphisms in ESR1 as well as the RsaI (1082A > G) and AluI (1730A > G) polymorphisms in ESR2 were assessed by polymerase chain reaction- restriction fragment length polymorphism (PCR-RFLP). A 1374 base pair (bp) fragment was amplified for the PvuII (c454-397 T > C) and XbaI (c454-351A > G) polymorphisms using the following primer pair: upstream, 5′-CTGCCACCCTATCTGTATC TTTTCCTATTCTCC-3′; downstream, 5′-TCTTTCTCT GCCACCCTGGCGTCGATTATCTGA-3′. A 476-bp fragment for the RsaI (1082A > G) polymorphism was amplified using the following primer pair: upstream, 5′-TTCT GAGCCGAGGTCGTAGT-3′; downstream, 5′-CCAGGA CTTTGTTCCCACTC-3′. A 391-bp fragment for the AluI (1730A > G) polymorphism was amplified with the following primer pair: upstream, 5′-GCACCTTTTTGTCC

CCATAGTAAC-3′; downstream, 5′-CTATGGCTTCC TCACACCGAC-3′. PCR was carried out on an ABI Prism 7500 sequence system (Applied Biosystems, USA) in 25 µl reactions, containing 5 µl genomic DNA, 10 µl of Taq PCR Master mix (2×), 2 µl of each primer, and 8 µl PCR buffer (Tiangen Biotech, China), as follows: 94 °C (4 min); 35 cycles of 94 °C (30 s), 57 °C (40 s) and 72 °C (40 s); 72 °C (7 min). Digestion of PCR products was performed overnight using XbaI (expected fragments of 1374, 393, and 981 bp), PvuII (expected fragments of 1374, 438, and 936 bp), RsaI (expected fragments of 476, 183, and 293 bp), and AluI (expected fragments of 391, 144, and 247 bp) (Biolabs, New England) at 37 °C. All the digested fragments were electrophoresed on 2% agarose gels containing Goldview. The genotypes of 10% specimens were verified by direct sequencing.

Statistical analysis

SPSS 20.0 was employed for statistical analyses. Normally distributed continuous data are mean ± standard deviation (SD). Genotype differences were assessed in MetS patients by analysis of variance. Baseline features between the MetS and control groups were evaluated by Student t-test. Comparisons among multiple groups were performed by ANOVA with Bonferroni correction. Hardy–Weinberg equilibrium test, allele genotype frequency assessment, and haplotype evaluation were carried out online with the SHEsis platform. Genotype frequency, allele frequency, and haplotype were analyzed by the chi-square test and odds ratio (OR) assessment. Multivariable logistic regression was performed to adjust ORs for possible confounders. $p < 0.05$ indicated statistical significance. The function pwr.chisq.test() in the R package was used to calculate statistical power.

Results

Demographic and clinical variables

The MetS and control groups included postmenopausal women, with similar ages in both groups. All clinical parameters in Table 1 showed statistically significant differences between the MetS and control groups. Elevated BMI values and waist circumferences were observed in MetS patients, who also showed higher mean systolic and diastolic BPs compared with controls. In addition, the MetS group had markedly higher FBG, hemoglobin A1c, fasting serum insulin and HOMA-IR levels, and worse lipid profile. Furthermore, prevalence of nonalcoholic fatty liver disease was far higher in MetS patients compared with controls.

Allele frequencies and genotype distribution

Genotype distribution for each of the four SNPs was compatible with the Hardy–Weinberg equilibrium ($p > 0.05$) in MetS and control patients. The Chi-square test of XbaI genotype's frequencies in the case and control groups can be used to calculate statistical power. The test power was calculated (power = 1), indicating that the allele frequencies and genotype distributions of MetS patients and controls (Table 2) led to credible conclusions.

Table 1 Patient clinico-biochemical features

Variables	Metabolic syndrome ($n = 150$)	No metabolic syndrome ($n = 154$)	P
Age (years)	63.0 ± 4.1	62.9 ± 4.8	0.751
BMI (kg/m²)	25.4 ± 2.9	22.5 ± 3.0	<0.001
Waist circumference (cm)	88.3 ± 5.2	81.9 ± 2.5	0.001
FBG (mM)	7.1 ± 1.4	5.2 ± 0.7	<0.001
HbA1C (%)	6.7 ± 0.9	5.2 ± 0.4	0.003
Systolic blood pressure (mmHg)	148.1 ± 6.9	122.1 ± 4.9	<0.001
Diastolic blood pressure (mmHg)	92.3 ± 4.5	71.8 ± 5.7	0.002
Triglycerides (mM)	2.4 ± 1.1	1.8 ± 1.2	<0.001
Total cholesterol (mM)	5.1 ± 1.0	4.6 ± 1.1	<0.001
HDL-C (mM)	1.0 ± 0.1	1.3 ± 0.1	<0.001
LDL-C (mM)	3.1 ± 0.9	2.8 ± 0.6	0.008
NAFLD (%)	110(73.3)	33 (21.4)	<0.001
Fasting serum insulin (µIU/mL)	14.3 ± 7.2	9.2 ± 5.0	<0.001
Estradiol (pg/ml)	23.2 ± 7.2	27.0 ± 7.2	<0.001
HOMA-IR	3.5 ± 1.8	2.1 ± 1.3	<0.001

Abbreviations BMI body mass index, *FBG* fasting blood glucose, *HbA1C* hemoglobin A1C, *HDL* high density lipoprotein, *LDL* low-density lipoprotein, *NAFLD* nonalcoholic fatty liver disease
Data are mean ± SD. Comparisons were performed by *t*-test
p < 0.05 indicates a significant difference from the normal control

Table 2 Allele frequencies and genotype distributions of ESR1 and ESR2 gene polymorphisms in the metabolic syndrome (MetS) and control groups

Variables	MetS n (%) ($n = 150$)	Control n (%) ($n = 154$)	P	OR(95 % CI)[a]
ESR1				
XbaI (A > G)				
A allele	131 (43.7)	171 (55.5)		
G allele	169 (56.3)	137 (44.5)	0.004	1.610 (1.169, 2.18)
1 (AA)	29 (19.3)	45 (29.2)		
2 (AG)	73 (48.7)	81 (52.6)	0.894	1.044 (0.556, 1.960)
3 (GG)	48 (32.0)	28 (18.2)	0.109	2.660 (0.874, 3.829)
PVUII (T > C)				
T allele	143 (47.7)	157 (52.3)		
C allele	158 (51.3)	150 (48.7)	0.223	1.219 (0.887, 1.676)
1 (TT)	31 (20.7)	38 (24.7)		
2 (TC)	79 (52.7)	84 (54.5)	0.012	2.440 (1.216, 4.897)
3 (CC)	40 (26.7)	32 (20.8)	0.038	2.288 (1.045, 5.009)
ESR2				
RsaI (B5) (1082A > G)				
A allele	101 (33.7)	99 (32.1)		
G allele	199 (66.3)	209 (67.9)	0.689	1.071 (0.764, 1.503)
1 (AA)	20 (13.3)	18 (11.7)		
2 (AG)	61 (40.7)	63 (40.9)	0.863	1.074 (0.476, 2.426)
3 (GG)	69 (46.0)	73 (47.4)	0.834	0.851 (0.412, 2.044)
AluI (B8) (1730A > G)				
A allele	100 (33.3)	96 (31.2)		
G allele	200 (66.7)	212 (68.8)	0.568	1.104 (0.786, 1.552)
1 (AA)	21 (14.0)	20 (13.0)		
2 (AG)	58 (38.7)	56 (36.4)	0.225	0.592 (0.254, 1.382)
3 (GG)	71 (47.3)	78 (50.6)	0.172	0.567 (0.251, 1.281)

Abbreviations: *CI* confidence interval, *OR* odds ratio, *NA* not available
OR OR value of rectified BMI and waist circumference for every allele
[a]95% of the 95% CI for the OR CI
p < 0.05 indicated statistical significance

G allele frequency in the XbaI polymorphism was markedly elevated in MetS patients compared with control individuals ($p = 0.004$; OR = 1.610, 95%CI 1.169–2.18).

Genotype distributions of the XbaI, PvuII, RsaI and AluI polymorphisms, and allele frequencies of the PvuII, RsaI and AluI polymorphisms were comparable between MetS patients and controls ($p > 0.05$).

Haplotype distributions of the four SNPs
LD assessment of all SNP pairs revealed XbaI and PvuII of ESR1 were associated, as well as RsaI (B5) and AluI (B8) of ESR2 (Additional file 1: Table S1). Haplotype distributions of the 4 SNPs (PvuII, XbaI, RsaI and AluI) are shown in Table 3. The exclusion criteria was set as frequency < 0.03.

ESR1 and ESR2 haplotype frequency distributions were greater than 3%. Analysis showed that XbaI–PvuII based haplotypes were associated with MetS (global $p = 0.022$), while those constructed from RsaI–AluI had no significant associations with MetS ($p > 0.05$). The haplotypes A–T ($p = 0.015$; OR = 0.638, 95%CI 0.443–0.919) and G–C ($p = 0.024$; OR = 1.512, 95%CI 1.055–2.168) obtained from XbaI–PvuII showed significant differences.

Associations of genotypes with clinical characteristics
Associations of the XbaI polymorphism with MetS components are shown in Table 4. Patients harboring the G allele in both homozygous and heterozygous forms (i.e. GG or AG) had elevated BMI, waist circumference,

Table 3 Estimated haplotype distributions in the metabolic syndrome (MetS) and control groups

SNP	Haplotype	MetS (freq.)	Control (freq.)	Global p-value	p-value
ESR1	A-C	65.15 (0.217)	76.73 (0.249)	0.022	0.351
XbaI-PvuII	A-T	65.85 (0.220)	94.27 (0.306)		0.015
	G-C	93.85 (0.313)	71.27 (0.231)		0.024
	G-T	75.15 (0.250)	65.73 (0.213)		0.279
ESR2	A-A	37.99 (0.127)	25.20 (0.082)	0.271	0.070
1082A > G-1730A > G	A-G	63.01 (0.210)	73.8 (0.240)		0.383
	G-A	62.01 (0.207)	70.8 (0.230)		0.489
	G-G	136.99 (0.457)	138.20 (0.44)		0.845

Abbreviation: *SNP* single-nucleotide polymorphism
Haplotypes have frequencies ≥3% in the MetS and control groups
$p < 0.05$ indicated statistical significance

systolic and diastolic BPs, FBG, HOMA-IR, TC, TG, LDL-C and NAFLD (%), and lower HDL-C. Among subjects with the PvuII polymorphism, those harboring the minor C allele in both homozygous and heterozygous forms (i.e. CC or TC) showed elevated BMI, fasting serum insulin and HOMA-IR (Additional file 1: Table S5). Associations of XbaI, PvuII and MetS were confirmed by multivariable regression analysis (Table 5). Among subjects with the RsaI polymorphism, those harboring the minor G allele in both homozygous and heterozygous forms showed elevated TG, LDL-C, fasting serum insulin and HOMA-IR (Additional file 1: Table S3). Among subjects with the AluI polymorphism, those carrying the minor G allele in both homozygous and heterozygous forms (AG or GG) showed elevated TC and LDL-C (Additional file 1: Table S4).

Regarding XbaI, the control group showed significantly different FBG, TG, TC, HDL-C and LDL-C among the three genotypes (all $p < 0.05$). In MetS patients, BMI, TG, TC and LDL-C were markedly different (Additional file 1: Table S2). As for RsaI (B5), the control group showed significant differences in fasting insulin and HOMA-IR among the three genotypes (all $p < 0.05$); in MetS patients, LDL-C and HOMA-IR were significantly different (Additional file 1: Table S3). As for AluI (B8), BMI and TC significantly differed among the three genotypes in control patients (all $p < 0.05$); in MetS patients, age and TG significantly differed (Additional file 1: Table S4). Regarding

Table 4 Associations of XbaI genotypes with various clinical characteristics

Variables	AA (n = 74)	AG (n = 154)	GG (n = 76)
Age (years)	62.14 ± 4.24	63.24 ± 4.85	63.11 ± 3.75
BMI (kg/m²)	22.97 ± 2.99	23.98 ± 3.40*	24.71 ± 3.18*
Waist circumference (cm)	84.26 ± 5.36	84.92 ± 5.13	86.07 ± 4.96*
FBG (mM)	4.95 ± 0.88	5.21 ± 1.41*	5.70 ± 1.10*#
HbA1C (%)	5.89 ± 1.00	5.94 ± 1.05	6.09 ± 0.98
Systolic blood pressure (mmHg)	132.31 ± 14.39	134.15 ± 13.96	139.05 ± 14.12*#
Diastolic blood pressure (mmHg)	79.95 ± 11.96	81.14 ± 11.39	85.86 ± 10.69*#
Triglycerides (mM)	1.84 ± 0.92	2.08 ± 1.20*	2.38 ± 1.16*
Total cholesterol (mM)	4.29 ± 1.20	4.72 ± 0.83*	5.53 ± 1.12*#
HDL-C (mM)	1.25 ± 0.26	1.15 ± 0.21*	1.06 ± 0.20*#
LDL-C (mM)	2.74 ± 0.64	2.83 ± 0.67	3.39 ± 0.83*#
NAFLD (%)	28 (37.8)	70 (45.5)	45 (59.2)*
Fasting serum insulin (μIU/mL)	11.15 ± 5.68	11.54 ± 6.23	12.54 ± 8.31
Estradiol (pg/ml)	26.82 ± 6.99	24.66 ± 7.48	24.49 ± 7.67
HOMA-IR	2.47 ± 1.32	2.72 ± 1.77*	3.20 ± 1.70*

Measurement data are mean ± SD, and were assessed by one way ANOVA with post-hoc SNK test
*Significant difference from patients harboring AA ($p < 0.05$)
#Significant difference from patients harboring AG ($p < 0.05$). Enumeration count data were described as rate, and assessed by the chi-square test

Endocrine and Metabolic Disorders

Table 5 Multivariable logistic regression analysis with MetS as the dependent variable

Risk factor	OR (95%CI)	P
BMI	6.541 (2.537,16.864)	< 0.001
Triglycerides	2.386 (1.238,4.599)	0.009
XbaI		
AA (reference)	–	–
AG	1.505 (0.819,2.764)	0.188
GG	2.330 (1.161,4.679)	0.017
PVUII		
TT (reference)	–	–
TC	2.235 (1.120,4.461)	0.023
CC	2.679 (1.225,5.855)	0.014

Abbreviations: BMI body mass index, *CI* confidence interval, *OR* odds ratio
p < 0.05 indicated statistical significance

PvuII, estradiol levels were significantly different among the three genotypes in control patients (all *p* < 0.05); in MetS patients, age, BMI, systolic BP, HDL-C and HOMA-IR were significantly different (Additional file 1: Table S5).

Discussion

Changing lifestyles, socioeconomic status, and dietary habits have likely contributed to a rapid increase in the incidence of MetS, which is currently considered a major threat to human health worldwide [21]. High MetS prevalence is found among postmenopausal women [22]. Associations of several polymorphisms in the ESR1 and ESR2 genes with MetS or related components have been described [23]. These associations were also reported in the Study of Women's Health Across the Nation (SWAN) trial of perimenopausal African-American, Caucasian, Chinese, and Japanese women between 42 and 52 years old [24]. The current study revealed positive associations of ESR1 polymorphisms with MetS in postmenopausal Chinese Han women. Subjects harboring the G allele of XbaI, or the A-T and G-C haplotypes of XbaI–PvuII polymorphisms of ESR1, showed elevated risk of MetS. Similar results were obtained in studies of women of different ages [25, 26]. Two ESR2 subtypes, including RsaI and AluI, were not significantly associated with Mets in this study.

ERb−/− mice show normal or improved glucose tolerance and insulin release compared with wild type counterparts [27]. Meanwhile, ERa−/− animals display glucose intolerance and insulin resistance [12]. ESR1 and ESR2 are widely distributed in various organs and tissues related to sugar metabolism. Associations of ESR1 polymorphisms and (T2DM) were demonstrated [28]. ESR2 polymorphisms are associated with MetS in Chinese and Japanese populations; in addition, SNPs in the ESR1 show associations with insulin sensitivity in Asian

women [24]. ER-α can exert co-modulatory functions with insulin receptor substrate 1 (IRS1) to modulate insulin signaling [29]. Previous studies suggested an inhibitory effect of ERb on glucose transporter four (GLUT4) expression, and revealed that unchecked ERb activity could result in diabetes [25, 30]. As shown above, patients harboring the minor alleles of XbaI and PvuII gene polymorphisms, in both homozygous (GG and CC) or heterozygous (AG and TC) forms, had higher FBG, fasting serum insulin and HOMA-IR. Meanwhile, those carrying the RsaI polymorphism of ESR2 (homozygous or heterozygous) had lower fasting serum insulin and HOMA-IR.

Estrogens have critical functions in lipoprotein metabolism. An imbalance between ESR1 and ESR2 in the adipose tissue could therefore affect the development of metabolic diseases. Epidemiological studies showed hyperlipidemia is a significant risk factor for atherosclerosis, stroke, CAD, and MI [31]. In mice, ERb absence inhibit triglyceride accumulation, maintains normal insulin signaling in the liver and skeletal muscle, and ameliorates whole body insulin sensitivity as well as glucose tolerance [32]. ESR1 polymorphisms are associated with LDL particle size, reduced LDL cholesterol, and TC in adolescent female individuals [33]. SNPs in ESR1 show associations with the degree of adiposity, BMI, and waist circumference [34]. The PvuII T allele of ESR1 and associated genotypes and haplotypes are associated with risk of hyperlipidemia in postmenopausal Chinese Han females [35]. In addition, women with the PvuII T allele show elevated amounts of small LDL particles [36]. Furthermore, postmenopausal women with the T allele have reduced HDL-C and elevated TG, and are more vulnerable to lipid metabolism disorders [37]. These findings were corroborated by several other reports showing associations of ESR1 polymorphisms with BMI; however, associations of ESR2 polymorphisms with hyperlipidemia remain unclear. A study showed that homozygotes for the AluI (rs4986938) of ESR2 have higher BMI, serum TG and apolipoprotein B, and reduced HDL-C [38]. In mice, ESR2 deficiency is associated with abnormal vascular function and hypertension [39]. ESR2 polymorphisms are also associated with hypertension in postmenopausal Japanese women [40]. As shown above, positive associations were obtained of the G allele of XbaI polymorphism of the ESR1 gene with elevated TG, TC, LDL-C levels, as well as lower HDL-C, in postmenopausal Chinese women. The RsaI and AluI polymorphisms of ESR2 exhibited associations with TG, TC and LDL-C amounts.

Conclusion

Currently, MetS incidence is higher in postmenopausal women compared with age—matched males. Interventions to halt the rapidly increasing MetS incidence are of great clinical interest. Several studies have assessed associations of ESR1 and ESR2 with MetS or related components in different populations, but have often yielded conflicting findings. Furthermore, very few such studies have evaluated Chinese subjects. We here demonstrated associations of ESR1 and ESR2 polymorphisms with MetS and related components, especially obesity, and lipid and glucose metabolism, in postmenopausal Chinese Han females. Meanwhile, the G allele frequency of the XbaI polymorphism was markedly elevated in MetS patients compared with the control group. The RsaI and AluI polymorphisms of the ESR2 gene were not associated with MetS. In addition, XbaI and PvuII polymorphisms of ESR1 were associated with some MetS components. The current findings could include biases related to sample size, age, and ethnicity. Nevertheless, the present data could provide valuable insights into MetS epidemiology, particularly in Han Chinese individuals, providing a basis for the development of novel therapeutic interventions.

Additional files

Additional file 1: Table S1. Linkage disequilibrium tests (D' and r^2). **Table S2.** Relationship between Xba1 genotypes and clinical indicators within each group. **Table S3.** Relationship between Rsal (B5) genotypes and clinical indicators in each group. **Table S4.** Relationship between AluI (B8) genotypes and clinical indicators of each group. **Table S5.** Relationship between PVUII genotypes and clinical indicators in each group. **Figure S1.** Genotype validation by direct sequencing for PvuII and XbaI. **Figure S2.** Genotype validation by direct sequencing for RsaI. **Figure S3.** Genotype validation by direct sequencing for AluI. (DOCX 430 kb)

Abbreviations

ATP III: Adult Treatment Panel III; BMI: Body mass index; BP: Blood pressure; CVD: Cardiovascular disease; DM: Diabetes mellitus; E2: Estradiol; ER: Estrogen receptor; ESR: Estrogen receptor; FBG: Fasting blood glucose; GLUT4: Glucose transporter four; HbA1C: Hemoglobin A1C; HDL-C: High-density lipoprotein cholesterol; HOMA-IR: Homeostasis model assessment of insulin resistance; IRS1: Insulin receptor substrate 1; LDL-C: Low density lipoprotein; MetS: Metabolic syndrome; MI: Myocardial infarction; NAFLD: Non-alcoholic fatty liver disease; SNPs: Single-nucleotide polymorphisms; SWAN: Study of Women's Health Across the Nation; T2DM: Type 2 diabetes mellitus; TC: Total cholesterol; TG: Triglyceride

Acknowledgments

We express our gratitude to Dayi Hospital Affiliated to Shanxi Medical University and Shanxi Medical University for technical support in this study, as well as the participants, data collectors, and all who contributed to the current work.

Funding

This project was funded by the ShanXi Science and Technology Department [no. 2015021194].

Authors' contributions

ZLX and ZGP supervised data generation and analysis, and drafted the manuscript. FXM and XGX were responsible for data collection. GQ contributed to study design and carried out statistical analyses. ZL and SXL interpreted the acquired data. ZZY and ZJL performed PCR. All authors were involved in study conception and design, as well as data acquisition. All authors read and approved the final manuscript.

Competing interests

The authors declare that they have no competing interest.

Author details

[1]Department of Biochemistry and Molecular Biology, Shanxi Medical University, Taiyuan, No.56, Xinjian South Road, Taiyuan, Shanxi 030001, People's Republic of China. [2]Department of Endocrinology Medicine, Dayi Hospital Affiliated to Shanxi Medical University, Taiyuan, Shanxi 030032, People's Republic of China. [3]Department of Physiology, Shanxi Medical University, Taiyuan, Shanxi 030001, People's Republic of China. [4]Department of Medical Statistics, School of Public Health of Shanxi Medical University, Taiyuan, Shanxi 030001, People's Republic of China. [5]Renal Division, Shanxi Medical University Second Hospital, Shanxi Kidney Disease Institute, Taiyuan, Shanxi 030001, People's Republic of China. [6]Centre for Transplantation and Renal Research, University of Sydney at Westmead Millennium Institute, Sydney, NSW 2145, Australia.

References

1. Fahed AC, El-Hage-Sleiman AK, Farhat TI, et al. Diet, genetics, and disease: a focus on the Middle East and North Africa region. J Nutr Metab. 2012;2012: 109037.
2. Li R, Li W, Lun Z, et al. Prevalence of metabolic syndrome in mainland China: a meta-analysis of published studies. BMC Public Health. 2016;16:296.
3. Navaneethan SD, Schold JD, Kirwan JP, et al. Metabolic syndrome, ESRD, and death in CKD. Clin J Am Soc Nephrol. 2013;8(6):945–52.
4. Wang Y, Jiang T, Wang X, et al. Association between insomnia and metabolic syndrome in a Chinese Han population: a cross-sectional study. Sci Rep. 2017;7(1):10893.
5. Grundy SM, Cleeman JI, Daniels SR, et al. Diagnosis and management of the metabolic syndrome: an American Heart Association/National Heart, Lung, and Blood Institute Scientific Statement. Circulation. 2005; 112(17):2735–52.
6. Westerman S, Wenger NK. Women and heart disease, the underrecognized burden: sex differences, biases, and unmet clinical and research challenges. Clinical Science 2016;130(8):551–63.
7. Hidalgo LA, Chedraui PA, Morocho N, et al. The metabolic syndrome among postmenopausal women in Ecuador. Gynecol Endocrinol. 2006; 22(8):447–54.
8. Salpeter SR, Walsh JM, Ormiston TM, et al. Meta-analysis: effect of hormone-replacement therapy on components of the metabolic syndrome in postmenopausal women. Diabetes Obes Metab. 2006;8(5): 538–54.
9. Shakir YA, Samsioe G, Nyberg P, et al. Do sex hormones influence features of the metabolic syndrome in middle-aged women? A population-based study of Swedish women: the Women's health in the Lund area (WHILA) study. Fertil Steril. 2007;88(1):163–71.
10. Arnal JF, Fontaine C, Abot A, et al. Lessons from the dissection of the activation functions (AF-1 and AF-2) of the estrogen receptor alpha in vivo. Steroids. 2013;78(6):576–82.
11. Mendelsohn ME, Karas RH. The protective effects of estrogen on the cardiovascular system. N Engl J Med. 1999;340(23):1801–11.
12. Heine PA, Taylor JA, Iwamoto GA, et al. Increased adipose tissue in male and female estrogen receptor-alpha knockout mice. Proc Natl Acad Sci U S A. 2000;97(23):12729–34.
13. Takeda K, Toda K, Saibara T, et al. Progressive development of insulin resistance phenotype in male mice with complete aromatase (CYP19) deficiency. J Endocrinol. 2003;176(2):237–46.
14. Barros RPA, Gustafsson J-Å. Estrogen receptors and the metabolic network. Cell Metab. 2011;14(3):289–99.

15. Zheng Y, Huo D, Zhang J, et al. Microsatellites in the estrogen receptor (ESR1, ESR2) and androgen receptor (AR) genes and breast cancer risk in African American and Nigerian women. PLoS One. 2012;7(7):e40494. https://doi.org/10.1371/journal.pone.0040494.

16. Hayes DF, Skaar TC, Rae JM, et al. Estrogen receptor genotypes, menopausal status, and the effects of tamoxifen on lipid levels: revised and updated results. Clin Pharmacol Ther. 2010;88(5):626–9.

17. Nilsson M, Naessén S, Dahlman I, et al. Association of estrogen receptor beta gene polymorphisms with bulimic disease in women. Mol Psychiatry. 2004;9(1):28–34.

18. Goulart AC, Zee RY, Pradhan A, et al. Associations of the estrogen receptors 1 and 2 gene polymorphisms with the metabolic syndrome in women. Metab Syndr Relat Disord. 2009;7(2):111–7.

19. Chinese Diabetes Society. China guideline for type 2 diabetes (2013). Chin J Endocrinol Metab. 2014;30(10):893–942.

20. Farrell GC, Chitturi S, Lau GK, et al. Guidelines for the assessment and management of non-alcoholic fatty liver disease in the Asia-Pacific region: executive summary. J Gastroenterol Hepatol. 2007;22(6):775–7.

21. Zimmet P, Magliano D, Matsuzawa Y, et al. The metabolic syndrome: a global public health problem and a new definition. J Atheroscler Thromb. 2005;12(6):295–300.

22. Ponholzer A, Temml C, Rauchenwald M, et al. Is the metabolic syndrome a risk factor for female sexual dysfunction in sexually active women? Int J Impot Res. 2008;20(1):100–4.

23. Lo JC, Zhao X, Scuteri A, et al. The association of genetic polymorphisms in sex hormone biosynthesis and action with insulin sensitivity and diabetes mellitus in women at midlife. Am J Med. 2006;119(9 Suppl 1):S69–78.

24. Sowers MR, Wilson AL, Karvonen-Gutierrez CA, et al. Sex steroid hormone pathway genes and health-related measures in women of 4 races/ethnicities: the study of Women's health across the nation (SWAN). Am J Med. 2006;119(9 Suppl 1):S103–10.

25. Ramos RG, Olden K. The prevalence of metabolic syndrome among US women of childbearing age. Am J Public Health. 2008;98(6):1122–7.

26. Ghattas MH, Mehanna ET, Mesbah NM, et al. Association of estrogen receptor alpha gene polymorphisms with metabolic syndrome in Egyptian women. Metabolism. 2013;62(10):1437–42.

27. Bryzgalova G, Lundholm L, Portwood N, et al. Mechanisms of antidiabetogenic and body weight-lowering effects of estrogen in high-fat diet-fed mice. Am J Physiol Endocrinol Metab. 2008;295(4):E904–12.

28. Huang Q, Wang TH, Lu WS, et al. Estrogen receptor alpha gene polymorphism associated with type 2 diabetes mellitus and the serum lipid concentration in Chinese women in Guangzhou. Chin Med J. 2006;119(21):1794–801.

29. Andò S, Panno ML, Salerno M, et al. Role of IRS-1 signaling in insulin-induced modulation of estrogen receptors in breast cancer cells. Biochem Biophys Res Commun. 1998;253(2):315–9.

30. Barros RP, Machado UF, Warner M, et al. Muscle GLUT4 regulation by estrogen receptors ERbeta and ERalpha. Proc Natl Acad Sci U S A. 2006;103(5):1605–8.

31. National Cholesterol Education Program (NCEP) Expert Panel on Detection, Evaluation, and Treatment of High Blood Cholesterol in Adults (Adult Treatment Panel III). Third report of the National Cholesterol Education Program (NCEP) expert panel on detection, evaluation, and treatment of high blood cholesterol in adults (adult treatment panel III) final report. Circulation. 2002;106(25):3143–421.

32. Foryst-Ludwig A, Clemenz M, Hohmann S, et al. Metabolic actions of estrogen receptor beta (ERbeta) are mediated by a negative cross-talk with PPARgamma. PLoS Genet. 2008;4(6):e1000108.

33. Nordström P, Glader CA, Dahlén G, et al. Oestrogen receptor alpha gene polymorphism is related to aortic valve sclerosis in postmenopausal women. J Intern Med. 2003;254(2):140–6.

34. Gallagher CJ, Langefeld CD, Gordon CJ, et al. Association of the estrogen receptor-alpha gene with the metabolic syndrome and its component traits in African-American families: the insulin resistance atherosclerosis family study. Diabetes. 2007;56(8):2135–41.

35. Zhao T, Zhang D, Liu Y, et al. Association between ESR1 and ESR2 gene polymorphisms and hyperlipidemia in Chinese Han postmenopausal women. J Hum Genet. 2010;55(1):50–4.

36. Demissie S, Cupples LA, Shearman AM, et al. Estrogen receptor-alpha variants are associated with lipoprotein size distribution and particle levels in women: the Framingham heart study. Atherosclerosis. 2006;185(1):210–8.

37. Lamon-Fava S, Asztalos BF, Howard TD, et al. Association of polymorphisms in genes involved in lipoprotein metabolism with plasma concentrations of remnant lipoproteins and HDL subpopulations before and after hormone therapy in postmenopausal women. Clin Endocrinol. 2010;72(2):169–75.

38. Mansur Ade P, Nogueira CC, Strunz CM, et al. Genetic polymorphisms of estrogen receptors in patients with premature coronary artery disease. Arch Med Res. 2005;36(5):511–7.

39. Zhu Y, Bian Z, Lu P, et al. Abnormal vascular function and hypertension in mice deficient in estrogen receptor beta. Science. 2002;295(5554):505–8.

40. Ogawa S, Emi M, Shiraki M, et al. Association of estrogen receptor beta (ESR2) gene polymorphism with blood pressure. J Hum Genet. 2000;45(6):327–30.

10

Community based study to assess the prevalence of diabetic foot syndrome and associated risk factors among people with diabetes mellitus

S. P. Vibha[1], Muralidhar M. Kulkarni[1*], A. B. Kirthinath Ballala[1], Asha Kamath[2] and G. Arun Maiya[3]

Abstract

Background: Diabetic foot is one of the most significant and devastating complication of diabetes. The objective of this study was to assess the prevalence of diabetic foot syndrome (DFS) and the associated risk factors among people with diabetes mellitus.

Methods: A community based cross-sectional study was carried out among 620 subjects with diabetes mellitus (DM) in rural areas of Udupi district. The Michigan Neuropathy Screening Instrument was used to identify peripheral neuropathy. Ankle brachial index was used to identify peripheral arterial disease (PAD). Subjects with diabetic foot syndrome were classified according to the International Working Group on Diabetic Foot (IWGDF) classification system.

Results: The overall prevalence of DFS was 51.8%. Among them 31.3, 11.9 and 8.5% belonged to category 1, 2 and 3 respectively. Multivariate logistic regression analysis showed advancing age, low socio-economic status, sedentary physical activity and longer duration of DM were significant independent correlates of DFS.

Conclusion: The overall prevalence of DFS was high among the study population; hence the screening for foot complications should start at the time of diagnosis of diabetes integrated with sustainable patient education at primary care level by training of health care providers at primary care level.

Keywords: Diabetic foot syndrome, Diabetic peripheral neuropathy, MNSI, Prevalence, Community based study

Background

Diabetes mellitus is a major public health problem with rising prevalence worldwide and in the year 2015 around 415 million people were known to have diabetes. This estimate is expected to increase to 642 million of the population by 2040 [1]. Further, it is the 6th leading cause of death [2], attributing to 5 million deaths globally in 2015. According to recent estimates, 69.2 million people are affected with diabetes in India [1].

Along with the raising prevalence of diabetes, an increase in its complications is also expected. Diabetes along with its complications is expected to result in increasing morbidity, mortality and health expenditure due to the requirement of specialized care [3].

Diabetic foot is one of the most significant and devastating complication of diabetes and is defined as a group of syndromes in which neuropathy, ischemia and infection lead to tissue breakdown, and possible amputation [4]. Around 15% of diabetic patients will develop foot ulcers in their life time and this is known to precede amputation in 85% of the cases [5]. Every 20 s a lower limb is lost to diabetes in the world and it is the most common cause of non-traumatic lower limb amputation [6]. It is estimated that approximately 45,000 lower limbs are amputated every year in India and the vast majority of these are probably preventable [5].

Prevention of diabetic foot ulceration is critical in order to reduce the associated high morbidity and mortality

* Correspondence: murali.kulkarni@manipal.edu
[1]Department of Community Medicine, Kasturba Medical College, Manipal Academy of Higher Education, Manipal, Karnataka 576104, India
Full list of author information is available at the end of the article

rates, and the danger of amputation. A number of contributory factors work together to cause foot ulceration in patients with diabetes. These include peripheral neuropathy; mechanical stress and peripheral vascular disease [7].

Regular comprehensive foot examination, patient education on foot care like simple hygienic practices, provision of appropriate footwear, and prompt treatment of minor injuries and a multi-disciplinary team approach can decrease ulcer occurrence by 50% and amputations by up to 85%. [3, 8].

Identification of diabetics with DFS and its associated factors is the key to reduce further complications and to have baseline information to initiate appropriate interventions. There is a dearth of community based studies in Coastal Karnataka, which assess the prevalence of diabetic foot syndrome and associated risk factors among diabetics. Hence the present study was planned to find the prevalence of foot problems and determine the risk factors leading to DFS.

Methods
Approval of institutional ethics committee was taken prior to conducting the study. All reported cases of diabetes mellitus aged more than 18 years, residing at least for the past 1 year in the study area were included in the study. Patients with gestational diabetes mellitus, stroke, bilateral below knee amputation, Hansen's disease and foot deformities secondary to other causes were excluded.

This is a community based cross-sectional study carried out during August 2015 to September 2017 among reported cases of diabetes mellitus currently residing in field practice area of Department of Community Medicine, Kasturba Medical College (KMC), Manipal. It is situated along the coastal belt of Udupi District of Karnataka state, India covering a population of 45,246 spread out over 13 villages. The healthcare services are provided by both public and private sectors. The area has good collaboration between two sectors with primary, secondary and tertiary care facilities in the vicinity. These villages have a homogenous population in terms of occupation, SES and food habits. The detailed information of the population in the field practice area is captured and fed into the central database in e-RMCWH portal which can be accessed any time.

According to previous study done by George H [9] et al. the prevalence of peripheral neuropathy, a component of DFS, among people with diabetes was reported to be 47%. Thus, with 10% precision on prevalence of 47%, sample size of 433 subjects was obtained. Considering 40% non-response, sample size was estimated to be 721. The list of all diabetes patients residing at field practice area was obtained from e- database. Complete enumeration of reported cases of diabetes in a given locality was done,

those available at the time of survey were included and adjacent locality was selected till the sample size was met.

The identification of households having patients with diabetes in the community was done with the help of health worker. A home visit was conducted and the purpose of the visit was explained. An informed written consent was taken. Subjects were interviewed using pre-structured questionnaire to collect data on socio-demographic details, history of diabetes mellitus including treatment and associated risk factors for development of diabetic foot including dietary habits, physical activity [10], tobacco use and alcohol consumption [11].

Physical activity was assessed according to a survey questionnaire used by Ramachandran et al. [10]. This tool is validated for Indian settings and uses a scoring system to grade the physical activity. Four categories of occupation are considered. (i) Manual labourers (including masons, carpenters and those who carry loads, agricultural work, e.g. ploughing and tilling); (ii) Office jobs or desk work; (iii) Housewives and retired persons; (iv) Persons unable to work. Duration of activities for each day and number of working days in a week were considered to calculate the score which gives a minimum score of one and maximum of 70. Based on the scores physical activity was graded as sedentary (score: 1–17); light (score: 18–34); moderate (score: 35–51) and strenuous (score: > 51).

Anthropometric measurements were noted as per WHO standard guidelines [12]. Blood pressure of the subject was measured as high blood pressure is considered as a risk factor for diabetic foot syndrome [13].

Michigan Neuropathy Screening Instrument (MNSI) [14] was used to screen for diabetic peripheral neuropathy. It had two components, the history and the physical assessment. The first part of the screening instrument comprises of 15 self-administered "yes or no" questions on foot sensation including pain, numbness, and temperature sensitivity. A higher score (out of a maximum of 13 points) indicates more neuropathic symptoms. The second part of the MNSI is a brief physical examination involving 1) inspection of the feet for deformities, dry skin, hair or nail abnormalities, callous, or infection; 2) semi-quantitative assessment of vibration sensation at the dorsum of the great toe; 3) grading of ankle reflexes; and 4) monofilament testing. Patients screening positive on the clinical portion of the MNSI (greater than 2.5 points on a 10 point scale) were considered neuropathic.

Vascular assessment [15] of feet was done by manual assessment of foot pulses in both lower limbs for posterior tibial and dorsalis pedis pulses and manual measurement of ankle-brachial index (ABI). Absence of peripheral pulses and ABI ≤ 0.9 was considered as peripheral arterial disease (PAD) [16].

The subjects found to be having foot problems were classified according to The International Working Group on Diabetic Foot (IWGDF) Risk Classification System [15]. Glycated hemoglobin (HbA1c) was estimated in sub sample population, taking equal number of subjects with foot at risk category 0, 1, 2 and 3 as identified from the survey matched for age and gender. Health education regarding foot care practices was given to all subjects. If the subjects were found to be category 1 or 2 were referred to nearest RMCW home for timely screening and subjects with category 3 risk were referred to Diabetic Foot clinic at KMC, Manipal.

The collected data was tabulated and analysed by using software SPSS (Statistical Package for Social Sciences) V.15.0 (SPSS South Asia, Bangalore) for windows. The data was cross checked for data entry errors. Findings were described in terms of proportions and their 95% confidence intervals. Continuous data was summarized using mean, and standard deviation or median and inter quartile range depending on skewness of data. Chi-square test was used to find the association and p-value < 0.05 was considered significant. Multiple logistic regression was used to find the risk factors.

Results

Socio-demographic details
In the study, there was a favourable response and the non-response rate was 13.7% with 620 diabetics consenting to participate in the study. The mean age of the participants was 63.37 years (SD 10.8) with 61.2% of subjects being in the age group above 60 years. There was female preponderance (57.4%) and majority of the study participants were Hindus. An overall literacy rate among study participants was 85.8%, with 57.6% having education up to high school. Housewives accounted for 46.9% of the study participants, skilled workers 11.7 and 10.8% were currently unemployed and 9.5% were retired.

SES was assessed as per modified Udai Pareek scale and majority (70%) of the study population belonged to middle class, 28.1% to low class and only 1.6% belonged to high class.

Details of DM and health seeking behaviour
Of the 620 participants, all were having type 2 DM with median duration of 7 years (IQR 3, 13) and 42.4% of the study population was diagnosed within the last 5 years. Half (53.2%) of the participants gave a family history of DM and only 6.3% gave a history of foot complications related to DM among their first degree relatives.

Majority (96.4%) were on allopathic treatment, among them 89.6% were on oral hypoglycemic agents (OHAs), 3.5% were on insulin and rest 6.8% were on combination of OHAs and insulin. Over 96.1% were regular on medications as prescribed by the treating physician. Of all the

subjects, 81.3% were going for regular consultation. Among them, 86.8 and 89.9% were monitoring their Fasting blood sugar (FBS) and Post prandial blood glucose (PPBS) regularly while only 6.1% monitored HbA1c. One third of the subjects got their Renal function test (RFT) done regularly and 21% underwent yearly ophthalmic evaluation and very meagre proportion of 0.6% underwent regular comprehensive foot assessment. Among the participants who sought regular consultation 57.2, 33.4 and 9.4% were predominantly approaching primary, secondary and tertiary health care facilities respectively.

Most commonly reported co-morbidity was hypertension (64.5%), followed by hypercholesterolemia (17.4%) and IHD (12.6%).

Lifestyle factors
The most commonly used substance was smokeless tobacco (21.1%), followed by consumption of alcohol (18.1%) and smoking (6.5%). Half of the study participants (51%) were sedentary, 46 and 2.4% were doing light and moderate physical activity. None were involved in heavy physical activity.

Majority (86.5%) of the study participants consumed mixed diet. Among 98.5% people advised on diabetic diet by the treating physician, only 20.3% were following it always and 59.1% were following it most of the times.

Prevalence of DFS
The overall prevalence of DFS was 51.8% in our population. According to IGWDF Risk Classification, Out of the study population, 48.2% were normal (category 0) while the remaining 51.8% had foot at risk. (Table 1).

About 51.8% subjects had foot at risk, 31.3% had foot at risk category 1; 11.9% patients had foot at risk category 2, in which 10.8% PAD and 10.4% patients had deformity. Only 8.5% of them belonged to category 3, in which 9 had an amputation.

As per MNSI, most common neuropathic symptom perceived by study population was numbness in the feet (51.5%), followed by burning pain (38.7%) and feet being

Table 1 Prevalence of diabetic foot syndrome according to IWGDF Risk Classification System ($n = 620$)

Risk category	Characteristics	N	%
Category 0	No peripheral neuropathy	299	48.2
Category 1	Peripheral neuropathy	194	31.4
Category 2	Peripheral neuropathy with peripheral artery disease and/or a foot deformity	74	11.9
Category 3	Peripheral neuropathy and a history of foot ulcer or lower-extremity amputation	53	8.5

too sensitive to touch (32.9%) and 26.5% subjects responded that symptoms worse at night. Among the participants, 9.8% had a history of previous foot ulceration with 1.5% of them going in for toe amputation.

On inspection of feet, 74.5% of the study subjects had abnormalities in foot appearance which include dry skin (41.9%), deformities (10.5%) including amputation (1.5%), callus (14.5%), infection (15.8%) and ingrown nail (7.6%). Among the study subjects, 1.5% currently presented with foot ulceration. On examination, 45.5% of the study

subjects had reduced/absent vibration perception with 128 Hz tuning fork, 34.7% had loss of protective sensation on 10 g SW monofilament testing and 15% had abnormal ankle reflexes. Prevalence of diabetic peripheral neuropathy in the study population was 51.8% based on MNSI examination score.

Risk factors for DFS

Table 2 describes the association of socio-demographic and lifestyle factors with DFS. Among subjects with

Table 2 Univariate analysis for association of socio-demographic and lifestyle factors with diabetic foot syndrome ($n = 620$)

Variables	Diabetic foot syndrome		Unadjusted OR 95% CI	P value
	Absent ($n = 299$) n (%)	Present ($n = 321$) n (%)		
Gender				
Male	116 (38.8)	148 (46.1)	1.35 (0.98–1.85)	0.066
Female	183 (61.2)	173 (53.9)	1	
Age in years				
< 50 years	64 (21.4)	18 (5.6)	1	< 0.001
51–60 years	96 (32.1)	62 (19.3)	2.29 (1.24–4.23)	
61–70 years	105 (35.1)	130 (40.5)	4.40 (2.45–7.88)	
> 70 years	34 (11.4)	111 (34.6)	11.60 (6.06–22.21)	
Socio-economic status				
Low	69 (23.1)	105 (32.7)	1	0.028
Middle	225 (75.2)	211 (65.7)	0.61 (0.43–0.88)	
High	5 (1.7)	5 (1.6)	0.65 (0.18–2.35)	
Literacy				
Illiterate	36 (12.0)	52 (16.2)	2.09 (1.15–3.78)	0.018
Primary	31 (10.4)	51 (15.9)	2.38 (1.29–4.37)	
High school	177 (59.2)	180 (56.1)	1.47 (0.92–2.38)	
PUC and above	55 (18.4)	38 (11.8)	1	
Occupation				
Professional/White collared	29 (9.7)	29 (8.7)	1	< 0.001
Skilled/Semiskilled	55 (18.4)	57 (17.8)	1.07 (0.56–2.03)	
Unskilled	13 (4.3)	21 (6.5)	1.67 (0.70–3.97)	
Housewife	152 (50.9)	139 (43.3)	0.94 (0.53–1.67)	
Unemployed	17 (5.7)	50 (15.6)	3.04 (1.42–6.49)	
Retired	33 (11.0)	26 (8.1)	0.81 (0.39–1.69)	
Habits				
Smoking	16 (5.4)	24 (7.5)	1.42 (0.74–2.74)	0.284
Smokeless tobacco use	48 (16.1)	83 (25.9)	1.82 (1.22–2.71)	0.003
Alcohol use	49 (16.4)	63 (19.6)	1.24 (0.82–1.88)	0.295
Physical Activity				
Sedentary	116 (38.8)	200 (62.3)	2.29 (0.77–6.78)	< 0.001
Light	175 (58.5)	115 (35.8)	0.87 (0.29–2.59)	
Moderate	8 (2.7)	6 (1.9)	1	

$p < 0.05$ is considered to be statistically significant

DFS, only 5.6% were < 50 years age and increasing proportions of DFS was observed with advancing age of the participants (> 70 years, OR 11.60; 95% CI: 6.06–22.21). The significant association of DFS was observed with low SES (high SES, OR: 0.65; CI: 0.18–2.35), low literacy (Illiterate OR: 2.09; CI: 1.15–3.78), unemployment (OR: 3.04; CI: 1.42–6.49), smokeless tobacco use (OR: 1.82; CI: 1.22–2.71) and sedentary physical activity (OR: 2.29; CI: 0.77–6.78). However other demographic factors like gender and religion did not show any significant association with DFS.

As depicted in Tables 3 and 4, a significant increase in proportion of DFS was observed among subjects with an increasing duration of DM. Subjects having DM for > 10 years are 3.7 times more likely to develop DFS compared to subjects with duration < 5 years. (OR: 3.77, CI: 2.53–5.62). Univariate analysis revealed presence of IHD (OR: 1.67; CI: 1.02–2.73), use of insulin (OR: 4.50; CI: 1.50–13.47) and level of care (OR: 1.55, CI: 1.09–2.21) was significantly associated with DFS. Anthropometric measurements like BMI, waist circumference; clinical parameters like blood pressure, glycated hemoglobin; presence of comorbidities like hypertension, hypercholesterolemia and health seeking behaviours like adherence to medications, frequency of consulting physician was not significantly associated with DFS.

Table 5 shows multivariate logistic regression analysis for association of factors of diabetic foot syndrome. Advancing age, low socio-economic status, sedentary physical activity and longer duration of DM were significant independent correlates of DFS.

Discussion

Diabetic foot syndrome is defined as a group of syndromes in which neuropathy, ischemia and infection lead to tissue breakdown, and possible amputation [4]. It is essential to identify the "foot at risk", through careful inspection and physical examination of the foot followed by neuropathy and vascular tests.

The overall prevalence of DFS was 51.8%. Similar results were observed in a study carried out by Shyam Kishore et al. [17] at Delhi, about 52% patients had foot at risk

Table 3 Univariate analysis for association of clinical and biochemical parameters with diabetic foot syndrome (N = 620)

Variables	Diabetic foot syndrome		Unadjusted OR 95% CI	P value
	Absent (n = 299) n (%)	Present (n = 321) n (%)		
Duration of DM				
0–5 years	168 (56.2)	95 (29.5)	1	< 0.001
6–10 years	72 (24.1)	100 (31.2)	2.45 (1.65–3.64)	
> 10 years	59 (19.7)	126 (39.3)	3.77 (2.53–5.62)	
Family h/o DM	169 (56.5)	161 (50.2)	0.77 (0.56–1.06)	0.112
Co-morbidities				
Hypertension	187 (62.5)	213 (66.4)	1.18 (0.85–1.64)	0.321
Ischemic heart disease	29 (9.7)	49 (15.3)	1.67 (1.02–2.73)	0.037
Hypercholesterolemia	56 (18.7)	52 (16.2)	0.89 (0.55–1.27)	0.407
BMI (kg/m^2)				
Underweight (< 18.5)	11 (3.7)	13 (4.1)	1	0.736
Normal (18.5–24.9)	141 (47.1)	157 (49.1)	0.94 (0.41–2.18)	
Overweight (25–29.9)	111 (37.1)	106 (33.1)	0.80 (0.34–1.88)	
Obese (≥ 30)	36 (12.1)	44 (13.8)	1.03 (0.41–2.58)	
Waist circumference (cm)				
Normal	72 (24.1)	96 (29.9)	1	0.103
High (Males > 90; Female > 80)	227 (75.9)	225 (70.1)	0.74 (0.52–1.06)	
Blood pressure (mmHg)				
Normal	136 (45.5)	147 (45.8)	1	0.938
High (BP ≥ 140/90)	163 (54.5)	174 (54.2)	0.98 (0.72–1.35)	
HbA1c (mean + SD)[a] (n = 146)	7.7 ± 1.8	7.8 ± 1.8		0.086

[a]Unpaired t-test
p < 0.05 is considered to be statistically significant

Table 4 Univariate analysis for association of health seeking behaviour with diabetic foot syndrome ($n = 620$)

Variables	Diabetic foot syndrome		Unadjusted OR 95% CI	P value
	Absent ($n = 299$) n (%)	Present ($n = 321$) n (%)		
System of medicine ($n = 617$)				
Allopathy	286 (96.0)	309 (96.9)	1	0.510
Ayurveda	9 (3.0)	5 (1.6)	0.51 (0.17–1.55)	
Both	3 (1.0)	5 (1.6)	1.54 (0.36–6.51)	
Medications for DM ($n = 603$)				
Oral hypoglycemic agents	270 (93.4)	270 (86.0)	1	< 0.001
Insulin	4 (5.2)	26 (8.3)	4.50 (1.50–13.47)	
Combined (OHAs+Insulin)	15 (1.4)	18 (5.7)	1.73 (0.89–3.34)	
Adherence to medications[a]				
Yes	286 (95.7)	310 (96.6)	1	0.917
No	13 (4.3)	11 (3.4)	1.28 (0.56–2.90)	
Frequency of consultation[b]				
Regular	246 (82.3)	258 (80.4)	1	0.607
Irregular	53 (17.7)	63 (19.6)	1.13 (0.75–1.69)	
Level of care ($n = 605$)				
Primary	182 (61.7)	105 (52.9)	1	0.043
Secondary	84 (28.5)	68 (38.1)	1.55 (1.09–2.21)	
Tertiary	29 (9.8)	12 (9.0)	1.07 (0.61–1.87)	

[a]Adherence to medication: Subject was considered adherent to medication, if he/she is taking prescribed medicines for 6 days or more in a week
[b]Physician consultation was considered regular if he/she is consulting physician once in 3 months or less
$p < 0.05$ is considered to be statistically significant

Table 5 Multivariate logistic regression analysis for association of factors of diabetic foot syndrome

Variable	Diabetic foot syndrome		Intercept	SE	Wald X^2	Adjusted OR 95% CI
	Absent ($n = 299$) n(%)	Present ($n = 321$) n(%)				
Age in years						
< 50 years	64 (21.4)	18 (5.6)			30.56	1
51–60 years	96 (32.1)	62 (19.3)	0.57	0.34	2.79	1.77 (0.90–3.45)
61–70 years	105 (35.1)	130 (40.5)	1.04	0.32	9.50	2.75 (1.44–5.25)
> 70 years	34 (11.4)	111 (34.6)	1.84	0.37	24.67	6.32 (3.05–13.08)
Socio-economic status						
Low	69(23.1)	105 (32.7)			8.40	1
Middle	225 (75.2)	211 (65.7)	−0.60	0.21	8.11	0.54 (0.36–0.82)
High	5 (1.7)	5 (1.6)	−0.81	0.70	1.32	0.44 (0.11–1.77)
Physical Activity						
Sedentary	116 (38.8)	200 (62.3)			11.46	1
Light	175 (58.5)	115 (35.8)	−0.65	0.19	11.37	0.51 (0.35–0.75)
Moderate	8 (2.7)	6 (1.9)	−0.14	0.68	0.47	0.86 (0.22–3.32)
Duration of DM						
0–5 years	168 (56.2)	95 (29.6)			17.74	1
6–10 years	72 (24.1)	100 (31.2)	0.74	0.22	10.51	2.10 (1.34–3.29)
> 10 years	59 (19.7)	126 (39.3)	0.87	0.23	14.59	2.40 (1.53–3.78)

(category 1 and 2) in which 33 and 19% were in category 1 and 2 respectively.

A study carried out by Lawrence A. Lavery et al. [18], where they have used International Diabetic Foot Classification System which is similar to IWGDF risk classification system. Among 1666 study subjects, 58.6% were in category 0 and 41.4% had foot at risk. Among them, 5.9% had DPN (category 1), 24.7% patients had foot at risk category 2 and about 10.8% of them belonged to category 3. In a study done by Edgar J.G. Peters et al. [19], subjects were stratified as per IWGDF classification and during 3 years of follow-up, ulceration occurred in 5.1, 14.3, 18.8 and 55.8% of the patients in categories 0, 1, 2, and 3, respectively (linear-by-linear association, $P < 0.001$) and all amputations were found in Groups 2 and 3 (3.1 and 20.9%, $P < 0.001$). Thus, it provides evidence that the foot risk classification of the IWGDF foresees ulceration and amputation and can function as a tool to guide prevention of lower extremity complications of diabetes.

DPN is one of the significant components of DFS. Diagnosis of diabetic neuropathy is done through many methods including neurological examination and electrophysiology to detect at its earliest stage.

The MNSI is a rapid, simple and reliable test, validated for Indian settings for screening diabetic peripheral neuropathy in both diabetes clinics and epidemiological surveys [20]. It investigates aspects of both small (pain and hyperesthesia) and large (numbness and muscular) nerve fibre patency. The sensitivity and specificity of MNSI with a cut-off value of 2.5 were 50 and 91%, respectively [21].

Prevalence of diabetic peripheral neuropathy using MNSI in the study population was 51.8%. Similar results were observed in Indian studies done by George H et al. [9] in Tamil Nadu and Mackson Nongmaithem et al. [22] in Maharashtra, where prevalence was found to be 47%. The present study results were similar to studies done outside India, studies done by Rodica Pop-Busui et al. [23] in USA and Gashaw Jember et al. [24] in Ethiopia showed 51 and 52.2% prevalence respectively.

The prevalence of DPN varied from 12 to 60% in different studies done at various parts of India [9, 25–30]. This could be attributed to genetic predisposition, duration of diabetes, existing healthcare facilities, study settings and different diagnostic criteria used.

Advancing age was found to be significantly associated with DFS in many studies in various parts India, Dipika Bansal et al. [25] at Chandigarh, Sailesh K Shahi et al. [31] in Varanasi, Monisha D'Souza et al. [27] in Mangalore, Padmaja Kumari Rani et al. [30], Vijay Viswanathan et al. [32] in Chennai.

A study done by Dipika Bansal et al. [25] showed significant association of low SES with foot complications which are similar to current study. This may be due to lack of awareness, low health seeking behaviour and

non-affordability for treatment which makes them prone to develop diabetic complications.

Among subjects with DFS, higher proportions (15.6%) were unemployed compared to subjects without DFS (5.6%). The odds of developing DFS among unskilled workers was 1.67 compared to professionals/white collared job holders and could be ascribed to more exposure to occupational trauma among the former group.

A higher proportion of subjects with DFS were smokers compared to subjects without DFS. Similar observations were made with respect to use of smokeless forms of tobacco and it was significantly associated with DFS. Smoking is an established risk factor for PAD and was identified as a risk factor for DFS in the present study too, in accordance with the research done by Shailesh K Shahi [31] in Varanasi, Mohammad Zubir et al. [33] at Aligarh, Mackson Nongmaithem et al. [22] at Pune, Mamta Jaiswal et al. [34] in USA and Juma M Al-Kaabi et al. [35] in UAE.

Longer duration of diabetes was identified as a risk factor in the study which is in accordance with many neuropathy prevalence studies carried out across the world [25, 26, 31, 35]. BMI and DFS had no significant association. However, obese subjects are 1.03 times more likely to develop DFS compared to underweight subjects (OR 1.03, CI: 0.41–2.58). Similar results were found in studies carried out by Mackson Nongmaithem et al. [22] in Pune and Mamta Jaiswal et al. [34] in USA. Present study did not show any association with HbA1c, this observation is supported in other studies done by Dipika Bansal et al. [25] in north India, RP Agrawal et al. [36] in west India.

Medications taken for the treatment of DM had a significant association with DFS. The subjects with DFS were 4.5 times more likely to be using insulin compared to OHAs (OR 4.50 CI: 1.50–13.47). This could be attributed to the fact that initiation of insulin therapy implies later stages in the natural history of DM. This also correlates with association of DFS with longer duration of DM. Insulin use was associated with severity of DFS in studies conducted by Shilesh K Shahi et al. [31] in north India, Reginald Alex et al. [37], Padmaja Kumari Rani et al. [30] in south India.

The healthcare level the subjects were approaching for treatment showed a significant association with DFS in the present study, similar results are observed in a study carried out by Shyam Kishore et al. [17].

Multivariate logistic regression revealed that advancing age, low socio-economic status, sedentary physical activity and longer duration of DM were significant correlates of DFS.

The strengths of study are; it is a community based study to report the prevalence of DFS while many studies reported prevalence based on hospital patients and we have ensured an adequate sample size and use of validated questionnaire coupled with thorough clinical examination for comprehensive foot evaluation. Limitations of the study include HbA1c not being done for the entire study population due to financial constraints, though we used subset drawn from all DFS risk categories which gives ample evidence about attributes of DFS. Besides DM the study could not assess other co-existing factors which might have led to peripheral neuropathy like autoimmune diseases and nutritional deficiencies as study is done among diabetic patients only. However other causes of neuropathy are considerably less.

Conclusion

The overall prevalence of diabetic foot syndrome was high among the study population and significantly associated with advancing age, low socio-economic status, sedentary physical activity and longer duration of DM. It can therefore be concluded that the screening for foot complications should start at the time of diagnosis of diabetes and integrated with sustainable patient education at primary care level by training of health care providers at primary care level.

Abbreviations

ABI: Ankle brachial index; DFS: Diabetic foot syndrome; DM: Diabetes mellitus; DPN: Diabetic peripheral neuropathy; IWGDF: The international working group on the diabetic foot; PAD: Peripheral arterial disease; SES: Socio-economic status

Acknowledgements

We acknowledge Indian Council of Medical Research, New Delhi and Manipal Academy of Higher Education, Manipal for financial assistance and World Diabetes Foundation project: "Diabetic Foot care Stepping ahead:WDF-15/941" for technical support in carrying out this study. The authors also thank the support of laboratory technicians and health workers in the smooth conduct of the study. The co-operation from all study participants is also appreciated.

Funding

This study was funded by Indian Council of Medical Research [No.3/2/March – 2016/PG-Thesis-HRD (7)].

Authors' contributions

MMK conceived the idea for the research, wrote the framework and drafted the manuscript. VSP participated in the design of the study and contributed in acquisition, analysis and interpretation of data. KBAB made framework, design and interpretation of data. AK was responsible for the study design, data analysis, interpretation and revision of the paper. GAM helped in design of the study, interpretation of data. All authors read and approved the final manuscript.

Competing interests

The authors declare that they have no competing interests.

Author details

[1]Department of Community Medicine, Kasturba Medical College, Manipal Academy of Higher Education, Manipal, Karnataka 576104, India. [2]Department of Statistics, Prasanna School of Public Health, Manipal Academy of Higher Education, Manipal, Karnataka 576104, India. [3]Department of Physiotherapy, School of Allied Health Sciences, Manipal Academy of Higher Education, Manipal, Karnataka 576104, India.

References

1. IDF. Diabetes Atlas. International Diabetes Federation, Brussels. 2015. https://www.idf.org/e-library/epidemiology-research/diabetes-atlas.html .Accessed 10 Sept 2017.
2. WHO. Top 10 causes of death. World health Organization 2017 http://www.who.int/mediacentre/factsheets/fs310/en/ . Accessed 10 Sept 2017.
3. Alexiadou K, Doupis J. Management of Diabetic Foot Ulcers. Diabetes Ther. 2012;3:4.
4. Forlee M. What is the diabetic foot? The rising prevalence of diabetes worldwide will mean an increasing prevalence of complications such as those of the extremities. Continuing Medical Education. 2010;28:152–6.
5. Jain AKC, Vishwanath S. Studying major amputations in a developing country using Amit Jain's typing and scoring system for diabetic foot complications - time for standardization of diabetic foot practice. Int Surg J. 2015;2:26–30.
6. The International Working Group on the Diabetic Foot 2017. http://iwgdf.org/ Accessed 10 Sept 2017.
7. Katsilambros N, Dounis E, Makrilakis K, Tentolouris N, Tsapogas P. Atlas of the diabetic foot. John Wiley & Sons. 2010.
8. Bakkar K, Foster A, Houtum WV, Riley P. Diabetes and Foot Care: Time to act. 4th edition. Netherlands: 2005.
9. George H, Rakesh PS, Krishna M, Alex R, Abraham VJ, George K, Prasad JH. Foot care knowledge and practices and the prevalence of peripheral neuropathy among people with diabetes attending a secondary care rural hospital in southern India. J Fam Med Primary Care. 2013;2:27–32.
10. Ramachandran A, Snehalatha C, Baskar ADS, Mary S, Sathish Kumar CK, Selvam S, Catherine S, Vijay V. Temporal changes in prevalence of diabetes and impaired glucose tolerance associated with lifestyle transition occurring in the rural population in India. Diabetologia. 2004;47:860–5.
11. Kulkarni MM, Shetty RS, Kamath A, Kamath VG, Varun N, Ramprasad VP. Tobacco use among adults in a rural area of coastal Karnataka. Indian Journal of Preventative Medicine. 2015;3:63–6.
12. World Health Organization. Waist circumference and waist-hip ratio. Geneva: Report of a WHO expert consultation; 2008.
13. Chobanian AV, Bakris GL, Black HR, Cushman WC, Green LA, Izzo JL Jr, Jones DW, Materson BJ, Oparil S, Wright JT Jr, Roccella EJ. The seventh report of the joint national committee on prevention, detection, evaluation, and treatment of high blood pressure: the JNC 7 report. JAMA. 2003;289:2560–71.
14. University of Michigan. How to Use the Michigan Neuropathy Screening Instrument. Michigan.http://diabetesresearch.med.umich.edu/peripherals/profs/documents/svi/MNSI_howto.pdf. Accessed on 18th Sept 2017.
15. Bus SA, Netten JJ, Lavery LA, Monteiro-Soares M, Rasmussen A, Jubiz Y, Price PE. IWGDF guidance on the prevention of foot ulcers in at-risk patients with diabetes. Diabetes Metab Res Rev. 2016;32:16–24.
16. Potier L, Khalil CA, Mohammedi KA, Roussel R. Use and Utility of ankle brachial index in patients with diabetic. Eur J Vasc Endovasc Surg. 2011;41:110–6.
17. Kishore S, Upadhyay AD, Jyotsna VP. Categories of foot at risk in patients of diabetes at a tertiary care center: insights into need for foot care. Indian J Endocrinol Metab. 2015;19:405–9.
18. Lavary LA, Armstrong DG, Wunderlich RP, Terdwell J, Boulton A. Evaluation the prevalence and incidence of foot pathology in Mexican-Americans and Nonhispanic whites from a diabetes disease management cohort. Diabetes Care. 2003;23:1435–8.
19. Peters EJ, Lavery LA. Effectiveness of the diabetic foot risk classification

system of the international working group on the diabetic foot. Diabetes Care. 2001;24:1442–7.

20. Feldman EL, Stevens MJ, Thomas PK, Brown MB, Canal N, Greene DA. A practical two-step quantitative clinical and electrophysiological assessment for the diagnosis and staging of diabetic neuropathy. Diabetes Care. 1994;17:1281–9.

21. Moghtaderi A, Bakhshipour A, Rashidi H. (2006). Validation of Michigan neuropathy screening instrument for diabetic peripheral neuropathy. Clin Neurol Neurosurg. 2006;108:477–1.

22. Nongmaithem M, Bawa APS, Pithwa AK, Bhatia SK, Singh G, Gooptu S. A study of risk factors and foot care behavior among diabetics. J Family Med Prim Care. 2016;5:399.

23. Pop-Busui R, Lu J, Lopes N, Jones TL. Prevalence of diabetic peripheral neuropathy and relation to glycemic control therapies at baseline in the BARI 2D cohort. J Peripher Nerv Syst. 2009;14:1–3.

24. Jember G, Melsew YA, Fisseha B, Sany K, Gelaw AY, Janakiraman B. Peripheral sensory neuropathy and associated factors among adult diabetes mellitus patients in Bahr Dar, Ethiopia. J Diabetes Metab Disord. 2017;16:16–20.

25. Bansal D, Gudala K, Muthyala H, Esam HP, Nayakallu R, Bhansali A. Prevalence and risk factors of development of peripheral diabetic neuropathy in type 2 diabetes mellitus in a tertiary care setting. J Diabetes Investig. 2014;5:714–21.

26. Gous SS, Suhail M, Hussain SAA, Shafee M. Prevalence of diabetic peripheral neuropathy and associated risk factors in type 2 diabetes patients attending a diabetes care Centre in Maharashtra. International journal of recent trends in. Sci Technol. 2015;16:620–3.

27. D'Souza M, Kulkarni V, Bhaskaran U, Ahmed H, Naimish H, Prakash A. Diabetic peripheral neuropathy and its determinants among patients attending a tertiary health care Centre in Mangalore, India. J Public Health Res. 2015;4:120–4.

28. Nagaraj C, Ramakuri M, Konapur KS. Burden of foot problems in diabetic subjects-a community-based study among urban poor in Bangalore. India Education. 2014;48:73–85.

29. Vaz NC, Ferreira AM, Kulkarni MS, Vaz FS, Pinto NR. Prevalence of diabetic complications in rural Goa, India. Indian J Community Med. 2011;36:283–6.

30. Rani PK, Raman R, Rachapalli SR, Pal SS, Kulothungan V, Sharma T. Prevalence and risk factors for severity of diabetic neuropathy in type 2 diabetes mellitus. Indian J Med Sci. 2010;64:51–7.

31. Shahi SK, Kumar A, Kumar S, Singh SK. Prevalence of diabetic foot ulcer and associated risk factors in diabetic patients from North India. Age. 2012;47:55–6.

32. Viswanathan V, Madhavan S, Rajasekar S, Chamukuttan S, Ambady R. Urban-rural differences in the prevalence of foot complications in south-Indian diabetic patients. Diabetes Care. 2006;29:701–3.

33. Zubair M, Malik A, Ahmad J. Incidence, risk factors for amputation among patients with diabetic foot ulcer in a north Indian tertiary care hospital. Foot. 2012;22:24–30.

34. Jaiswal M, Lauer A, Martin CL, Bell RA, Divers J, Dabelea D, Pettitt DJ, Saydah S, Pihoker C, Standiford DA, Rodriguez BL. Peripheral neuropathy in adolescents and young adults with type 1 and type 2 diabetes from the SEARCH for diabetes in youth follow-up cohort. Diabetes Care. 2013;36:3903–8.

35. Al-Kaabi JM, Al Maskari F, Zoubeidi T, Abdulle A, Shah SM. Prevalence and determinants of peripheral neuropathy in patients with type 2 diabetes attending a tertiary care center in the United Arab Emirates. J Diabetes Metab Disord. 2014;5:2–9.

36. Agrawal R, Ola V, Bishnoi P, Gothwal S, Sirohi P, Agrawal R. Prevalence of micro and macrovascular complications and their risk factors in type-2 diabetes mellitus. J Assoc Physicians India. 2014;62:504–8.

37. Alex R, Ratnaraj B, Winston B, Devakiruba DN, Samuel C, John J, Mohan VR, Prasad JH, Jacob KS. (2010). Risk factors for foot ulcers in patients with diabetes mellitus-a short report from Vellore, South India. Indian J Community Med. 2010;35:183–5.

11

Determining the joint effect of obesity and diabetes on functional disability at 3-months and on all-cause mortality at 1-year following an ischemic stroke

Colleen Bauza[1,2]* (iD), Sharon D. Yeatts[1], Keith Borg[3], Gayenell Magwood[4], Renee' H. Martin[1], Anbesaw Selassie[1] and Marvella E. Ford[1]

Abstract

Background: Obesity and diabetes mellitus, or diabetes, are independently associated with post-ischemic stroke outcomes (e.g., functional disability and all-cause mortality). Although obesity and diabetes are also associated with post-ischemic stroke outcomes, the joint effect of obesity and diabetes on these post-ischemic stroke outcomes has not been explored previously. The purpose of the current study was to explore whether the effect of obesity on post-ischemic stroke outcomes differed by diabetes status in a cohort of acute ischemic stroke subjects with at least a moderate stroke severity.

Methods: Data from the Interventional Management of Stroke (IMS) III clinical trial was analyzed for this post-hoc analysis. A total of 656 subjects were enrolled in IMS III and were followed for one year. The joint effects of obesity and diabetes on functional disability at 3-months and all-cause mortality at 1-year were examined.

Results: Of 645 subjects with complete obesity and diabetes information, few were obese (25.74%) or had diabetes (22.64%). Obese subjects with diabetes and non-obese subjects without diabetes had similar odds of functional disability at 3-months following an ischemic stroke (adjusted common odds ratio, 1.038, 95% CI: 0.631, 1.706). For all-cause mortality at 1-year following an ischemic stroke, obese subjects with diabetes had a similar hazard compared with non-obese subjects without diabetes (adjusted hazard ratio, 1.005, 95% CI: 0.559, 1.808). There was insufficient evidence to declare a joint effect between obesity and diabetes on either the multiplicative scale or the additive scale for both outcomes.

Conclusions: In this post-hoc analysis of data from the IMS III clinical trial of acute ischemic stroke patients with at least a moderate stroke severity, there was not sufficient evidence to determine that the effect of obesity differed by diabetes status on post-ischemic stroke outcomes. Additionally, there was not sufficient evidence to determine that either factor was independently associated with all-cause mortality. Future studies could differentiate between metabolically healthy and metabolically unhealthy patients within BMI categories to determine if the effect of obesity on post-stroke outcomes differs by diabetes status.

Keywords: Joint effect, Obesity, Diabetes, All-cause mortality, Functional disability

* Correspondence: cbauza1@jhmi.edu
[1]Department of Public Health Sciences, Medical University of South Carolina, Charleston, SC, USA
[2]Department of Health Informatics, Johns Hopkins All Children's Hospital, 601 5th Street South, Suite 707, St. Petersburg, FL 33701, USA
Full list of author information is available at the end of the article

Background

Obesity and diabetes mellitus, or diabetes, are not only highly prevalent in both the general US and international populations [1–4], but these factors are also prevalent among individuals who have been diagnosed with an ischemic stroke [5]. It is estimated that between 18 and 44% of individuals who previously had an ischemic stroke are obese, and between 25 and 45% of individuals who previously had an ischemic stroke have diabetes [5].

Stroke is a leading cause of long-term disability and death [6]. As a result, it is important to target modifiable factors in order to reduce the burden of these post stroke outcomes. Obesity and diabetes are independently associated with functional disability [7–12] and all-cause mortality [7, 13–26] following an ischemic stroke. Although obesity is a modifiable risk factor for ischemic stroke [27, 28], the reported effects of obesity on post-stroke outcomes of functional disability and of all-cause mortality have been conflicting. Whereas studies of the general population have found that increasing body mass concurrently increases the risk of functional disability [29] and of all-cause mortality [30, 31], a number of observational studies in a stroke population have reported that obesity is associated with a decreased risk of functional disability [7–9] and all-cause mortality [7, 13–18, 20]; this apparent discrepancy is referred to as the obesity paradox. As a result of these findings, the American Heart Association and American Stroke Association recommend all individuals who are diagnosed with an ischemic stroke be screened for obesity [5]. However, these agencies do not recommend weight reduction for overweight or obese individuals due to the null results of the Look Action for Health in Diabetes trial, a clinical trial that randomized overweight and obese individuals with type 2 diabetes to intensive behavioral intervention or usual care to compare the risk of vascular events (e.g., stroke, myocardial infarction, or vascular death) [5, 32]. Despite evidence supporting the obesity paradox in the stroke literature as well as in the literature of other chronic diseases such as myocardial infarction, heart failure, and renal disease [33, 34], several investigators have questioned the validity of studies supporting the 'obesity paradox,' citing methodological issues (e.g., the measurement of obesity, duration of obesity, treatment and/or selection bias due to the study population) or residual confounding as potential explanations [33–36]. In contrast to the conflicting reported effects of obesity on functional disability and all-cause mortality following a stroke, prior studies have established that diabetes is consistently associated with higher rates of functional disability [10–12] and higher risk of all-cause mortality [21–26] following a stroke.

Although obesity is a strong predictor of diabetes [37, 38], it is unknown whether diabetes modifies the inflammatory effects of obesity on functional disability or on all-cause mortality after an ischemic stroke. Research has recently supported the heterogeneity of the metabolic profile among obese individuals [39, 40], which suggests that the effect of obesity on functional disability and all-cause mortality following an ischemic stroke may differ according to diabetes status. The primary objective of this post-hoc analysis was to explore whether the effect of obesity on functional disability and all-cause mortality following an ischemic stroke differed by diabetes status.

Methods

Study population

This present study used data from the Interventional Management of Stroke (IMS) III clinical trial (IMS III, ClinicalTrials.gov number NCT00359424) [41]. Details of the scientific rationale, eligibility requirements, and baseline characteristics of the IMS III subjects have been published elsewhere [41, 42]. Briefly, the objective of the IMS III trial was to determine if subjects treated with a combined approach of intravenous recombinant tissue plasminogen activator (IV rt-PA) and endovascular therapy were more likely to have a better functional outcome than subjects treated with standard IV rt-PA alone [41, 42]. Eligibility was restricted to subjects between 18 and 80 years old, initiated with IV rt-PA within 3 h of ischemic stroke onset, and with a moderate-to-severe ischemic stroke, defined by a baseline National Institutes of Health Stroke Scale (NIHSS) score of at least 8 [41, 42]. Prior to enrollment, written informed consent was obtained from subjects (or a legal representative) [41, 42]. Subjects were followed for one year after onset of the ischemic stroke [41]. The Data and Safety Monitoring Board recommended the trial to stop in April 2012, after 656 subjects were randomized, due to crossing the pre-specified boundary for futility [42]. Specifically, the trial failed to show a benefit in functional outcome for the combined approach of IV rt-PA and endovascular therapy compared with standard IV rt-PA alone [42].

Exposures of interest

Obesity and diabetes are the exposures of interest for this study. Based on source documentation and the IMS III Case Report Form Guidelines, obesity (yes, no) and diabetes (yes, no) were collected at the baseline visit. No further information was included in the Case Report Form Guidelines regarding the source for identifying this information (i.e. medical record documentation, patient reported history of disease, medically documented history of disease, lab test).

Outcomes

The outcomes of interest for this study include functional disability at 3-months and all-cause mortality at 1-year following an ischemic stroke. Functional disability was measured using the modified Rankin scale (mRS), a 7-point ordinal scale that measures a subject's degree of functional disability in daily activities after suffering from a stroke [43]. The mRS ranges from 0 to 6, with higher scores indicating greater functional disability [43]. For the current study, the full scale of the mRS was analyzed in order to incorporate response information from all categories. The mRS categories of 5 and 6 were collapsed into a single category based on the opinions of stroke subjects who indicated that being severely disabled (i.e., category 5) is just as bad as or worse than death (i.e., category 6) [44]. All-cause mortality at 1-year was defined as death due to any cause.

Baseline data

A number of potential confounders were considered in the modeling approach on the basis of prognostic value or consistency within the literature [7–19, 21–26]. Multivariable models for each outcome were fit including pre-specified variables that were forced into the final model in addition to potential confounders, which are shown in Table 1.

Statistical analysis

All subjects were followed from the date of enrollment until the date of death, loss to follow-up, or the end of their 1-year follow-up, whichever occurred first. The relationship between functional disability at 3-months following an ischemic stroke and exposures of obesity and diabetes was modeled via proportional odds regression. A cross-product interaction term was used to derive adjusted common odds ratios (OR) and 95% confidence intervals (CI). The proportional odds assumption was assessed for all exposure variables and potential confounders using the Score test. The relationship between all-cause mortality at 1-year following an ischemic stroke and exposures of obesity and diabetes was modeled via Cox proportional hazards regression. A cross-product interaction term was used to derive adjusted hazard ratios (HR) and 95% CIs. The proportional hazards assumption was verified for all exposure variables and potential confounders using Schoenfeld residuals and time-dependent covariates [45]. For both models, multicollinearity between covariates was assessed by calculating individual variance inflation factors for each of the exposure variables and the potential confounders.

The joint effect of obesity and diabetes was examined on both the multiplicative and additive scales. The likelihood ratio test of the cross-product interaction term

Table 1 Variables and Definitions of Pre-Specified Variables and Potential Confounders for Analysis

Variables	Definition
Pre-Specified Variables	
Age[a,b]	≤ 65 years, > 65 years
Gender[a,b]	Male, Female
Race/ethnicity [a,b]	White, Black/Other
Treatment assignment [a,b]	IV rt-PA + Endovascular therapy, IV rt-PA
Baseline stroke severity [a,b]	NIHSS < 20, NIHSS ≥20
Ischemic stroke sub-type [a,b]	Large-artery atherosclerosis, Cardioembolic, Small-artery occlusion/Other/Unknown
Potential Confounders	
Baseline systolic blood ressure [a,b]	< 140 mmHg, ≥ 140 mmHg
Baseline diastolic blood pressure [a,b]	in mmHg
Baseline glucose [a,b]	in mmol/L
History of previous stroke [a,b]	Yes, No
History of atrial fibrillation [a,b]	Yes, No
History of coronary artery disease [a,b]	Yes, No
History of hypertension [a,b]	Yes, No
Smoking status [a,b]	Current smoker, Former/Never smoker
Alcohol use [a,b]	Current drinker, Former/Never drinker

[a]Potential confounder for functional disability; [b]Potential confounder for all-cause mortality

was used to determine the significance of the joint effect on the multiplicative scale. The joint effect on the additive scale, or the biologic interaction, was evaluated by two indices: the relative excess risk because of the interaction (RERI); and the attributable proportion because of the interaction (AP) [46]. RERI is an estimate of the excess risk attributable to the joint effect of obesity and diabetes and AP is defined as the proportion of risk attributable to the joint effect of obesity and diabetes [46]. These indices, along with their 95% CIs, were constructed using the approach of Li and Chambless [47]. A value of 0 indicates that there is no biologic interaction present [47, 48].

All statistical tests were two-sided and used an alpha-level of 0.05 with the exception of the joint effect on the multiplicative scale. For the joint effect on the multiplicative scale, statistical significance was defined at an alpha-level of 0.10, rather than 0.05, because clinical trials are not designed to detect a joint effect, only a main effect [49]. Statistical analyses were conducted using SAS software package version 9.4 (SAS Institute, Cary, NC). Institutional Review Board approval for this analysis was obtained from the Medical University of South Carolina (Pro00063231).

Results

Baseline characteristics of the IMS III study sample

Of the 656 IMS III subjects who were enrolled and randomized, obesity or diabetes information was not available for 11 (1.68%) subjects. Baseline characteristics according to obesity and diabetes information are shown in Table 2. Among these 645 subjects with complete obesity and diabetes information, few subjects were obese (25.74%) or had diabetes (22.64%). The majority of subjects were older than 65 years (58.45%), male (51.78%), white (84.50%), had a history of hypertension (74.73%), and were former/never smokers (75.19%). Among subjects without diabetes, obese subjects were more likely to have the following characteristics: be younger than 65 years, female, have a history of hypertension, have a baseline systolic blood pressure of at least 140 mmHg, and have a higher baseline median glucose. Among subjects with diabetes, obese subjects were also more likely to be younger than 65 years and have a higher baseline median glucose but were more likely to be male, white, and have a baseline systolic blood pressure of at least 140 mmHg.

Joint effect of obesity and diabetes on functional disability at 3-months

The adjusted joint effect of obesity and diabetes on functional disability at 3-months following an ischemic stroke is shown in Table 3. Obese subjects with diabetes had similar odds of functional disability at 3-months compared with the reference group (common OR, 1.038, 95% CI: 0.631, 1.706). Similarly, there was not sufficient evidence to declare a joint effect between obesity and diabetes on either the multiplicative scale ($P_{interaction}$, 0.6746) or the additive scale (RERI, 0.078, 95% CI: -0.260, 0.416; AP = 0.075, 95% CI: -0.169, 0.319). To further illustrate the distribution of functional disability at 3-months following an ischemic stroke, the mRS scores according to obesity and diabetes are displayed using Grotta bars in Fig. 1.

Main effects of obesity and diabetes on functional disability at 3-months

There was insufficient evidence to demonstrate that obesity was associated with increased odds of functional disability at 3-months following an ischemic stroke (Table 4, common OR: 0.740, 95% CI: 0.524, 1.044), after adjusting for diabetes and other factors. Similarly, there was also not sufficient evidence to determine that diabetes was not associated with increased odds of functional disability at 3-months following an ischemic

stroke (common OR, 1.339, 95% CI: 0.924, 1.941), after adjusting for obesity and other factors.

Joint effect of obesity and diabetes on all-cause mortality at 1-year

The adjusted joint effects of obesity and diabetes on all-cause mortality at 1-year following an ischemic stroke are shown in Table 5. Obese subjects with diabetes had a similar hazard of all-cause mortality at 1-year following an ischemic stroke compared with the reference group (HR, 1.005, 95% CI: 0.559, 1.808). Furthermore, there was not sufficient evidence to declare a joint effect between obesity and diabetes on either the multiplicative scale ($P_{interaction}$, 0.5311) or the additive scale (RERI, – 0.257, 95% CI: -0.842, 0.327; AP = – 0.256, 95% CI: -0.557, 0.045).

Main effects of obesity and diabetes on all-cause mortality at 1-year

There was insufficient evidence to demonstrate that obesity was associated with an increased hazard of all-cause mortality at 1-year following an ischemic stroke (Table 4, HR, 1.092, 95% CI: 0.744, 1.602), after adjusting for diabetes and other factors. Similarly, there was also not sufficient evidence to determine that diabetes was not associated with an increased hazard of all-cause mortality at 1-year following an ischemic stroke (HR, 0.983, 95% CI: 0.638, 1.514), after adjusting for obesity and other factors.

Discussion

The purpose of this post-hoc analysis of data from the IMS III clinical trial of acute ischemic stroke patients with at least a moderate stroke severity was to explore the presence of a joint effect of obesity and diabetes on functional disability and on all-cause mortality following an ischemic stroke. Overall, there was not sufficient evidence to determine that the effect of obesity differed by diabetes status on functional disability at 3-months, or on all-cause mortality at 1-year, following an ischemic stroke on either the multiplicative scale or the additive scale. In addition, although obesity [7, 13–19] and diabetes [21–26] have been previously shown to be independently associated with all-cause mortality following a stroke, there was not sufficient evidence to determine that each factor was independently associated with all-cause mortality after adjusting for potential confounders in this cohort of acute ischemic stroke patients with at least a moderate stroke severity. In contrast, the point estimates for the independent associations between each factor and functional disability at 3-months following an ischemic stroke were consistent with the findings from the literature [7–12].

Table 2 Baseline Characteristics of IMS III Subjects and by Obesity Categories and Diabetes Status

Characteristic	All subjects	No Diabetes		Diabetes	
		Non-Obese	Obese	Non-Obese	Obese
	No. (%)	No. (%)	No. (%)	No. (%)	No. (%)
No. of subjects [a]	645	398	101	81	65
Obese					
Yes	166 (25.74)				
No	479 (74.26)				
Diabetes					
Yes	146 (22.64)				
No	499 (77.36)				
Sociodemographic Characteristics					
Age					
> 65 years	377 (58.45)	230 (57.79)	48 (47.52)	64 (79.01)	35 (53.85)
Gender					
Male	334 (51.78)	222 (55.78)	37 (36.63)	37 (45.68)	38 (58.46)
Race/ethnicity					
White	545 (84.50)	339 (85.18)	87 (86.14)	61 (75.31)	58 (89.23)
Black/Other	100 (15.50)	59 (14.82)	14 (13.86)	20 (24.69)	7 (10.77)
Clinical Characteristics					
Qualifying stroke subtype					
Large vessel atherosclerosis	127 (19.69)	70 (17.59)	24 (23.76)	18 (22.22)	15 (23.08)
Cardioembolic	299 (46.36)	185 (46.48)	46 (45.54)	37 (45.68)	31 (47.69)
Small vessel disease/Other/Unknown	219 (33.95)	143 (35.93)	31 (30.69)	26 (32.10)	19 (29.23)
Baseline stroke severity					
Severe (NIHSS ≥20)	198 (30.99)	6.3 (5.6-7.5)	6.7 (5.9-7.4)	8.2 (6.2-10.0)	8.8 (6.9-12.5)
Baseline glucose (median, IQR)	6.7 (5.7-8.1)	6.3 (5.6-7.4)	6.7 (5.9-7.4)	8.2 (6.1-10.0)	8.8 (6.9-12.3)
Baseline systolic blood pressure					
≥ 140 mmHg	386 (60.60)	219 (55.73)	67 (67.68)	62 (77.50)	38 (58.46)
Baseline diastolic blood pressure (median, IQR)	81 (71-94)	80 (70-93)	85 (70.5-98)	85 (73-96)	80 (71-91)
Treatment assignment					
IV rt-PA+ Endovascular therapy	429 (66.51)	274 (68.84)	61 (60.40)	50 (61.73)	44 (67.69)
IV rt-PA	216 (33.49)	124 (31.16)	40 (39.60)	31 (38.27)	21 (32.31)
Risk Factors and Comorbidities					
Smoking status					
Current smoker	160 (24.81)	106 (26.63)	30 (29.70)	14 (17.28)	10 (15.38)
Alcohol use					
Current drinker	251 (38.91)	165 (41.46)	43 (42.57)	21 (25.93)	22 (33.85)
History of a previous stroke					
Yes	86 (13.33)	46 (11.56)	9 (8.91)	21 (25.93)	10 (15.38)
History of hypertension					
Yes	482 (74.73)	269 (67.59)	79 (78.22)	72 (88.89)	62 (95.38)
History of coronary artery disease					
Yes	170 (26.36)	90 (22.61)	22 (21.78)	37 (45.68)	21 (32.31)
History of atrial fibrillation					
Yes	192 (29.77)	120 (30.15)	30 (29.70)	22 (27.16)	20 (30.77)

[a]11 subjects were excluded due to missing obesity or diabetes information
IMS III Interventional Management of Stroke III, *NIHSS* National Institutes of Health Stroke Scale, *IV rt-PA* Intravenous recombinant tissue plasminogen activator, *IQR* Interquartile range

Table 3 Adjusted Common ORs for Functional Disability at 3-months in Relation to Obesity and Diabetes

Functional Disability at 3-months following the ischemic stroke	Obesity Categories	
	Non-obese	Obese
	OR (95% CI)	OR (95% CI)
Diabetes		
No	1.00	0.704 (0.466, 1.063)
Yes	1.256 (0.780, 2.020)	1.038 (0.631, 1.706)
Joint effect (additive):		
RERI (95% CI)		0.078 (-0.260, 0.416)
AP (95% CI)		0.075 (-0.169, 0.319)
Joint effect on the multiplicative scale: *p*-value		P=0.6746

ORs are adjusted for age, gender, race/ethnicity, ischemic stroke sub-type, baseline stroke severity, baseline glucose, treatment assignment, smoking status, alcohol use, history of previous stroke, history of hypertension, and history of coronary artery disease
RERI Relative excess risk due to interaction, *AP* Attributable proportion due to interaction

In comparison to some of the studies that cite the obesity paradox on post-stroke outcomes, there are several potential reasons for the discrepant results in the present study. First, the population only consisted of acute ischemic stroke subjects [33, 35, 50]. Some of the results from this study are consistent with several other studies that included only ischemic stroke subjects whereas the majority of the studies that support the obesity paradox included different patient populations (i.e., only hemorrhagic [20], only ischemic [8, 9, 11–14, 16, 50, 51], stroke or TIA [7, 17], or both

ischemic and hemorrhagic strokes [10, 15, 18, 19]). It is important to point out these differences in the study population because the pathogenesis of ischemic stroke is markedly different from that of hemorrhagic stroke, thus the effect of obesity on post-stroke outcomes may not be the same [52]. However, results of this study were similar to several other studies that only included recent ischemic stroke subjects [8, 9, 51]. Second, the outcomes of interest in studies that support the association between obesity and a decreased risk of all-cause mortality post-stroke were assessed at widely varying periods ranging from a week to 10 years [33, 35, 50]. However, the studies that had time points similar to the time points of acute stroke trials (IMS III, for example) determined that there was no functional or survival benefit for obese subjects [8, 50, 53]. Third, the inclusion of important prognostic factors, such as stroke severity and smoking use, as potential confounders differed across studies [33, 35, 50]. It is critical to account for these important confounders to reduce residual confounding, however many of the studies that assessed these associations did not account for these confounding variables. Lastly, the measure of obesity is nearly always body mass index (BMI). Although BMI is the most commonly used diagnostic tool for obesity in clinical practice [5, 54], BMI is unable to differentiate between body fat percentage and lean mass which leads to misclassification [55] nor does it tell the distribution of body fat. Rather than using BMI to measure obesity, it is critical to determine alternative

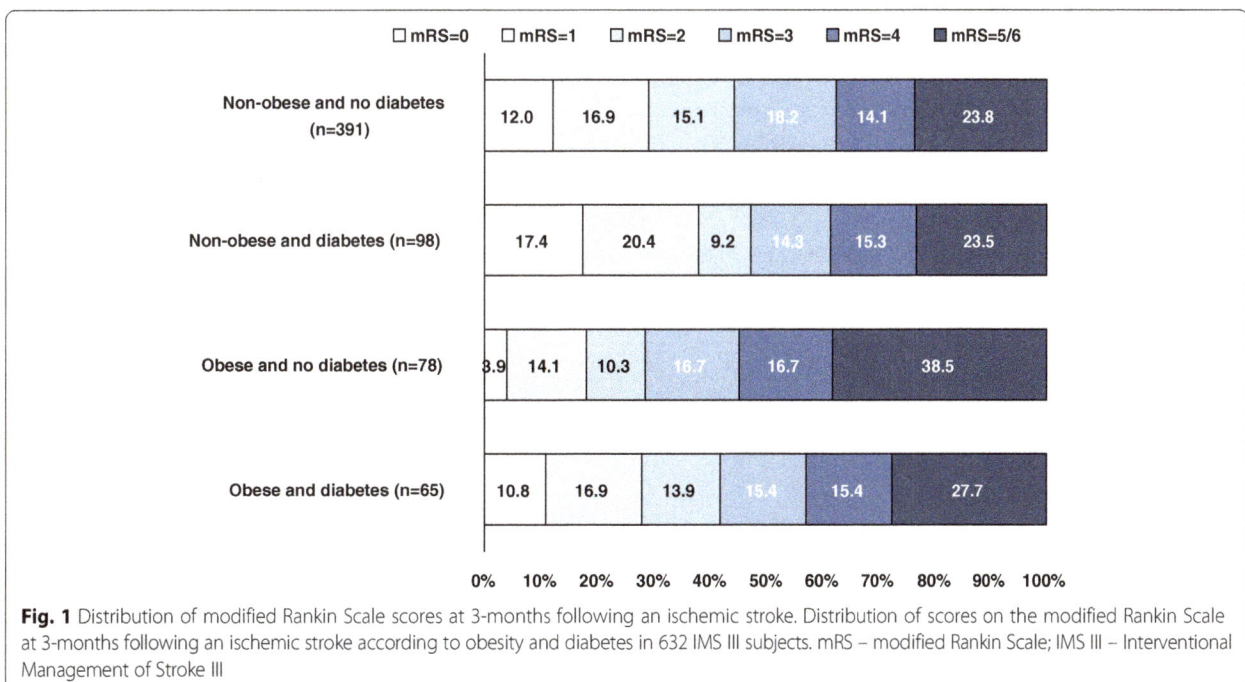

Fig. 1 Distribution of modified Rankin Scale scores at 3-months following an ischemic stroke. Distribution of scores on the modified Rankin Scale at 3-months following an ischemic stroke according to obesity and diabetes in 632 IMS III subjects. mRS – modified Rankin Scale; IMS III – Interventional Management of Stroke III

Table 4 Adjusted Effect Measures for Associations between Obesity, Diabetes and Outcomes of Interest

Outcome	
3-month functional disability[a]	OR (95% CI)
Obesity	0.740 (0.524, 1.044)
Diabetes	1.339 (0.924, 1.941)
All-cause mortality[b]	HR (95% CI)
Obesity	1.092 (0.744, 1.602)
Diabetes	0.983 (0.638, 1.514)

[a]ORs are adjusted for age, gender, race/ethnicity, ischemic stroke sub-type, baseline stroke severity, baseline glucose, treatment assignment, smoking status, alcohol use, history of previous stroke, history of hypertension, and history of coronary artery disease
[b]HRs are adjusted for age, gender, race/ethnicity, ischemic stroke sub-type, baseline stroke severity, baseline glucose, baseline diastolic blood pressure, treatment assignment, smoking status, alcohol use, history of hypertension, and history of previous stroke

diagnostic tools capable of differentiating risk of poor clinical outcomes following an ischemic stroke such as waist circumference or waist-to-hip ratio [33, 56].

The present study has a number of limitations that could influence the interpretation of the study results. Due to the restrictive criteria of the IMS III clinical trial, the results of the present study may not be generalizable to all acute ischemic stroke patients. For example, patients were excluded if they had mild stroke severity (NIHSS < 8). The generalizability of the results of this study is therefore limited to ischemic stroke patients with at least a moderate stroke severity who met all of the study eligibility criteria. Thus, the potential for selection bias cannot be excluded. Future research could be performed to determine if the results demonstrated among a cohort of acute ischemic stroke subjects with at least a moderate stroke severity would be similar to the results among a cohort of acute ischemic stroke subjects.

Additional identified limitations are associated with the measurement of the exposures of interest. Results of this study were limited in the interpretability of the results partially due to how obesity and diabetes information were captured (i.e., binary summary measures). There may be measurement error based on the how obesity and diabetes information was ascertained. Specifically, no further definition of these variables was provided in the IMS III Case Report Form Guidelines. Therefore, we were not able to accurately define obesity or diabetes based on their BMI or fasting blood glucose levels, respectively. Although these measures are based on high-quality data, the degree of obesity or diabetes could not be determined at baseline. Thus, the potential for measurement bias cannot be excluded. Future studies could capture multiple measures of obesity, specifically BMI, waist circumference, and/or waist-to-hip ratio, rather than a summary indicator for obesity and/or utilize the World Health Organization's public health action points [57] to further define subjects' degree of obesity. These alternative measures would allow for greater interpretability. Additionally, the exposures of interest are only snapshots of subjects' history of obesity and/or diabetes. As a result, it was not possible to determine the cumulative effect, or allostatic load, of either exposure of interest. Future studies could collect information on subjects' weight histories in addition to the duration of diabetes to accurately determine whether the effect of obesity on post-ischemic stroke outcomes differs by diabetes status.

Additionally, IMS III was not designed to answer the research questions of the present study. Examining joint effects, or interactions, is challenging because tests for interactions are typically underpowered [58]. Despite these limitations and the confines of statistical power, this study was able to demonstrate the joint effect of obesity and diabetes on functional disability and on all-

Table 5 Adjusted HRs for All-Cause Mortality at 1-year in Relation to Obesity and Diabetes

All-Cause Mortality at 1-year	Obesity Categories			
	Non-obese		Obese	
	Deaths/total	HR (95% CI)	Deaths/total	HR (95% CI)
Diabetes				
No	85/398	1.00	24/101	1.198 (0.743, 1.932)
Yes	27/81	1.064 (0.642, 1.761)	17/65	1.005 (0.559, 1.808)
Joint effect (additive):				
RERI (95% CI)				-0.257 (-0.842, 0.327)
AP (95% CI)				-0.256 (-0.557, 0.045)
Joint effect on the multiplicative scale: p-value				P=0.5311

HRs are adjusted for age, gender, race/ethnicity, ischemic stroke sub-type, baseline stroke severity, baseline glucose, baseline diastolic blood pressure, treatment assignment, smoking status, alcohol use, history of hypertension, and history of previous stroke
RERI Relative excess risk due to interaction, *AP* Attributable proportion due to interaction

cause mortality following an ischemic stroke is insignificant. Although other analytical strategies were applied to offset these problems, it is imperative to strive for sufficient power to examine the potential joint effect of obesity and diabetes on clinical outcomes following an ischemic stroke. Thus, it is critical to utilize a national or international ischemic stroke registry that would provide sufficient resources and power for future studies to address these research questions.

Despite some limitations, the present study includes several notable strengths. First, this is the first study to explore the potential multiplicative and additive joint effects of obesity and diabetes on functional disability and all-cause mortality following an ischemic stroke. Results of this research provide evidence for generating hypotheses for future studies investigating how obesity and diabetes could potentially interact with one another to affect the clinical outcomes following an ischemic stroke. Second, the rigorous data collection of the IMS III trial reduced information bias. Rather than relying on subjects self-reporting their medical history, the use of source documentation to verify sociodemographic characteristics, clinical characteristics, and risk factors and comorbidities prevented bias that may have resulted from self-reporting. Third, IMS III investigators followed strict study procedures, which minimized the potential bias from incorrect documentation of the trial's outcomes.

Conclusions
Overall, it is important to continue to study joint effects of these common modifiable factors to identify susceptible subgroups of individuals that would potentially benefit from effective interventions targeted at reducing the burden of functional disability and all-cause mortality [58]. This topic is of high public health priority. Obesity and diabetes are not only highly prevalent in both the general US and international populations [1, 3, 4, 59], but they are also prevalent among individuals who have been diagnosed with a stroke [5]. It is estimated that between 18 and 44% of individuals who previously had an ischemic stroke are obese, and between 25 and 45% of individuals who previously had an ischemic stroke have diabetes [5]. Recent research has supported the heterogeneity of the metabolic profile among obese individuals [39, 40]. Overall, the underlying mechanisms by which obesity and diabetes may interact to affect functional disability or all-cause mortality following an ischemic stroke remain unclear. Thus, future studies should differentiate between metabolically healthy and metabolically unhealthy patients within BMI categories (or other diagnostic tools for obesity) to determine if the effect of obesity on post-ischemic stroke outcomes differs by diabetes (or some other metabolic health measure).

Abbreviations
AP: The attributable proportion because of the interaction; CI: Confidence interval; HR: Hazard ratio; IMS III: Interventional Management of Stroke III; IV rt-PA: Intravenous recombinant tissue plasminogen activator; mRS: Modified Rankin Scale; NIHSS: National Institutes of Health Stroke Scale; OR: Odds ratio; RERI: The relative excess risk because of the interaction

Funding
This work was supported by National Institute of Health/National Cancer Institute Grant Number: 5P20CA157071-02; and by National Institute of Health/National Institute on Minority Health and Health Disparities Grant Number: 4R01MD005892-05. These funding bodies had no role in the design of the study and collection, analysis, and interpretation of data nor in the writing of this manuscript.

Authors' contributions
CB, SDY, KB, GM, RHM, AS, and MEF contributed in the conceptualization of this study. CB analyzed the data and prepared the manuscript. CB, SDY, RHM, and AS interpreted the data. SDY, RHM, AS, and MEF revised the manuscript for important intellectual content. CB, SDY, KB, GM, RHM, AS, and MEF read and approved the final manuscript.

Competing interests
The authors declare that they have no competing interests.

Author details
[1]Department of Public Health Sciences, Medical University of South Carolina, Charleston, SC, USA. [2]Department of Health Informatics, Johns Hopkins All Children's Hospital, 601 5th Street South, Suite 707, St. Petersburg, FL 33701, USA. [3]Department of Emergency Medicine, Medical University of South Carolina, Charleston, SC, USA. [4]Department of Nursing, Medical University of South Carolina, Charleston, SC, USA.

References
1. Ogden CL, Carroll MD, Fryar CD, Flegal KM. Prevalence of obesity among adults and youth: United States, 2011-2014. NCHS Data Brief. 2015;219:1–8.
2. World Health Organization. Global status report on noncommunicable diseases 2010. 2011.
3. World Health Organization. Global report on diabetes. 2016.
4. Centers for Disease Control and Prevention. National Diabetes Statistics Report, 2017: estimates of diabetes and its burden in the epidemiologic estimation methods. Atlanta: US Dep. Heal. Hum. Serv; 2017.
5. Kernan WNW, Ovbiagele B, Black HHR, Bravata DMD, Chimowitz MI, Ezekowitz MD, et al. Guidelines for the prevention of stroke in patients with stroke and transient ischemic attack: a guideline for healthcare professionals from the American Heart Association/American Stroke Association. Stroke. 2014;45:2160–236.
6. Mozaffarian D, Benjamin E, Go A, Arnett D, Blaha M, Cushman M, et al. Heart disease and stroke statistics-2015 update: a report from the American Heart Association. Circulation. 2015;131:e29–322.
7. Doehner W, Schenkel J, Anker SD, Springer J, Audebert H. Overweight and obesity are associated with improved survival, functional outcome, and stroke recurrence after acute stroke or transient ischaemic attack: observations from the tempis trial. Eur Heart J. 2013;34:268–77.

8. Zhao L, Du W, Zhao X, Liu L, Wang C, Wang Y, et al. Favorable functional recovery in overweight ischemic stroke survivors: findings from the China National Stroke Registry. J Stroke Cerebrovasc Dis. 2014;23:e201–6.

9. Jang S, Shin Y, Kim D, Sohn M, Lee J, Oh G, et al. Effect of obesity on functional outcomes at 6 months post-stroke among elderly Koreans: a prospective multicenter study. BMJ Open. 2015;5:e008712–8.

10. Megherbi S, Milan C, Minier D, Couvreur G, Osseby G-V, Tilling K, et al. Association between diabetes and stroke subtype on survival and functional outcome 3 months after stroke. Stroke. 2003;34:688 LP–694.

11. Tziomalos K, Spanou M, Bouziana SD, Papadopoulou M, Giampatzis V, Kostaki S, et al. Type 2 diabetes is associated with a worse functional outcome of ischemic stroke. World J Diabetes. 2014;5:939–44.

12. Spratt N, Wang Y, Levi C, Ng K, Evans M, Fisher J. A prospective study of predictors of prolonged hospital stay and disability after stroke. J Clin Neurosci. 2003;10:665–9.

13. Olsen TS, Dehlendorff C, Petersen HG, Andersen KK. Body mass index and poststroke mortality. Neuroepidemiology. 2008;30:93–100.

14. Skolarus LE, Sanchez BN, Levine DA, Baek J, Kerber KA, Morgenstern LB, et al. Association of body mass index and mortality after acute ischemic stroke. Circ Cardiovasc Qual Outcomes. 2014;7:64–9.

15. Andersen KK, Olsen TS. The obesity paradox in stroke: lower mortality and lower risk of readmission for recurrent stroke in obese stroke patients. Int J Stroke. 2015;10:99–104.

16. Vemmos K, Ntaios G, Spengos K, Savvari P, Vemmou A, Pappa T, et al. Association between obesity and mortality after acute first-ever stroke: the obesity-stroke paradox. Stroke. 2011;42:30–6.

17. Towfighi A, Ovbiagele B. The impact of body mass index on mortality after stroke. Stroke. 2009;40:2704–8.

18. Bell CL, LaCroix A, Masaki K, Hade EM, Manini T, Mysiw WJ, et al. Prestroke factors associated with poststroke mortality and recovery in older women in the women's health initiative. J Am Geriatr Soc. 2013;61:1324–30.

19. Bazzano L, Gu D, Whelton M, Wu X. Al. E. Body mass index and risk of stroke among Chinese men and women. Ann Neurol. 2010;67:11–20.

20. Kim B, Lee S, Ryu W, Kim C, Lee J, Al E. Paradoxical longevity in obese patients with intracerebral hemorrhage. Neurology. 2011;76:567–73.

21. Kamalesh M, Shen J, Eckert GJ. Long term postischemic stroke mortality in diabetes: a veteran cohort analysis. Stroke. 2008;39:2727–31.

22. Sprafka J, Virnig B, Shahar E, McGovern P. Trends in diabetes prevalence among stroke patients and the effect of diabetes on stroke survival: the Minnesota heart survey. Diabet Med. 1994;11:678–84.

23. Icks A, Claessen H, Morbach S, Glaeske G, Hoffman F. Time-dependent impact of diabetes on mortality in patients with stroke. Diabetes Care. 2012;35:1868–75.

24. Eriksson M, Carlberg B, Eliasson M. The disparity in long-term survival after a first stroke in patients with and without diabetes persists: the northern Sweden MONICA study. Cerebrovasc Dis. 2012;34:153–60.

25. Winell K, Paakonen R, Pietila A, Reunanen A, Niemi M, Salomaa V. Prognosis of ischaemic stroke is improving similarly in patients with type 2 diabetes in nondiabetic patients in Finland. Int J Stroke. 2011;6:295–301.

26. Tuomilehto J, Rastenyte D, Jousilahti P, Sarti C, Vartiainen E, Rastenytė D, et al. Diabetes mellitus as a risk factor for death from stroke. Stroke. 1996;27:210–5.

27. Allen CL, Bayraktutan U. Risk factors for ischaemic stroke. Int J Stroke. 2008;3:105–16.

28. Sacco R, Benjamin E, Broderick J, Dyken M, Easton D, Feinberg W, et al. Risk factors. Stroke. 1997;28:1507–17.

29. Bell J, Sabia S, Singh-Manoux A, Hamer M, Kivimäki M. Healthy obesity and risk of accelerated functional decline and disability. Int J Obes. 2017;41:866–72.

30. Calle E, Thun M, Petrelli J, Rodriguez C, Al E. Body mass index and mortality in a prospective cohort of US adults. N Engl J Med. 1999;341:1097–105.

31. Adams K, Schatzkin A, Harris T, Kipnis V, Al E. Overweight, obesity, and mortality in a large prospective cohort of persons 50 to 71 years old. N Engl J Med. 2006;355:763–78.

32. Meschia JF, Bushnell C, Boden-Albala B, Braun LT, Bravata DM, Chaturvedi S, et al. Guidelines for the primary prevention of stroke: a statement for healthcare professionals from the American heart association/American stroke association. Stroke. 2014;45:3754–832.

33. Oesch L, Tatlisumak T, Arnold M, Sarikaya H. Obesity paradox in stroke-myth or reality? A systematic review. PLoS One. 2017;12:e0171334.

34. Stevens J, Bradshaw PT, Truesdale KP, Jensen MD. Obesity paradox should not interfere with public health efforts. Int J Obes (Lond). 2014;39:80–1. Nature Publishing Group

35. Standle E, Erbach M, Schnell O. Defending the con side: obesity paradox does not exist. Diabetes Care. 2013;36:S282–6.

36. Dixon J, Egger G, Finkelstein E, Kral J, Lambert G. "Obesity paradox" misunderstands the biology of optimal weight throughout the life cycle. Int J Obes. 2014;39:82–4. Nature Publishing Group

37. Golay A, Ybarra J. Link between obesity and type 2 diabetes. Best Pract Res Clin Endocrinol Metab. 2005;19:649–63.

38. Al-Goblan A, Al-Alfi M, Khan M. Mechanism linking diabetes mellitus and obesity. Diabetes Metab Syndr Obes. 2014;7:587–91.

39. Appleton SL, Seaborn CJ, Visvanathan R, Hill CL, Gill TK, Taylor AW, et al. Diabetes and cardiovascular disease outcomes in the metabolically healthy obese phenotype: a cohort study. Diabetes Care. 2013;36:2388–94.

40. Primeau V, Coderre L, Karelis AD, Brochu M, Lavoie M-EM, Al E, et al. Characterizing the profile of obese patients who are metabolically healthy. Int J Obes. 2011;35:971–81. Nature Publishing Group

41. Khatri P, Hill MD, Palesch YY, Spilker J, Jauch EC, Carrozzella JA, et al. Methodology of the interventional Management of Stroke III trial. Int J Stroke. 2008;3:130–7.

42. Broderick JP, Palesch YY, Demchuk AM, Yeatts SD, Khatri P, Hill MD, et al. Endovascular therapy after intravenous t-PA versus t-PA alone for stroke. N Engl J Med. 2013;368:893–903.

43. Rankin J. Cerebral vascular accidents in patients over the age of 60. Scott Med J. 1957;2:200–15.

44. Samsa G, Matchar D, Goldstein L, Al E. Utilities for major stroke:results from a survey of preferences among persons at increased risk for stroke. Am Heart J. 1998;136:703–13.

45. Kleinbaum DGKM. Survival analysis: a self-learning text. 3rd ed. New York: Springer; 2012.

46. Rothman K. Modern Epidemiology. 1st ed. Boston: Little, Brown and Company; 1986.

47. Li R, Chambless L. Test for additive interaction in proportional hazards models. Ann Epidemiol. 2007;17:227–36.

48. Hosmer D, Lemeshow S. Confidence interval estimation of interaction. Epidemiology. 1992;3:452–6.

49. Fleiss J. Analysis of data from multiclinic trials. Control Clin Trials. 1986;7:267–75.

50. Sun W, Huang Y, Xian Y, Zhu S, Jia Z, Liu R, et al. Association of body mass index with mortality and functional outcome after acute ischemic stroke. Sci Rep. 2017;7:2507.

51. Ryu W, Lee S, Kim C, Kim B, Yoon B. Body mass index, initial neurological severity and long-term mortality in ischemic stroke. Cerebrovasc Dis. 2011;32:170–6.

52. Andersen K, Olsen T, Dehlendorff C, Kammersgaard L. Hemorrhagic and ischemic strokes compared stroke severity, mortality, and risk factors. Stroke. 2009;40:2068–72.

53. Kim B, Lee S, Jung K, Yu K, Lee B, Roh J. Dynamics of obesity paradox after stroke related to time from onset, age, and causes of death. Neurology. 2012;79:856–63.

54. Stevens J, McClain J, Truesdale K. Selection of measures in epidemiologic studies of the consequences of obesity. Int J Obes. 2008;32:S60–6.

55. Shah N, Braverman E. Measuring adiposity in patients: the utility of body mass index (BMI), percent body fat, and leptin. PLoS One. 2012;7:e33308.

56. Romero-Corral A, Somers VK, Sierra-Johnson J, Thomas RJ, Collazo-Clavell ML, Korinek J, et al. Accuracy of body mass index in diagnosing obesity in the adult general population. Int J Obes. 2008;32:959–66.

57. World Health Organization. Obesity 2016 [Internet]. [cited 2016 Jun 4]. Available from: http://www.who.int/topics/obesity/en/.

58. Greenland S, Lash TL, Rothman KJ. Concepts of interaction. In: Rothman K, Greenland S, Lash TL, editors. Mod Epidemiol. 3rd ed. Philadelphia: Lippincott Williams and Wilkins; 2008.

59. Bonora E, Tuomilehto J. The pros and cons of diagnosing diabetes with A1C. Diabetes Care. 2011;34(Suppl 2):S184–90.

12

Effect of duration of diabetes on bone mineral density: a population study on East Asian males

Miso Jang[1], Hyunkyung Kim[2], Shorry Lea[3], Sohee Oh[4], Jong Seung Kim[5] and Bumjo Oh[5*] (iD)

Abstract

Background: The aim of the present study is to evaluate the association between BMD and type 2 DM status in middle-aged and elderly men. To investigate a possible correlation, the present study used the BMD dataset of the Korea National Health and Nutrition Examination Survey (KNHANES) from 2008 to 2011.

Methods: In total, 37,753 individuals participated in health examination surveys between 2008 and 2011. A total of 3383 males aged ≥50 years were eligible. They underwent BMD measurement through dual-energy X-ray absorptiometry (DXA). The fasting plasma glucose and insulin levels of participants were also measured.

Results: Men with prediabetes and diabetes had significantly higher mean BMD at all measured sites than control men did, irrespective of DM status. This was confirmed by multivariable linear regression analyses. DM duration was an important factor affecting BMD. Patients with DM for > 5 years had lower mean BMD in the total hip and femoral neck than those with DM for ≤5 years. Per multivariable linear regression analyses, patients with DM for > 5 years had significantly lower mean BMD at the femoral neck than those with DM ≤5 years.

Conclusions: DM duration was significantly associated with reduced femoral neck BMD.

Keywords: Diabetes mellitus, Prediabetic state, Bone mineral density, Dual-energy X-ray absorptiometry, Osteoporosis, Korea National Health and nutritional examination survey

Background

Type 2 diabetes mellitus (DM) is a common metabolic disease with an increasing worldwide prevalence rate of 8.3% [1], and with 11% among Korean male adults. Considering that more than 9 million osteoporotic fractures are recorded annually worldwide, osteoporosis is a significant contributor to morbidity and lost life years globally [2]. Osteoporosis and type 2 DM share many common characteristics in that they are both chronic diseases with an increasingly global medical burden.

Although individuals with type 1 DM show decreased bone mass density (BMD), those with type 2 DM often have normal or even slightly elevated BMD compared with an age-matched control population [3]. Bone fragility results from decreased bone mineral mass and alterations in bone microstructure. Multiple mechanisms can contribute to increased fractures in type 2 DM patients. Glucose toxicity, lack of insulin and other factors affects bone metabolism. A substantial number of studies examined the association between type 2 DM and fracture risk [4, 5]. Longer type 2 DM duration increases diabetic complications, insulin usage, and fracture risk and results in inadequate glucose control. Clinically, assessing the bone microstructure of type 2 DM patients is difficult because CT or MRI should be used [3]. Therefore determining the BMD is the best approach for now.

The prevention of fractures is an important goal for studies concerning older adults. Many studies focus on osteoporosis in women. However, as many as one in four men aged > 50 years will develop at least one osteoporosis-related fracture in his lifetime, highlighting the need for more studies on osteoporosis in men [6]. One in three men die in within a year after a hip fracture, another one in three experience a subsequent

---

* Correspondence: bumjo.oh@gmail.com
[5]Department of Family Medicine, SMG-SNU Boramae Medical Center, 20, Boramae-ro 5-gil, Dongjak-gu, Seoul 07061, Republic of Korea
Full list of author information is available at the end of the article

fracture again [7]. Generally, men have worse smoking and alcohol drinking habits and higher risk of fall than women [8], which may contribute to bone health deterioration. Furthermore, men are approximately 70% less frequently screened for osteoporosis than women [9]. For individuals aged ≥50 years in Korea, the prevalence rates of osteoporosis and osteopenia are 7.3% and 38.0% in men and 46.5% and 48.7% in women, respectively [10]. In another Korean study, only 7.6% of men found out that they had osteoporosis, and only 5.7% of them had their disease treated [11].

In light of public health, male osteoporosis associated with type 2 DM should be carefully considered. The present study aimed to assess the association between BMD and type 2 DM status by considering several confounding factors such as age, body mass index (BMI), and fasting insulin and glucose level. We hypothesized that participants with longer duration of type 2 DM may have lower BMD because of poor disease control and insulin deficiency.

Methods
Study design and participants
The Korea National Health and Nutritional Examination Survey (KNHANES) is a nationwide survey representing the non-institutionalized civilian population of South Korea. The Division of Health and Nutritional Survey of the Korea Centers have periodically conducted it for Disease Control and Prevention (KCDCP) since 1998. The data from KNHANES is open data for research purposes. A complex, stratified, multilevel probability sampling design was used, and sampling units were selected based on geographical area, age and sex [12]. Each sampled participant is assigned a numerical sample weight that measures the number of populations represented by that specific participant [12]. A complex sampling design and sample weights facilitate the production of nationally representative data [13]. The KNHANES consists of three components: a health interview, a nutrition survey, and a health examination. Until the first half of 2008, data were gathered through household interviews and direct standardized physical examinations conducted at simple checkup centers at city government offices and town halls [14]. From the second half of 2008 to 2011, the survey was conducted by introducing mobile inspection vehicles. In July 2008, the whole-body dual-energy x-ray absorptiometry (DXA) survey was newly introduced and tested until May 2011. People who were tested before July 2008 and after May 2011 have not received the DXA. From 2008 to 2011, the KNHANES included 37753 individuals. Of the 5872 male participants who were aged ≥50 years, 2489 were eliminated from the study based on the following exclusion criteria: missing data, fasting time of <8 h, taking prescription medication for osteoporosis, and the questionnaire answered with having been diagnosed and treated by physicians for the conditions

affecting bone metabolism, such as all types of cancer, chronic kidney disease, liver cirrhosis, thyroid disease, or rheumatoid arthritis (Fig. 1). After all exclusions, 3383 participants were finally included in this analysis.

Associated factors
As described previously [12], the demographic and behavior variables were age, monthly house income, smoking (never, past, or current smoker), alcohol drinking (grams of alcohol per day), and physical activity (low, moderate, or high). The average alcoholic beverage intake was assessed by self-reported questionnaire and then converted to the amount of pure alcohol (in grams) consumed per day. Physical activity was quantified as the metabolic equivalent of task (MET) minutes per week calculated using the Korean version score calculation of the short-form International Physical Activity Questionnaire. Therefore, physical activity levels were then classified as low (< 600 MET minutes per week), moderate (600 ≤ – < 3000 MET minutes per week), or high (≥3000 MET minutes per week) [12].

Standardized techniques and equipment were used to measure height and weight, and body mass index (BMI) was calculated by dividing body weight by the square of height (kg/m^2) [14]. Blood pressure (BP) was measured by a standard method using a sphygmomanometer in a sitting position. The following definition for hypertension was obtained from the Division of Health and Nutritional Survey under the KCDCP: either by a self-reported history of hypertension diagnosis and current usage of antihypertensive drug or by ≥140 mmHg systolic BP or ≥ 90 mmHg diastolic BP.

Laboratory examinations
During the survey, in the morning, blood samples were collected and analyzed by a certified central laboratory. Plasma total cholesterol (milligrams per deciliter), high-density lipoprotein (HDL) cholesterol (milligram per deciliter), triglycerides (milligrams per deciliter) and fasting glucose levels (milligrams per deciliter) were enzymatically measured using a Hitachi Modular 7600 automatic analyzer (Hitachi Ltd., Tokyo, Japan). The fasting insulin (micro-International units per milliliter) and serum vitamin D (nanograms per milliliter) concentrations were measured using immunoradiometric and radioimmunoassays using a gamma-counter (1470 Wizard; PerkinElmer, Waltham, MA, USA). The direct measurement of low-density lipoprotein (LDL) cholesterol was limited, and it was mainly calculated using the Friedewald equation (i.e., LDL cholesterol = total cholesterol – HDL cholesterol – triglyceride/5) [15]. Insulin resistance was evaluated using the homeostasis model assessment: estimated insulin resistance (HOMA-IR) index (i.e., HOMA-IR = [fasting plasma glucose] × [fasting plasma

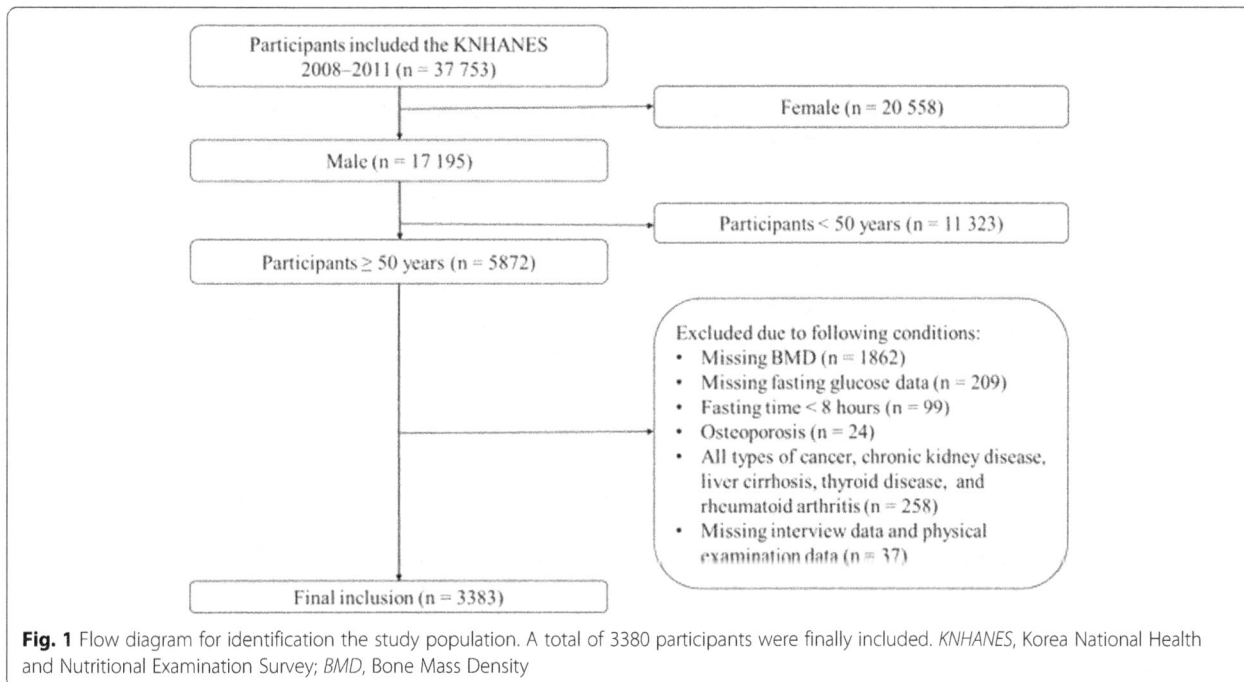

Fig. 1 Flow diagram for identification the study population. A total of 3380 participants were finally included. *KNHANES*, Korea National Health and Nutritional Examination Survey; *BMD*, Bone Mass Density

insulin] × 0.055 /22.5) and homeostasis model assessment: estimated beta cell function (HOMA-beta) index (i.e., HOMA-beta = 20 × [fasting plasma insulin / ([fasting plasma glucose] × 0.055–3.5)] [16].

Assessment of BMD

The whole-body dual-energy x-ray absorptiometry (DXA) survey begin in July 2008 and ended in May 2011. The BMDs of the lumbar spine, left total hip, and left femoral neck, and body composition including percent fat mass, were measured using DXA (Discovery-W; Hologic Inc., Waltham, MA, USA). As described previously [14], for the lumbar spine, the mean value of BMDs of L1–L4 was selected for analysis according to the recommendation of the International Society for Clinical Densitometry [17]. The BMD of the right femur was used when the left femur could not be measured (e.g., postoperative state, fracture, deformity, or malformation). The technicians performing the BMD measurements tested the precision based on duplicate or triplicate measurements in 30 or 15 participants, respectively. The precision error was calculated as the percentage coefficient of variation (CV %). The precision errors allowed for the total hip, femur neck, and lumbar vertebrae were 1.8%, 2.5%, and 1.9%, respectively [14].

Assessments and definition of DM/prediabetes and duration of DM

The following definitions were obtained from the Division of Health and Nutritional Survey of the KCDCP. DM was defined by either a self-reported history of DM diagnosis

and current usage of insulin or oral hypoglycemic agents, or by a ≥ 126 mg/dL fasting blood glucose level or ≥ 6.5% glycated hemoglobin (HbA1c) level. Prediabetes was defined as ≥100–125 mg/dL fasting blood glucose, or ≥ 5.7–6.5 HbA1c levels. DM duration was calculated by subtracting the age at the time of DM diagnosis from the age at the time of the investigation. Data without time-diagnosed diabetes were excluded.

Statistical analysis

Statistical analyses were carried out using STATA 14.0 (StataCorp, College Station, TX, USA) with the SVY commands to account for the complex sampling design and include sample weight, which enabled the results to represent the entire national male population > 50 years [13]. All continuous data were presented as the mean ± standard error (SE). All categorical data were presented as numbers and percentages. To compare the participants' characteristics of the study among control, groups with prediabetes and DM, the analysis of variance (ANOVA) test and χ^2 test for continuous and categorical variables, respectively, were used. Multivariable linear regression analyses were performed to determine whether the BMD at each measured site differed based on the DM status and duration. In model 1, we adjusted for major factors, such as age and BMI. Model 2 was also adjusted for alcohol consumption; serum vitamin D concentration; smoking status; triglyceride levels, HDL cholesterol levels and total cholesterol levels, hypertension diagnosis, physical activity level, and HOMA-IR index scores. LDL cholesterol was not included as a covariate in model 2 because a significant collinearity was found between LDL and total cholesterol levels. Bonferroni's correction was performed for comparisons between the control group and groups with prediabetes and DM. The reported probability values are two-sided, and results with a p-value < 0.05 were considered statistically significant.

Results
Baseline characteristics of the participants based on type 2 DM status

Among all participants aged ≥50 years of the 2008–2011 KNHANES, 1037 (29.76%) men had prediabetes, and 644 (18.57%) men had DM. Table 1 shows the baseline characteristics of the control, participants with prediabetes and DM. Patients with diabetes were slightly older

Table 1 Weighted baseline characteristics of study participants from the KNHANES (2008–2011)

	Men (n = 3383, N = 4 370 109)			p-value
	Normal $n=1702(51.67)^{b}$	Prediabetes $n=1037(29.76)^{b}$	Diabetes $n=644(18.57)^{b}$	
Age (years)	60.46 ± 0.27	60.63 ± 0.32	61.59 ± 0.41	0.03
Weight (kg)	65.40 ± 0.29	68.25 ± 0.40	68.97 ± 0.51	<0.001
Height (cm)	167.11 ± 0.18	167.46 ± 0.24	166.72 ± 0.29	0.53
BMI (kg/m2)	23.39 ± 0.09	24.29 ± 0.11	24.78 ± 0.16	<0.001
Fat mass (%) (n = 3298)	21.74 ± 0.15	23.03 ± 0.18	23.49 ± 0.25	<0.001
Low income (n = 3342) n, (%)	484 (11.87)	246 (5.83)	217 (5.53)	0.003
Physical activity n, (%)[a]				
low	429 (25.90)	259 (23.59)	159 (24.23)	
moderate	663 (36.97)	417 (40.40)	272 (43.13)	
high	608 (37.12)	360 (36.01)	211 (32.64)	
	1700	1036	642	0.65
Smoking history n, (%)				
never	305 (18.11)	191 (16.41)	101 (14.28)	
past	817 (45.87)	525 (48.27)	327 (47.22)	
current	580 (36.02)	321 (35.33)	216 (38.50)	
	1702	1037	644	0.397
alcohol consumption (g/day)	13.42 ± 0.56	16.24 ± 0.77	15.23 ± 1.14	0.043
hypertension[a]	848(44.13)	705(34.1)	446(21.7)	<0.001
fasting glucose (mg/dl)	90.99 ± 0.17	107.03 ± 0.27	141.38 ± 1.96	<0.001
fasting insulin (IU/mL) (n = 2927)	8.74 ± 0.13	10.40 ± 0.19	10.83 ± 0.33	<0.001
HbA1c (n = 1001)	5.45 ± 0.02	5.91 ± 0.03	7.21 ± 0.07	<0.001
HOMA-IR (n = 2927)[a]	1.95 ± 0.03	2.75 ± 0.05	3.74 ± 0.12	<0.001
HOMAbeta (n = 2927)[a]	120.59 ± 1.89	86.18 ± 1.53	58.97 ± 6.70	<0.001
DM duration (years) (n = 505)			8.43 ± 0.34	
total cholesterol (mg/dl)	186.99 ± 1.09	192.80 ± 1.40	181.16 ± 2.00	0.168
HDL-C (mg/dl)	45.26 ± 0.36	45.72 ± 0.43	42.27 ± 0.49	<0.001
LDL-C (mg/dl)	111.77 ± 1.15	111.11 ± 1.46	99.98 ± 2.03	<0.001
Triglyceride (mg/dl)	149.80 ± 4.87	179.85 ± 5.37	194.53 ± 7.85	<0.001
serum vitamin D (ng/mL)	21.38 ± 0.29	21.17 ± 0.34	20.52 ± 0.41	0.062

[a]The data are presented as n (%) or the means ± standard error (SE). n = unweighted; N = the size of Korean population estimated using sample weights; physical activity level = low (<600 MET minutes per week), moderate (≥600-<3000 MET minutes per week), high (≥3000 MET minutes per week); hypertension = diagnosis and current usage of antihypertensive drug or ≥140 mmHg systolic BP, or ≥90 mmHg diastolic BP; HOMA-IR = [fasting plasma glucose] × [fasting insulin] ×0.055/22.5; HOMA-beta = 20 × [fasting plasma insulin / ([fasting plasma glucose] × 0.055-3.5); HbA1c = glycated hemoglobin; LDL-C = low-density lipoprotein cholesterol; HDL-C = high-density lipoprotein cholesterol
[b]The prevalence (%) are presented weighted value

than men in other groups. Men who had prediabetes and diabetes were more likely to be overweight or obese have hypertension; have higher fasting glucose levels, HOMA-IR index scores, HDL and LDL cholesterol levels, triglyceride levels, and alcohol consumption; and have lower HOMA-beta index scores, than those in the control group ($p < 0.05$). The control, prediabetic, and diabetic groups differed in terms of BMD based on the World Health Organization's criteria.

Association between BMD and DM status

The BMDs at various measured sites in the control, prediabetic, and diabetic groups were compared. Men with prediabetes and diabetes had higher lumbar spine and total hip BMDs than controls in the crude analysis. The prediabetic group had higher femoral neck BMDs than the control group. No significant differences in three BMD sites were found between the prediabetic and diabetic groups. In model 1, after adjusting for age and BMI, the prediabetic group had higher lumbar spine and total hip BMDs than the control group. After further adjustments for all clinically relevant covariates (model 2), the men with DM and men with prediabetes had higher lumbar spine, total hip, and femoral neck BMDs than controls. Similarly, no significant difference at three BMD sites were found between the prediabetic and diabetic groups in both models 1 and 2 (Table 2).

Baseline characteristics of the participants based on DM duration

Table 3 shows the baseline characteristics of the participants with diabetes duration of ≤ 5 years and those with

a disease duration of > 5 years. A total of 505 people were identified for type 2 DM duration: 235 participants with a disease duration of ≤ 5 years and 270 with longer DM duration. No significant differences between the two groups were found in terms of insulin-associated factors, BMI, fat mass, total cholesterol levels, and HDL and LDL cholesterol levels. However, longer DM duration participants were slightly older with a lower percentage of current smokers and had higher fasting glucose and HbA1c levels than those with shorter DM duration.

Association between BMD and DM duration

The BMDs at various measured sites were compared between the participants with DM duration of ≤ 5 years and those with disease duration of > 5 years. The group with longer DM durations had lower total hip and femoral neck BMDs than those with shorter DM durations in the crude analysis. The strength of the association between total hip BMD and DM duration declined after further adjustments; however, the group with longer DM durations had lower femoral neck BMDs than those with shorter DM durations in both models 1 and 2 (Table 4).

Discussion

In the present study, the prediabetic and diabetic groups had higher mean BMDs at all measured sites than the control group. The BMDs in men with prediabetes were similar to those in men with diabetes in all cases. However, men with diabetes with a disease duration of > 5 years had lower mean femoral neck BMDs than those with a

Table 2 Comparison of BMDs (g/cm^2) at various measured sites

	Men (n = 3383, N = 4 370 109)[c]			Normal vs. preDM	Normal vs. DM	PreDM vs. DM
	Normal	PreDM	DM	p-value	p-value	p-value
	n = 1702 (51.67%)	n = 1037 (29.76%)	n = 644 (18.57%)			
Crude						
lumbar spine (n = 3215)	0.928 ± 0.004	0.966 ± 0.006	0.973 ± 0.008	<0.001*	<0.001*	0.478
total hip	0.924 ± 0.003	0.951 ± 0.005	0.950 ± 0.006	<0.001*	<0.001*	0.872
femoral neck	0.751 ± 0.003	0.768 ± 0.005	0.762 ± 0.006	0.004*	0.091	0.448
Model 1[a]						
lumbar spine	0.923 ± 0.001	0.962 ± 0.001	0.967 ± 0.002	0.001*	0.006*	0.994
total hip	0.911 ± 0.002	0.940 ± 0.002	0.936 ± 0.003	0.014*	0.226	0.434
femoral neck	0.738 ± 0.001	0.757 ± 0.002	0.749 ± 0.002	0.228	0.702	0.222
Model 2[b]						
lumbar spine	0.922 ± 0.001	0.967 ± 0.002	0.969 ± 0.002	<0.001*	0.001*	0.765
total hip	0.912 ± 0.002	0.944 ± 0.002	0.939 ± 0.002	<0.001*	<0.001*	0.316
femoral neck	0.738 ± 0.002	0.760 ± 0.002	0.752 ± 0.003	0.046	0.034	0.707

[a]Model 1: adjusted for age and BMI
[b]Model 2: adjusted for age, BMI, alcohol consumption, serum vitamin D, smoke status, triglyceride, HDL-cholesterol, total cholesterol, hypertension, physical activity, and HOMA-IR
[c]The data are presented as means ± SE. n = unweighted; N = the size of Korean population estimated using sample weights
*P<0.0167 compared to 3 groups by Bonferroni's correction

Table 3 Weighted baseline characteristics of the diabetes group based on diabetic duration

	Men (n = 505, N = 618 430)		p-value
	DM duration ≤ 5 years	DM duration > 5 years	
	n = 235 (51.01)[b]	n = 270 (48.99)[b]	
Age (years)	60.45 ± 0.60	62.79 ± 0.64	0.008
Weight (kg)	70.25 ± 0.90	68.06 ± 0.69	0.054
Height (cm)	167.24 ± 0.56	166.33 ± 0.43	0.199
BMI (kg/m2)	25.06 ± 0.26	24.56 ± 0.21	0.132
Fat mass (%) (n = 495)	23.66 ± 0.43	23.58 ± 0.37	0.879
Low income (n = 497) n, (%)	79 (26.95%)	93 (34.15%)	0.124
Physical activity n, (%)[a]			
low	59 (21.82)	66 (27.29)	
moderate	95 (44.34)	115 (40.35)	
high	80 (33.84)	88 (32.38)	
	234	269	0.5099
Smoker (%)			
never	45 (18.62)	40 (12.41)	
past	100 (34.80)	153 (55.73)	
current	90 (46.58)	77 (31.86)	
	235	270	0.0005
alcohol (g/day)	15.96 ± 1.78	12.90 ± 1.61	0.204
Hypertension (%)[a]	34.98	30.29	0.201
fasting glucose	134.42 ± 2.98	144.06 ± 3.82[b]	0.047
fasting insulin (n = 432)	10.24 ± 0.49	10.66 ± 0.45	0.528
HbA1c (n = 488)	6.97 ± 0.09	7.54 ± 0.11	<0.001
HOMA-IR (n = 432)[a]	3.39 ± 0.21	3.70 ± 0.16	0.243
HOMAbeta (n = 432)[a]	67.94 ± 5.39	51.60 ± 17.91	0.383
total cholesterol (mg/dl)	175.71 ± 2.79	179.53 ± 3.21	0.37
HDL-C (mg/dl)	42.53 ± 0.78	41.79 ± 0.76	0.498
LDL-C (mg/dl)	98.73 ± 2.56	100.91 ± 2.58	0.549
Triglyceride (mg/dl)	172.25 ± 9.44	182.15 ± 9.12	0.365
serum vitamin D (ng/mL)	20.27 ± 0.55	20.60 ± 0.59	0.69

[a]The data are presented as n (%) or the means ± standard error (SE). n = unweighted; N = the size of Korean population estimated using sample weights; physical activity level = low (<600 MET minutes per week), moderate (≥600-<3000 MET minutes per week), high (≥3000 MET minutes per week); hypertension = diagnosis and current usage of antihypertensive drug or ≥140 mmHg systolic BP, or ≥90 mmHg diastolic BP; HOMA-IR = [fasting plasma glucose] × [fasting insulin] ×0.055 /22.5; HOMA-beta = 20 × [fasting plasma insulin / ([fasting plasma glucose] × 0.055-3.5); HbA1c = glycated hemoglobin; LDL-C = low-density lipoprotein cholesterol; HDL-C = high-density lipoprotein cholesterol
[b]The prevalence (%) are presented weighted value

disease duration of ≤5 years after adjustment for all clinically relevant covariates.

Asian people develop diabetes at a lower degree of obesity and at younger ages and experience chronic diabetic complications [18]. In addition, some studies in Japan [19] and Korea [20] have showed that Asian patients with type 2 DM have lower BMI and decreased β-cell function compared with European and American patients. Current study showed that each groups had similar BMI in overweight range, but not obesity. Therefore a study on the relationship between type 2 diabetes

and osteoporosis in Asian population would be good in isolating the effect of obesity.

The association between BMD and type 2 DM remains unclear. However, the results of the current study are consistent with those of previous studies in that DM patients have higher BMDs [21–23]. This study showed that men with prediabetes had higher BMDs than controls. Moreover, in this study, men with prediabetes and DM showed similar fasting insulin levels. Excessively high insulin level in the blood has been reported to be associated with increased bone mass [24] because of the

Table 4 Comparison of BMDs (g/cm^2) at various measured sites based on diabetes duration

	Men (n = 505, N = 618 430)[c]		p-value
	diabetic duration ≤ 5 years	diabetic duration > 5 years	
	n=235(51.01)	n=270(48.99)	
Crude			
lumbar spine (n = 481)	0.979 ± 0.013	0.977 ± 0.012	0.906
total hip	0.968 ± 0.009	0.940 ± 0.008	0.026*
femoral neck	0.786 ± 0.009	0.746 ± 0.008	0.001*
Model 1[a]			
lumbar spine	0.976 ± 0.002	0.976 ± 0.002	0.914
total hip	0.953 ± 0.004	0.930 ± 0.003	0.258
femoral neck	0.770 ± 0.004	0.735 ± 0.003	0.026*
Model 2[b]			
lumbar spine	0.976 ± 0.003	0.977 ± 0.003	0.896
total hip	0.955 ± 0.005	0.933 ± 0.004	0.337
femoral neck	0.773 ± 0.004	0.738 ± 0.004	0.018*

[a]Model 1: adjusted for age and BMI
[b]Model 2: adjusted for age, BMI, alcohol consumption, serum vitamin D, smoke status, triglyceride, HDL-cholesterol, total cholesterol, hypertension, physical activity, and HOMA-IR
[c]Data are presented as means ± SE. n = unweighted; N = the size of Korean population estimated using sample weights.
*Statistically significant (p<0.05) on the basis of the multivariable linear regression test

anabolic effects of insulin [25] and increase in free sex hormone levels [26]. Although prediabetes is not considered a disease, insulin resistance in prediabetes will affect bone mass and microstructure [12].

Bone fragility results from decreased BMD and alterations in bone microstructure [3]. Assessing the macrogeometry of cortical bone and the microarchitecture of the trabecular bone is difficult owing to the use of quantitative CT or MRI. In clinical setting, the gold standard of bone strength measurement is DXA and BMD remains a significant predictor of fracture risk in type 2 DM, that is, independent of trabecular bone score and DM itself [27].

Elevated fasting insulin levels play a key role in DM development, and they mostly result in increased bone mass. In complicated conditions, such as advanced type 2 DM, elevated insulin levels have an unexpected effect. As insulin resistance increases, the fasting insulin levels are inversely related to BMD, and this relationship becomes more significant as the degree of insulin resistance increases [12]. In advanced type 2 DM requiring insulin, pancreatic ß- cell function certainly decreased. However, the exact timing of this phenomenon remains to be determined. A Korean prospective cohort study [20] reported on the role of ß-cell dysfunction on DM development, focusing on Asian populations. Insulin levels possibly increased and then decreased at some point, and the bone density may have become weak at this point.

In the present study, insulin levels were similar in prediabetes and diabetes and in two groups with different duration

of disease. It was significantly different that fasting glucose levels in prediabetes and diabetes, and HbA1c levels between men with diabetes duration of ≤5 years and those with diabetes duration > 5 years. High blood glucose induces formation of advanced glycation end-products (AGE), with negative effects on structural proteins such as type I collagen, the main bone matrix protein. AGE may also reduce bone strength by impairing bone formation [28]. Most of the recent studies have confirmed decreased levels of bone turnover markers in patients with DM [3]. The previous research on mechanisms of type 2 DM showed that action on bone with long-term high glucose levels could lower the turnover, resulting in unfavorable bone balance.

Researchers have generally neglected osteoporosis in men for some time, and many studies have focused on women as participants. One study showed that non-obese women with type2 DM had lower BMD than control participants matched for BMI [29]. In the present study, we investigated the correlation between BMD and BMI in the group with DM. Our results confirmed the absence of such a correlation. Obese patients with type 2 DM have increased BMD, and evidence indicates that older white women, but not men or black women, with diabetes exhibited more rapid bone loss at the femoral neck and total hip than those with normal glucose homoeostasis [30]. Type 2 DM has been associated with higher bone loss at the femoral neck than at the total hip in white women even after adjusting for weight loss. Although white women with type 2 DM had higher baseline BMDs, they still exhibited increased bone loss rate, particularly at the femoral neck, than those with normal glucose homoeostasis. This seemingly contradictory finding of higher cross-sectional BMD being associated with more rapid bone loss may reflect the net result of the positive effects of excessive weight and hyperinsulinemia on bones combined with the negative effects of longer diabetes duration [31].

Possible explanations for significant reduction of femoral BMD are existing literature on bone loss and cortical porosity. Pentosidine is the best-studied AGEs to date. The content of pentosidine in cortical and trabecular bone was higher in patients with femoral neck fractures than in age-matched controls [3]. These women with prior fractures have significantly lower femoral neck volumetric BMD, a trend towards larger bone volume and thinner cortices on quantitative CT, and higher serum levels of sclerostin than women with diabetes without fractures and nondiabetic controls with fractures(increases of 31.4% and 25.2%, respectively) [32].

Patients with type 2 DM have a significantly higher fracture risk than the general population [3, 5]. Men with type 2 DM have lower muscle mass and strength, contributing to the higher incidence of falls and fractures observed in type 2 DM patients [33]. Hip fracture is the most serious osteoporotic fracture, and our study shows that the femoral neck BMD was lower in the group with a DM duration of > 5 years than in those with a DM duration of ≤5 years. Previous studies showed that patients with type 2 DM have an increased fracture risk in the hip [5, 22]. Furthermore, another study revealed that women with a DM duration of ≥10 years have particularly high major osteoporotic and hip fracture risks [33].

This study used relatively large sample sizes representing national population-based data. The sample design and size were also estimated using the methods described in the KNHANES. Therefore, the results can be generalized to whole Korean diabetics. This study is the first to indicate decreased femoral neck BMD in long-time DM in Asia, which is consistent with the findings of previous studies. Current study demonstrated decreased BMD by DXA with duration of type 2 DM different from the earlier studies. However, several limitations should be considered when interpreting the results of this study. The intrinsic nature of cross-sectional design studies precludes this study from conclusively determining any potential causal relationships. The KNHANES was conducted annually, and the subjects were those who were not able to undergo DXA between 2008 and 2011, despite the introduction of DXA in 2008. This study did not consider the anti-diabetic medication in the group with DM; therefore, the effects of drugs are unknown. The reduction in BMD associated with type 2 DM duration requires further study. Five-year type 2 DM duration is a very short period to evaluate its effects on BMD. Moreover, femoral neck BMD decreased in participants with relatively short-term type 2 DM; thus, caution is needed when interpreting the results.

Conclusions

This study aimed to assess the association between BMD and type 2 DM status in middle-aged or older men based on a nationwide survey. DM duration was significantly associated with reduced femoral neck BMD in men after adjusting for associated factors, such as age, BMI, and serum vitamin D level.

Abbreviations

AGE: Advanced glycation end-products; BMD: bone mineral density; BMI: body mass index; BP: Blood pressure; CV: Coefficient of variation; DM: diabetes mellitus; DXA: Dual-energy X-ray absorptiometry; HbA1c: Glycated hemoglobin; HDL: High-density lipoprotein; HOMA-beta: Homeostasis model assessment: estimated beta cell function; HOMA-IR: Homeostasis model assessment: estimated insulin resistance; KCDCP: Korea Centers for Disease Control and Prevention; KNHANES: Korea National Health and Nutritional Examination Survey; LDL: Low-density lipoprotein; MET: Metabolic equivalent of task

Acknowledgments

We are grateful to all study participants for their contributions.

Authors' contributions

All authors read and approved the final manuscript. Conceptualization: MJ, HK, SL, JSK, BO. Data curation: MJ, HK, SL, SO.Formal analysis: MJ, HK, JSK, BO. Investigation: MJ, HK, BO. Methodology: MJ, SO, JSK, BO.Software: MJ, HK, SL, SO. Supervision: SO, JSK, BO. Validation: SO, JSK, BO. Writing – original draft: MJ. Writing – review & editing: SO, JSK, BO.

Competing interests

Miso Jang, Hyunkyung Kim, Shorry Lea, Sohee Oh, Jong Seung Kim, and Bumjo Oh declare that they have no competing of interest.

Author details

[1]Department of Family Medicine and Center for Cancer Prevention and Detection, Hospital, National Cancer Center, 323, Ilsan-ro, Ilsandong, Goyang-si, Gyeonggi-do 10408, Republic of Korea. [2]Department of Family Medicine, DDH Hospital, 60, Hi park 2-ro, Ilsanseo-gu, Goyang-si, Gyeonggi-do 10234, Republic of Korea. [3]Center for Health Promotion, Cheil General Hospital, 17, Seoae-ro 1-gil, Jung-gu, Seoul 04619, Republic of Korea. [4]Department of Biostatistics, SMG-SNU Boramae Medical Center, 20, Boramae-ro 5-gil, Dongjak-gu, Seoul 07061, Republic of Korea. [5]Department of Family Medicine, SMG-SNU Boramae Medical Center, 20, Boramae-ro 5-gil, Dongjak-gu, Seoul 07061, Republic of Korea.

References

1. Federation ID. *IDF diabetes atlas*. Brussels: International Diabetes Federation; 2013.
2. Johnell O, Kanis JA. An estimate of the worldwide prevalence and disability associated with osteoporotic fractures. Osteoporos Int. 2006;17(12):1726–33.
3. Napoli N, et al. Mechanisms of diabetes mellitus-induced bone fragility. Nat Rev Endocrinol. 2017;13(4):208–19.
4. Yamaguchi T, Sugimoto T. Bone metabolism and fracture risk in type 2 diabetes mellitus [review]. Endocr J. 2011;58(8):613–24.
5. Schwartz AV, et al. Association of BMD and FRAX score with risk of fracture in older adults with type 2 diabetes. JAMA. 2011;305(21):2184–92.
6. Willson T, et al. The clinical epidemiology of male osteoporosis: a review of the recent literature. Clin Eng. 2015;7:65.
7. McGuigan FE, Besjakov J, Åkesson K. Hip fracture in men—survival and subsequent fractures: a cohort study with 22-year follow-up. J Am Geriatr Soc. 2011;59(5):806–13.
8. Byrnes JP, Miller DC, Schafer WD. Gender differences in risk taking: A meta-analysis. Am Psychol Assoc. 1999;
9. Alswat K, Adler SM. Gender differences in osteoporosis screening: retrospective analysis. Arch Osteoporos. 2012;7:311–3.
10. Park EJ, et al. Prevalence of osteoporosis in the Korean population based on Korea National Health and nutrition examination survey (KNHANES), 2008-2011. Yonsei Med J. 2014;55(4):1049–57.
11. Kim Y, Kim JH, Cho DS. Gender difference in osteoporosis prevalence, awareness and treatment: based on the Korea National Health and nutrition examination survey 2008~ 2011. J Korean Acad Nurs. 2015;45(2)
12. Shin D, et al. Association between insulin resistance and bone mass in men. J Clin Endocrinol Metab. 2014;99(3):988–95.
13. Kweon S, et al. Data resource profile: the Korea national health and nutrition examination survey (KNHANES). Int J Epidemiol. 2014;43(1):69–77.
14. Lim Y, et al. Association of bone mineral density and diabetic retinopathy in diabetic subjects: the 2008-2011 Korea National Health and nutrition examination survey. Osteoporos Int. 2016;27(7):2249–57.
15. Friedewald WT, Levy RI, Fredrickson DS. Estimation of the concentration of low-density lipoprotein cholesterol in plasma, without use of the preparative ultracentrifuge. Clin Chem. 1972;18(6):499–502.
16. Matthews D, et al. Homeostasis model assessment: insulin resistance and β-cell function from fasting plasma glucose and insulin concentrations in man. Diabetologia. 1985;28(7):412–9.
17. Simonelli C, et al. Dual-energy x-ray absorptiometry technical issues: the 2007 ISCD official positions. J Clin Densitom. 2008;11(1):109–22.
18. Yoon K-H, et al. Epidemic obesity and type 2 diabetes in Asia. Lancet. 2006;368(9548):1681–8.
19. Morimoto A, et al. Impact of impaired insulin secretion and insulin resistance on the incidence of type 2 diabetes mellitus in a Japanese population: the Saku study. Diabetologia. 2013;56(8):1671–9.
20. Ohn JH, et al. 10-year trajectory of beta-cell function and insulin sensitivity in the development of type 2 diabetes: a community-based prospective cohort study. Lancet Diabet Endocrinol. 2016;4(1):27–34.
21. Ma L, et al. Association between bone mineral density and type 2 diabetes mellitus: a meta-analysis of observational studies. Eur J Epidemiol. 2012;27(5):319–32.
22. Vestergaard P. Discrepancies in bone mineral density and fracture risk in patients with type 1 and type 2 diabetes--a meta-analysis. Osteoporos Int. 2007;18(4):427–44.
23. Leidig-Bruckner G, et al. Prevalence and determinants of osteoporosis in patients with type 1 and type 2 diabetes mellitus. BMC Endocr Disord. 2014;14:33.
24. De Liefde I, et al. Bone mineral density and fracture risk in type-2 diabetes mellitus: the Rotterdam study. Osteoporos Int. 2005;16(12):1713–20.
25. Thrailkill KM, et al. Is insulin an anabolic agent in bone? Dissecting the diabetic bone for clues. Am J Physiol Endocrinol Metab. 2005;289(5):E735–45.
26. Dennison E, et al. Type 2 diabetes mellitus is associated with increased axial bone density in men and women from the Hertfordshire cohort study: evidence for an indirect effect of insulin resistance? Diabetologia. 2004;47(11):1963–8.
27. Leslie WD, et al. TBS (trabecular bone score) and diabetes-related fracture risk. s. 2013;98(2):602–9.
28. Napoli N, et al. The alliance of mesenchymal stem cells, bone, and diabetes. Int J Endocrinol. 2014, 2014.
29. Zhou Y, et al. Prevalence and predictors of osteopenia and osteoporosis in postmenopausal Chinese women with type 2 diabetes. Diabetes Res Clin Pract. 2010;90(3):261–9.
30. Schwartz AV, et al. Diabetes and bone loss at the hip in older black and white adults. J Bone Miner Res. 2005;20(4):596–603.
31. Sellmeyer DE, et al. Skeletal metabolism, fracture risk, and fracture outcomes in type 1 and type 2 diabetes. Diabetes. 2016;65(7):1757–66.
32. Heilmeier U, et al. Volumetric femoral BMD, bone geometry, and serum sclerostin levels differ between type 2 diabetic postmenopausal women with and without fragility fractures. Osteoporos Int. 2015;26(4):1283–93.
33. Majumdar SR, et al. Longer duration of diabetes strongly impacts fracture risk assessment: the Manitoba BMD cohort. J Clin Endocrinol Metab. 2016;101(11):4489–96.

13

Associations among IGF-1, IGF2, IGF-1R, IGF-2R, IGFBP-3, insulin genetic polymorphisms and central precocious puberty in girls

Hua-Pin Chang[1,2], Shun-Fa Yang[3,4], Shu-Li Wang[5,6] and Pen-Hua Su[7,8]*

Abstract

Background: Insulin and insulin-like growth factor (IGF)-1 coupled with growth hormone helps control timing of sexual maturation. Mutations and variants in multiple genes are associated with development or reduced risk of central precocious puberty (CPP).

Methods: We assessed single nucleotide polymorphisms (SNPs) in the *IGF-1, IGF-2, IGF-3*, IGF-1 receptor (*IGF1R*), IGF-2 receptor (*IGF2R*), and IGF -binding protein 3 (*IGFBP-3*) genes, and their association with demographics and metabolic proteins in girls with CPP. Z-scores of height, weight, and body mass index (BMI) were calculated with the WHO reference growth standards for children.

Results: IGF-1 serum levels of CPP group exhibited a higher correlation with bone age, z-scores of height and weight, and luteinizing hormone (LH) than those of control group, regardless of BMI adjustment. In the CPP group, height was associated with *IGF-2(3580)*, an adenine to guanine (A/G) SNP at position + 3580. BMI in the CPP group was associated with *IGF-2(3580), IGF1R*, and the combinations of [*IGF-2(3580) + IGF2R*], and [*IGF-2(3580) + IGFBP-3*]. Body weight in the CPP group was associated with the combination of [*IGF-2(3580) + IGFBP-3*] ($p = 0.024$). Weight and BMI were significantly associated with the combination of [*IGF-2(3580) + IGF2R + IGFBP-3*] in the CPP group. These associations were not significantly associated with z-scores of weight, height, or BMI. The distribution of these genotypes, haplotypes, and allele frequencies were similar between control and CPP groups.

Conclusions: These known SNPs of these IGF-1 axis genes appear to play minor roles in the risk for development of CPP.

Keywords: Insulin-like growth factor 1, Insulin-like growth factor 2, Central precocious puberty, Single nucleotide polymorphism, Insulin-like growth factor binding protein 3, Insulin-like growth factor receptor

Background

Precocious puberty (PP) is defined as early development of puberty in females and males (before 8 years and 9 years of age, respectively). The two types of PP, central precocious puberty (CPP) and pseudo or peripheral precocious puberty (PPP) differ in their etiology. Secondary sex characteristics of PPP develop early due to excessive hormonal secretion from reproductive tumors or adrenal hyperplasia, and PPP is considered gonadotropin-independent. In contrast, CPP is gonadotropin-dependent and involves the premature maturation of the hypothalamic-pituitary-gonadal axis which induces the early secretion of testosterone from boys' testes and estrogens from girls' ovaries. Although the cause of CPP is not elucidated in most cases, CPP can be associated with obesity, brain structural abnormalities, head injuries, and products that contain compounds which mimic hormones including cosmetic products, some insecticides, and some foods [1]. CPP causes early onset of menarche and initial breast development in girls, psychosocial challenges, and early epiphyseal fusion in bones which reduces further growth spurts and thus may lower final height.

---

* Correspondence: jen@csh.org.tw
[7]Department of Pediatrics, Chung Shan Medical University Hospital, Taichung, Taiwan
[8]School of Medicine, Chung Shan Medical University, Number 110, Section 1, Chien-Kou North Road, Taichung 402, Taiwan
Full list of author information is available at the end of the article

Treatment has the goal of preserving growth and height potential and can involve gonadotropin-releasing hormone (GnRH) analogs [2]. Treatment for CPP did not significantly affect the risk of cancer death, obesity, or metabolic disorders in 30- to 50-year-old women who had had CPP [3].

Environmental and metabolic factors may influence the initiation of puberty in 20 to 50% of cases [4]. Poor nutrition may delay puberty while obesity promotes earlier initiation of puberty in girls [5–9].

The hormones, insulin, insulin-like growth factor-1 (IGF-1), and growth hormone (GH) are linked to precocious puberty [10–12]. GH and the IGF signaling pathways play major roles in regulating endocrine secretions involved in growth and sex maturation. The complex IGF network involves several growth factors (IGF-1, IGF-2), high affinity insulin-like growth factor binding proteins (IGFBP3, IGFALS) and cell surface receptors (IGF-1R). Girls with CPP have higher insulin and IGF-1 blood levels than girls without PP [11–13]. In animal studies, insulin or IGF-1 stimulation augments GnRH secretion, confirming that insulin receptors (IRs) and IGF-IR are present on GnRH neurons. Furthermore, puberty is delayed in female mice lacking IGF-1R, but not in males [14], suggesting a role of IGF-1 signaling in timing of puberty in females.

Mutations in the *MKRN3* gene and the *KISS* gene are highly associated with CPP [15, 16]. However, the influence of the IGF axis genes on puberty in humans, especially CPP, is unclear. As tangential evidence, girls diagnosed with PP have a higher risk for developing breast cancer than girls without PP [17]. Abnormalities in the IGF signaling pathways affect progression of breast cancer [18].

The hypothesis of this study is that polymorphisms in one or more of the IGF genes may influence sex hormonal changes and affect the development of precocious puberty. Since members of the IGF family are involved in the onset of puberty, we aimed to identify polymorphisms in insulin (*INS*), *IGF-1*, *IGF-2*, IGF-1 receptor (*IGF1R*), *IGR2R*, and IGF binding protein 3 (*IGFBP-3*) that may alter the risk for development of central precocious puberty.

Methods
Study population
This two-cohort study assessed ≤8 year old girls who showed development of secondary sex characteristics and sought care in the genetic/metabolic outpatient department at the Hospital of Chung Shan Medical University. The study included a total of 489 girls with 264 girls in the CPP group, and 225 girls in the early puberty (EP) control group. During the study's implementation period, all girls received treatment and consultation. All girls were examined for bone age (BA), weight, and

height; their blood samples were collected for estradiol (E2), luteinizing hormone (LH), and luteinizing hormone-releasing hormone (LHRH) analysis; and their BA/CA (bone age/chronological age) ratio and BMI were calculated during their first visit. Follow-up visits occurred every 3 months.

Girls were diagnosed with CPP if the girls' bone age examination results were greater than their age growth, estradiol was ≥10 pg/ml, and highest LHRH and LH values were ≥ 10 ml U/ml [19]. Girls with CPP received consultation, health education, and treatment from a genetic/metabolic counselor. Eligibility criteria for the CPP group included continuing outpatient treatment at this hospital after outpatient examination and diagnosis with CPP.

Exclusion criteria for the CPP group consisted of refusal to sign a consent form or having a disease that may have caused CPP, such as a chromosome anomaly; a noncancerous tumor in the brain or pituitary gland, brain injury; an infection in the brain (e.g. meningitis); radiation or chemotherapy for cancer treatment.

If the girls' bone age, estradiol, LH, and LHRH test results did not fully meet the diagnostic standard in the first visit and they only had emergent secondary sex characteristics, they were considered to have EP. The girls with EP received consultation and health education from a genetic/metabolic counselor and continued to receive outpatient follow-up. Exclusion criteria for the EP group were a GnRH homolog treatment, failure to continue to receive follow-ups, refusal of family members to sign the participation consent forms, or the aforementioned diseases or treatments in the exclusion criteria for CPP.

Ethical considerations
The study protocol was approved by the Human Investigations Committee of the Hospital of Chung Shan Medical University before the study started. Because all participating girls were 8 years old or younger, the parents or guardians of the participating girls uniformly provided signed informed consent.

Bone age, body mass index (BMI)
Left-hand X-rays were performed on all subjects, and bone age (BA) was determined using the method of Greulich and Pyle [20]. Three replicate measurements of standing height were made using a wall-mounted stadiometer. BMI was calculated by dividing body weight (kg) by the square of height in meters (m^2). Tanner stage standards were used to assess breast and pubic hair development [21, 22].

Blood and data collection
After girls fasted eight-hours, blood specimens were collected for measurement of basal E2 (pmol/L), follicle

stimulating hormone (FSH, U/L), LH (U/L), growth hormone (GH), IGF-1, and insulin-like growth factor binding protein 3 (IGFBP-3).

GnRH test
After the subjects had fasted overnight, venous access was secured with a three-way stopcock and heparinized saline for the GnRH test. After baseline blood samples (2 mL) were drawn for LH & FSH or estradiol measurements, GnRH (range for children: 2.5 mcg/kg to 100 mcg/kg) was administered intravenously as a bolus. After 20 min and 60 min, blood samples (2 mL) for LH & FSH assessments were drawn and serum was harvested [23, 24].

Immunoassays
Serum E2 levels were measured using a commercial radioimmunoassay kit (Diagnostic Systems Laboratories). Sensitivity was 2.2 pg/ml, with intra- and inter-assay coefficients of variation (CV) at 7.5 and 9.3%, respectively. Serum FSH and LH levels were measured by enzyme immunoassay (FSH: Abbott Laboratories, Rome, Italy; LH: Dade Behring, Milan, Italy). Sensitivity for both assays was 0.2 mIU/ml. Intra- and inter-assay CVs were 4.7 and 8.9%, respectively, for FSH, and 3.1 and 4.0%, respectively, for LH.

Quantification of serum GH, IGF-1 and IGFBP-3 levels
After acid extraction, serum GH, IGF-I and IGFBP-3 levels were measured using the commercial radioimmunoassay (RIA) kits (Diagnostic Systems Laboratories, Webster, TX, USA). The sensitivities were 0.01 ng/mL, 0.9 mg/L and 0.01 ng/mL for GH, IGF-1 and IGFBP-3, respectively. The intra- and interassay CVs were 5.3 and 5.7% for GH; 7.2 and 9.8% for IGF-1; and 5.8 and 8.2% for IGFBP-3.

Genomic DNA extraction
Venous blood from each subject was drawn into Vacutainer tubes containing EDTA and stored at 4 °C. Genomic DNA was extracted by QIAamp DNA Blood Mini Kits (Qiagen, Valencia, CA, USA) according to the manufacturer's instructions. DNA was dissolved in Tris-EDTA buffer (10 mM Tris (pH 7.8) and 1 mM EDTA) and then quantitated by a measurement of optical density at 260 nm. The final preparation was stored at – 20 °C and used as a template for PCR.

Polymerase chain reaction-restriction fragment length polymorphism (PCR-RFLP)
The IGF-1R, IGF-2, IGF-2R and INS gene polymorphisms were determined by PCR-RFLP assay. The sequences of primers used to amplify the related genotype and restriction enzyme for digestion as well as PCR

products after digestion were listed in Table 1. PCR was performed in a 10 µL volume containing 100 ng DNA template, 1.0 µL 10´ PCR buffer (Invitrogen, Carslbad, CA, USA), 0.25 U Taq DNA polymerase (Invitrogen), 0.2 mM dNTPs (Promega, Madison, WI, USA), and 200 nM primer (MDBio Inc., Taipei, Taiwan). The PCR products of gene polymorphisms were subjected to enzymatic digestion by incubation with related restriction enzyme for 4 h at 37 °C and were then submitted to electrophoresis in 3% agarose gels.

Real-time PCR
The IGF-1 + 1770, + 6093, and IGFBP-3 -202 genes polymorphisms were determined by real-time PCR assay. Real-time PCR based on VIC (green) and FAM (blue) fluorescent dyes were applied for accurate quantification of the target sequence. The sequences of IGF-1 + 1770, + 6093, and IGFBP-3 -202-specific primers and PCR conditions were listed in Table 1. Strength of fluorescence for each sample was detected in each reaction cycle and plotted the fluorescent values against cycle number. The quantity and polymorphisms of each gene were observed by the intensity and color of fluorescence.

Statistical analysis
Subjects' demographics and characteristics data were represented as mean ± standard deviations (SD). The height, weight, and BMI values were used to calculate the z-scores with the WHO Child Growth Standards for subjects 5 years and younger [25] and the WHO 2007 reference for ages 5 years to 19 years [26]. The comparison of the subjects' demographic and characteristic data between groups was performed using Mann-Whitney U test because the data were not normally distributed. Moreover, a Kruskall-Wallis test was conducted for to assess associations between two or more than two types of genotypes or combinations of genotypes and the subjects' demographic and characteristics data. A Spearman correlation analysis was applied for identifying the correlation between serum IGF-1 and IGFBP-3 levels with subjects' demographic and characteristic data; the coefficient of correlation r was calculated. A Pearson's correlation was also applied for the correlation analysis with adjusted subjects' BMI. All statistical analyses were carried out with IBM SPSS statistical software version 22 for Windows (IBM Corp., Armonk, NY, USA).

Results
This study enrolled a total of 489 girls who were classified into the CPP (n = 264) and EP control (n = 225) groups. Demographics and characteristics of CPP and control groups are summarized in Table 2. The mean chronological age of all subjects was 8.61 yrs. (SD = 1.36) and was not significantly different between groups. There

Table 1 Sequences of primers used to amplify related genotypes, restriction enzymes for digestion, and sizes of PCR products after digestion

Gene name	Primers	Annealing temperature	Enzyme	Polymorphism
IGF-1R[a]	5'-TGCTTTAATTACGGTTTCTTC-3'	60 °C	MnI I	G:132, 77, 50, 20 bp
	5'-GCTTTTCAGGAACTTTCTCTT-3'			A:132, 97, 50 bp
IGF-2				
+ 3123[a]	5'-CCCCAGGTCACCCCATGTGA-3'	65 °C	ApaI	G: 173, 63 bp
	5'-GGGCTGGAGGCAGCTGAGTG –3'			A: 236 bp
+ 3580[a]	5'-CCACCCCTTCTGGGAAGCTAAAAG-3'	56 °C	MspI	A: 122, 118 bp
	5'-CCCTCGGTCCTCCAGGAATGGACA-3'			G: 122, 118, 34 bp
IGF-2R[a]	5'-AACAATGGTTAAAGCCGGATTG-3'	67 °C	Nci I	A: 456 bp
	5'-GGCCCGGGTGCAGCCAGGCACTG-3'			G: 307, 149 bp
INS[a]	5'-GGGTCCCCTGCAGAAGCGTGGCA-3'	65 °C	PstI	T: 562 bp
	5'-CTCCCTCCACAGGGACTCCATC-3'			C: 470, 92 bp
IGF-1				
+ 1770[b]	5'-tagaatattatttatagtattaaac [a/g]aggttttactagatatgtagtaact –3'	60 °C	–	T:VIC dye C:FAM dye
+ 6093[b]	5'-acagataaaagatgtaagtagacag [c/t]ttgaggtttcagagtccctcctgc – 3'	60 °C	–	G: VIC dye A: FAM dye
IGFBP-3				
-202[b]	5'-tcgcccgggcacctgctcctcgtgc [g/t]cacgcccggagcccgggtcaccttg	60 °C	–	C: VIC dye A: FAM dye

[a]using PCR-RFLP methods; [b]using real-time PCR methods

Table 2 Demographic and clinical characteristics of CPP and control groups

Variables	Total (n = 489)	Control group (n = 225)	CPP group (n = 264)	p-value
Chronological age (CA), years	8.61 ± 1.36	8.75 ± 1.55	8.49 ± 1.16	0.199
Bone age (BA), years	9.70 ± 1.98	8.75 ± 2.14	10.51 ± 1.39	< 0.001*
BA/CA ratio	1.13 ± 0.18	1 ± 0.17	1.24 ± 0.08	< 0.001*
Age of onset, years	7.63 ± 1.18	7.99 ± 1.44	7.32 ± 0.77	< 0.001*
Height, cm	136.20 ± 10.76	131.3 ± 10.07	140.38 ± 9.5	< 0.001*
Z-scores of height[a]	130.12 ± 8.24	0.09 ± 1.02	1.86 ± 1.40	0.078
Weight, kg	34.00 ± 9.44	30.44 ± 8.7	37.03 ± 8.99	< 0.001*
Z-scores of weight[a]	26.26 ± 3.24	26.26 ± 3.11	26.71 ± 3.33	0.137
BMI	18.02 ± 3.14	17.4 ± 3.3	18.55 ± 2.91	< 0.001*
Z-scores of BMI[a]	16.02 ± 0.58	16.10 ± 0.72	15.96 ± 0.41	0.008*
E2, pmol/l	32.74 ± 35.39	32.07 ± 48.24	33.31 ± 18.58	< 0.001*
FSH, U/l	14.40 ± 9.23	10.12 ± 8.03	18.05 ± 8.61	< 0.001*
LH, U/l	23.54 ± 30.70	5.62 ± 12.61	38.82 ± 33.23	< 0.001*
GH, ng/ml	3.43 ± 5.05	3.3 ± 5.22	3.55 ± 4.91	0.320
IGF-1, ng/ml	321.56 ± 125.87	257.46 ± 104.08	376.18 ± 116.88	< 0.001*
IGFBP-3, ng/ml	2282.02 ± 1167.12	1873.12 ± 1441.39	2630.51 ± 702.17	< 0.001*

*p < 0.05

[a]Z-scores calculated with WHO Child Growth Standards for children up to 5 years old [25] and WHO 2007 reference for children older than 5 years [26]

were significant differences between the CPP and control groups in most demographics and characteristics, except for GH levels (Table 2).

We assessed the correlation of serum IGF-1 (Table 3) and IGFBP-3 (Table 4) levels with subjects' characteristics. The serum IGF-1 level in the total population was positively correlated with most characteristics, especially bone age and LH. The IGF-1 levels in the CPP group showed a higher correlation with bone age, z-scores of height, z-scores of weight, z-scores of BMI, and LH compared to the control group. After adjusting for subjects' BMI which differed significantly between the control and CPP groups, the IGF-1 levels in the CPP group also showed a higher correlation with bone age, CPP onset age, z-scores of height and weight, and LH levels compared to the control group (Table 3). The correlations between IGF-1 levels and the different demographic and pathological features after adjusting for bone age are summarized in Table 5.

The serum IGFBP-3 level of the total population was significantly and positively correlated to bone age, BA/CA ratio, and FSH (Table 4). The serum IGFBP-3 level was positively correlated to FSH in the control group but not in the CPP group (Table 4), both prior to and after adjusting for the subjects' BMI (Table 4).

There were no significant differences in the distribution of genotypes and allele frequency of IGF1R, IGF-1(6093), IGF-1(1770), IGF-2(3123), IGF2R, IGF-2(3580), IGFBP-3, and insulin between the control and CPP groups (Additional file 1: Table S1). There were also no significant differences in genotype distribution of combinations of two SNPs in two distinct genes between the CPP and control groups (Additional file 1: Tables S2–1; S2–2).

We evaluated the association of demographic and pathological features with SNP genotype in both the control and CPP groups. In the control group, bone age was significantly associated with IGF1R (p = 0.033) and IGF-2(3580) (p = 0.046); E2 levels were significantly associated with insulin (p = 0.019); and the LH levels were significantly associated with IGF-1(1770) (p = 0.020). IGF-1 levels were significantly associated with IGFBP-3 (p = 0,014) (Fig. 1; Additional file 1: Table S3–1). IGF-1 levels were significantly associated with IGFBP-3 in the CPP group (p = 0.038) (Fig. 2; Additional file 1: Table S3–2).

We compared the association of demographic and pathological features with a combination of two genotypes in the control (Fig. 3; Additional file 1: Table S4–1) and CPP (Fig. 4; Additional file 1: Table S4–2) groups. For the control group, the serum IGF-1 level was associated with the combinations of [IGF-1(1770) + IGFBP-3] (p = 0.038), [IGF-1(6093) + IGFBP-3] (p = 0.013), and [IGF-2(3580) + IGFBP-3] (p = 0.036). The z-scores of BMI were associated with the combination, [IGF-2(3123) + IGF-2R] (p = 0.012) (Fig. 3). For CPP group, the age of onset was shown associated with combination [IGF-2(6093) + IGFBP-3] (p = 0.039) (Fig. 4). However, none of the other demographic or pathological features were significantly associated with the combination of two SNP genotypes (Additional file 1: Table S4–2).

Furthermore, we compared the association between demographic and pathological features and a combination of the IGFBP-3 genotypes with two additional genes, in the control (Additional file 1: Table S5–1) and CPP (Additional file 1: Table S5–2) groups. In the control group, there was a significant association between IGF-1 levels and the combination, [IGF-1(6093) + IGF1R + IGFBP-3] (p = 0.026), and [IGF-2(3580) + IGF2R + IGFBP-3] (p = 0.010). The z-scores of weight was associated with the gene combination, [IGF-2(3123) + IGF2R +

Table 3 Correlations of IGF-1 levels with demographic and pathological features with and without BMI adjustment by group

Variables	r with IGF1 (ng/ml)			[a]Adjusted r' with IGF1 (ng/ml)		
	Total (n = 489)	Control (n = 225)	CPP (n = 264)	Total (n = 485)	Control (n = 221)	CPP (n = 261)
Chronological age, years	0.275[c]	0.276[c]	0.466[c]	0.247[c]	0.259[c]	0.434[c]
Bone age, years	0.429[c]	0.172[c]	0.423[c]	0.386[c]	0.159[e]	0.390[c]
BA/CA ratio	0.292[c]	−0.015	−0.113	0.253[c]	−0.023	− 0.113
Age of onset, years	−0.019	0.141[e]	0.224[c]	0.053	0.225[d]	0.266[c]
Z-scores of height[a]	0.276[c]	0.160[e]	0.486[c]	0.289[c]	0.147[e]	0.411[c]
Z-scores of weight[a]	0.293[c]	0.151	0.475[c]	0.299[c]	0.120	0.435[c]
Z-scores of BMI[a]	0.263[c]	0.157[e]	0.464[c]	–	–	–
E2, pmol/l	0.165[c]	0.165[e]	0.273[c]	0.159[c]	0.164[e]	0.254[c]
FSH, U/l	0.045	−0.283[c]	−0.136[e]	0.037	−0.303[c]	− 0.115
LH, U/l	0.523[c]	0.172[c]	0.447[c]	0.496[c]	0.101	0.425[c]
GH, ng/ml	0.176[d]	0.281[d]	0.111	0.199[c]	0.297[c]	0.131[e]

[a]Adjusted r': correlation with adjustment for BMI
[b]Z-scores calculated with WHO Child Growth Standards for children up to 5 years old [25] and WHO 2007 reference for children older than 5 years [26]
[c, d, e]Correlations are significant at the 0.001, 0.01, and 0.05 levels (2-tailed)

Table 4 Correlations of IGFBP-3 levels with demographic and pathological features with and without BMI adjustment by group

Variables	r with IGFBP-3 (ng/ml)			Adjusted r' with IGFBP-3 (ng/ml)[a]		
	Total (n = 489)	Control (n = 225)	CPP (n = 264)	Total (n = 485)	Control (n = 221)	CPP (n = 261)
Chronological age, years	0.096[e]	0.148[e]	0.110	0.077	0.134[e]	0.100
Bone age, years	0.343[c]	0.266[c]	0.157[e]	0.314[c]	0.240[c]	0.148[e]
BA/CA ratio	0.360[c]	0.227[d]	0.096	0.335[c]	0.199[d]	0.098
Age of onset, years	−0.057	0.170[e]	−0.033	−0.102[e]	−0.053	0.009
Z-scores of height[b]	0.131[e]	0.171[e]	0.121[e]	0.012	−0.049	0.087
Z-scores of weight[b]	0.078	0.019	0.103	0.028	−0.023	0.087
Z-scores of BMI[b]	0.124[d]	0.170[e]	0.102	–	–	–
E2, pmol/l	0.042	0.043	0.018	0.036	0.041	0.012
FSH, U/l	0.395[c]	0.584[c]	−0.106	0.395[c]	0.593[c]	−0.102
LH, U/l	0.262[c]	0.274[c]	0.066	0.240[c]	0.308[c]	0.057
GH, ng/ml	0.026	−0.018	0.090	0.036	−0.005	0.093

[a]Adjusted r': correlation with BMI adjustment
[b]Z-score calculated with WHO Child Growth Standards for children up to 5 years old [25] and WHO 2007 reference for children older than 5 years [26]
[c, d, e]Correlations are significant at the 0.001, 0.01, and 0.05 levels (2-tailed)

IGFBP-3] (*p* = 0.035) (Additional file 1: Table S5–1; Fig. 5). The CPP group showed a significant association between age of onset and the combination [*IGF-2(3580) + IGF2R + IGFBP-3*] (*p* = 0.020; Fig. 6). However, none of the other demographic or pathological features were significantly associated with the combination of three SNP genotypes (Additional file 1: Table S5–2).

Discussion

Our findings showed that the IGF-1 serum levels of the CPP group exhibited a higher correlation with bone age, z-scores of height, z-scores of weight, and LH than those of the control group, regardless of adjustment for BMI. The height of the CPP group, but not the z-score of the

height, was associated with *IGF-2(3580)*. The BMI of the CPP group, but not the z-score of the BMI, was associated with *IGF-2(3580)*, *IGF1R*, and the combinations of [*IGF-2(3580) + IGF2R*], and [*IGF-2(3580) + IGFBP-3*]. The weight of the CPP group, but not the z-score of the weight, was associated with the combination of [*IGF-2(3580) + IGFBP-3*] (*p* = 0.024). The CPP group showed a significant association between weight and BMI with the combination of [*IGF-2(3580) + IGF2R + IGFBP-3*]. The distribution of genotypes and allele frequency in *IGF1R*, *IGF-1(6093)*, *IGF-1(1770)*, *IGF-2(3123)*, *IGF2R*, *IGF-2(3580)*, *IGFBP-3*, and *insulin* between control and CPP groups were similar. Likewise, the distributions of the gene SNP combinations were similar.

Table 5 Correlations between IGF-1 levels and demographic and pathological features after adjusting for bone age by group

Variables	[a]r'' with IGF1 (ng/ml)		
	Total (n = 489)	Control (n = 225)	CPP (n = 264)
Chronological age, years	0.016	0.143[e]	0.204[d]
Bone age, years	–	–	–
BA/CA ratio	−0.035	− 0.118	− 0.195[d]
Age of onset, years	− 0.170	0.143[e]	− 0.067
Z-scores of height[b]	0.021	0.145[e]	0.185[d]
Z-scores of weight[b]	0.041	0.109	0.244[c]
Z-scores of BMI[b]	0.069	0.015	0.233[c]
E2, pmol/l	0.112[e]	−0.141[e]	0.160[e]
FSH, U/l	0.049	−0.297[c]	0.040
LH, U/l	0.419[c]	−0.222[c]	0.362[c]
GH, ng/ml	0.159[d]	0.221[d]	0.080

[a]Adjusted r'': correlation with adjustment for BA (bone age)
[b]Z-scores calculated with WHO Child Growth Standards for children up to 5 years old [25] and WHO standards for children older than 5 years [26]
[c,d,e]Correlations are significant at the 0.001, 0.01, and 0.05 levels (2-tailed)

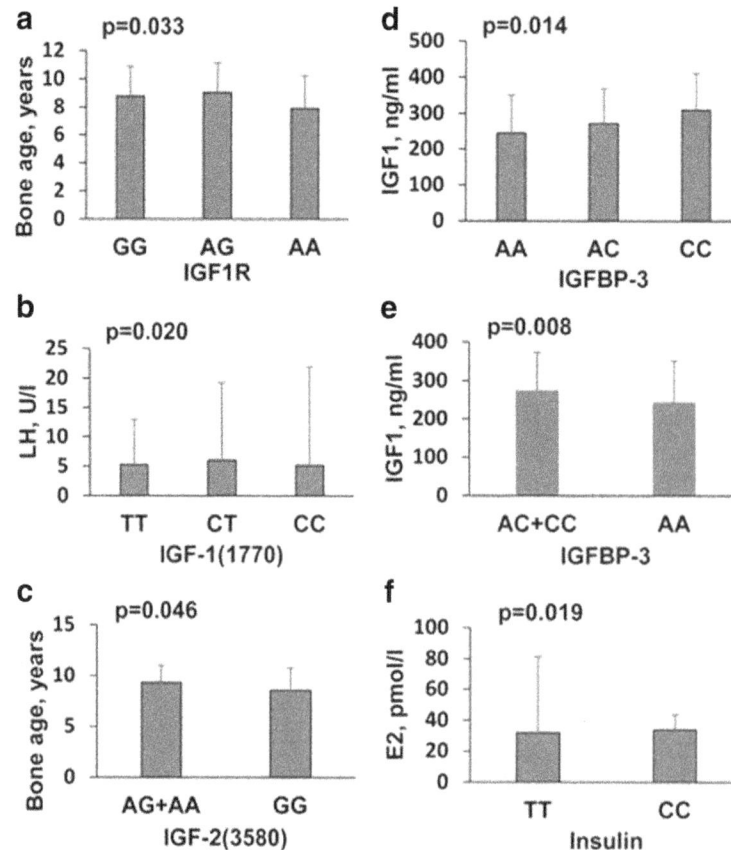

Fig. 1 Data were presented as mean +-SD given SNP genotype (**a**. Bone age v.s IGF1R; **b**. LH v.s IGF-1(1770); **c**. Bone age v.s IGF-2(3580); **d**. IGF-1 v.s IGFBP-3(AA, AC, CC); **e**. IGF-1 v.s IGFBP-3(AC+CC, AA); **f**. E2 v.s Insulin)

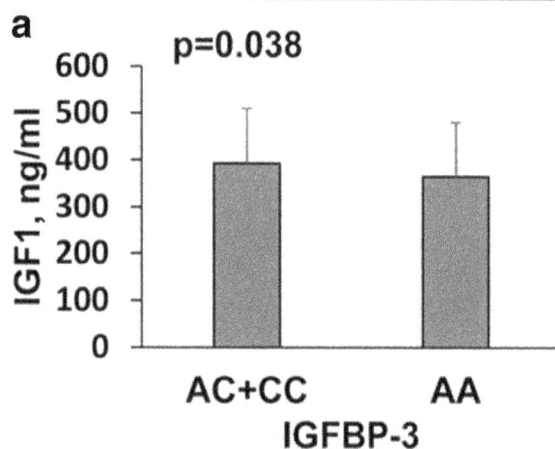

Fig. 2 Demographic and pathological features significantly associated with SNP genotype in CPP group. Data were presented as mean ± SD given SNP genotype and p-value was presented form difference among genotypes

A number of studies have previously investigated the relationship between various IGF family SNPs and variables such as age, BMI, and weight. The IGF family plays an important role in stimulating skeletal growth, cell differentiation and metabolism, and has been shown to influence body composition [27]. IGF-2 has been reported to play a role in fetal development, while IGF-1 is expressed after birth [28]. A polymorphism in the IGF-1 promoter was reported to be associated with IGF-1 serum levels, birth weight and body height in girls with CPP, as well as in adults. This polymorphism was also shown to be associated with higher body weight, BMI, fat mass, and waist circumference in young subjects [27]. A SNP in IGF-1R was shown to influence free IGF-1 plasma concentrations. This A → G variant was predicted to generate a silent mutation, E1013E, and was associated with higher IGF-1 concentrations in Italian adults [29]. Homozygosity for the A variant was associated with the lowest mean IGF-1 concentration, whereas heterozygosity was associated with a slightly higher mean IGF-1 concentration. Homozygosity for the G variant was associated with the highest mean IGF-1 concentration. These data suggested that IGF-1 concentrations were influenced by the IGF-1R genotype at codon 1013 [29].

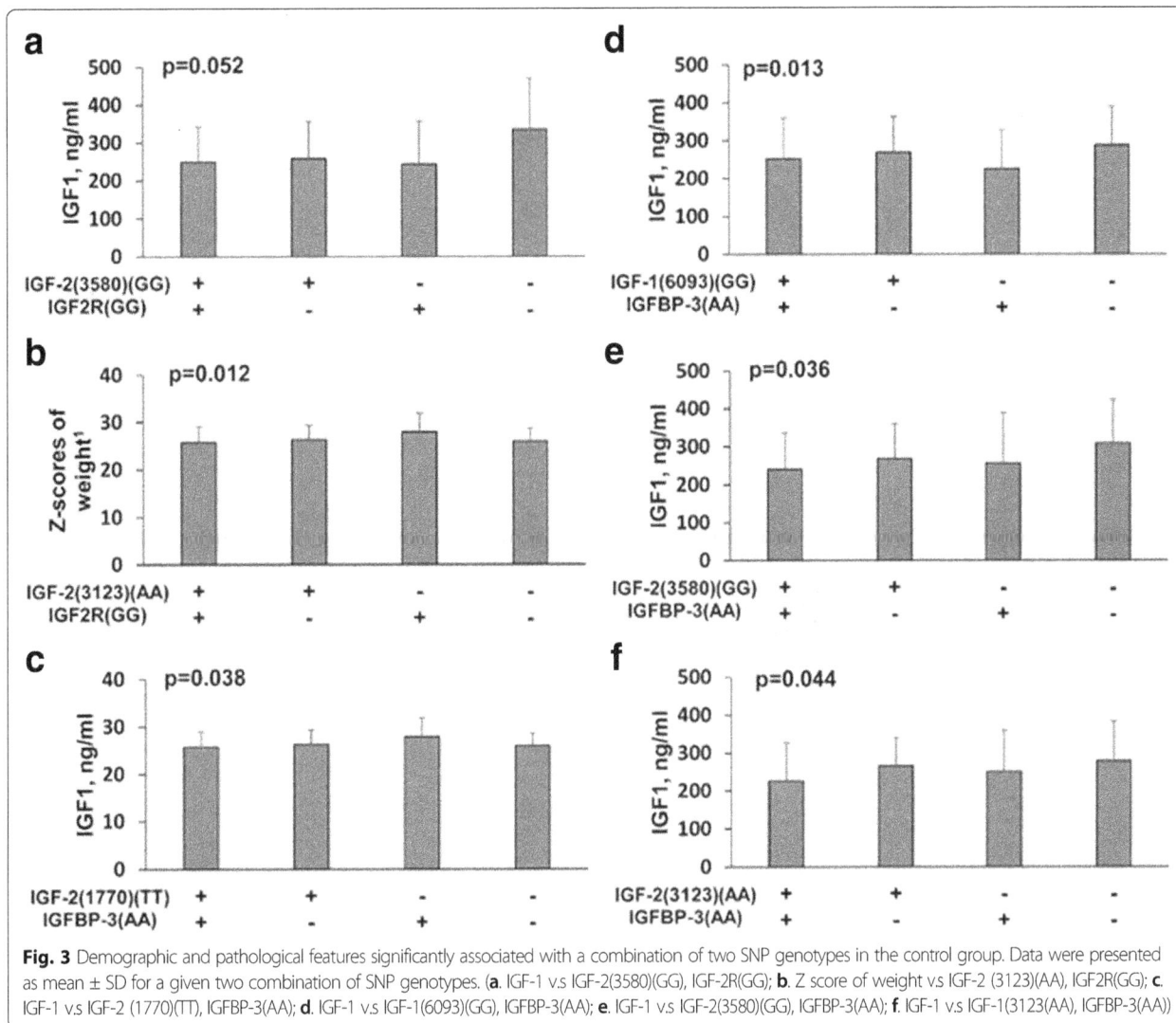

Fig. 3 Demographic and pathological features significantly associated with a combination of two SNP genotypes in the control group. Data were presented as mean ± SD for a given two combination of SNP genotypes. (**a**. IGF-1 v.s IGF-2(3580)(GG), IGF-2R(GG); **b**. Z score of weight v.s IGF-2 (3123)(AA), IGF2R(GG); **c**. IGF-1 v.s IGF-2 (1770)(TT), IGFBP-3(AA); **d**. IGF-1 v.s IGF-1(6093)(GG), IGFBP-3(AA); **e**. IGF-1 v.s IGF-2(3580)(GG), IGFBP-3(AA); **f**. IGF-1 v.s IGF-1(3123(AA), IGFBP-3(AA))

The AA, AG, and GG have been reported there have a dramatic difference in birth weight standard deviation scores (SDSs) in neonatal + 3123/ApaI genotypes of IGF-2 [30]. AA homozygotes had a mean birth weight SDS of 0.18 lower than that of GG homozygotes ($p = 0.01$), while

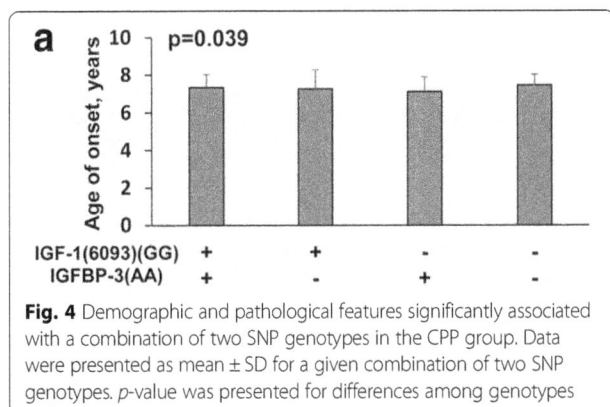

Fig. 4 Demographic and pathological features significantly associated with a combination of two SNP genotypes in the CPP group. Data were presented as mean ± SD for a given combination of two SNP genotypes. *p*-value was presented for differences among genotypes

heterozygotes showed an intermediate mean value. In contrast, there was no significant difference in birth weight SDSs between the AA, AG and GG maternal + 3123/ApaI genotypes. There was also no significant difference in birth weight SDSs between the AA, AG, and GG + 3580/MspI genotypes in both neonatal and maternal samples. However, the association between IGF-2 polymorphisms and size at birth remains controversial [30]. Analysis of the + 3123/ApaI genotype in 693 Hertfordshire adults showed that birth weight was highest for the GG genotype but the differences were not statistically significant [31]. Other data showed that the IGF-2 genotype was not significantly associated with BMI and/or birth weight in 294 healthy volunteers, but there was a statistically significant correlation between birth weight and BMI in subjects with the GG genotype whose birth weight was higher than 3.5 kg [32]. One reason for these different findings regarding the association between + 3123/ApaI polymorphism and size at birth may be differences in race and

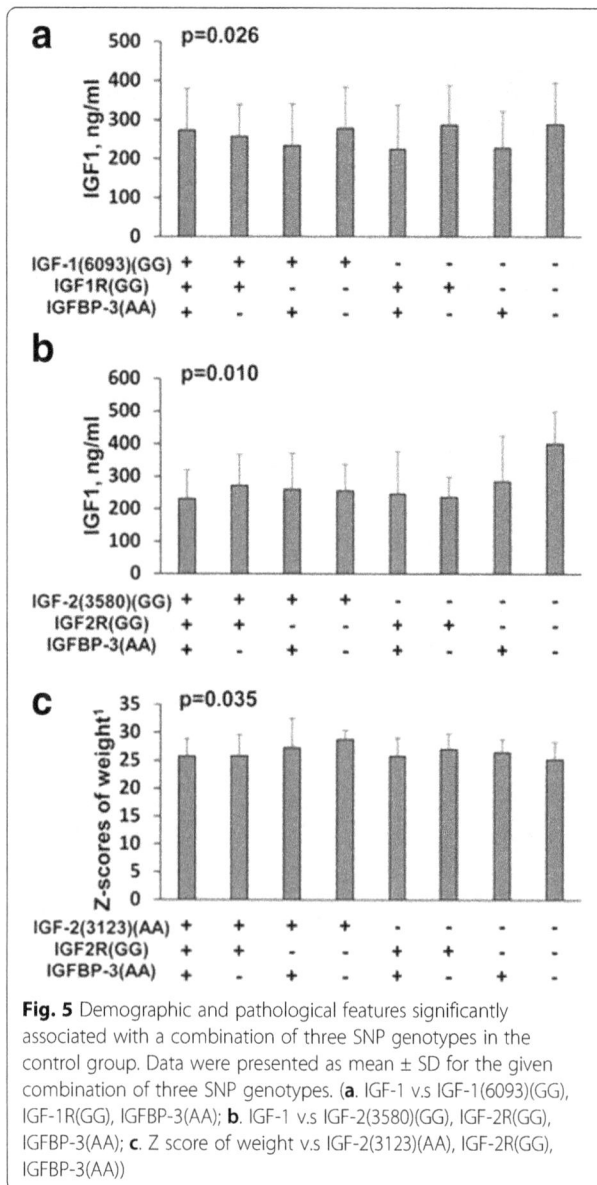

Fig. 5 Demographic and pathological features significantly associated with a combination of three SNP genotypes in the control group. Data were presented as mean ± SD for the given combination of three SNP genotypes. (**a**. IGF-1 v.s IGF-1(6093)(GG), IGF-1R(GG), IGFBP-3(AA); **b**. IGF-1 v.s IGF-2(3580)(GG), IGF-2R(GG), IGFBP-3(AA); **c**. Z score of weight v.s IGF-2(3123)(AA), IGF-2R(GG), IGFBP-3(AA))

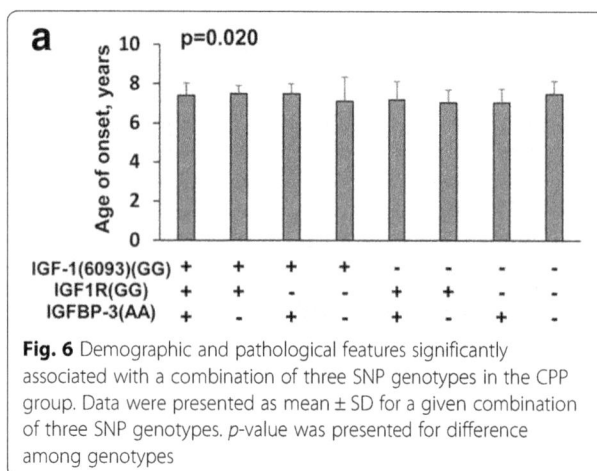

Fig. 6 Demographic and pathological features significantly associated with a combination of three SNP genotypes in the CPP group. Data were presented as mean ± SD for a given combination of three SNP genotypes. p-value was presented for difference among genotypes

size of the study population, or differences in handling of the somatoscopic characteristics [32].

A recent study found a significant difference between the experimental and control groups in the distribution frequency of the IGF-2 + 3580 polymorphism. Additionally, multiple regression model analyses showed that the presence of the IGF-2R AA or AG genotypes may exert a protective effect against hepatitis C [odds ratio (OR) = 0.35, 95% confidence interval (CI) = 0.15–0.82]. The combination of IGF-2 + 3580 AA genotype and IGF-2R GG genotype may be associated with a significantly lower risk of HCC (OR = 0.20, 95% CI = 0.05–0.87). No polymorphisms of any IGF genes were associated with liver-related clinicopathological markers in serum [33]. Comparison of allele frequencies between the premature pubarche (PP), hyperandrogenism (HA), and healthy control subjects showed a significantly higher frequency of the G allele in the PP group compared to the other groups, ($P = .0781$). However, allele frequencies were comparable in the HA and the healthy control subjects [34].

IGF-1 levels are significantly higher in girls of any age undergoing puberty than those in prepubertal girls. Our results suggest that the known variants in the genes of the IGF-1 axis play minor roles in the timing of elevation of IGF-1 and IGFBP-3 protein levels during puberty, similar to the role that SNPs in IGF-1 axis genes play in breast cancer [35]. In a similar manner, although the CPP group had significantly higher leptin levels than the control group, the differences in timing and expression level of leptin could not be explained by single nucleotide polymorphisms in either leptin or the leptin receptor [36].

The similar distribution of SNPs of the genes in the IGF-1 axis between CPP and control groups were in contrast to the skewed distribution of mutations and SNPs of four genes that were more prevalent in patients with CPP: the autosomal dominant *GPR54 R386P* mutation [37, 38], several polymorphisms (55,648,184; 55,648,186) in the *KISS1* gene [39], the intron 4 (TTTA)$_{13}$ repeat in the cytochrome *P450 19A1* gene *CYP19A1* gene [40], and a haplotype in the 5' promoter region of the *LH* β gene [41]. In addition, eight unrelated girls with CPP at age 6 had one of five novel heterozygous loss-of-function mutations in the makeorin ring finger 3 (*MKRN3*), which normally suppresses or delays GnRH secretion [42]. Conversely, the mutations and SNPs of four genes were less prevalent in patients with CPP than in controls: the polymorphism (55648176) in the *KISS1* gene [39], the AC haplotype of *Lin28B* in two positions (SNPs *rs4946651, RS369065*) [43], and the cytochrome P450 *CYP1B1 Eco571* variant (V432 L) [44]. In addition, leptin levels were significantly higher in the CPP group than those in the control group but SNPs in either the leptin receptor or leptin genes were not able to explain the differences [36]. Taken together, these studies indicate that multiple genes can influence the onset of puberty, and specific genotypes and haplotypes can increase the risk for development of CPP [39–43].

In our present study, we found no significant association between the SNPs evaluated and z-scores of height, weight, or BMI in either the EP or CPP groups. However, our data showed that the bone ages of subjects in the IGF-1R + 1013 (AG) and IGF-2 + 3580 (AG + AA) groups were more advanced in the EP group. This could possibly be because although the girls did not appear to have entered puberty, their bone age had already acquired the characteristics of puberty. It is possible that differences between our data and previous studies could be due to ethnic or other demographic differences in our study population. Although our data did not directly prove that IGF-1R and IGF-2 + 3580 were related to precocious puberty in girls, our results showed that the IGF-1R G variant and the IGF-2 + 3580 A variant were associated with CPP. In addition, we also believe that the interaction between IGF-I and IGF-II polymorphisms could play an important role, and warrants further investigation.

Some important limitations of this study were 1) healthy subjects were not included, 2) IGF-2 levels were not measured, and 3) the role of other genetic pathways which could play a role in CPP were not investigated.

Conclusion

In conclusion, specific genotypes from several genes (GPR54, *KISS, CYP19A1, and Lin28B)* can accelerate or slow the onset of puberty and have been associated with higher or lower prevalence in girls with CPP. The IGF-1 protein levels coupled with human GH levels affect timing of menarches [45–47]. This study showed that single SNPs of the genes in the IGF-1 axis (*IGF-1(6093), IGF-1(1770), IGF1R, IGF-2(3123), IGF-2(3580), IGF2R, IGFBP-3(– 202)*) did not appear to exert a significant role in the risk for development of CPP. However, several combinations were significantly associated with higher IGF-1 blood levels. Whether epigenetic modulation of the genes in the IGF axis plays a more prominent role in the risk for CPP than SNPs will require further research. Alternatively, other genes [37–40] or environmental factors [48, 49]) appear to play a more prominent role in triggering the development of CPP.

Additional file

Additional file 1: Table S1. Distribution of SNPs in *IGF1R, IGF-1(6093), IGF-1(1770), IGF-2(3123), IGF2R, IGF-2(3580), IGFBP-3,* and *insulin* in CPP and control groups. **Table S2–1** Summary of genotype distribution of two SNP combinations in two distinct genes by group. **Table S2–2.** (continued) Summary of genotype distribution in two SNP combinations in two distinct genes by group. **Table S3–1.** Associations between demographic and pathological features and SNP genotypes in control group. **Table S3–2.** Associations between demographic and pathological features and SNP genotypes in CPP group. **Table S4–1.** Comparison of associations between demographic and pathological features with two SNP genotype combinations in the control group. **Table S4–2.** Associations between

demographic and pathological features and two SNP genotype combinations in the CPP group. **Table S5–1.** Associations between demographic and pathological features and combinations of IGFBP-3 and two additional genes in the control group. **Table S5–2.** Associations between demographic and pathological features and combinations of IGFBP-3 and two additional genes in the CPP group. **Table S6.** Summary of the power for given control and CPP groups. (DOCX 144 kb)

Abbreviations

BA: Bone age; BMI: Body mass index; CPP: Central precocious puberty; CV: Coefficients of variation; E2: Estradiol; EP: Early puberty; FSH: Follicle stimulating hormone; GH: Growth hormone; GnRH: Gonadotropin-releasing hormone; IGF-1: Insulin-like growth factor-1; IGF-1R: Insulin-like growth factor 1 receptor; IGFALS: Insulin-like growth factor binding protein, acid labile subunit; IGFPB3: Insulin-like growth factor-binding protein 3; IRs: Insulin receptors; LH: Luteinizing hormone; LHRH: Luteinizing hormone-releasing hormone; MKRN3: Makeorin ring finger 3; PCR: Polymerase chain reaction; PP: Precocious puberty; PPP: Pseudo or peripheral precocious puberty; RFLP: Restriction fragment length polymorphism; RIA: Radioimmunoassay; SD: Standard deviation

Funding

This study was supported by Chung Shan Medical University Hospital (Grant No.: CSH-2015-C-017 and CSH-2016-C-029).

Authors' contributions

CH participated in the design of the study, performed in the acquisition of data and analysis and interpretation of data, helped to draft the manuscript. YS participated in the design of the study, performed in the acquisition of data and analysis and interpretation of data, helped to draft the manuscript. WS participated in the design of the study, performed in the acquisition of data and analysis and interpretation of data. SP participated in the design of the study, performed in the acquisition of data. All authors read and approved the final manuscript.

Competing interests

The authors declare that they have no competing interests.

Author details

[1]Department of Nursing, Asia University, Taichung, Taiwan. [2]Department of Nursing, Asia University Hospital, Taichung, Taiwan. [3]Institute of Medicine, Chung Shan Medical University, Taichung, Taiwan. [4]Department of Medical Research, Chung Shan Medical University Hospital, Taichung, Taiwan. [5]National Institute of Environmental Health Sciences, Zhuman, Taiwan. [6]The Department of Public Health, China Medical University, Taichung, Taiwan. [7]Department of Pediatrics, Chung Shan Medical University Hospital, Taichung, Taiwan. [8]School of Medicine, Chung Shan Medical University, Number 110, Section 1, Chien-Kou North Road, Taichung 402, Taiwan.

References

1. Berberoglu M. Precocious puberty and normal variant puberty: definition, etiology, diagnosis and current management. J Clin Res Pediatr Endocrinol. 2009;1:164–74.

2. Chen M, Eugster EA. Central precocious puberty: update on diagnosis and treatment. Paediatr Drugs. 2015;17:273–81.

3. Lazar L, Lebenthal Y, Yackobovitch-Gavan M, Shalitin S, de Vries L, et al. Treated and untreated women with idiopathic precocious puberty: BMI evolution, metabolic outcome, and general health between third and fifth decades. J Clin Endocrinol Metab. 2015;100:1445–51.

4. Palmert MR, Boepple PA. Variation in the timing of puberty: clinical spectrum and genetic investigation. J Clin Endocrinol Metab. 2001;86:2364–8.

5. Euling SY, Herman-Giddens ME, Lee PA, Selevan SG, Juul A, et al. Examination of US puberty-timing data from 1940 to 1994 for secular trends: panel findings. Pediatrics. 2008;121(Suppl 3):S172–91.

6. Biro FM, Khoury P, Morrison JA. Influence of obesity on timing of puberty. Int J Androl. 2006;29:272–7. discussion 286-90

7. Slyper AH. The pubertal timing controversy in the USA, and a review of possible causative factors for the advance in timing of onset of puberty. Clin Endocrinol. 2006;65:1–8.

8. Kaplowitz PB. Link between body fat and the timing of puberty. Pediatrics. 2008;121(Suppl 3):S208–17.

9. Kaplowitz PB, Slora EJ, Wasserman RC, Pedlow SE, Herman-Giddens ME. Earlier onset of puberty in girls: relation to increased body mass index and race. Pediatrics. 2001;108:347–53.

10. Veldhuis JD, Roemmich JN, Richmond EJ, Bowers CY. Somatotropic and gonadotropic axes linkages in infancy, childhood, and the puberty-adult transition. Endocr Rev. 2006;27:101–40.

11. Anderson CA, Zhu G, Falchi M, van den Berg SM, Treloar SA, et al. A genome-wide linkage scan for age at menarche in three populations of European descent. J Clin Endocrinol Metab. 2008;93:3965–70.

12. Veldhuis JD, Roemmich JN, Richmond EJ, Rogol AD, Lovejoy JC, et al. Endocrine control of body composition in infancy, childhood, and puberty. Endocr Rev. 2005;26:114–46.

13. Renehan AG, Frystyk J, Flyvbjerg A. Obesity and cancer risk: the role of the insulin-IGF axis. Trends Endocrinol Metab. 2006;17:328–36.

14. Divall SA, Williams TR, Carver SE, Koch L, Bruning JC, et al. Divergent roles of growth factors in the GnRH regulation of puberty in mice. J Clin Invest. 2010;120:2900–9.

15. Silveira LG, Noel SD, Silveira-Neto AP, Abreu AP, Brito VN, et al. Mutations of the KISS1 gene in disorders of puberty. J Clin Endocrinol Metab. 2010;95: 2276–80.

16. Abreu AP, Dauber A, Macedo DB, Noel SD, Brito VN, et al. Central precocious puberty caused by mutations in the imprinted gene MKRN3. N Engl J Med. 2013;368:2467–75.

17. Hamilton AS, Mack TM. Puberty and genetic susceptibility to breast cancer in a case-control study in twins. N Engl J Med. 2003;348:2313–22.

18. Mu L, Tuck D, Katsaros D, Lu L, Schulz V, et al. Favorable outcome associated with an IGF-1 ligand signature in breast cancer. Breast Cancer Res Treat. 2012;133:321–31.

19. Garibaldi L, Chemaitilly W. Chapter 556, Disorders of pubertal development. In: Kliegman RM, BMD S, editors. Nelson textbook of pediatrics. 2. 19th ed. Philadelphia: Elsevier Saunders; 2011. p. 1886–1894.e1883.

20. Greulich W, Pyle S. Radiographic Altas of skeletal development of hand and wrist. Stanford: Stanford University Press; 1999.

21. Tanner JM, Whitehouse RH, Takaishi M. Standards from birth to maturity for height, weight, height velocity, and weight velocity: British children, 1965. I. Arch Dis Child. 1996;41:454–71.

22. Tanner JM, Whitehouse RH, Takaishi M. Standards from birth to maturity for height, weight, height velocity, and weight velocity: British children, 1965. II. Arch Dis Child. 1966;41:613–35.

23. Wu FC, Butler GE, Kelnar CJ, Sellar RE. Patterns of pulsatile luteinizing hormone secretion before and during the onset of puberty in boys: a study using an immunoradiometric assay. J Clin Endocrinol Metab. 1990;70:629–37.

24. Yen SS, VandenBerg G, Rebar R, Ehara Y. Variation of pituitary responsiveness to synthetic LRF during different phases of the menstrual cycle. J Clin Endocrinol Metab. 1972;35:931–4.

25. World health Organization. WHO child growth standards length/height-for-age, weight-for-age, weight-for-length, weight-for-height and body mass index-for-age methods and development. Geneva, Switzerland: World Health Organization,; 2007.

26. de Onis M, Onyango AW, Borghi E, Siyam A, Nishida C, et al. Development of a WHO growth reference for school-aged children and adolescents. Bull World Health Organ. 2007;85:660–7.

27. Voorhoeve PG, van Rossum EFC, te Velde SJ, Koper JW, Kemper HC, et al. Association between an IGF-I gene polymorphism and body fatness: differences between generations. Eur J Endocrinol. 2006;154:379–88.

28. Randhawa R, Cohen P. The role of the insulin-like growth factor system in prenatal growth. Mol Genet Metab. 2005;86:84–90.

29. Bonafè M, Barbieri M, Marchegiani F, Olivieri F, Ragno E, et al. Polymorphic variants of insulin-like growth factor I (IGF-I) receptor and phosphoinositide 3-kinase genes affect IGF-I plasma levels and human longevity: cues for an evolutionarily conserved mechanism of life span control. J Clin Endocrinol Metab. 2003;88:3299–304.

30. Kaku K, Osada H, Seki K, Sekiya S. Insulin-like growth factor 2 (IGF2) and IGF2 receptor gene variants are associated with fetal growth. Acta Paediatr. 2007; 96:363–7.

31. Sayer AA, Syddall H, O'Dell SD, Chen XH, Briggs PJ, et al. Polymorphism of the IGF2 gene, birth weight and grip strength in adult men. Age Ageing. 2002;31:468–70.

32. Gomes MV, Soares MR, Pasqualim-Neto A, Marcondes CR, Lobo RB, et al. Association between birth weight, body mass index and IGF2/Apal polymorphism. Growth Hormon IGF Res. 2005;15:360–2.

33. Weng CJ, Hsieh YH, Tsai CM, Chu YH, Ueng KC, et al. Relationship of insulin-like growth factors system gene polymorphisms with the susceptibility and pathological development of hepatocellular carcinoma. Ann Surg Oncol. 2010;17:1808–15.

34. Roldan MB, White C, Witchel SF. Association of the GAA1013→GAG polymorphism of the insulin-like growth factor-1 receptor (IGF1R) gene with premature pubarche. Fertil Steril. 2007;88:410–7.

35. Canzian F, McKay JD, Cleveland RJ, Dossus L, Biessy C, et al. Polymorphisms of genes coding for insulin-like growth factor 1 and its major binding proteins, circulating levels of IGF-I and IGFBP-3 and breast cancer risk: results from the EPIC study. Br J Cancer. 2006;94:299–307.

36. Su PH, Yang SF, Yu JS, Chen SJ, Chen JY. Study of leptin levels and gene polymorphisms in patients with central precocious puberty. Pediatr Res. 2012;71:361–7.

37. Teles MG, Bianco SD, Brito VN, Trarbach EB, Kuohung W, et al. A GPR54-activating mutation in a patient with central precocious puberty. N Engl J Med. 2008;358:709–15.

38. Luan X, Yu H, Wei X, Zhou Y, Wang W, et al. GPR54 polymorphisms in Chinese girls with central precocious puberty. Neuroendocrinology. 2007;86: 77–83.

39. Rhie YJ, Lee KH, Ko JM, Lee WJ, Kim JH, et al. KISS1 gene polymorphisms in Korean girls with central precocious puberty. J Korean Med Sci. 2014;29: 1120–5.

40. Lee HS, Kim KH, Hwang JS. Association of aromatase (TTTA)n repeat polymorphisms with central precocious puberty in girls. Clin Endocrinol. 2014;81:395–400.

41. Zhao Y, Chen T, Zhou Y, Li K, Xiao J. An association study between the genetic polymorphisms within GnRHI, LHbeta and FSHbeta genes and central precocious puberty in Chinese girls. Neurosci Lett. 2010;486:188–92.

42. Macedo DB, Abreu AP, Reis AC, Montenegro LR, Dauber A, et al. Central precocious puberty that appears to be sporadic caused by paternally inherited mutations in the imprinted gene makorin ring finger 3. J Clin Endocrinol Metab. 2014;99:E1097–103.

43. Park SW, Lee ST, Sohn YB, Cho SY, Kim SH, et al. LIN28B polymorphisms are associated with central precocious puberty and early puberty in girls. Korean J Pediatr. 2012;55:388–92.

44. Matsuzaki CN, Junior JM, Damiani D, de Azevedo Neto RS, Carvalho KC, et al. Are CYP1A1, CYP17 and CYP1B1 mutation genes involved on girls with precocious puberty? A pilot study. Eur J Obstet Gynecol Reprod Biol. 2014;181:140–4.

45. Gamba M, Pralong FP. Control of GnRH neuronal activity by metabolic factors: the role of leptin and insulin. Mol Cell Endocrinol. 2006;254-255:133–9.

46. Sorensen K, Mouritsen A, Mogensen SS, Aksglaede L, Juul A. Insulin sensitivity and lipid profiles in girls with central precocious puberty before and during gonadal suppression. J Clin Endocrinol Metab. 2010;95:3736–44.

14

Quality improvement strategies at primary care level to reduce inequalities in diabetes care: an equity-oriented systematic review

Natalie Terens[1], Simona Vecchi[2]* iD, Anna Maria Bargagli[2], Nera Agabiti[2], Zuzana Mitrova[2], Laura Amato[2] and Marina Davoli[2]

Abstract

Background: There is evidence that disparities exist in diabetes prevalence, access to diabetes care, diabetes-related complications, and the quality of diabetes care. A wide range of interventions has been implemented and evaluated to improve diabetes care. We aimed to review trials of quality improvement (QI) interventions aimed to reduce health inequities among people with diabetes in primary care and to explore the extent to which experimental studies addressed and reported equity issues.

Methods: Pubmed, EMBASE, CINAHL, and the Cochrane Library were searched to identify randomized controlled studies published between January 2005 and May 2016. We adopted the PROGRESS Plus framework, as a tool to explore differential effects of QI interventions across sociodemographic and economic factors.

Results: From 1903 references fifty-eight randomized trials met the inclusion criteria (with 17.786 participants), mostly carried out in USA. The methodological quality was good for all studies. Almost all studies reported the age, gender/sex and race distribution of study participants. The majority of trials additionally used at least one further PROGRESS-Plus factor at baseline, with education being the most commonly used, followed by income (55%). Large variation was observed between these studies for type of interventions, target populations, and outcomes evaluated. Few studies examined differential intervention effects by PROGRESS-plus factors. Existing evidence suggests that some QI intervention delivered in primary care can improve diabetes-related health outcomes in social disadvantaged population subgroups such as ethnic minorities. However, we found very few studies comparing health outcomes between population subgroups and reporting differential effect estimates of QI interventions.

Conclusions: This review provides evidence that QI interventions for people with diabetes is feasible to implement and highly acceptable. However, more research is needed to understand their effective components as well as the adoption of an equity-oriented approach in conducting primary studies. Moreover, a wider variety of socio-economic characteristics such as social capital, place of residence, occupation, education, and religion should be addressed.

Keywords: Type 2 diabetes, Quality improvement strategies, Equity, Systematic review

* Correspondence: s.vecchi@deplazio.it
[2]Department of Epidemiology, Lazio Region- ASL Rome1, Rome, Italy
Full list of author information is available at the end of the article

Background

Diabetes is a complex, chronic disease recognized as an important cause of premature death and disability [1] and disproportionately affects socially and economically disadvantaged populations [2–4]. According the National Institute for Health and Care Excellence guidelines [5], patients with type 2 diabetes should receive a clear gamut of care to be provided by primary care providers. Annual routine monitoring of health indicators such as urinary albumin, BMI, cholesterol, blood creatinine, HbA1c and BP measured, eyes and feet examined and a smoking review, forms a major part of patient diabetes care. In addition patients should expect to receive an evidenced-based education and access to specialist healthcare professionals including ophthalmologists, podiatrists and dieticians.

Quality of care among diabetic patient can be influenced by a range of factors that has been already described. Previous systematic reviews showed that low individual socio-economic status and residential area deprivation are often associated with both worse process indicators and worse intermediate outcomes among patients with type 2 diabetes [6]. These differences are present even in countries with a significant level of economic development that have a universal health care system. Moreover, disparities in diabetes care exist among racial or ethnic minority groups, independent of economic status [7].

To improve diabetes care, it might be important to focus on quality management (QM), especially because the complexity of healthcare system and patients complexities has dramatically increased. QM comprises procedures to monitor, assess, and enhance the quality of care. In the last years many countries have developed quality improvement interventions (QI) to improve both patient outcomes and the quality of diabetes care [8, 9]. A meta-analysis of studies investigating QI strategies [10] found that interventions targeting the entire system of disease management (team changes, case management, promotion of self-management) along with patient-mediated QI activities were important components of strategies to improve diabetes care. However, the studies included in this review were targeted to the general population, irrespective of socio-demographic characteristics or socio-economic status.

Acknowledging the existence of such disparities, our aims are to: a) describe the extent to which effects on social inequalities are considered in randomized controlled trials (RCTs) evaluating the effects of QI interventions to improve quality of diabetes care and b) synthesize evidence on the effectiveness of QI strategies to reduce health inequities in diabetes care in the primary care setting. We conducted an equity-oriented systematic review including RCTs only, using an international taxonomy of QI interventions, and assessing the quality of included studies with a methodological rating tool.

Methods

For the purpose of the review, a "socially disadvantaged group" is defined by differences that place the group at distinct levels in a social hierarchy. To explicitly consider health equity and to capture characteristics possibly indicating disadvantaged status, we adopted the PROGRESS-Plus framework recommended by the Campbell and Cochrane Equity Methods Group and the Cochrane Public Health Group to identify studies with a focus on reducing health inequalities [11]. PROGRESS-Plus stands for place of residence, race/ethnicity/culture/language, occupation, gender/sex, religion, socioeconomic status and social capital. This systematic review was conducted in accordance with PRISMA-E 2012 (Preferred Reporting Items for Systematic Reviews and Meta-Analyses, Equity 2012 Extension), a validated tool to improve both the reporting and conducting of equity focused systematic reviews, were upheld in this review [12].

Data sources and searches

We searched all relevant biomedical databases such as Pubmed, EMBASE, CINAHL, and the Cochrane Library for relevant published RCTs and cluster-RCTs published in English. We limited the search from 1 January 2005 to 31 May 2016. A combination of MeSH terms and keywords were chosen to reflect selection criteria tailored to each database. Details of the full search strategy for PubMed are included in supplemental material (Additional file 1). In addition, we scanned the reference lists of relevant reviews to track relevant RCTs.

Study selection

Two authors (NT, AMB) independently screened all title and abstracts of all studies obtained from electronic searches. For studies meeting the inclusion criteria, we retrieved full texts and the same authors independently evaluated them for inclusion. Any disagreements were resolved through consensus or in discussion with the extended authorial group.

We used the "population, intervention, comparison, outcome, setting" (PICOS) logic to guide the systematic review (Additional file 2). We included randomized controlled trials (RCTs) and cluster-randomized trials, evaluating all QI interventions designed to improve health outcomes in social disadvantaged people with type 2 diabetes and designed to reduce inequalities in diabetes care. We considered studies that reported quantitative estimates of total effect of treatment and differential effects for the PROGRESS-Plus factors.

We used the Agency for Healthcare Research and Quality [13] taxonomy to identify QI strategies (Additional file 3). QI strategies can be delivered to specific levels of influence:

- Patient level (e.g. patient education, patient reminders, or promotion of self-management);
- Health care provider level (e.g. electronic medical record reminders, audit & feedback, cultural competency training);
- Health care system level (e.g. change in the health system structure or delivery, adjusting roles of care team members, nurse care management model).

Data extraction and quality assessment

Two authors independently extracted data (NT, SV), and disagreements were resolved by discussion. Data from multiple publications of the same study was considered as a single study. A data extraction form was designed to document the following study details: trials characteristics; participants (total number at baseline, age range, gender, clinical features); type of intervention and comparator; clinical and no clinical outcomes; timing; risk of bias; study results. For continuous outcomes, we extracted the mean change from baseline (with the standard deviation) and the mean difference, if available, with the corresponding 95% confidence interval (CIs). Relative risk (RR), and absolute risk differences, with the corresponding 95% CI, was extracted for binary primary outcomes. If studies reported data for more than one time point, we extracted data for the longest-term outcomes.

Baseline population characteristics relevant for addressing potential issues in health equity were extracted using the PROGRESS-Plus framework. We extracted data on outcome assessed, according to whether PROGRESS-Plus factors were considered as control variables (e.g., by adjusting in regression analyses) and the methods utilized to investigate differential effects (stratified analysis or modification/interaction analysis). We also extracted details on the duration of intervention, duration of follow up, health professional group involved, details of the strategy being implemented (i.e. modality, delivery format).

Two authors independently assessed risk of bias of included studies using the Cochrane 'Risk of bias' tool for RCTs [14]. We considering the following domains: sequence generation, allocation concealment, blinding of participants and personnel, blinding of outcome assessment, incomplete data, selective reporting, and other biases. For each domain, risk of bias was classified as "high," "low," or "unclear". Since we included cluster-randomized controlled trials, additional items were considered: (1) recruitment bias: did recruitment of diabetes patients take place before or after randomization of the clusters?, (2) did the intervention and control group differ in baseline characteristics?, (3) did any of the clusters drop out during follow-up, (4) was clustering accounted for in the statistical analyses? We investigated detection bias separately for objective and subjective outcome measures. We defined clinical and laboratory measures, process indicators, diabetes complications, hospital admissions, emergency admissions and all-cause mortality as objective outcome measures. We defined measures of self-management/adherence to recommendations as subjective outcome measures. With respect to missing data, we judged individual trials at high risk of bias if data from more than 10% of participants were not available. We used the quality criteria for descriptive purposes only to highlight differences between studies. We used RevMan 2014 software [15] to generate figures related to risk of bias.

Data synthesis

We synthesized findings from the included studies by intervention level (patients, health care provider, and health care system). The wide variety of interventions (in terms of mode of delivery, frequency and duration of follow up assessment) and population groups considered in the included studies did not allow for a meaningful meta-analysis to be conducted. We summarized results using narrative methods. We described in more detail studies reporting differences in QI interventions effects across subgroups.

Results

The search strategy generated 1903 citations after removing duplicates. Upon reviewing titles and abstracts, we retrieved full text articles for 247 studies that were screened by two authors independently (NT, AMB). We excluded 189 trials. Most common reasons for exclusion were not addressing a socially disadvantaged group, an evaluation of primary prevention intervention, and being conducted in a setting other than primary care. Fifty-eight RCTs met eligibility criteria. PRISMA Flow Diagram Fig. 1 shows the details of study selection process.

Overview of the included studies

A substantial synthesis of the characteristics of all 58 studies included in this review is reported in Table 1. Overall the majority of studies (n = 54) used a parallel RCT design while four trials were cluster RCTs [16–19]. Follow-up periods varied in duration from less than 1 month to 5 years, with the majority lasting 6 to 12 months. Most of trials were conducted in the USA (n = 47); the remaining studies were carried out in Canada [20], Asia [21], the United Kingdom [16], New Zealand [22], Australia [19], Trinidad and American Samoa [18, 23].

Almost all studies reported the age, gender/sex and race distribution of study participants. The majority of studies additionally used at least one further PROGRESS-Plus factor for the description of participants' baseline characteristics.

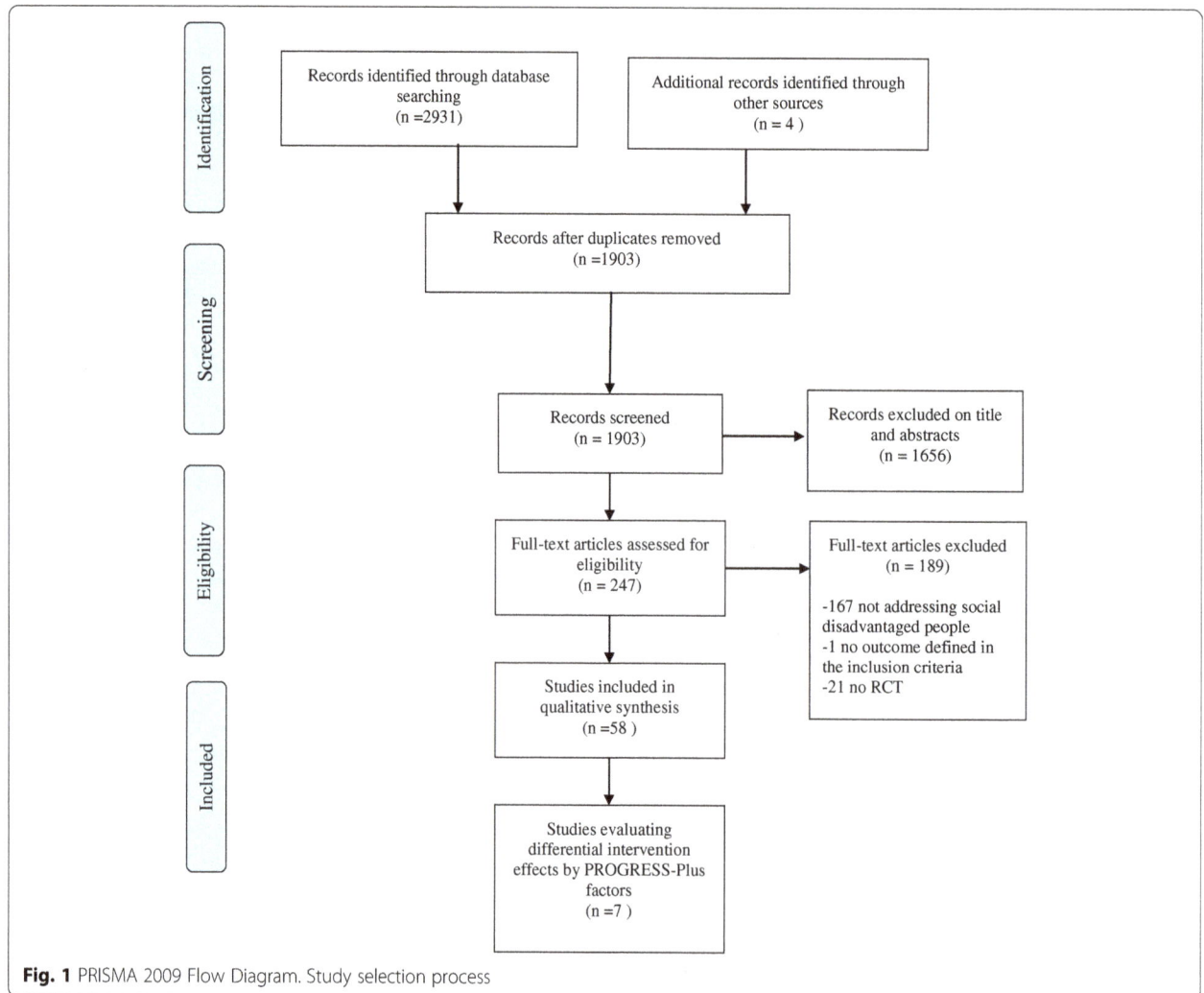

Fig. 1 PRISMA 2009 Flow Diagram. Study selection process

Among these, education was the most commonly reported factor ($n = 45$), followed by income ($n = 32$). Twenty-six studies considered at least one PROGRESS-Plus factor as control variable when measuring intervention effects (e.g., by adjusting in multivariate analyses). Again, age ($n = 23$) and gender/sex ($n = 20$) were the factors most commonly controlled for, followed by education ($n = 9$). Seven (12%) trials used at least one PROGRESS-Plus factors for examining differential intervention effects, and gender, age, race and education were those most often considered.

Detailed descriptions of the QI interventions were not always clearly provided in the trials. In order of frequency, were twenty-nine studies (50%) focused on interventions delivered at the patient level [17, 20, 21, 24–27, 29, 32–39, 41, 42, 55, 61–70], and twenty-six at the health care organization level (45%) [16, 18, 19, 22, 23, 28, 30, 31, 40, 45–54, 56–60, 72, 73]. The remaining three studies (5%) [43, 44, 71] described interventions at the provider level. In the majority of studies comparators were "usual" or "standard" care (69%), five studies reported waiting list,

delayed intervention or no intervention. Health professionals who participated in studies included physicians, specialist nurses, social workers, dietitians, diabetes educators, community health workers, general practitioners, practice nurses and home care nurses.

The majority of trials (96%) provided data on change in HbA1c. Thirty-seven trials (63%) reported BMI outcome; blood pressure and cholesterol data in 38 and 30 trials, respectively. Process measures including diabetic foot exam, dilated eye exam and attendance at office appointments were seldom reported.

For secondary outcomes, data were available for patient-reported measures including diet and physical activity ($n = 28$) using a considerable variety of instruments. Medication adherence and home glucose monitoring were measured less consistently (in 17 and 15 studies, respectively) as were diabetes complications and hospital admissions.

A detailed description of trials characteristics and intervention components by intervention level is presented in Additional file 4.

Table 1 Synthesis of the characteristics of the included studies by level of intervention and PROGRESS factors

Level of intervention	Patient level		Provider level		Health care systems level		Total QI strategies	
Total of studies	29		3		26		58	
	N	%	N	%	N	%	N	%
Sample characteristics								
Age	55.13	-	55.37	-	53.82	-	55.06	-
Sex, female (%)		64.05		58.69		57.84		60.20
Baseline HgA1c (%; mmol/mol)	8.88; 74	7.0–11.8; 53–105	9.53; 81	8.1–12.05; 31–109	8.51; 70	7.6–10.5; 60–91	8.88; 74	7.0–12.05; 53–109
Progress factors reported at baseline								
Place of residence	29	50	3	5.2	26	44.8	58	-
Race/ethnicity	26	49.1	3	5.7	24	45.3	53	-
Occupation	12	54.5	–	-	10	45.5	22	-
Gender/sex	24	46.2	3	5.8	25	48.1	52	-
Religion	–	-	–	-	–	-	–	-
Education	26	57.7	1	2.2	18	40.1	45	-
Socioeconomic status (SES)	–		–		–		–	
Income	20	62.5	–	-	12	37.5	32	-
Social capital	10	62.5	–	-	6	37.5	16	-
Age	28	50.0	3	5.4	25	44.7	56	-
Disability	–	-	–	-	–	-	–	-
Sexual orientation	–	-	–	-	–	-	–	-
Study characteristics								
Year of publication								
2005–2010	11	19	2	3.5	11	19	24	41.4
2011–2016	18	31	1	1.7	15	25.9	34	58.6
Study location								
North America	25	86.2	3	100	22	85	47	
UK	1	3.4	–	-	1	3.8	2	3.4
Australia	–	–	–	-	2	-	2	3.4
Asia	3	10.4	–	-	1	7.7	4	6.9
Duration of study (months)	10	3–26	4.5	0.25–36	12	6–60	8.9	0.25–60
Average sample size (range)	190 (56–526)		1573 (182–4138)		290 (65–1665)		684 (50–4138)	

Risk of bias in included studies

A summary of 'risk of bias' for each study and comparative data across the studies is reported in Figs. 2 and 3 . All studies were described as individual RCT ($n = 54$) or cluster-RCTs ($n = 4$). None of the randomized studies had uniformly low risk of bias. The allocation sequence was adequately reported in 48% of the studies (28/58), with random number tables or a computer-generated randomized list as the most commonly used methods. One study was categorized as high risk due to the use of a gender-based randomization procedure [24]. Most RCTs (40/58) did not describe or described in sufficient detail the allocation concealment to allow a judgment and were evaluated to be at unclear risk of bias.

In the majority of the trials, all participants were aware of the treatment they were receiving, and only eight studies blinded providers [20, 21, 25–30]. For studies reporting objective outcomes with standardized collection methods (e.g. automated blood test), we assigned a low risk of detection bias (79%), as knowledge of treatment assignment was considered unlikely to affect the outcome. Twenty-eight studies reporting subjective outcomes, those that used self-reported measures (i.e. questionnaire on dietary habits or physical activities) were at high risk of bias due to the lack of blinding of outcome assessment (24 studies). In the remaining 30 studies, independent research personnel who were not involved in the intervention performed outcome assessments, which we evaluated as low risk of detection bias.

Thirty studies were at low risk of incomplete outcome data due to a low attrition rate ($< 10\%$) or an intention-to-treat (ITT) analysis for primary outcomes.

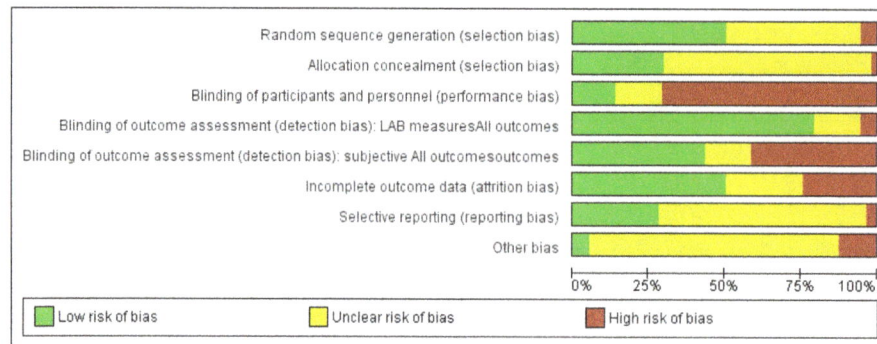

Fig. 2 Risk of bias graph

Thirteen studies were at high risk of bias because a high proportion of participants were lost to follow-up or were missing outcome measurements. Selective reporting bias was difficult to detect in most studies because published protocols were often unavailable. Most trials reported all outcomes. One study [30] collected a large quantity of baseline data but did not adequately describe follow-up data. One paper [31] did not report some subjective measures listed in the published protocol. Risk of contamination was high in most of the studies because patients receiving interventions and those receiving usual care or other interventions were seen within the same health center. Among cluster RCTs, three accounted for the effects of clustering in their results analysis.

Study evaluating the effect of QI strategies by intervention level (n = 51)

Patient level

More than half (n = 17) of the studies showed significant effect in at least one of the outcomes considered in this review; most (n = 11) of these interventions include group education sessions or visits and principles of self-management.

Twenty-seven out of 29 trials reported data on glycemic control measured as HbA1c level. Ten studies reported an improvement in HbA1c levels in the experimental group compared to the control group.

An education program based on telephone calls [32] was found to be associated with a decrease in HbA1c both in the unadjusted ($-0.23 \pm 0.11\%$ vs $0.13 \pm 0.13\%$, $p < 0.04$, $n = 526$) and adjusted analysis (MD = 0.40, 95% CI 0.10–0.70; $p = 0.009$).

Rosal et al. [27] evaluated a nutritionist or health educator-led self-management education program supported by counseling and a self-monitoring device. The study showed a difference between groups in HbA1c level at 4 months (MD = -0.53, 95% CI-0.92 to -0.14; $p > 0.008$, $n = 252$) but not sustained at 12 months.

An intensive training group intervention addressing both diabetes and cardiovascular diseases, combined with problem-solving training sessions [29], was effective in improving glycemic control (MD = -0.72, 95% CI -1.42 to -0.01, $p = 0.02$, $n = 56$).

Two studies (n = 265) showed an improvements in glycemic control as measured by HbA1c (8.2% ± 0.4 vs 8.6% ± 0.3, $p = 0.004$ and 7.6 ± 1.8 vs 8.2 ± 2.5; $p = 0.006$, respectively), comparing behavioral education programs via telehealth [33] or using a computerized self-management program [26] vs standard care.

Berry et al. [17] reported a greater improvement in HbA1c levels in low-income participants receiving sessions led by a multidisciplinary team than in the control group (7.6% vs 9.3%; $p = 0.001$, $n = 80$).

One study [21] found that an education program with incentives and self-monitoring devices produced a significant reduction in HbA1c (7.29% ± 0.58 vs 7.73% ± 0.57; $p < 0.05$, $n = 132$).

Philis-Tsimikas et al. [34] did not report difference between groups but a significant decrease of HbA1c from baseline to follow-up (-1.5%, $p < 0.01$) was observed in the experimental group.

Finally, two trials [35, 36] did not find a significant decrease in HbA1c in the study population, but reported a positive association for a subgroup of participants. Brown et al. [35] (n = 460) found that for those who attended ≥50% of the self-management patient education sessions, the reduction of HbA1c was -0.6% for the "compressed" group and -1.7% for the "extended" group. In Gerber et al. [36] (n = 244), the intervention resulted in significant improvement in HbA1c among low–health literacy subjects with poor glycemic control.

Eighteen trials reported data on change in BMI, three found a significant improvement in the experimental group.

Anderson-Loftin et al. [37] reported that the group exposed to the dietary self-management intervention had a decrease in BMI while the control group showed an increase in BMI control group (-0.81 kg/m2 vs $+0,57$ Kg/m^2; $p = 0.009$, $n = 97$). Tang et al. [38] reported a decrease in BMI in the intervention group receiving behavioral

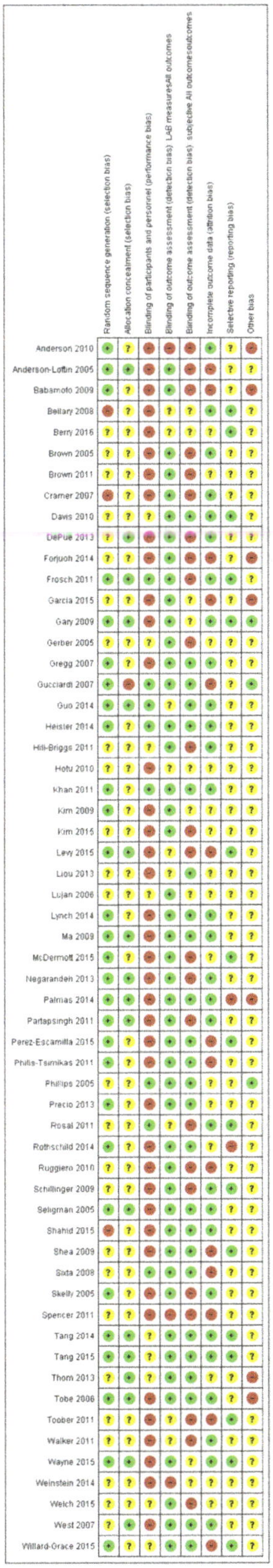

Quality improvement strategies at primary care level to reduce inequalities in diabetes care: an equity-oriented...

123

Fig. 3 Risk of bias summary

support delivered by a peer leader compared with the control group; the benefit was observed at different follow-up times and maintained at the longest one (15 months) (MD = $-$ 0.8 Kg/m^2 95CI%-1.6 to $-$ 0.1; $p = 0.032$, $n = 106$). Toobert et al. [39] showed a significant difference in BMI (MD of $-$ 0.40 Kg/m^2; $p < 0.05$, $n = 280$) in an underserved and high-risk Latino population treated with a long-term multiple-behavior-change program.

Fifteen of the 26 studies examining healthcare interventions in diabetes care considered blood pressure among the outcomes. Two studies showed differences favoring the experimental intervention. In the study conducted by Hill-Briggs et al. [29], participants receiving a self-management training adapted for low literacy experienced an individual improvement in DBP and SBP (median reduction = $-$ 7.17 mmHg, $n = 8$, median reduction of $-$ 14.67 mmHg, $n = 9$, respectively). Tang et al. [40] also reported a greater reduction in the group that received a combination of self-management and peer support interventions than the control group, both in SBP (MD = $-$ 10.0 mmHg (95% CI -17.6 to $-$ 2.4, $p = 0.01$) and DBP (MD = $-$ 8.3 mmHg (95% CI -13.2 to $-$ 3.4, $p = 0$ .001).

A significant improvement ($p < 0.001$) in hypertension in both groups was found by Shahid et al. [24] ($n = 440$) but between-group differences were not reported.

Eighteen studies reported data on diet adherence. Seven studies [22, 25, 31, 35, 39, 44, 51] observed between group differences although using different instruments and scales.

Anderson-Loftin et al. [37] used the Food Habits Questionnaire (FHQ) adapted for southern African Americans to measure dietary pattern. The intervention was a patient education program delivered by nurse case manager with nutrition focus combined with support groups, and weekly telephone follow-up. The authors reported a significant improvement in the experimental group with a decrease in high-fat diet while the control group continued previous high-fat dietary behaviors (MD =0.2 points, $p = 0.005$).

One trial [20] used the Summary of Diabetes Self-care Activities Questionnaire (SDCA) to assess the nutrition adherence in Canadian Portuguese-speaking adults. There was an improvement in self-reported nutrition adherence at 3 months in favor of the experimental intervention (MD = 0.42 ± 0.14, $p < 0.05$, $n = 87$).

Negarandeh [41] evaluated patient education program based on different format (Pictorial or teach back strategy) compared to usual care. Adherence to dietary pattern was measured through a self-structured nine-item scale. The score improved in all study participants ($n = 130$) in follow up measurements but the improvement was more pronounced for the intervention groups than the control group ($p < 0.05$). The mean difference between groups was $-$ 2.24 (95% CI- 2.67 to1.81) for the Pictorial format group, and – 2.52 (95% CI:-2.95 to – 2.09) for the Teach back format group.

A culturally tailored self-management intervention adapted for a low income Latino group [27], improved the quality of diet as measured by the Alternative Healthy Eating Index. Significant between group differences were found at 12 months (MD = 2.83 95% CI 0.58 to 5.08, $p = 0.014$, $n = 252$).

A similar intervention was evaluated by Shahid et al. [24] among people residing in rural areas in Pakistan. In the intervention group there was a significant increase in the proportion of participants compliant to the diet plan (17.3% at baseline to 43.6% at follow up, $p < 0.01$) while in the control group there was no significant increase (13.6% at baseline to 15.9% follow up, $p = 0.522$).

Weinstein's trial [42] assessed fruit and vegetable consumption self-reported daily following brief educational intervention. At 12 weeks, the percentage of participants who reported ever purchasing from a produce market increased significantly in the intervention group (81% vs 48%; $p = 0.003$, $n = 79$). Moreover, there was an overall decrease of the percentage of participants reporting difficulty affording fresh fruits and vegetables (55% vs 74% at baseline, $p = 0.008$). This decrease was not significantly different between arms.

Toobert et al. [39] reported the percent of calories from saturated fat measured using a food frequency questionnaire following a culturally adapted Mediterranean lifestyle intervention. He found an improvement of 0.33 points at the 24-month follow-up.

Provider level

Two studies evaluating reminder and reminder+feedback interventions [43, 44] showed an improvement in glycemic control (HbA1c) compared to the usual care or no intervention group (0.6% vs 0.2%, $p < 0.02$, $n = 399$; MD = – 0.80 $p < 0.001$, $n = 2046$, respectively). Both of these interventions utilized computerized systems to produce physician reminders. One study [43] found an improvement for LDL cholesterol for all intervention arms, with the greater change observed in the reminders +feedback group (– 18 mg/dl). No studies reported differences between intervention and control arms for blood pressure and BMI.

Health care system level

The majority of studies that evaluated interventions targeting the health care system ($n = 20$), showed significant effect in at least one of the outcomes considered in this review.

As far HbA1c, nine studies reported a significant reduction of HbA1c values [18, 23, 30, 45–50] with a mean difference ranging from – 0.29% to – 0.8%. The studies considered a range of health care system-based

strategies including interventions such as individualized case management activities [23], and culturally tailored counseling delivered by a CHW [46, 47, 49][2] and/or NCM [18, 45], and promotoras [50]. Three RCTs included additional activities, in particular home visits to support patient's progress [30, 47, 48].

Seven studies found a significantly greater reduction in HbA1c levels in the experimental group between baseline and follow up. One study [51] evaluating individual culturally tailored care provided by NCM and CHW compared to minimal care, showed a significant decrease in HBA1c levels. The effect was significant only in the group of participants receiving a higher number of home visits (– 0.68% vs 0.43%, $p = 0.03$, $n = 522$). Another study conducted with Korean Americans immigrants [52] found that a culturally tailored program including psycho-behavioral education, home glucose monitoring with tele-transmission, and bilingual nurse telephone counseling, was associated with a greater improvement in HbA1c values (– 1.3% vs – 0.4%; $p = 0.01$, $n = 79$).

A study conducted in a rural setting [53], showed an improvement in HbA1c levels among patients exposed to diabetes education with interactive online sessions, delivered by a multidisciplinary team (0.7 ± 1.3% vs 0.1 ± 1.0%; $p < 0.03$ after adjustment for baseline HbA1c, $n = 95$).

A significant decrease of HbA1c was observed following a case management program delivered by a CHW with the support of a clinical outreach team that included home visits [19] (– 1.0% vs – 0.2%, $p = 0.02$, $n = 233$). Lujan et al. [54] tested the effectiveness of a multi-component education program led by promotoras showing a mean change of HbA1c in the intervention group significantly greater than that of the control group at 6 months ($p < 0.001$, $n = 149$).

A multicenter study [55] considered a composite outcome measure based on the achievement of target values for HbA1c, SBP, and LDL. Participants assigned to the intervention arm (health coaching group) showed higher proportions of people reaching all clinical goals (46.4% vs 34.3%, $p = 0.02$, $n = 389$) compared to usual care.

A study evaluated an education program [56] supervised by a nurse specifically trained for case management (DPP Lifestyle Program) where participants in the experimental group also received an evidence-based medication algorithm. The authors observed a significant improvement in HbA1c levels in the experimental group compared to the control (– 1.87% ± 0.81 vs – 0.54% ± 0.55; $p = 0.011$). However, no information on sample size and participant characteristics were reported.

Significant differences in blood pressure were found between groups in three studies [16, 22, 45]. A difference in means of change from baseline in diastolic blood pressure significantly favored the intervention in a multicenter study [16] where participants received intensive disease management led by practice nurse supported by link workers and a diabetes specialist (adjusted MD = − 1.91 mmHg; $p < 0.001$, $n = 1486$). In the study of Hotu et al. [22], Maori and Pacific patients with diabetes and chronic kidney diseases who received twelve months of home visits by a nurse, achieved a significant lower systolic blood pressure compared to usual care group (149 mmHg vs 140 mmHg; $p < 0.05$, $n = 55$). In a long-term follow-up study [45] (60 months, $n = 1665$), a significant reduction in SBP (MD = − 4.32 mmHg, 95% CI -6.72 to − 1.92] and DPB (MD = − 2.63 mmHg, 95% CI -3.74 to − 1.52] was detected among ethnically diverse, medically underserved patients receiving a self-management intervention with the support of home telemedicine and a nurse case manager.

Of the 14 trials reporting BMI outcome, only one [45] showed an adjusted MD of 0.40 kg/m^2 (95% CI 0.20 to 0.60) when enhanced care through a diabetes-specialist nurse and link worker were compared to usual care.

One [56] of the two studies reporting data on weight change from baseline found a significant decrease at the end of the nine-month intervention of − 2.47 kg (±1.87) in the experimental group and + 0.88 kg (±1.84) in the control group ($p = 0.01$).

Seventeen trials assessed the impact of QI interventions on total cholesterol and/or HDL cholesterol, LDL cholesterol, and triglycerides. In three studies there were significant differences in change from baseline between groups.

At six months follow-up, Garcia et al. [57] reported statistically significant differences between the control and intervention group for total cholesterol ($p = 0.003$) and LDL cholesterol ($p = 0.014$), although not for triglycerides ($p = 0.179$).

A significant effect on total cholesterol and triglycerides was found in Kim et al. [52]. The intervention group showed significantly lower levels of total cholesterol (− 24.7 mg/dl vs 7.2 mg/dl; $p = 0.03$) and triglyceride (− 84.6 mg/dL vs − 4.2 mg/dL; $p < 0.05$) when compared with the control group. The intervention group also showed a trend toward a lower HDL, but this difference was not statistically significant ($p = 0.059$).

In Shea et al. [45], the intervention group experienced net improvement in LDL cholesterol level relative to usual care; a significant between groups difference was reported at 5 years (MD = − 3.84; 95% CI -7.77 to − 0.08).

Glucose monitoring was considered in four studies [19, 36, 46, 48]. The study conducted by McDermott et al. [19] showed that participants in the control group (waiting-list group) were more likely to self-monitor their glucose level than the experimental group.

Nine trials reported adherence to diet but measures and scores used varied between trials. Three studies found a difference between groups.

Babamoto et al. [58] found that the proportion of patients consuming two or more servings of fruits and vegetables daily increased significantly in the CHW and case management groups but not in the standard provider care group. Patients' self-reported intake of fatty foods decreased significantly from 29 to 16% ($p < 0.05$) in the CHW group but remained unchanged in the other groups.

Cramer et al. [56] used the Dietary Questionnaire to measure eating habits and observed a significant improvement in the experimental group compared with the usual care group ($p < 0.001$). Lynch et al. [59] also observed a significant increase in the number of days following a general and specific diet among participants receiving a culturally-oriented self-management program (MD = 1.9, 95% CI 0.6 to 3.1; MD = 1.2, 95% CI 0.2 to 2.2, respectively, $n = 61$), measured by the Block Food frequency Questionnaire.

Eight trials studied physical activity using different measures, and two reported an effect following the experimental intervention. One study [59] reported results from the CHAMPS (Community Healthy Activities model for Seniors) physical activity questionnaire modified for use among African Americans. At study endpoint there was a statistically significant difference between groups (MD = 2.517 Kcal/week; $p < 0.01$).

Comparing usual care with two educational programs provided by a different case manager (CHW or NCM), Babamoto et al. [58] found a significant improvement in physical activity with an increase from 28 to 63% ($p < 0.05$) in the CHW group, and from 17 to 35% ($p < 0.05$) in the standard provider care group, without any change in the case management group.

Six studies reported data on diabetes knowledge measured by validated instruments such as the Diabetes Knowledge Questionnaire [28, 54, 58], the Spoken Knowledge in Low Literacy in Diabetes Scale [57], and the Diabetes Knowledge Test [46, 52]. A significant improvement in patient's skills was observed in three studies [46, 54, 58].

In one out of three studies considering emergency and/ or hospital admissions [51, 58, 60], there was a reduction in emergency visits from baseline to 24 months among patients receiving a culturally tailored care provided by a NCM and a CHW (RR = 0.77, 95% CI, 0.59–1.00) [60].

One study [45] investigated the effect of telemedicine compared with usual care on all cause mortality but no differences between groups were reported (HR 1.01, 95% CI 0.82, 1.24).

Studies evaluating differential intervention effects by PROGRESS factors (n = 7)

Seven studies conducted sub-analyses to explore a differential intervention effects across PROGRESS-Plus factors ($n = 7$) and all were conducted in developed countries.

They used a parallel study design with a follow up of 12–24 months.

Table 2 gives the details of studies and results. Females, age ≥ 50, African-Americans and those with low education showed a better improvement in glycemic control. Patient education based on low-fat dietary strategies delivered by discussion groups and supported by phone contacts, produced a greater decrease in BMI, weight, and dietary behaviors among women than men [37]. At healthcare organization level, diabetes self-management supported by CHW was associated with a greater BMI reduction and an increase in exercise frequency among participants aged ≥50. One study analyzed intervention differential effect by levels of health literacy [36]. The experimental program aimed to supply information and promote diabetes self-management skills by computer multi-media including audio/video sequences. Among low literacy subjects with poor glycemic control, the authors found a greater decrease in HbA1C in the group exposed to computer multi-media education program than in the control group (– 2.1 vs. -0.3%, $p = 0.036$). No significant difference was found among high-literacy subjects. Moreover, the multimedia users with low health literacy demonstrated gains in knowledge, self-efficacy, and perceived susceptibility to complications compared with those having higher health literacy.

Discussion

Applying an equity-oriented approach, this review identified 58 RCTs (17.786 participants) evaluating QI strategies to improve the quality of diabetes care in a primary care setting.

Forty-seven studies were from USA and evaluated interventions specifically designed to reach population subgroups mainly defined on the basis of race or ethnicity. A narrow subset of these studies ($n = 7$) considered other dimensions of disadvantage as defined by the PROGRESS framework, such as socio-economic status and place of residence.

The RCTs included in this systematic review covered a wide assortment of QI strategies, varying from patient-mediated interventions with sessions of self-management supported by healthcare professionals, to provider education and other more complex programs based on changes in healthcare organization. Twenty-nine studies considered QI interventions conducted at the patient level, three at the provider level, and twenty-six at the health care organization level.

Pooling of results and quantitative synthesis was precluded by marked heterogeneity (mainly clinical), because study population, types of interventions, outcome measures, outcome assessment tools, duration of follow-up and risk of bias varied widely between studies.

QI strategies based on patient education and self-management strategies improved HbA1c levels among racial and ethnic minority participants but heterogeneity and complexity of interventions made difficult to identify the effective components of these interventions. The evidence on the effect of patient level interventions on improving other clinical and laboratory parameters, such as blood pressure, cholesterol levels and BMI, as well as self-management behaviours is scant. Few studies explored the effectiveness of other patient level strategies, including incentives and reminders. The only study included in this review [34] testing a rewards-based incentive intervention, showed effective results.

With regard to interventions at provider level, only one study reported a significant between groups difference in HbA1c reduction while no significant impact on blood pressure or BMI was observed.

Many of the studies included in this systematic review were designed to evaluate the effectiveness of changing, expanding, or integrating the roles of healthcare professionals combined with patient education to improve diabetes care and outcomes. QI interventions based on multidisciplinary teams including trained nurses or local community health workers providing culturally competent care, were associated with a significant reduction of HbA1c values. Changes in the role of health care professionals have been shown to produce an improvement in glucose control in ethnic minority communities on ethnic minority communities showed.

As far other primary outcomes considered in this review, a significant improvement in cholesterol levels was reported while n differences were found for secondary outcome measures, except for an increase in physical activity and diabetes knowledge.

Seven studies reported data on the differential effect by at least one PROGRESS factor. We did not find evidence of a differential effect by gender and race of any intervention on HbA1c levels reduction. One study reported an improvement in glucose control among a low literacy population subgroup, exposed to a culturally competent education program delivered through multi-media tools. We found some evidence of effectiveness of QI interventions in weight loss and BMI among females and weight loss among African-Americans.

In general, the heterogeneity of baseline HbA1c values and mean age of participants can affect intervention outcomes due to the biomedical challenge of lowering HbA1c from a higher baseline value. Moreover, some studies defined a minimum A1C value as inclusion criterion possibly considering patients which may not be representative of diabetic population receiving care in a real world clinical setting. Rather than implementing minimum A1C values for participant inclusion, as many of the studies reviewed incorporated, it is important (it may be worthwhile) to maintain the integrity of studying quality improvement interventions in real-life clinical

Table 2 Evidence synthesis on differential effect analyses by PROGRESS-Plus factors

Study, country	PROGRESS-factor	Intervention type	Outcome	Method of analysis	Overall intervention effect	Differential effect
Anderson 2010 [61] USA	Spanish speaking only, education level	Patient level Number of experimental conditions: 2 (1 intervention, 1 control) Intervention: • telephonic disease management (weekly, bi-weekly, or monthly) based on: 1. brief clinical assessment 2. self-management: including diet, exercise, stress reduction, smoking cessation, readiness assessment, and development of specific self-management goals 3. medication adherence 4. glucose monitoring and review of home glucose monitoring results • educational materials Personnel involved: nurse Control group: • Usual care at Community Health Center	A1c, DBP,SBP, BMI, LDL, diet behavior (BDA); physical activity (RAPA); depression measured Patient Health questionnaire (PHQ-9)	Subroups analysis and interaction analysis	No significant differences between groups for any outcomes *Retention rate* 79% vs 64%	*A1C* Spanish speakers (yes vs no) MD = − 0.10(− 0.53, 0.33) vs 0.35 (− 0.17, 0.88) Educational level: (high level vs low level) MD = 0.14(− 0.30, 0.57) vs 0.00 (− 0.52, 0.52) None of the interactions was significant
Anderson-Loftin 2005 [37] USA	Gender	Patient level Number of experimental conditions: 2 (1 intervention, 1 control) Intervention: • Education in low fat dietary strategies (4 weekly classes) • 1-h peer-professional discussion groups (5 monthly) • Additional educational support by phone (weekly) • Incentives for attendance Personnel involved: nurse case manager Control group: • Usual care including a referral to a local 8-h traditional diabetes class (information on nature and complications of diabetes) • Incentives for attendance	A1c, BMI, LDL, weight, dietary fat behaviors assessed by FHQ, physical activity, psychological status	Stratification by gender	A1c No significant differences Mean weight Significant effect I: - 4 lb. C: +4.2 lb. BMI I: − 0.81 kg/mm2 C: + 0.57 kg/mm2 MD = 1.38 kg/mm2 *p* = 0.009 Dietary behaviors (FHQ score) I: 2.5 ± 0.4 C: -2.6 ± 0.4 MD = 0.2 *p* = 0.005	Men *vs* women A1c No significant differences Mean weight Significant effect + 5.4 lb. vs − 1.5 lb.; MD = 6.9 lb. BMI + 2 kg/mm2 vs 0.16 kg/mm2 *p* = 0.02 Dietary behaviors Significant effect (FHQ score) − 0.24 vs − 0.17
Babamoto 2009 [58] USA	Age	Healthcare level Number of experimental conditions: 3 (2 intervention, 1 control) Intervention: • Group A, CHW program, Amigos en Salud (Friends in Health): education through individual session and monitoring services; individual	BMI, A1C, medication adherence, diet, physical activity, emergency department admission (ED)	Logistic regression models	Mean A1c Within group CHW = 8.6 to 7.2%; *p* < 0.05 CM =8.5 to 7.4%; *p* < 0.05 Standard care = 9.5 to 7.4%*p* < 0.05 No significant differences were found between groups	Patients aged≥50 were less likely to have reduced BMI at follow-up OR[a] = 0.4 (95% CI = 0.2–0.8) Exercise frequency[b] 3 times or more per week vs 2 times or fewer per week OR = 2.2 (95% CI = 1.1–4.1)

Table 2 Evidence synthesis on differential effect analyses by PROGRESS-Plus factors *(Continued)*

Study, country	PROGRESS-factor	Intervention type	Outcome	Method of analysis	Overall intervention effect	Differential effect
		sessions with participants and family member; telephone calls to participants to monitor self-management, to help participants improve their diabetes self-management skills • Group B, case management: education from two linguistically competent and culturally sensitive. Patients case management were usually seen on a monthly basis + follow-up calls. Personnel involved: bilingual, trained community health workers, nurse case manager Setting: Community, home, clinic Control group Standard Provider Care: standardized clinical care by physicians and nurse practitioners, without case management or CHW services			BMI Significantly greater decrease for the CHW group compared with the standard care group OR = 2.9 (95% CI 1.1–6.6) ED Change from baseline CHW: total visit decrease 11% Case management: total visit increase 40% Standard care: increase 15% between groups at 6-month follow-up $p < 0.05$ Diet CHW group were more likely (OR = 2.43; 95% CI =1. 13–5.23) to report having two or more servings of fresh fruit per day than standard care Physical activity CHW group was more likely (OR = 2.87, 95% CI = 1.34–6.17) than standard care to report exercising three or more times per week	
Brown, 2011 [63] USA	Gender	Patient level Number of experimental conditions: 2 (1 intervention, 1 control) Intervention: • Diabetes self-management education (DSME) including 8 consecutive weeks of education followed by a support group session at 3 and 6 months • Experienced NCM providing: culturally tailored diabetes self-management education; individualized health guidance and assistance with overcoming cultural and environmental barriers to improving health; guidance on locating, accessing, and navigating healthcare services; enhanced coordination of health care and communication with physicians and other healthcare providers • Random observations visits	A1c, FBG, lipids, BP, BMI, diabetes-related knowledge, health behaviors (physical activity, dietary intake, glucose monitoring)	Interaction terms in hierarchical linear and nonlinear models to test for differential impact of treatment by gender	Over time, both the experimental and control groups showed improvements in FBG levels at three and At six months For A1c the control group had greater clinical improvements at both intervals Self-reported physical activity and fat intake Improvement for both experimental and control groups	FBG, BMI: No significant differences between gender The rate of change in A1c over time did not differ significantly by gender (coefficient^ = − 0.06, t ratio = 0.25, $p = 0.806$)

Table 2 Evidence synthesis on differential effect analyses by PROGRESS-Plus factors (Continued)

Study, country	PROGRESS-factor	Intervention type	Outcome	Method of analysis	Overall intervention effect	Differential effect
Forjuoh 2014 [64] USA	Race/ethnicity	Personnel involved: bilingual NCM, nurses, dietitians, and CHWs Control Group: DSME intervention only. Patient level Number of experimental conditions: 4 (3 intervention, 1 control) Intervention: • Group A. self-management through personal digit assistant (PDA). Dia betes Pilot Chronic Disease Self Management Program (CDSMP): 6 week group education program to increase self efficacy • Group B. self-management through PDA • Group C. combination of A + B Personnel involved: trained facilitator, project coordinators Setting: outpatient clinic, community Control group: usual clinical diabetes care, along with patient education materials	A1C, physical activity, BMI, BP, diet	Interaction terms in multilevel models to test for differential impact of treatment by race/ethnicity	BMI and BP: Modest reductions from baseline to 12 months of follow-up for all four groups. No significant difference for other outcomes. Self care activities: Hispanic washing feet significantly more than other racial/ethnic groups (P = 0.02) Retention rate: CDSMP: 85%; PDA 64%, CDSMP + PDA 64%; Control 78%	A1c Modest reductions occurred in A1c from baseline to 12 months of follow-up for all/ethnic groups. There was no significant difference in A1c change over time by race/ethnicity.
Gerber 2005 [36] USA	Health literacy	Patient level Number of experimental conditions: 2 (1 intervention, 1 control) Intervention: Education by computer multi-media including audio/video sequences ("Living Well with Diabetes") to communicate information, provide psychosocial support and promote self-management. Subject received compensation based on computer usage. Lessons in English and Spanish. Navigation provided through a simplified interface, including forward/backward buttons for user control. Advanced features included "pop-up" supplementary text information or additional testimonials related to the concurrent screen concept Personnel involved: bilingual research assistant Setting: urban outpatient clinics Control group: simple multiple-choice quizzes on diabetes-related concepts	A1c, BMI, BP, eye exam, diabetes knowledge, self-efficacy, self-reported medical care, and per-ceived susceptibility to complications	Stratification by level of health literacy	No significant differences for all outcomes but perceived susceptibility to diabetes complications	Lower literacy group % change A1c − 0.21 ± 2.0 vs − 0.1% ± 1.3 MD = − 0.10 [− 0.67, 0.47] People with A1c > 9% − 2.1 vs − 0.3 (p = 0.036) Perceived susceptibility to complications % change score= 1.48 ± 2.7 vs 0.19 ± 2.5 (p = 0.016) Self-efficacy trend toward greater improvement in self-efficacy 1.51 ± 1.5 vs. 0.99 ± 1.4 (p = 0.113) Higher literacy % change A1c + 0.3% ± 1.6 vs. -0.5 ± 1.5 MD = 0.80 [0.22, 1.38] Perceived susceptibility to complications 0.76 ± 2.5 vs. 0.29 ± 2.4 (p = 0.267) Medical care Improvement over time (p < 0.012 for time interaction) but no effect for either lower- or higher-literacy groups

Table 2 Evidence synthesis on differential effect analyses by PROGRESS-Plus factors (*Continued*)

Study, country	PROGRESS-factor	Intervention type	Outcome	Method of analysis	Overall intervention effect	Differential effect
Sixta 2008 [28] USA	age	Healthcare level Number of experimental conditions: 2 (1 intervention, 1 control) Intervention: Diabetes culturally self-management education with group sessions Personnel involved: promotores in consultation with a care team Control group: Usual care delivered by provider at the clinic or to a self-care management	A1C, knowledge, beliefs	Stratified analysis by age	A1C, knowledge, beliefs	A1C No difference between groups DKQ, HBQ. No difference between groups DKQ, HBQ, and HbA1c results were significantly affected by age; Slightly negative effect on DKQ scores per year of age. Slightly negative effect on HBQ scores and HbA1c levels per year of age
West 2007 [70] USA	Race/ethnicity	Patient level Number of experimental conditions: 2 (1 intervention, 1 control) Intervention: • 42 group session of behavioral weight control program focusing on attainable and sustainable changes in dietary and physical activity habits • Motivational interviewing: 5 individual sessions lasted 45 min Personnel involved: Behaviorist, nutritionist, diabetes educator, trained clinical psychologist Setting: outpatient clinic Control group: health education sessions with focus on women's health topics	A1C, glucose monitoring	The weight patterns over time by race were examined using a two-factor repeated measures ANOVA stratified by treatment	Weight At 6 months Means: − 4.7 ± 5.4 kg vs − 3.1 ± 3.9 kg ($p = 0.03$) Over 18 months: Means: − 3.5 ± 6.8 Kg vs − 1.7 ± 5.7Kg ($p = 0.04$) A1C Decrease in both groups ($p < 0.0001$) at 6 months but not sustained at 18 months Greater decrease in the intervention than in the control group ($p = 0.002$)	Weight at 6 months regardless treatment: African-American vs White -3 kg ± 3.9 vs. -4.5 ± 5.1 kg ($p = 0.03$) Weight at 12 months regardless treatment: − 2.3 kg ± 4.4 vs − 4.6 ± 6.8 kg ($p = 0.09$) Weight at 18 months regardless treatment: − 1.4 kg ± 4.7 vs − 3.3 ± 7.1 kg ($p = 0.09$) For African-American experimental intervention produced greater weight loss than control group at 3 and 6 months. The benefit was not sustained after 12 months A1c African American had high A1c values regardless of treatment assignment. No interaction by race Attendance between groups was comparable.

Data are means ± SD; *I* intervention group, *C* control group, *OR* odds ratio, A1c, Glycated hemoglobin; *BMI* Body Mass Index, *LDL* low density cholesterol, *BP* blood pressure, *SBP* systolic blood pressure, *DBP* diastolic blood pressure, *MD* mean difference, *FHQ* food habit questionnaire, *PHQ-9* Patient Health Questionnaire, *DSME* Diabetes self-management education, *DKQ* diabetes knowledge questionnaire, *HBQ* Health Beliefs Questionnaire

[a]multivariate analysis adjusted for study group, gender, dietary, exercise activity (did not persist after the other covariates were controlled for); ^b = regression coefficient

settings and therefore address differences in baseline A1C values across studies in ways other than restricting patient participant inclusion.

Another relevant issue in the evaluation of QI strategies is that the control groups received a wide range of interventions, from basic education materials, usual care, to individualized coaching from community health workers. Furthermore, in many of these studies, the control group intervention was not described in detail. This is important as the usual or routine care in different settings varies by a multitude of variables including payment system, geographic location, country, and more generally, the resources and quality of services routinely provided to patients. In addition, type and quality of usual care at a health center can impact baseline values, especially HbA1c. Moreover, biases may exist depending on previous improvement activities implemented and general commitment of medical staff and organizational leadership to reducing disparities and improving care.

The conclusions of this systematic review are largely in accord with those in a previous review on this topic among socially disadvantaged population living in industrialized countries published in 2006 [74]. The review identified 17 studies, seven trials were with low SES populations, and ten focused on etno-racial groups. The small number of studies in Glazier's review provided limited and inconclusive evidence on intervention attributes that improved diabetes quality of care and health outcomes, underlining the potential effect of some features in reducing health disparities.

Our review provides an update and a more complete overview of the available evidence considering three specific aspects: use of PROGRESS framework to capture different socio-economic dimensions; assessment of the risk of bias of included studies; and the inclusion of studies evaluating QI strategies defined according to international classification.

Using an equity oriented approach, we identified a large number of randomized studies showing that considerable strides have been made to test interventions to address health inequities in diabetes care and outcomes. Despite the increase of the number of trials, the methodological quality resulted to be low. This finding is consistent with a previous review [75] reporting that the increase in the number of RCTs on QI strategies runs parallel to the proportion of trials having at least one domain with high risk of bias. Most included trials did not report the method of randomization and description of the allocation process. The area of the greatest potential risk of bias was the inadequate blinding of participants and outcome assessors, and poor follow up. In some of included trials the general lack of reporting of methods made it difficult to assess methodological quality and thereby judge risk of bias, independently of year of publication. The issue of small sample size extends beyond the quality of those studies included in this review. There were a number of studies, both pilot and not, that were excluded from this review because they had a sample size smaller than 50. Furthermore, since most studies were carried out in USA, their degree of external validity is uncertain. Results from these studies may be less transferrable to other countries and settings due to their being tested in a market-based health care system. It is likely that the patients' population covered by universalistic care is more heterogeneous with regard to socio-demographic and clinical characteristics. For example, those countries with universal health care systems may have more heterogeneous patient populations in a single community. It is therefore necessary to plan trials in other countries. By the same token, interventions addressing health disparities in other countries are likely to involve groups of varying social advantage or disadvantage being served under the same health center or system. The approach to addressing inequity becomes more about reducing health disparities on a more granular level requiring tools such as health equity audit.

Although the PROGRESS framework provides a vast array of disadvantage categories, there was limited heterogeneity in the dimensions of disadvantage considered in RCTs. The most common PROGRESS factor were age and race/ethnicity, this underlines the needs of further research with a focus on other characteristics such as socioeconomic status, social capital, place of residence, occupation, education, and religion. Researchers studying populations at social disadvantage must also describe the study population and the nature of their disadvantage more specifically. This is of further importance because a lack of description or definition of a socially disadvantaged group was a common reason for study exclusion in this review and others.

There is also a clear need for more RCTs at the provider level, especially those evaluating interventions based on computerized provider reminder systems. With the widespread uptake of recognition and certification programs in primary care (e.g. medical home, diabetes recognition programs,), it is likely that audit and feedback strategies using benchmarking are common among primary care practices, but are less frequently reported for effectiveness among disadvantaged patient populations.

This research reveals an overall lack of focus on interventions that address outcomes related to adherence to guidelines where disparities are stark according to the literature. The paucity of studies measuring process of care may be a reflection of the few number of QI interventions at the provider level who, in conjunction with other members of the primary care team, are responsible for performing or referring to these services. Clinical outcomes should derived from electronic health record systems, but may not be as recurrently funded as bio-chemical diabetes outcomes. Process outcomes or adherence to guidelines is crucial to measure and address due to the evidence of disparities that exist on the level of clinical quality and care. It is also important to note that several studies measured diabetes "self-care" or "self-management" activities but did not report results on distinct components such as medication adherence or glucose monitoring. As these clinical outcome measures are crucial in measuring effectiveness of diabetes intervention, it is important to report on these components as distinctive measures.

We see many studies that aim to evaluate interventions to improve care and/or outcomes among a disadvantaged group, but seldom do we find studies investigating the effect of QI interventions disentangled by different levels of indicators of socio-economic position or relevant socio-demographic factors. This may because practices are not disaggregating data to identify disparities within patient populations and are therefore not initiating action to address them. It should be necessary to promote and sustain a different approach including audit activities to identify inequities in care and outcomes, and then work to address these disparities. Moreover, an "equity lens" approach should be adopted by the scientific community when identifying research priorities aimed at contrasting socioeconomic differentials. This equity-oriented approach is necessary to identify and describe the appropriate target population, to define inequalities indicators, and select process and outcome indicators useful for assessing the differential effect of an intervention.

Conclusions

Because of the methodological differences and weaknesses that precluded meta-analytic synthesis, we can draw no strong conclusions concerning the potential benefits or harms of QI strategies to reduce inequalities in access to care for patients with diabetes in primary care. Moreover, the included studies did not allow for an analysis of the differential effects of interventions across population sub-groups.

This review highlights some QI strategies for consideration and in need of further study. Health care professionals and policy makers need the best available evidence to administer and support those interventions most likely to be effective to reduce disparities in diabetes care.

Additional files

Additional file 1: Search strategy for PubMed. (DOCX 17 kb)

Additional file 2: Table S1. Inclusion and exclusion criteria (PICOS). (DOCX 14 kb)

Additional file 3: Table S2. Quality improvement strategies: level and description. (DOCX 13 kb)

Additional file 4: Table S3. Characteristics of eligible studies assessing the efficacy of QI interventions in participants with type 2 diabetes. (DOCX 71 kb)

Authors' contributions

NT, AB, and NA made substantial contributions to the conception and design of this systematic review. ZM completed the literature search. NT and AB screened studies against eligibility criteria, extracted data, and analysed and interpreted data. All authors contributed to writing and revising the final manuscript. All authors read and approved the final manuscript LA and MD contributed to the critical revision.

Competing interests

The authors declare that they have no competing interests.

Author details

[1]Trenton Health Team, Trenton, New Jersey, USA. [2]Department of Epidemiology, Lazio Region- ASL Rome1, Rome, Italy.

References

1. World Health Organization. Global Report on Diabetes 2016. http://apps.who.int/iris/bitstream/handle/10665/204871/9789241565257_eng.pdf;jsessionid=45F529CEFB7FB49CB7EE39B0F63BA11F?sequence=1. Accessed 20 Feb 2016.
2. Agardh E, Allebeck P, Hallqvist J, Moradi T, Sidorchuk A. Type 2 diabetes incidence and socio-economic position: a systematic review and meta-analysis. Int J Epidemiol. 2011;40:804–18.
3. Redle EE, Atkins D. The applicability of quality improvement research for comparative effectiveness. Implement Sci. 2013;8(Suppl 1):S6.
4. Espelt A, Arriola L, Borrell C, Larrañaga I, Sandín M, Escolar-Pujolar A. Socioeconomic position and type 2 diabetes mellitus in Europe 1999-2009: a panorama of inequalities. Curr Diabetes Rev. 2011;7(3):148–58.
5. NICE. Type 2 diabetes in adults: management 2015. https://www.nice.org.uk/guidance/ng28/evidence/full-guideline-pdf-78671532569. Accessed 20 Feb 2016.
6. Grintsova O, Maier W, Mielck A. Inequalities in health care among patients with type 2 diabetes by individual socio-economic status (SES) and regional deprivation: a systematic literature review. Int J Equity Health. 2014;13:43. https://doi.org/10.1186/1475-9276-13-43.
7. Heidemann DL, Joseph NA, Kuchipudi A, Perkins DW, Drake S. Racial and economic disparities in Diabetes in a Large Primary Care Patient Population. Ethn Dis. 2016;26(1):85–90. https://doi.org/10.18865/ed.26.1.85.
8. Calvert M, Shankar A, McManus RJ, Lester H, Freemantle N. Effect of the quality and outcomes framework on diabetes care in the United Kingdom: retrospective cohort study. BMJ. 2009;338:b1870. https://doi.org/10.1136/bmj.b1870. Erratum in: BMJ. 2009;339:b2768
9. Rossi MC, Candido R, Ceriello A, Cimino A, Di Bartolo P, Giorda C, et al. Trends over 8 years in quality of diabetes care: results of the AMD annals continuous quality improvement initiative. Acta Diabetol. 2015;52(3):557–71. https://doi.org/10.1007/s00592-014-0688-6.
10. Tricco AC, Ivers NM, Grimshaw JM, Moher D, Turner L, Galipeau J, et al. Effectiveness of quality improvement strategies on the management of diabetes: a systematic review and meta-analysis. Lancet. 2012;379(9833):2252–61. https://doi.org/10.1016/S0140-6736(12)60480-2.
11. O'Neill J, Tabish H, Welch V, Petticrew M, Pottie K, Clarke M, et al. Applying an equity lens to interventions: using PROGRESS ensures consideration of socially stratifying factors to illuminate inequities in health. J Clin Epidemiol. 2014;67(1):56–64. https://doi.org/10.1016/j.jclinepi.2013.08.005.

12. Welch V, Petticrew M, Petkovic J, Moher D, Waters E, White H, et al. PRISMA-equity Bellagio group. Extending the PRISMA statement to equity-focused systematic reviews (PRISMA-E 2012): explanation and elaboration. J Clin Epidemiol. 2016;70:68–89. https://doi.org/10.1016/j.jclinepi.2015.09.001.

13. McPheeters ML, Kripalani S, Peterson NB, Idowu RT, Jerome RN, Potter SA, et al. Quality improvement interventions to address health disparities. In: Closing the quality gap: revisiting the state of the science. Evidence report no. 208. (prepared by the Vanderbilt University evidence-based practice center under contract no. 290–2007-10065.) AHRQ publication no. 12-E009-EF. Rockville: Agency for Healthcare Research and Quality; 2012. https://effectivehealthcare.ahrq.gov/sites/default/files/pdf/disparities-quality-improvement_research.pdf.

14. Higgins JP, Altman DG, Gøtzsche PC, Jüni P, Moher D, Oxman AD, et al. Cochrane Bias methods group; Cochrane Statistical Methods Group The Cochrane Collaboration's tool for assessing risk of bias in randomised trials. BMJ. 2011;343:d5928. https://doi.org/10.1136/bmj.d5928.

15. RevMan 2014. The Nordic Cochrane Centre, The Cochrane Collaboration. Review Manager (RevMan). Version 5.3. Copenhagen: The Nordic Cochrane Centre, The Cochrane Collaboration; 2014.

16. Bellary S, O'Hare JP, Raymond NT, Gumber A, Mughal S, Szczepura A, et al. Enhanced diabetes care to patients of south Asian ethnic origin (the United Kingdom Asian Diabetes Study): a cluster randomised controlled trial. Lancet. 2008;371(9626):1769–76.

17. Berry DC, Williams W, Hall EG, Heroux R, Bennett-Lewis T. Imbedding interdisciplinary diabetes group visits into a community-based medical setting. Diabetes Educ. 2016;42(1):96–107.

18. DePue JD, Rosen RK, Seiden A, Bereolos N, Chima ML, Goldstein MG, et al. Implementation of a culturally tailored diabetes intervention with community health workers in American Samoa. Diabetes Educat. 2013;39(6): 761–71.

19. McDermott RA, Schmidt B, Preece C, Owens V, Taylor S, Li M, et al. Community health workers improve diabetes care in remote Australian indigenous communities: results of a pragmatic cluster randomized controlled trial. BMC Health Serv Res. 2015;15:68.

20. Gucciardi E, DeMelo M, Lee RN, Grace SL. Assessment of two culturally competent diabetes education methods: individual versus individual plus group education in Canadian Portuguese adults with type 2 diabetes. Ethn Health. 2007;12(2):163–87.

21. Guo H, Tian X, Li R, Lin J, Jin N, Wu Z, Yu D. Reward-based, task-setting education strategy on glycemic control and self-management for low-income outpatients with type-á2 diabetes. J Diabetes Investig. 2014;5(4):410–7.

22. Hotu C, Collins J, Harwood L, Whalley G, Doughty R, Gamble G, Braatvedt G. A community-based model of care improves blood pressure control and delays progression of proteinuria, left ventricular hypertrophy and diastolic dysfunction in Maori and Pacific patients with type 2 diabetes and chronic kidney disease: a randomized controlled trial. Nephrol Dial Transplant. 2010; 25(10):3260–6.

23. Partapsingh VA, Maharaj RG, Rawlins JM. Applying the Stages of Change model to Type 2 diabetes care in Trinidad: A randomised trial. J Negat Results Biomed. 2011;10(1):13.

24. Shahid M, Mahar SA, Shaikh S, Shaikh Z-U-D. Mobile phone intervention to improve diabetes care in rural areas of Pakistan: a randomized controlled trial. J Coll Physicians Surg Pak. 2015;25(3):166–71.

25. Frosch DL, Uy V, Ochoa S, Mangione CM. Evaluation of a behavior support intervention for patients with poorly controlled diabetes. Arch Intern Med. 2011;171(22):2011–7.

26. Khan MA, Shah S, Grudzien A, Onyejekwe N, Banskota P, Karim S, et al. A diabetes education multimedia program in the waiting room setting. Diabetes Ther. 2011;2(3):178–88. https://doi.org/10.1007/s13300-011-0007-y. Epub 2011 Aug 22

27. Rosal MC, Ockene IS, Restrepo A, White MJ, Borg A, Olendzki B, et al. Randomized trial of a literacy-sensitive, culturally tailored diabetes self-management intervention for low-income latinos: latinos en control. Diabetes Care. 2011;34(4):838–44.

28. Sixta CS, Ostwald S. Texas-Mexico border intervention by promotores for patients with type 2 diabetes. Diabetes Educ. 2008;34(2):299–309.

29. Hill-Briggs F, Lazo M, Peyrot M, Doswell A, Chang YT, Hill MN, et al. Effect of problem-solving-based diabetes self-management training on diabetes control in a low income patient sample. J Gen Intern Med. 2011;26(9):972–8.

30. Rothschild SK, Martin MA, Swider SM, Tumialán Lynas CM, Janssen I, Avery EF, et al. Mexican American trial of community health workers: a

randomized controlled trial of a community health worker intervention for Mexican Americans with type 2 diabetes mellitus. Am J Public Health. 2014; 104(8):1540–8.

31. Palmas W, Findley SE, Mejia M, Batista M, Teresi J, Kong J, et al. Results of the northern Manhattan diabetes community outreach project: a randomized trial studying a community health worker intervention to improve diabetes care in hispanic adults. Diabetes Care. 2014;37(4):963–9.

32. Walker EA, Shmukler C, Ullman R, Blanco E, Scollan-Koliopoulus M, Cohen HW. Results of a successful telephonic intervention to improve diabetes control in urban adults: a randomized trial. Diabetes Care. 2011;34(1):2–7.

33. Davis RM, Hitch AD, Salaam MM, Herman WH, Zimmer-Galler IE, Mayer-Davis EJ. TeleHealth improves diabetes self-management in an underserved community: diabetes TeleCare. Diabetes Care. 2010;33(8):1712–7.

34. Philis-Tsimikas A, Fortmann A, Lleva-Ocana L, Walker C, Gallo LC. Peer-led diabetes education programs in high-risk Mexican Americans improve glycemic control compared with standard approaches: a project Dulce promotora randomized trial. Diabetes Care. 2011;34(9):1926–31.

35. Brown SA, Blozis SA, Kouzekanani K, Garcia AA, Winchell M, Hanis CL. Dosage effects of diabetes self-management education for Mexican Americans: the Starr County border health initiative. Diabetes Care. 2005; 28(3):527–32.

36. Gerber BS, Brodsky IG, Lawless KA, Smolin LI, Arozullah AM, Smith EV, et al. Implementation and evaluation of a low-literacy diabetes education computer multimedia application. Diabetes Care. 2005;28(7):1574–80.

37. Anderson-Loftin W, Barnett S, Bunn P, Sullivan P, Hussey J, Tavakoli A. Soul food light: culturally competent diabetes education. Diabetes Educ. 2005; 31(4):555–63.

38. Tang TS, Funnell MM, Sinco B, Spencer MS, Heisler M. Peer-led, empowerment-based approach to self-management efforts in diabetes (PLEASED): a randomized controlled trial in an African American community. Ann Fam Med. 2015;13(Suppl 1):S27–35.

39. Toobert DJ, Strycker LA, King DK, Barrera M Jr, Osuna D, Glasgow RE. Long-term outcomes from a multiple-risk-factor diabetes trial for Latinas: -íViva Bien! Transl Behav Med. 2011;1(3):416–26.

40. Tang TS, Funnell M, Sinco B, Piatt G, Palmisano G, Spencer MS, Kieffer EC, Heisler M. Comparative effectiveness of peer leaders and community health workers in diabetes selfmanagement support: results of a randomized controlled trial. Diabetes Care. 2014;37(6):1525–34.

41. Negarandeh R, Mahmoodi H, Noktehdan H, Heshmat R, Shakibazadeh E. Teach back and pictorial image educational strategies on knowledge about diabetes and medication/dietary adherence among low health literate patients with type 2 diabetes. Prim Care Diabetes. 2013;7(2):111–8.

42. Weinstein E, Galindo RJ, Fried M, Rucker L, Davis NJ. Impact of a focused nutrition educational intervention coupled with improved access to fresh produce on purchasing behavior and consumption of fruits and vegetables in overweight patients with diabetes mellitus. Diabetes Educat. 2014;40(1): 100–6.

43. Phillips LS, Ziemer DC, Doyle JP, Barnes CS, Kolm P, Branch WT, et al. An endocrinologist-supported intervention aimed at providers improves diabetes management in a primary care site: improving primary care of African Americans with diabetes (IPCAAD) 7. Diabetes Care. 2005;28(10): 2352–60.

44. Welch G, Zagarins SE, Santiago-Kelly P, Rodriguez Z, Bursell SE, Rosal MC, et al. An internet-based diabetes management platform improves team care and outcomes in an urban Latino population. Diabetes Care. 2015; 38(4):561–7.

45. Shea S, Weinstock RS, Teresi JA, Palmas W, Starren J, Cimino JJ, et al. IDEATel consortium. A randomized trial comparing telemedicine case management with usual care in older, ethnically diverse, medically underserved patients with diabetes mellitus: 5 year results of the IDEATel study. J Am Med Inform Assoc. 2009;16(4):446–56.

46. Kim MT, Kim KB, Huh B, Nguyen T, Han H-R, Bone LR, et al. The effect of a community-based self-help intervention: Korean Americans with type 2 diabetes. Am J Prev Med. 2015 Nov;49(5):726–37.

47. Perez-Escamilla R, Damio G, Chhabra J, Fernandez ML, Segura-Perez S, Vega-Lopez S, et al. Impact of a community health workers-led structured program on blood glucose control among Latinos with type 2 diabetes: The DIALBEST Trial. Diabetes Care. 2015;38(2):197–205. // () *National Center for Advancing Translational Sciences*

48. Spencer MS, Rosland AM, Kieffer EC, Sinco BR, Valerio M, Palmisano G, et al. Effectiveness of a community health worker intervention among African

American and Latino adults with type 2 diabetes: a randomized controlled trial. Am J Public Health. 2011;101(12):2253–60.

49. Prezio EA, Cheng D, Balasubramanian BA, Shuval K, Kendzor DE, Culica D. Community diabetes education (CoDE) for uninsured Mexican Americans: a randomized controlled trial of a culturally tailored diabetes education and management program led by a community health worker. Diabetes Res Clin Pract. 2013;100(1):19–28. https://doi.org/10.1016/j.diabres.2013.01.027.

50. Thom DH, Ghorob A, Hessler D, Vore D, Chen E, Bodenheimer TA. Impact of peer health coaching on glycemic control in low-income patients with diabetes: a randomized controlled trial. Ann Fam Med. 2013;11(2):137–44.

51. Gary TL, Batts-Turner M, Yeh HC, Hill-Briggs F, Bone LR, Wang NY, et al. The effects of a nurse case manager and a community health worker team on diabetic control, emergency department visits, and hospitalizations among urban African Americans with type 2 diabetes mellitus: a randomized controlled trial. Arch Intern Med. 2009;169(19):1788–94.

52. Kim MT, Han HR, Song HJ, Lee JE, Kim J, Ryu JP, et al. A community-based, culturally tailored behavioral intervention for Korean Americans with type 2 diabetes. Diabetes Educat. 2009;35(6):986–94.

53. Liou J-K, Soon M-S, Chen C-H, Huang T-F, Chen Y-P, Yeh Y-P, et al. Shared care combined with telecare improves glycemic control of diabetes patients in a rural, underserved community. J Diabetes Sci Technol. 2013; 7(1):A82.

54. Lujan J, Ostwald SK, Ortiz M. Promotora diabetes intervention for Mexican Americans. Diabetes Educ. 2007;33(4):660–70.

55. Levy NK, Moynihan V, Nilo A, Singer K, Etiebet M-A, Bernik L, et al. The mobile insulin titration intervention (MITI) study: innovative chronic disease management of diabetes. J Gen Intern Med. 2015;30:S547–S8.

56. Cramer JS, Sibley RF, Bartlett DP, Kahn LS, Loffredo L. An adaptation of the diabetes prevention program for use with high-risk, minority patients with type 2 diabetes. Diabetes Educat. 2007;33(3):503–8.

57. Garcia AA, Brown SA, Horner SD, Zuniga J, Arheart KL. Home-based diabetes symptom self-management education for Mexican Americans with type 2 diabetes. Health Educ Res. 2015;30(3):484–96.

58. Babamoto KS, Sey KA, Camilleri AJ, Karlan VJ, Catalasan J, Morisky DE. Improving diabetes care and health measures among hispanics using community health workers: results from a randomized controlled trial. Health Educ Behav. 2009;36(1):113–26.

59. Lynch EB, Liebman R, Ventrelle J, Avery EF, Richardson D. A self-management intervention for African Americans with comorbid diabetes and hypertension: a pilot randomized controlled trial. Prev Chronic Dis. 2014;11:E90.

60. Tobe SW, Pylypchuk G, Wentworth J, Kiss A, Szalai JP, Perkins N, et al. Effect of nurse-directed hypertension treatment among first nations people with existing hypertension and diabetes mellitus: the diabetes risk evaluation and microalbuminuria (DREAM 3) randomized controlled trial. CMAJ. 2006; 174(9):1267–71.

61. Anderson DR, Christison-Lagay J, Villagra V, Liu H, Dziura J. Managing the space between visits: a randomized trial of disease management for diabetes in a community health center. J Gen Intern Med. 2010;25(10):1116–22.

62. Baradaran HR, Knill-Jones RP, Wallia S, Rodgers A. A controlled trial of the effectiveness of a diabetes education programme in a multi-ethnic community in Glasgow [ISRCTN28317455]. BMC Public Health. 2006;6:134.

63. Brown SA, García AA, Winter M, Silva L, Brown A, Hanis CL. Integrating education, group support, and case management for diabetic Hispanics. Ethn Dis. 2011;21(1):20–6.

64. Forjuoh SN, Bolin JN, Huber Jr JC, Vuong AM, Adepoju OE, Helduser JW, et al. Behavioral and technological interventions targeting glycemic control in a racially/ethnically diverse population: a randomized controlled trial. BMC Public Health. 2014;14:71.

65. Gregg JA, Callaghan GM, Hayes SC, Glenn-Lawson JL. Improving diabetes self-management through acceptance, mindfulness, and values: a randomized controlled trial. J Consult Clin Psychol. 2007;75(2):336–43.

66. Heisler M, Choi H, Palmisano G, Mase R, Richardson C, Fagerlin A, et al. Comparison of community health worker-led diabetes medication decision-making support for low-income Latino and African American adults with diabetes using e-health tools versus print materials: a randomized, controlled trial. Ann Intern Med. 2014;161(10 Suppl):S13–22.

67. Schillinger D, Hammer H, Wang F, Palacios J, McLean I, Tang A, et al. Seeing in 3-D: examining the reach of diabetes self-management support strategies in a public health care system. Health Educ Behav. 2008;35(5): 664–82.

68. Skelly AH, Carlson JR, Leeman J, Holditch-Davis D, Soward AC. Symptom-focused management for African American women with type 2 diabetes: a pilot study. J Nurs Scholarsh. 2005;18(4):213–20.

69. Wayne N, Perez DF, Kaplan DM, Ritvo P. Health coaching reduces HbA1c in type 2 diabetic patients from a lower-socioeconomic status community: a randomized controlled trial. J Med Internet Res. 2015;17(10):e224.

70. West DS, DiLillo V, Bursac Z, Gore SA, Greene PG. Motivational interviewing improves weight loss in women with type 2 diabetes. Diabetes Care. 2007; 30(5):1081–7.

71. Seligman HK, Wang FF, Palacios JL, Wilson CC, Daher C, Piette JD, et al. Physician notification of their diabetes patients' limited health literacy. A randomized, controlled trial. J Gen Intern Med. 2005;20(11):1001–7.

72. Ruggiero L, Moadsiri A, Butler P, Oros SM, Berbaum ML, Whitman S, et al. Supporting diabetes self-care in underserved populations: a randomized pilot study using medical assistant coaches. Diabetes Educ. 2010;36(1):127–31.

73. Willard-Grace R, Chen EH, Hessler D, DeVore D, Prado C, Bodenheimer T, et al. Health coaching by medical assistants to improve control of diabetes, hypertension, and hyperlipidemia in low-income patients: a randomized controlled trial. Ann Fam Med. 2015;13(2):130–8.

74. Glazier RH, Bajcar J, Kennie NR, Willson K. A systematic review of interventions to improve diabetes care in socially disadvantaged populations. Diabetes Care. 2006;29(7):1675–88.

75. Ivers NM, Tricco AC, Taljaard M, Halperin I, Turner L, Moher D, et al. Quality improvement needed in quality improvement randomised trials: systematic review of interventions to improve care in diabetes. BMJ Open. 2013;3(4): e002727. https://doi.org/10.1136/bmjopen-2013-002727.

15

Type 2 diabetes affects bone cells precursors and bone turnover

Francesca Sassi[1], Ilaria Buondonno[1], Chiara Luppi[1], Elena Spertino[1], Emanuela Stratta[1], Marco Di Stefano[1], Marco Ravazzoli[1], Gianluca Isaia[3], Marina Trento[2], Pietro Passera[2], Massimo Porta[2], Giovanni Carlo Isaia[1] and Patrizia D'Amelio[1]* ⓘ

Abstract

Background: Here we study the effect of type 2 diabetes (T2DM) on bone cell precursors, turnover and cytokines involved in the control of bone cell formation and activity.

Methods: We enrolled in the study 21 T2DM women and 21 non diabetic controls matched for age and body mass index (BMI). In each subject we measured bone cell precursors, Receptor Activator of Nuclear Factor κB (RANKL), Osteoprotegerin (OPG), Sclerostin (SCL) and Dickoppf-1 (DKK-1) as cytokines involved in the control of osteoblast and osteoclast formation and activity, bone density (BMD) and quality trough trabecular bone score (TBS) and bone turnover. T2DM patients and controls were compared for the analyzed variables by one way ANOVA for Gaussian ones and by Mann-Whitney or Kruskal-Wallis test for non-Gaussian variables.

Results: RANKL was decreased and DKK-1 increased in T2DM. Accordingly, patients with T2DM have lower bone turnover compared to controls. BMD and TBS were not significantly different from healthy controls. Bone precursor cells were more immature in T2DM. However the number of osteoclast precursors was increased and that of osteoblasts decreased.

Conclusions: Patients with T2DM have more immature bone cells precursors, with increased number of osteoclasts and decreased osteoblasts, confirming low bone turnover and reduced cytokines such as RANKL and DKK-1. BMD and TBS are not significantly altered in T2DM although, in contrast with other studies, this may be due to the match of patients and controls for BMI rather than age.

Keywords: Diabetes, Osteoblast, Osteoclast, Sclerostin, Receptor activator of nuclear factor κB, Bone density

Background

Type 2 diabetes mellitus (T2DM) increases the risk of fragility fractures [1], even though it is often associated with increased bone density [1, 2]. T2DM has been associated with poor bone quality [3] and this may lead to increased fracture risk. Nevertheless, how T2DM affects bone is still controversial. Several mechanisms may be involved, such as direct effects of insulin resistance and hyperglycemia on the bone and bone marrow microenvironment, advanced glycation end products of bone matrix proteins, abnormal cytokine production, and impaired neuromuscular/skeletal interactions [4, 5]. Obesity associated with

T2DM may be a confounder due to its controversial effect on bone per se (see Dolan et al., 2017 for a comprehensive review) [6]. Several studies suggest that obesity protects against bone loss in diabetic patients [7–9]. Moreover, recent data suggest that obesity, regardless of the presence of T2DM, is associated with a favorable bone microarchitecture and greater bone strength at the distal radius and distal tibia [10]. Serum markers of bone formation such as osteocalcin (OCN) and amino-terminal propeptide of procollagen type 1 (P1NP) have been found decreased in T2DM patients [11–13], supporting the hypothesis that bone formation is lower than in controls. Also bone resorption has been found reduced in T2DM by some authors [11, 14], however this data has not been confirmed by others [15]. T2DM may affect bone metabolism influencing osteoblast (OB) and osteoclast (OC) formation and

* Correspondence: patrizia.damelio@unito.it
[1]Department of Medical Science, Gerontology and Bone Metabolic Diseases, University of Torino, Corso Bramante 88/90, 10126 Torino, Italy
Full list of author information is available at the end of the article

activity by altering the cytokines involved in these processes other than having direct toxic effect on bone cells. OB formation and activity are mainly induced by the activation of the Wnt pathway, two of the most studied inhibitors of this pathway being sclerostin (SCL) and Dickoppf-1 (DKK-1) [16]. Otherwise, osteoclast formation and activity are mainly regulated by the Receptor Activator of Nuclear Factor κB (RANKL), its receptor (RANK) and its decoy receptor Osteoprotegerin (OPG) [17].

In vitro, in animal models and in humans it has been demonstrated that hyperglycemia increases the level of SCL [18–20] and DKK-1 [21–23], and that these cytokines blunt osteoblast formation and activity. As regards the RANKL/RANK/OPG pathway, this has been studied mainly in relation to cardiovascular damage and vascular calcification in T2DM [24]. Nowadays there are no human data on the relation between the cytokines involved in the control of bone cells and bone cell precursors in patients affected by T2DM. In this paper we show the effect of T2DM on bone turnover, bone precursors cells and cytokines involved in bone turnover taking into account the confounding factor of obesity and age.

Methods

Study population

We performed a case-control study enrolling 42 subjects, 21 women affected by T2DM and 21 non diabetic controls. Patients and controls had been in spontaneous menopause for, at least, one year. T2DM patients were matched with controls for Body Mass Index (BMI) ± 2 SD and age ± 5 years. Screening for micro-and macrovascular complications of diabetes was done yearly. Retinopathy was investigated by 45° digital retinal photography and graded according to the American Academy of Ophthalmology Simplified Classification [25]. Nephropathy was screened for by measuring albumin excretion rate and serum creatinine. Neuropathy was assessed according to the San Antonio Consensus [26]. Large vessel disease was screened for by examining peripheral pulses and history of coronary or peripheral artery disease. None of the T2DM patients included were affected by renal or macro-vascular complications, 4 were affected by retinopathy (19%). Of these patients,1 was also affected by neuropathy, and another 5 only had neuropathy (23.8%). (Table 1 shows the clinical characteristics of patients and controls). Five patients (23.8%) were treated by insulin, 11 by metformin and five by DPP4 inhibitors.

T2DM patients were recruited from the outpatient diabetes clinic of Medicina Interna 1 U. In Italy diabetic patients are managed by general practitioners and periodically referred to specialist centers to evaluate their disease state, hence the enrollment of patients from a tertiary referral center did not bias our results. Inclusion criteria for patients were:female genderin post-menopausal period and diagnosis of T2DM.

Table 1 Characteristics of subjects

	Patients (21)	Controls(21)	P value
Age (yrs)	71 ± 6	70 ± 6	–
Post-menopausalperiod (yrs)	22 ± 9	21 ± 7	NS
DMduration (yrs)	16 ± 2	–	–
HbA1C (mmol/mol)	57 ± 8.1	–	–
DM complications (%)	42.9%	–	–
Retinopathy (%)	14.3%	–	–
Neuropathy + retinopathy (%)	4.8%	–	–
Neuropathy (%)	23.8%	–	–
Insulin treatment (%)	23.8%		
Metformin treatment (%)	52.4%		
DPP4 inhibitors treatment (%)	23.8%		
Waist/hip ratio	0.92 (0.88–0.96)	0.88 (0.84–0.94)	NS
Fat mass (%)	39.4 (36.1–41.1)	39.1 (34.1–42.3)	NS
BMI (Kg/m^2)	29 ± 5	29 ± 5	–

Data depicted are mean ± SD for Gaussian variables and median with 25° and 75° percentiles for non-Gaussian variables, non-continuous variables are shown percentage. Statistical differences were analyzed by using ANOVA one-way or Mann-Whitney U test

Exclusion criteria were: mental inability to sign the informed consent; known secondary osteoporosis; treatment with drugs active on bone turnover within the previous six months including: biphosphonates, strontium ranelate, parathyroid hormone, thyroid hormones, raloxifene, denosumab, corticosteroids, estrogen, oral anticoagulants, calcium and vitamin D andimmunosuppressant (as cyclosporine, azathioprine) within the previous year; diagnosis of type 1 diabetes; use of thiazolidinediones; history of cancer; liver disease, kidney failure (stage II or higher); malabsorption; hyperthyroidism.

Glycemic control in patients was measured by Hemoglobin A1C (HbA1C) with high performance liquid chromatography (HPLC), the mean level was 57 ± 8.1 mmol/mol.

Controls were recruited from the general population starting from the database used for our previous study, fully described elsewhere [27]. Briefly, controls were enrolled from the general practitioner lists amongst non-diabetic women without diseases active on bone metabolism, matched for age and BMI to T2DM patients, as previously described. Exclusion criteria were the same used for the patients. The whole population was Caucasian.

Clinical evaluation of bone health

An accurate medical history, including the presence of fragility fractures, and physical examination was collected in all women. A bone scan was performed with a Hologic QDR 4500 X-ray densitometer to measure bone mineral density (BMD), both at lumbar spine and femur, and to evaluate the presence of vertebral fractures by morphometric DXA analyses. The spinal deformity index (SDI) [28] was calculated on DXA morphometry. Bone texture was analyzed by trabecular bone score (TBS) at lumbar vertebrae from DXA images with a dedicated software (TBS iNsight, Medimaps Group SA, Pessac, France). TBS is a textural index that evaluates pixel gray-level variations in the lumbar spine DXA image, providing an indirect index of trabecular micro-architecture. TBS is not a direct physical measurement of bone microarchitecture, but rather an overall score computed by the projection of the 3D structure onto a 2D plane that provides an indirect estimation of bone microarchitecture from spine DXA images [29].

Bone turnover markers, cytokines and bone cells precursors

Markers of bone formation, OCN (Life Technologies Corp, Frederick, MD), P1NP (USCN, Life Science Inc. Houston, TX), and of bone resorption serum Tartrate Resistant Acid Phosphatase 5b (TRAP5b, Quidel, San Diego, CA) were measured by ELISA.

RANKL (Biovendor Research and Diagnostic Products, BRNO, Czech Republic), OPG (R&D Systems Inc., Minneapolis, USA), SCL (R&D Systems Inc., Minneapolis, USA) and DKK-1 (R&D Systems Inc., Minneapolis, USA) were also measured by ELISA.

To evaluate the role of circulating OC and OB precursors in T2DM, we measured them in peripheral blood mononuclear cells (PBMCs) separated by Ficoll-Paque technique [30]. Briefly, OC precursors were evaluated by staining PBMCs with fluorescein (FITC, supplied by B&D) conjugated anti-vitronectin receptor (VNR), phycoerythrin (PE, supplied by B&D) conjugated anti-CD14 and allophycocyanin (APC, supplied by B&D) conjugated anti-CD11b mAb, or with the corresponding isotype control, followed by incubation at 4 °C for 30 min as previously described [30]. Triple-positive cells (CD14+/CD11b+/VNR+) were regarded as osteoclast precursors, according to the literature [30, 31]. OB precursors were evaluated by staining PBMCs with FITC conjugated anti-CD15 (in order to exclude granulocytes expressing alkaline phosphatase, supplied by e-Bioscience), APC conjugated anti-alkaline phosphatase (ALP, supplied by R&D System Inc), PE conjugated anti-OCN (supplied by R&D System Inc), or with the corresponding isotype control, followed by incubation at 4 °C for 30 min as previously described [30–32]. CD15-/ALP+/OCN+ cells were regarded as osteoblast precursors according to the literature [30–32]. Membrane antigen expression was analyzed with the CellQuest software (Becton Dickinson & Co).

Fat mass

In order to compare patients and controls for body fat mass and distribution, body fat was assessed by plicometry (Mahr GMBH Esslingen). The Pollock, Schmidt and Jackson's formula was used on three sites (triceps,

subscapular and abdomen) to calculate fat percentage [33]. In order to calculate BMI the women were weighted with a precision scale and their height recorded with a wall-mounted altimeter. BMI was measured as weight in Kg/ squared height in meters, to evaluate fat distribution the waist/hip ratio was measured.

Statistical analyses

The sample size was calculated to provide an 80% power ($p < 0.05$) to detect a 2-fold difference in SCL and DKK-1 in T2DM compared to healthy controls. The 2-fold difference was chosen based on previous papers [18–23]. In order to correctly weight the other data obtained the sample calculated post-hoc to evaluate differences in BMD to provide an 80% power ($p < 0.05$) to detect a 0.140 g difference in BMD in T2DM compared to healthy controls48 patients per group will be necessary. The 0.140 g difference was chosen based on previous papers [1, 2]. The sample size needed to evaluate differences in TBS to provide an 80% power ($p < 0.05$) to detect a 0.05difference in TBS in T2DM compared to healthy controls 100 patients per group will be necessary. The 0.05 difference was chosen on the basis of a previous paper [34]. The sample size needed to evaluate differences in bone turnover and in particular in P1NP to provide an 80% power ($p < 0.05$) to detect a 8 ng/mL difference in T2DM compared to healthy controls 33 patients per group will be necessary. The 8 ng/mL difference was chosen on the basis of previous paper [35].

T2DM patients and controls were compared by one-way ANOVA for Gaussian variables, by Mann-Whitney or Kruskal-Wallis test for non-Gaussian variables. Gaussian distribution was evaluated by kurtosis test. Gaussian variables were correlated by Pearson's coefficient, non-Gaussian with Spearman correlation. Data were tested for outliers with the ROUT method, no outliers were identify and removed from the analyses. Statistics were performed by means of SPSS 24.0 for windows, Graph Pad Prism 7.0 for windows was used to drawn the graphs. P values were considered significant if lower than 0.05.

Results

T2DM affects bone precursors cell

To evaluate if T2DM affects circulating bone precursors cells, we measured circulating OB and OC precursor cells and cytokines involved in osteoclastogenesis, osteoblastogenesis and in the regulation of bone turnover. We observed a significant reduction of circulating OB precursors cells in T2DM patients compared to controls (Fig. 1a), whereas OC precursors are increased (Fig. 1c). Both OC and OB precursors are more immature in diabetic patients; in particular OBs express lower levels of ALP and OCs express lower levels of VNR (Fig. 1b, d).

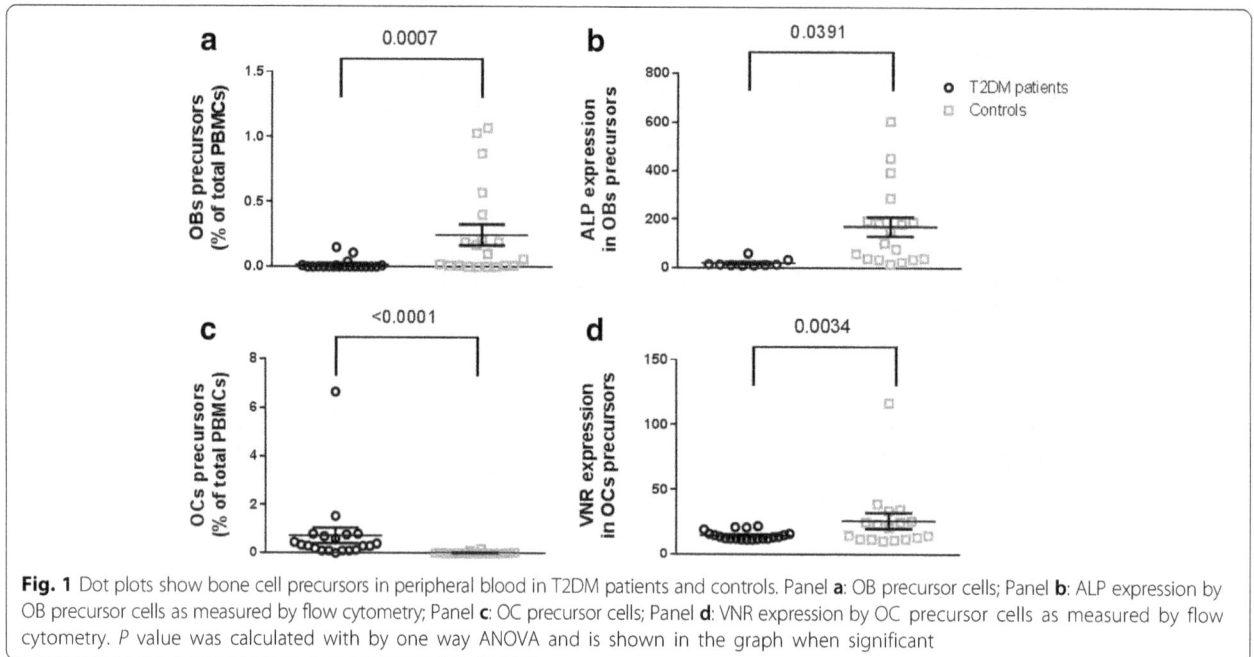

Fig. 1 Dot plots show bone cell precursors in peripheral blood in T2DM patients and controls. Panel **a**: OB precursor cells; Panel **b**: ALP expression by OB precursor cells as measured by flow cytometry; Panel **c**: OC precursor cells; Panel **d**: VNR expression by OC precursor cells as measured by flow cytometry. *P* value was calculated with by one way ANOVA and is shown in the graph when significant

Cytokines involved in the regulation of bone cells are altered in T2DM patients: DKK-1 was increased in patients compared to controls ($p = 0.04$), whereas RANKL was decreased in T2DM ($p = 0.0362$). DKK-1 was 1824 pg/mL (1345–2572 interquartile range (IQR)) in T2DM versus 1526 pg/mL (963.2–1792 IQR) in the control group; RANKL was 3590 pg/mL (1434–7154 IQR) in T2DM versus 5018 pg/mL (2632–9343 IQR) in the control group (Fig. 2a, c). OPG was not significantly altered 965.2 pg/mL (759.1-1346IQR) in T2DM versus 938 pg/mL (783–1207

IQR) in the control group (Fig. 2b). SCL was undetectable in the majority of both patients' and controls' sera 561.3 ± 73.4 pg/mL in T2DM versus 309.8 ± 31 pg/mL (Fig. 2d). In three T2DM and 5 controls SCL was detectable in the serum, in those subjects bone formation measured by P1NP was significantly lower (12,420.6 ± 6706.1 vs 24,025.2 ± 992.9, $p = 0.003$), no other differences in the tested variables were detectable. The increased level of SCL may be related to decreased bone formation measured by P1NP.

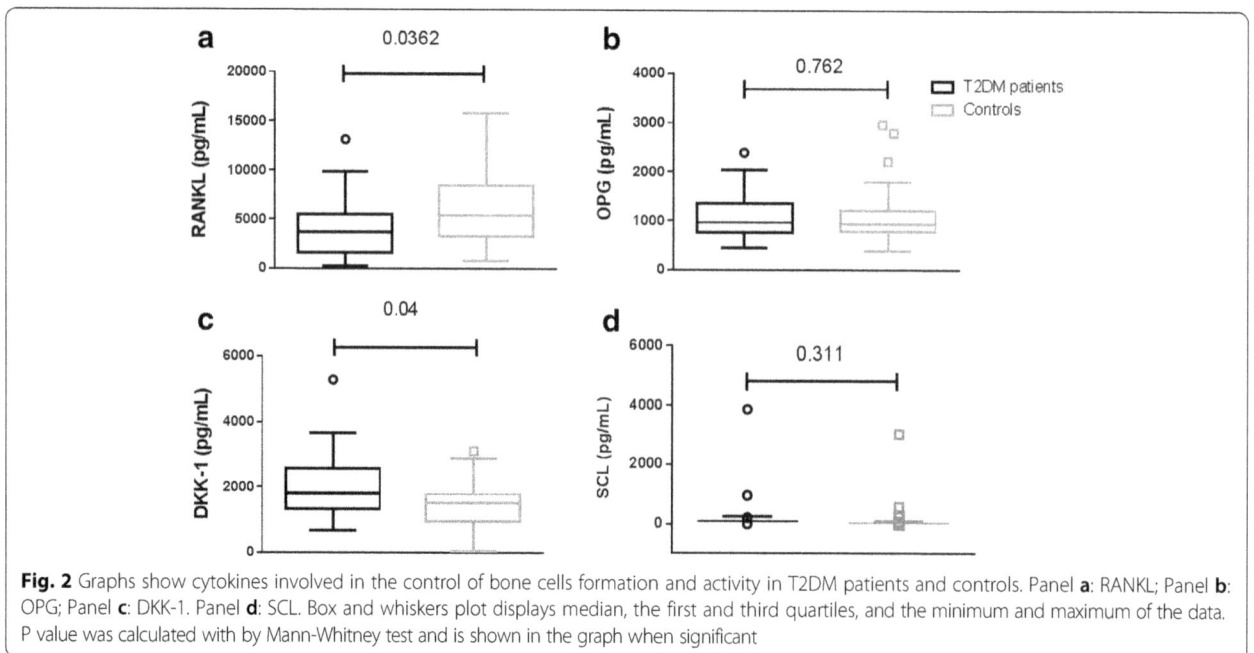

Fig. 2 Graphs show cytokines involved in the control of bone cells formation and activity in T2DM patients and controls. Panel **a**: RANKL; Panel **b**: OPG; Panel **c**: DKK-1. Panel **d**: SCL. Box and whiskers plot displays median, the first and third quartiles, and the minimum and maximum of the data. P value was calculated with by Mann-Whitney test and is shown in the graph when significant

Age per se is weakly correlated with RANKL ($R = 0.32$, $p = 0.047$) and with OB precursors maturation ($R = -0.384$, $p = 0.048$). Post-menopausal state is directly correlated with RANKL ($R = 0.323$, $P = 0.045$). Other parameters are not influenced by age, post-menopausal state or by BMI.

Glycemic control measured by HbA1C did not correlate with bone cell precursor percentage and maturation, nor with cytokines involved in the control of bone turnover. There were no significant differences in the parameters analyzed in patients with or without diabetic complications and between patients taking different anti-hyperglycaemic drugs (data not shown).

Bone metabolism is impaired in T2DM patients

BMD measured at lumbar spine, femoral neck and total femur was not significantly different between patients and controls; even though lumbar BMD was, on average, higher in T2DM than in controls. Bone structure measured by TBS, as well as SDI, were not altered in diabetic patients compared to controls (Table 2).

Obesity influences bone per se as there were significant correlations between BMI, BMD and TBS, the distribution of fat influenced only TBS (Table 3). Bone formation measured by P1NP as well as bone resorption measured by TRAP5b were significantly decreased in T2DM (Fig. 3). Glycemic control measured by HbA1C influenced bone structure but not bone density (Table 3). As regards bone turnover markers, HbA1C was inversely correlated with bone formation measured by OCN ($R = -0.59$, $p = 0.005$).

Discussion

The detrimental effect of T2DM on bone is well established [1, 2], but the possible mechanisms through which this happens have not been clearly elucidated. Here we evaluated the effect of T2DM on bone precursor cells and cytokines in patients and controls matched for BMI as well as age. One of the most confounding factor in the evaluation of diabetes effect on bone health is obesity, which is often associated with T2DM and has controversial effect on bone metabolism and fracture risk per se. Some studies suggest that obese subjects have a lower risk of proximal femur and vertebral fracture

Table 2 Bone health in T2DM patients and controls

	T2DM patients (21)	Controls (21)	P value
Lumbar BMD (g/cm2)	0.97 ± 0.16	0.92 ± 0.15	0.059
FemoralBMD (g/cm2)	0.71 ± 0.12	0.69 ± 0.11	0.275
SDI	0 (0–1)	0 (0–1)	0.982
TBS	0.926 (0.799–1.027)	0.965 (0.766–1.051)	0.875

Data depicted are mean ± SD for Gaussian variables and median with 25° and 75° percentiles for non-Gaussian variables. Statistical differences are analyzed by using ANOVA one-way or Mann-Whitney U test

Table 3 Correlations between bone density and structure, obesity and glycemic control

		BMI	Fat mass	Waist/hip	HbA1C
Lumbar BMD	r	**0.23**	0.84	0.91	−0.35
	p	**0.005**	0.338	0.276	0.286
Femoral BMD	r	**0.27**	0.154	0.10	−0.092
	p	**0.001**	0.078	0.904	0.701
TBS	r	−0.319	−0.36	**−0.34**	**−0.55**
	p	**< 0.0001**	0.693	**< 0.0001**	**0.016**

Pearson' coefficient correlations between BMD measured at lumbar spine and at femoral neck and BMI, Fat mass % and waist/hip ratio in the whole population under study, TBS was correlated by Spearman coefficient. Correlations between bone parameters and HbA1C were run only in T2DM patients. Significant values are in bold

compared to adults with normal BMI [36, 37]. However the risk of fracture in obese subjects is variable at different skeletal sites according to the difference in falling mechanisms in these patients; in particular the risk for proximal humerus, upper leg and ankle fracture is higher in obese than in non-obese adults [38]. Moreover, increased fat mass could be detrimental to bone due to increased inflammation and production of adipokines that affect bone turnover [39, 40]. For these reasons, we enclosed in this study controls matched with patients for BMI as well as for age. The use of obese controls may explain why, differently from other studies, we did not find significant differences in bone microarchitecture measured by TBS between T2DM patients and controls. Although our study was not powered to measure differences in TBS [3, 41], our data show that obesity is inversely correlated with bone quality measured by TBS.

Here we show that osteoblast precursors cells are decreased and more immature according with decreased bone formation and increased DKK-1, whereas OC precursors are increased in the peripheral blood of T2DM patients. Data on OCs seem to be in contrast with decreased bone resorption in patients. However, it should be underlined that these are immature cells, which may not be able to home in bone microenvironment. Low RANKL levels in patients may explain the low grade of OCs maturation and decreased bone resorption.

This is the first study to evaluate bone cell precursors in the peripheral blood of diabetic patients. Previous data ina diabetic mouse model suggested reduced osteoclast and osteoblast formation in bone microenvironment [42]. An elegant in vitro study suggests that osteoclastogenesis mediated by RANKL is impaired in the presence of high glucose levels [43].

The increase in DKK-1, a well-known negative regulator of bone formation, may explain the decrease in bone formation in T2DM and confirms previous reports [18–20]. On the contrary, SCL was mostly undetectablein our cohort of patients. In the patients with detectable level

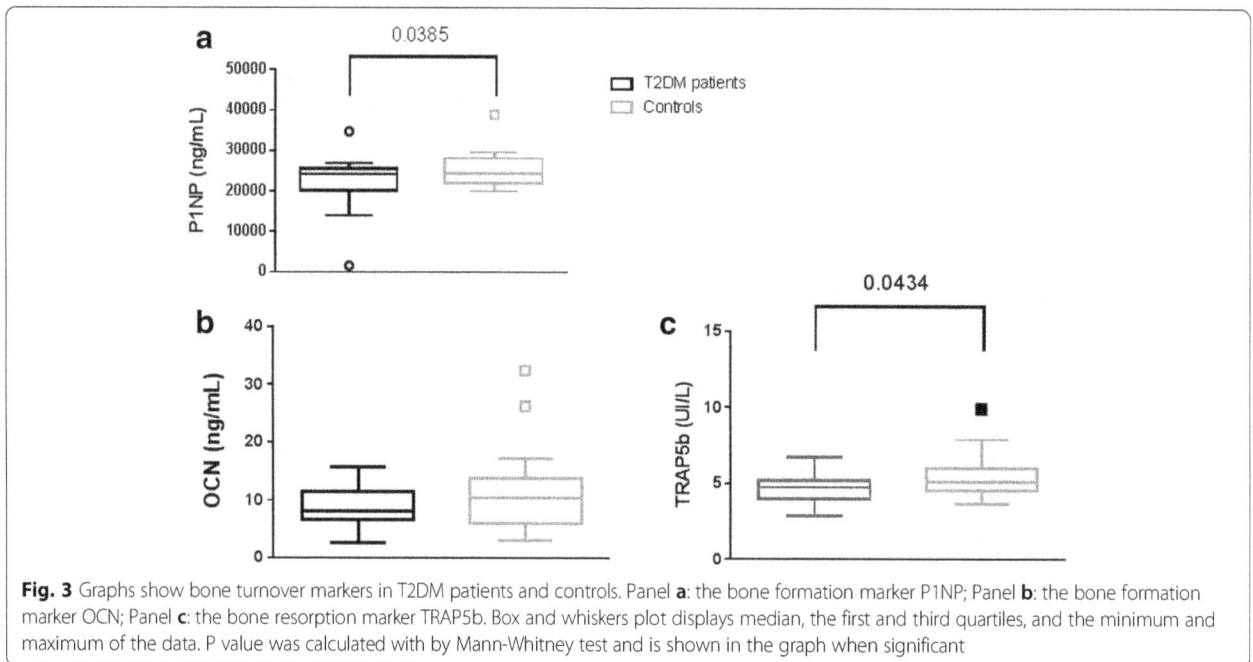

Fig. 3 Graphs show bone turnover markers in T2DM patients and controls. Panel **a**: the bone formation marker P1NP; Panel **b**: the bone formation marker OCN; Panel **c**: the bone resorption marker TRAP5b. Box and whiskers plot displays median, the first and third quartiles, and the minimum and maximum of the data. P value was calculated with by Mann-Whitney test and is shown in the graph when significant

we found a decreased bone formation without any other differences in the variables measured. Several studies investigated the levels of SCL in diabetic patients reporting conflicting results. Gennari et al. [44] showed increased levels of SCL in T2DM, but not in Type 1 diabetes mellitus (T1DM); other studies reported increased SCL in T2DM [45–47]. A recent study on post-menopausal women showed no difference between diabetic and non-diabetic patients in SCL levels [48]. In our study we evaluated only post-menopausal obese subjects, and this may be the reason why we achieved different results from other studies which included younger, leaner populations, also including men. Glycemic control, the use of different anti-hyperglycaemic drugs and the presence of diabetic complications did not appear to bias our results. Poor glycemic control may influence the levels and activity of cytokines active on bone turnover, some studies demonstrated that OPG is increased in T2DM and T1DM patients regardless to their glycemic control [49, 50], this finding is controversial as another study shows a reduction in OPG in T1DM patients [51], here we do not find any significant increase in OPG regardless to glycemic control. RANKL levels seem not to be influenced by glycemic control as shown by Lappin and colleagues [49], we found a decreased RANKL level without any correlation with glycemic control. SCL levels were not studied in relation with glycemic controls in previous studies [20, 44] here we do not find any relationship between glycemic control and SCL.

As regards clinical evaluation of bone health, we did not find a significant increase in BMD in T2DM compared to controls, in contrast to previous results [1, 2]. However, our cohort was small and the use of obese

controls may have influenced this result as BMI per se, regardless of T2DM, is directly correlated with BMD both at lumbar spine and femoral neck.

As regards bone turnover, we found a significant decrease in bone formation and bone resorption in T2DM, confirming other studies [22, 35, 52].

The study was not powered to detect differences in fracture prevalence, hence the similar SDI between T2DM and controls may be due to chance. Age was weakly correlated with RANKL, as expected, and – interestingly – inversely correlated with OB precursor maturation. Use of controls matched with patients for age and BMI excludes this as a confounding factor.

Our study has several strengths and limitations. The analyses of bone turnover and related controlling cytokines was performed in well-characterized cohorts of patients and matched controls. This is the first study evaluating the role of bone cell precursors in T2DM. The significance of our findings may be limited by the small sample size and lack of measurement of parameters related to inflammation and adipocytokines production, some of the results reported may be flawed by the insufficient power.

Conclusion

We show that bone precursor cells are affected by T2DM and, in particular there was a reduction of OB precursors and an increase in OC precursors. Both cell types appear to be more immature in T2DM, and this could be explained by increased levels of DKK-1 and decreased levels of RANKL.

Abbreviations

ALP: Alkaline Phosphatase; APC: Allophycocyanin; BMD: Bone Mineral Dansity; BMI: Body Mass Index; DKK-1: Dickkopf-related Protein 1; FITC: Fluorescein Isothiocyanate; HbA1C: Hemoglobin A1C; HPLC: High Performance Liquid Chromatography; IQR: Interquartile Range; OB: Osteoblast; OC: Osteoclast; OCN: Osteocalcin; OPG: Osteoprotegerin; P1NP: Procollagen Type 1 Amino-terminal Propeptide; PBMCs: Peripheral Blood Mononuclear Cells; PE: Phycoerythrin; RANK: Receptor Activator of Nuclear Factor Kappa-B; RANKL: Receptor Activator of Nuclear Factor Kappa-B Ligand; SCL: Sclerostin; SDI: Spinal Deformity Index; T1DM: Type 1 diabetes mellitus; T2DM: Type 2 diabetes mellitus; TBS: Trabecular Bone Score; TRAP5b: Tartrate-resistant Acid Phosphatase 5b; VNR: Vitronectin

Funding

This work has been founded by Italian Ministry for University and Research. FS is supported by a grant from MIUR PRIN 2015.
IB is supported by a grant from ERC CONSOLIDATOR GRANT -European Project "BOOST".

Authors' contributions

FS, MR and IB performed the lab experiments, acquired and analyzed the lab data. FS and IB partecipated in drafting and critically revising the manuscript. CL, ESpertino, EStratta, MDS, MR, GI, MT and PP performed the clinical evaluation of patients and managed the data set. MP and GCI participated in the study design and were major contributors in writing the manuscript. PD designed the study,performed the statistical analyses and wrote the paper. All authors read and approved the final manuscript.

Competing interests

The authors declare that they have no competing interests.

Author details

[1]Department of Medical Science, Gerontology and Bone Metabolic Diseases, University of Torino, Corso Bramante 88/90, 10126 Torino, Italy. [2]Department of Medical Science, Internal Medicine, University of Torino, Torino, Italy. [3]Geriatric Division, University of Turin, San Luigi Gonzaga Hospital, Orbassano, Turin, Italy.

References

1. Janghorbani M, Van Dam RM, Willett WC, Hu FB. Systematic review of type 1 and type 2 diabetes mellitus and risk of fracture. Am J Epidemiol. 2007; 166:495–505.
2. Bonds DE, Larson JC, Schwartz AV, et al. Risk of fracture in women with type 2 diabetes: the Women's health initiative observational study. J Clin Endocrinol Metab. 2006;91:3404–41.
3. Dhaliwal R, Cibula D, Ghosh C, Weinstock RS, Moses AM. Bone quality assessment in type 2 diabetes mellitus. Osteoporos Int. 2014;25:1969–73.
4. Starup-Linde J, Vestergaard P. Management of endocrine disease: diabetes and osteoporosis: cause for concern? Eur J Endocrinol. 2015;173:R93–9.
5. Xu F, Dong Y, Huang X, et al. Decreased osteoclastogenesis, osteoblastogenesis and low bone mass in a mouse model of type 2 diabetes. Mol Med Rep. 2014; 10:1935–41.
6. Dolan E, Swinton PA, Sale C, Healy A, O'Reilly J. Influence of adipose tissue mass on bone mass in an overweight or obese population: systematic review and meta-analysis. Nutr Rev. 2017; https://doi.org/10.1093/nutrit/nux046.
7. Bridges MJ, Moochhala SH, Barbour J, Kelly CA. Influence of diabetes on peripheral bone mineral density in men: a controlled study. Acta Diabetol. 2005;42:82–6.
8. Wakasugi M, Wakao R, TawataM,Gan N, Koizumi K,Onaya T Bone mineral density measured by dual energy x-ray absorptiometry in patients with non-insulin-dependent diabetes mellitus Bone1993;14:29–33.
9. Perez-Castrillon JL, De Luis D, Martin-EscuderoJC,Asensio T, del Amo R, Izaola O. Non-insulin-dependent diabetes, bone mineral density, and cardiovascular risk factors. J Diabetes Complicat 2004;18:317–321.
10. Evans AL, Paggiosi MA, Eastell R, Walsh JS. Bone density, microstructure and strength in obese and normal weight men and women in younger and older adulthood. J Bone Miner Res. 2015;30:920–8.
11. Rubin MR. Bone cells and bone turnover in diabetes mellitus. Curr Osteoporos Rep. 2015; https://doi.org/10.1007/s11914-015-0265-0.
12. Rosen CJ, Chesnut CH, Mallinak NJ. The predictive value of biochemical markers of bone turnover for bone mineral density in early postmenopausal women treated with hormone replacement or calcium supplementation. J Clin Endocrinol Metab. 1997; https://doi.org/10.1210/jcem.82.6.4004.
13. Shu A, Yin MT, Stein E, et al. Bone structure and turnover in type 2 diabetes mellitus. Osteoporos Int. 2012; https://doi.org/10.1007/s00198-011-1595-0.
14. Oz SG, Guven GS, Kilicarslan A, Calik N, Beyazit Y, Sozen T. Evaluation of bone metabolism and bone mass in patients with type-2 diabetes mellitus. J Natl Med Assoc. 2006;98:1598–604.
15. Achemlal L, Tellal S, Rkiouak F, et al. Bone metabolism in male patients with type 2 diabetes. Clin Rheumatol. 2005; https://doi.org/10.1007/s10067-004-1070-9.
16. Wang Y, Li YP, Paulson C, et al. Wnt and the Wnt signaling pathway in bone development and disease. In: Landmark Ed.Front Biosci; 2014. p. 379-407
17. Oikawa T, Kuroda Y, Matsuo K. Regulation of osteoclasts by membrane-derived lipid mediators. Cell Mol Life Sci. 2013;70:3341–53.
18. Hie M, Iitsuka N, Otsuka T, et al. Insulin-dependent diabetes mellitus decreases osteoblastogenesis associated with the inhibition of Wnt signaling through increased expression of Sost and Dkk1 and inhibition of Akt activation. Int J Mol Med. 2011;28:455–62.
19. Gaudio A, Privitera F, Battaglia K, et al. Sclerostin levels associated with inhibition of the Wnt/β-catenin signaling and reduced bone turnover in type 2 diabetes mellitus. J Clin Endocrinol Metab. 2012;97:3744–50.
20. García-Martín A, Rozas-MorenoP, Reyes-García R, et al. Circulating levels of sclerostin are increased in patients with type 2 diabetes mellitus. J Clin Endocrinol Metab. 2012;97:234–41.
21. Lin CL, Wang JY, Ko JY, Huang YT, Kuo YH, Wang FS. Dickkopf-1 promotes hyperglycemia-induced accumulation of mesangial matrix and renal dysfunction. J Am Soc Nephrol. 2010;21:124–35.
22. Garcia-Martín A, Reyes-Garcia R, García-Fontana B, et al. Relationship of Dickkopf1 (DKK1) with cardiovascular disease and bone metabolism in caucasian type 2 diabetes mellitus. PLoS One. 2014;9:e111703.
23. Gaudio A, Privitera F, Pulvirenti I, Canzonieri E, Rapisarda R, Fiore CE. The relationship between inhibitors of the Wntsignalling pathway (sclerostin and Dickkopf-1) and carotid intima-media thickness in postmenopausal women with type 2 diabetes mellitus. DiabVasc Dis Res. 2014;11:48–52.
24. Ndip A, Williams A, Jude EB, et al. The RANKL/RANK/OPG signaling pathway mediates medial arterial calcification in diabetic Charcot neuroarthropathy. Diabetes. 2011;60:2187–96.
25. Wilkinson CP, Ferris FL 3rd, Klein RE, et al. (Global Diabetic Retinopathy Project Group). Proposed international clinical diabetic retinopathy and diabetic macular edema disease severity scales. Ophthalmology. 2003; https://doi.org/10.1016/S0161-6420(03)00475-5.
26. Consensus statement: Report and recommendations of the San Antonio conference on diabetic neuropathy. American Diabetes Association American Academy of Neurology. Diabetes Care. 1988;11:592–7.
27. D'Amelio P, Spertino E, Martino F, Isaia GC. Prevalence of postmenopausal osteoporosis in Italy and validation of decision rules for referring women for bone densitometry. Calcif Tissue Int. 2013;92:437–43.
28. Kerkeni S, Kolta S, Fechtenbaum J, Roux C. Spinal deformity index (SDI) is a good predictor of incident vertebral fractures. Osteoporos Int. 2009;20:1547–52.
29. Silva BC, Leslie WD, Resch H, et al. Trabecular bone score: a noninvasive analytical method based upon the DXA image. Bone Miner Res. 2014;29: 518–30.
30. D'Amelio P, Cristofaro MA, Grimaldi A, et al. The role of circulating bone cell precursors in fracture healing. Calcif Tissue Int. 2010;86:463–9.
31. Eghbali-Fatourechi GZ, Lamsam J, Fraser D, Nagel D, Riggs BL, Khosla S. Circulating osteoblast-lineage cells in humans. N Engl J Med. 2005;352: 1959–66.
32. D'Amelio P, Tamone C, Sassi F, et al. Teriparatide increases the maturation of circulating osteoblast precursors. Osteoporos Int. 2012;23:1245–53.
33. Jackson AS, Pollock ML, Ward A. Generalized equations for predicting body density of women. Med Sci Sports Exerc. 1980;12:175–81.

34. Choi YJ, Ock SY, Chung YS. Trabecular bone score (TBS) and TBS-adjusted fracture risk assessment tool are potential supplementary tools for the discrimination of morphometric vertebral fractures in postmenopausal women with type 2 diabetes. J Clin Densitom. 2016; https://doi.org/10.1016/j.jocd.2016.04.001.

35. Purnamasari D, Puspitasari MD, Setiyohadi B, Nugroho P, Isbagio H. Low bone turnover in premenopausal women with type 2 diabetes mellitus as an early process of diabetes-associated bone alterations: a cross-sectional study. BMC Endocr Disord. 2017; https://doi.org/10.1186/s12902-017-0224-0.

36. Armstrong ME, Cairns BJ, Banks E, Green J, Reeves GK, Beral V. Different effects of age, adiposity and physical activity on the risk of ankle, wrist and hip fractures in postmenopausal women. Bone. 2012;50:1394–400.

37. De Laet C, Kanis JA, Oden A, et al. Body mass index as a predictor of fracture risk: a meta-analysis. Osteoporos Int. 2005;16:1330–8.

38. Prieto-Alhambra D, Premaor MO, Fina Aviles F, et al. The association between fracture and obesity is site-dependent: a population-based study in postmenopausal women. J Bone Miner Res. 2012;27:294–300.

39. Colaianni G, Brunetti G, Faienza MF, Colucci S, Grano M. Osteoporosis and obesity: role of Wnt pathway in human and murine models. World J Orthop. 2014;5:242–6.

40. Isaia GC, D'Amelio P, Di Bella S, Tamone C. Is leptin the link between fat and bone mass? J Endocrinol Invest. 2005;28Suppl 10:61–5.

41. Kim JH, Choi HJ, Ku EJ, et al. Trabecular bone score as an indicator for skeletal deterioration in diabetes. J ClinEndocrinol Metab. 2015; 100:475–82.

42. Xu J, Yue F, Wang J, Chen L, Qi W. High glucose inhibits receptor activator of nuclear factor-κB ligand-induced osteoclast differentiation via downregulation of v-ATPase V0 subunit d2 and dendritic cell-specific transmembrane protein. Mol Med Rep. 2015;11:865–70.

43. Christman MA, Goetz DJ, Dickerson E, et al. Wnt5a is expressed in murine and human atherosclerotic lesions. Am J Physiol Heart Circ Physiol. 2008; 294:H2864–70.

44. Gennari L, Merlotti D, Valenti R, et al. Circulating sclerostin levels and bone turnover in type 1 and type 2 diabetes. J Clin Endocrinol Metab. 2012; https://doi.org/10.1210/jc.2011-2958.

45. Gaudio A, Privitera F, Battaglia K, et al. Sclerostin levels associated with inhibition of the Wnt/β-catenin signaling and reduced bone turnover in type 2 diabetes mellitus. J Clin Endocrinol Metab. 2012; https://doi.org/10.1210/jc.2012-1901.

46. Napoli N, Strollo R, Defeudis G, et al. Serum Sclerostin and Bone Turnover in Latent Autoimmune Diabetes in Adults. J Clin Endocrinol Metab. 2018; https://doi.org/10.1210/jc.2017-02274.

47. Hygum K, Starup-Linde J, Harsløf T, Vestergaard P, Langdahl BL. MECHANISMS IN ENDOCRINOLOGY: Diabetes mellitus, a state of low bone turnover- a systematic review and meta-analysis. Eur J Endocrinol. 2017; https://doi.org/10.1530/EJE-16-0652.

48. Kalem MN, Kalem Z, Akgun N, Bakırarar B. The relationship between postmenopausal women's sclerostin levels and their bone density, age, body mass index, hormonal status, and smoking and consumption of coffee and dairy products. Arch Gynecol Obstet. 2017; https://doi.org/10.1007/s00404-017-4288-x.

49. Lappin DF, Eapen B, Robertson D, Young J, Hodge PJ. Markers of bone destruction and formation and periodontitis in type 1 diabetes mellitus. J Clin Periodontol. 2009; https://doi.org/10.1111/j.1600-051X.2009.01440.x.

50. Galluzzi F, Stagi S, Salti R, et al. Osteoprotegerin serum levels in children with type 1 diabetes: a potential modulating role in bone status. Eur J Endocrinol. 2005; https://doi.org/10.1530/eje.1.02052.

51. Abd El Dayem SM, El-Shehaby AM, Abd El Gafar A, Fawzy A, Salama H. Bone density, body composition, and markers of bone remodeling in type 1 diabetic patients. Scand J Clin Lab Invest. 2011; https://doi.org/10.3109/00365513.2011.573574.

52. D'Amelio P, Grimaldi A, Di Bella S, et al. Estrogen deficiency increases osteoclastogenesis up-regulating T cells activity: a key mechanism in osteoporosis. Bone. 2008;43:92–100.

16

Reintroducing testosterone in the *db/db* mouse partially restores normal glucose metabolism and insulin resistance in a leptin-independent manner

Koichi Yabiku[1][*] [iD], Keiko Nakamoto[2] and Akihiro Tokushige[3]

Abstract

Background: Testosterone signals through the androgen receptor (AR) and AR knockout mice develop obesity, suggesting a functional association between AR and leptin signaling. Furthermore, physiological blood concentrations of testosterone have been found to inhibit the development of arteriosclerosis, obesity and diabetes. However, these findings have not been verified by testosterone replacement in animal models and whether or not testosterone acts directly by activating AR to enhance leptin signaling, or indirectly by its conversion into estrogen remains unclear. Therefore, we investigated the effect of exogenously supplemented testosterone on glucose and lipid metabolism.

Methods: Four-week-old male leptin receptor-knockout *db/db* mice were used as controls for a model of obesity retaining low testosterone. Mice were divided into sham-operated, castrated, or castrated and testosterone-supplemented groups and fed a high-fat diet (HFD) for 2 weeks from 5 weeks of age. Testosterone concentrations, blood glucose, plasma insulin levels, and intraperitoneal glucose tolerance and insulin tolerance were measured. At 7 weeks, triglyceride and glycogen content were measured in the liver and muscle. Lipid accumulation in the liver and soleus muscle was determined by immunohistochemistry with Oil Red O. Statistical analyses were performed using the Student's *t*-test or ANOVA where applicable.

Results: Lower testosterone levels in *db/db* mice compared with wild type (WT) *db/+* mice were associated with glucose intolerance and fatty liver. Furthermore, castrated male *db/db* mice at 4 weeks of age progressively developed glucose intolerance accompanying a 15% increase in liver fat. Male mice fed a HFD had lower levels of testosterone compared with those fed a normal diet. We found that exogenous testosterone replacement injected subcutaneously into castrated male *db/db* mice alleviated the exacerbation of fatty liver and glucose intolerance, suggesting a leptin-independent mechanism. This mechanism is most likely mediated through gonadal axis suppression in this mouse model.

Conclusions: In summary, testosterone may use a novel pathway to complement leptin signaling to regulate glucose and lipid metabolism, and thus offers a new therapeutic target to treat metabolic disorders.

Keywords: Testosterone replacement, Leptin signal knockout, Aromatization, Impaired glucose tolerance, Fatty liver

* Correspondence: kyabiku@med.u-ryukyu.ac.jp
[1]Division of Endocrinology, Diabetes and Metabolism, Hematology, Rheumatology (Second Department of Internal Medicine), Graduate School of Medicine, University of the Ryukyus, 207 Uehara, Nishihara, Okinawa 903-0215, Japan
Full list of author information is available at the end of the article

Background

In addition to maintaining gametes, testosterone is responsible for maintaining and elevating daily activity levels in adult men. For example, not all men adapt to a decrease in testosterone with aging. A rapid decrease in testosterone levels with aging has been reported in many cases, leading to a marked impairment of quality of life (QOL) in middle-aged to elderly men [1–3]. A decrease in blood testosterone levels was recently shown to increase the incidence of all-cause mortality [4], in addition to metabolic syndrome (MetS) [5–7], type 2 diabetes [8–10] associated with the progression of visceral obesity and enhancement of insulin resistance, osteoporosis-associated fracture [11–13], and progression of arteriosclerosis [14–16]. Although testosterone was previously considered to be an arteriosclerosis-promoting hormone because endogenous testosterone was shown to decrease HDL-cholesterol levels, the action of testosterone within its physiological blood concentration range was demonstrated to have an inhibitory effect on the development and progression of lifestyle-related diseases such as arteriosclerosis, obesity and diabetes [8, 17]. However, whether a low testosterone level may be a potent predictor of clinically-important coronary arterial disease has not been confirmed in previous case-controlled and longitudinal studies [18, 19].

The results of animal studies on exogenous testosterone are varied, with both positive and negative effects being observed. For example, it has been shown to exacerbate hypertension and induce renal failure in male SHR rats [20], whereas amelioration of erectile dysfunction has been reported in castrated animals [21–24]. Testosterone is known to act through the androgen receptor (AR). In AR knockout (KO) mice, the development of male-specific delayed-onset obesity has been reported, and the activation of AR enhanced leptin-induced STAT3 nuclear translocation and transcription of leptin target genes, in an in vitro system [25–27]. Therefore, the functional association between AR and leptin signaling has recently attracted attention. Although more detailed evidence is needed, AR is assumed to exhibit an anti-obesity effect by enhancing leptin signaling, which has been shown to activate sympathetic nerves.

Whether the effect of endogenous testosterone is directly caused by testosterone or its active form, dihydrotestosterone (DHT), through AR, or by estrogen (testosterone is converted to estrogen by aromatase), has not yet been elucidated [28, 29]. Qiu Y et al. demonstrated that administration of a physiological level of the non-aromatized androgen, DHT, to an arteriosclerosis model prepared by feeding a high-cholesterol diet to orchidectomized rabbits directly acted against arteriosclerosis [30]. Furthermore, studies using aromatase KO mice confirmed close associations with, first, the energy metabolism-related factor,

leptin, and then with other factors such as PPARγ [31]. However, this has not yet been verified in animal studies by actual testosterone replacement.

In this study, we initially investigated testosterone and glucose metabolism in *db/db* mice relative to WT *db/+* controls and assessed a normal chow diet (NCD) and HFD. Changes in testosterone levels with aging were also investigated in each group of mice, as was the effect of diet (NCD or HFD). Subsequently, the influence of exogenously-supplemented testosterone on glucose and liver steatosis was investigated in *db/db* (castrated or sham-operated) mice. To confirm whether aromatisation is important for testosterone effects, we used its inhibitor, anastrozole. Conditions that elevated testosterone levels were simulated by keeping male and female mice in the same cage during the reproductive period to investigate how testosterone levels responded in male mice.

Methods

Animal experiments

Male and female *db/+* heterogeneous mice (10 weeks of age) were purchased from the Jackson Laboratory (Sacramento, CA) and housed in a temperature-controlled room (22–23 °C) with a 12 h light/dark cycle. All animal experiments were approved by the Institutional Animal Care Committee of the Faculty of Medicine at the University of the Ryukyus (No. 5115). Male *db/+* and *db/db* offspring were weaned at 4 weeks of age, divided into two groups at 5 weeks of age, and then fed a NCD or HFD for 2 weeks. To measure the blood testosterone level, tail vein blood was collected at 7 weeks of age. Blood samples were centrifuged, and the plasma testosterone concentrations were determined using an enzyme-linked immunosorbent assay (ELISA) kit (Endocrine Technologies, Inc. USA).

Castration of mice

Four-week-old male *db/db* mice were castrated according to the following procedure. Under barbiturate anesthesia, an incision was made approximately 2 cm cranial to the penis, and an approximately 1 cm incision was made in the exposed abdominal muscle layer. The testes, epididymides and vas deferentia were pulled out of the body while avoiding injury to the intestines. For each testis, the vas deferens was ligated at two sites and cut between ligations. The testes were then resected and the wound sutured. Testosterone replacement was initiated in 5-week-old mice.

Testosterone injection and measurement of plasma estradiol levels

Testosterone propionate (Wako, Osaka, Japan) was dissolved in sesame oil (Sigma-Aldrich, Tokyo, Japan) and its concentration was adjusted (20 μg/μl). Testosterone was injected subcutaneously into each group of castrated mice at 1, 10 or 100 µg/g body weight/2 days for 2 weeks from 5 weeks of age, and blood estradiol levels were measured at 7 weeks of age using an ELISA kit (Endocrine Technologies, Inc. USA).

Analysis of fuel homeostasis

Sham-operated, castrated, and castrated and testosterone-supplemented groups ($n = 8-14$ per group) were fed HFD for 2 weeks from 5 weeks of age, and then intraperitoneal glucose tolerance (ipGTT) and insulin tolerance (ipITT) tests were performed. At 7 weeks of age, triglyceride (TG) content and glycogen content were also measured in the liver and muscle. The mice were fasted overnight and injected intraperitoneally with glucose (1 g/kg) for ipGTT testing. Mice fasted for 4 h were injected intraperitoneally with REGULAR human insulin (Humulin R, 1.2 U/kg, Eli Lilly, Indianapolis, USA) for ipITT testing. Blood glucose values were determined using a Medisafe glucometer (Terumo, Tokyo, Japan) and plasma insulin levels were quantified using an ELISA kit (Shibayagi, Gunma, Japan). Tissue TG content was measured using an enzymatic assay method reported previously [32, 33]. To measure glycogen content, pieces of the liver were isolated from 7-week-old mice in a 16 h fasted or ad libitum-fed state, and then homogenized in 3% (w/w) perchloric acid on ice. An aliquot of the homogenate was incubated for 2 h at 40 °C with amyloglucosidase. The resulting glucose residues were quantified using an enzymatic glucose kit (Sigma-Aldrich, Tokyo, Japan), and the glycogen content was expressed as milligram (mg) per gram (g) of wet liver.

Histology and immunohistochemistry

To evaluate lipid accumulation in the liver and soleus muscle, frozen sections were stained with filtered Oil Red O (in isopropanol) and visualized with 0.1% lithium carbonate. Oil Red O-positive areas in the sections were measured as previously reported [33, 34]. To evaluate the pancreatic β cell mass, 4-µm sections were treated with guinea pig anti-porcine insulin (1:200). The sections were incubated with biotinylated secondary antibodies and the signals were visualized with 2,3′ diaminobenzidine (DAB). Images were captured using a ScanScope Digital Slide Scanner (Aperio, Vista, CA) and the β cell mass was estimated.

Immunoblotting and real-time PCR

Immunoblotting was performed as described previously [35]. Regular human insulin (5 units/kg mouse body weight) was injected into each group after a 16 h fast, and the liver and soleus muscle were excised 30 min after injection. The excised organs were frozen in liquid nitrogen and stored prior to immunoblotting. To prepare the samples for immunoblotting, the tissues were lysed at 4 °C in NP-40 lysis buffer (1% NP-40, 50 mM Tris-HCl (pH 8.0), 150 mM NaCl) containing proteinase and phosphatase inhibitors

(Sigma, Tokyo, Japan). Twenty micrograms (20 µg) of total protein from each sample were then separated by electrophoresis on 10% denaturing sodium dodecyl sulfate-polyacrylamide gels and transferred to nitro-cellulose membranes (Millipore, Billerica, MA, USA). After blocking with Tris-buffered saline containing 0.05% Tween 20, the membranes were incubated with an anti-phosphoserine Akt (Ser473) antibody (Cell Signaling Technology, Beverly, MA, USA) (RRID: AB_39825) followed by a horseradish peroxidase-conjugated anti-rabbit IgG. Bound antibodies were detected using an enhanced chemiluminescence (ECL) system (Amersham, Little Chalfont, UK). The bound antibodies were then stripped from the membranes, which were reprobed with an anti-Akt antibody (Cell Signaling Technology, Beverly, MA, USA) (RRID: AB_329827) to reveal the location and intensity of the 60-kDa-labelled band. Scion Image software (US National Institutes of Health) was used for quantitative analysis of the blots.

Liver and muscle tissues samples for real-time PCR were preserved in RNAlater (Qiagen, Tokyo, Japan) prior to the isolation of total RNA using the RNeasy Lipid Tissue Mini Kit (Qiagen, Tokyo, Japan). The RNA samples were treated with DNase and reverse-transcribed into cDNA using Superscript II (Life Technologies, Foster City, CA). The cDNA samples were treated with RNase and used for real-time RT-PCR with SYBR Green PCR Master Mix (Applied Biosystems, Foster City, CA) in an ABI StepOnePlus Real-time PCR System as described previously [36, 37]. The expression of mRNA for each target gene was normalized relative to that of glyceraldehyde 3-phosphate dehydrogenase (*Gapdh*). The sense and antisense primers were 5′-TCTGGGTGGCAGTGGTCGGA-3′ and 5′-TGGC CAGAGGGACTTCCTGGT-3′, respectively, for *G6pc*, 5′-CGCAGGACGCGGAACCATGT-3′ and 5′-CATGCT GCCAGCTGAGGGCT-3′ for *Pck1*, 5′-TGTCGCAGGT GGAGAGCGACT-3′ and 5′-TCACAGGCACGGCGCAC AAT-3′ for *Gck*, and 5′-TGTGTCCGTCGTGGATCTG A-3′ and 5′-TTGCTGTTGAAGTCGCAGGAG-3′, respectively, for *Gapdh*. The cycle number at which fluorescence exceeded the threshold of detection (CT) for *Gapdh* was subtracted from that of the target gene in each well (ΔCT). The percentage change in expression, relative to that of the vehicle-treated group, was defined as (2 − ΔΔCT × 100), where ΔΔCT = ΔCT for the intervention group − ΔCT for the vehicle-treated group.

Continuous anastrozole infusion using an osmotic pump and subcutaneous implantation of a testosterone pellet in the neck

To block the conversion of testosterone to estradiol (aromatization), the aromatase inhibitor, anastrozole (Astra-Zeneca, London, UK), was dissolved in 0.3% hydroxypropylcellulose and 0.9% NaCl, added to an osmotic

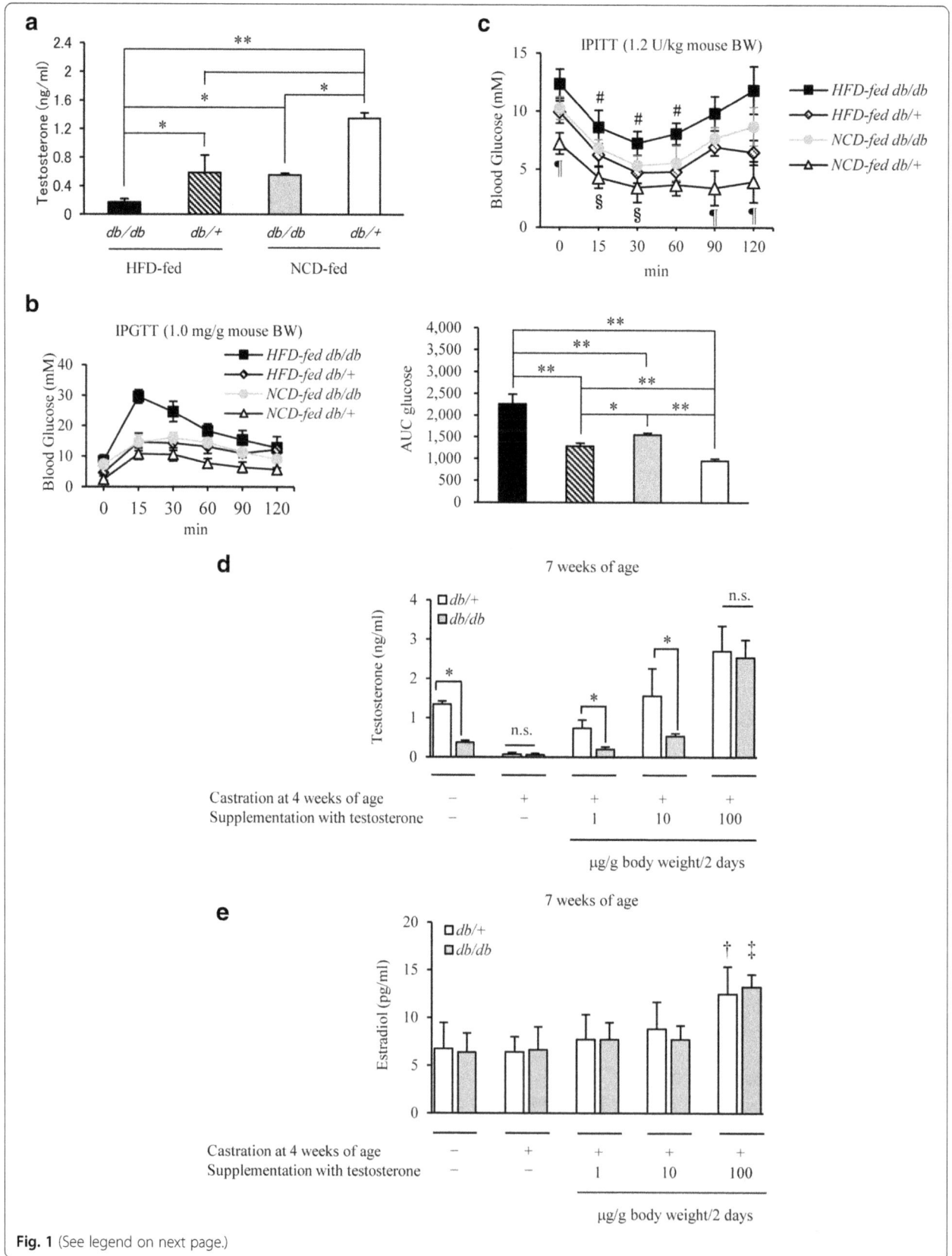

Fig. 1 (See legend on next page.)

(See figure on previous page.)

Fig. 1 Induction of low levels of testosterone by leptin receptor KO or HFD. **a** Comparison of testosterone levels in NCD-fed *db/+* and *db/db* male mice, and HFD-fed *db/+* and *db/db* male mice, at 7 weeks of age ($n = 14$/group). Testosterone levels were the lowest in HFD-fed *db/db* mice, and increased in the order, NCD-fed *db/db* > NCD-fed *db/+* mice. **b** IpGTT analysis in 7-week-old mice on NCD or HFD in each group ($n = 12-14$/group). The area under the curve (AUC glucose) is shown in the right panel. Glucose homeostasis was exacerbated by HFD feeding. **c** IpITT analysis in 7-week-old mice in each group ($n = 10-13$/group) as indicated. **d** The dose of exogenous testosterone replacement and blood testosterone levels in castrated mice ($n = 9-12$/group). Exogenous testosterone was administered once every 2 days. Blood testosterone levels increased with an increase in the dose of testosterone replacement. **e** The dose of exogenous testosterone replacement and blood estradiol levels in castrated mice ($n = 9-12$/group). Blood estradiol levels did not significantly increase until the dose of exogenous testosterone replacement was elevated to 100 μg/g body weight/2 days. Results are expressed as means ± s.e.m. *$P < 0.05$, **$P < 0.01$ between the indicated groups. #$P < 0.01$, ¶$P < 0.01$ versus the other group of mice at each time, 2-way ANOVA. §$P < 0.01$ versus the other group of mice on NCD at each time, 2-way ANOVA. †$P < 0.05$ versus another group of *db/+* mice. ‡$P < 0.01$ versus another group of *db/db* mice. n.s., no significant

mini-pump (Alzet, Cupertino, CA), and delivered under the skin via an indwelling catheter in the back of 4-week-old castrated mice (the continuous infusion rate of anastrozole was adjusted to 200 μg/day). To adjust the blood testosterone levels to a steady state, a testosterone pellet (15 mg/tablet) (Nacalai Tesque, Kyoto, Japan) was simultaneously implanted under the neck skin of 4-week-old castrated mice using a precision trochar (a placebo pellet was implanted in control mice). This testosterone treatment produces maximal stimulation of spermatogenesis [38]. Glucose and lipid metabolism were similarly evaluated in 7-week-old mice, at which time the blood estradiol levels were also measured to confirm that they were below the level of sensitivity.

Time-course evaluation of blood gonadotropin and testosterone levels and evaluation of testosterone using the hCG load test

Changes in blood testosterone and gonadotropin (luteinizing hormone (LH) and follicle stimulating hormone (FSH)) levels with aging were measured in male *db/db* and *db/+* mice from 4 weeks to 1 year of age and also according to the diet given (NCD and HFD) using an ELISA kit (CUSABIO, Wuhan, China). Ten-week-old male and female mice were kept in the same cage (separated by a fence to avoid copulation) for 2 weeks (male *db/db* mice × female *db/db* mice, male *db/db* × female *db/+*, male *db/+* × female *db/db*, and male *db/+* × female *db/+*), and blood testosterone levels were measured in the male mice. Control male mice were maintained without a female for 2 weeks from 10 weeks of age, and their testosterone levels were measured at 12 weeks of age. In addition, human chorionic gonadotropin (hCG) (Sigma, Tokyo, Japan) in PBS was administered (0.5 IU/g body weight) to 12-week-old mice, and increases in blood testosterone levels were compared between the groups.

Statistical analysis

Data are presented as means ± s.e.m. Statistical analyses were performed using Student's *t*-test or ANOVA with Tukey's HSD multiple comparisons as appropriate.

Differences were considered significant at $P < 0.05$. In addition, power calculations were performed based on average value differences and common standard deviations in each group, with the two-sided α-error set at 0.05.

Results

Influence of obesity and fatty foods on low circulating testosterone levels in mice

A significant decrease in blood testosterone levels was observed in the order: HFD-fed *db/db* > NCD-fed *db/db* > NCD-fed *db/+* mice (Fig. 1a), which was consistent with the order of glucose intolerance observed in response to ipGTT and assessed by measurement of glucose area under curve (AUC) (Fig. 1b). Similar findings were also observed for ipITT analysis (Fig. 1c). Testosterone is known to be converted to estrogen by aromatase (aromatization); therefore, whether the effect of endogenous testosterone was direct or through estrogen remained unclear. Thus, 4-week-old *db/db* mice were castrated and treated with testosterone at various concentrations (1, 10 and 100 μg/g body weight/2 days) for 2 weeks from 5 weeks of age, and blood testosterone and estradiol levels were measured to establish the dose for testosterone replacement. Blood testosterone levels increased with an increase in the dose of testosterone (Fig. 1d). No significant increase in blood estradiol levels was observed at exogenous testosterone doses up to 10 μg/g body weight/2 days; however, a significant increase was noted at 100 μg/g body weight/2 days (Fig. 1e). Thus, the dose for testosterone replacement was set at 10 μg/g body weight/2 days.

Impact of testosterone replacement on fuel homeostasis in castrated mice

IpGTT testing of the 4 HFD-fed groups—sham-operated, sham-operated+testosterone-supplemented, castrated, and castrated+testosterone-supplemented groups—at 7 weeks of age revealed that glucose tolerance was significantly lower in the castrated group than in the sham group, and also that testosterone replacement significantly reversed the exacerbation of glucose tolerance in castrated mice (glucose AUC: 2194 ± 295 in the sham group, 2101 ± 371

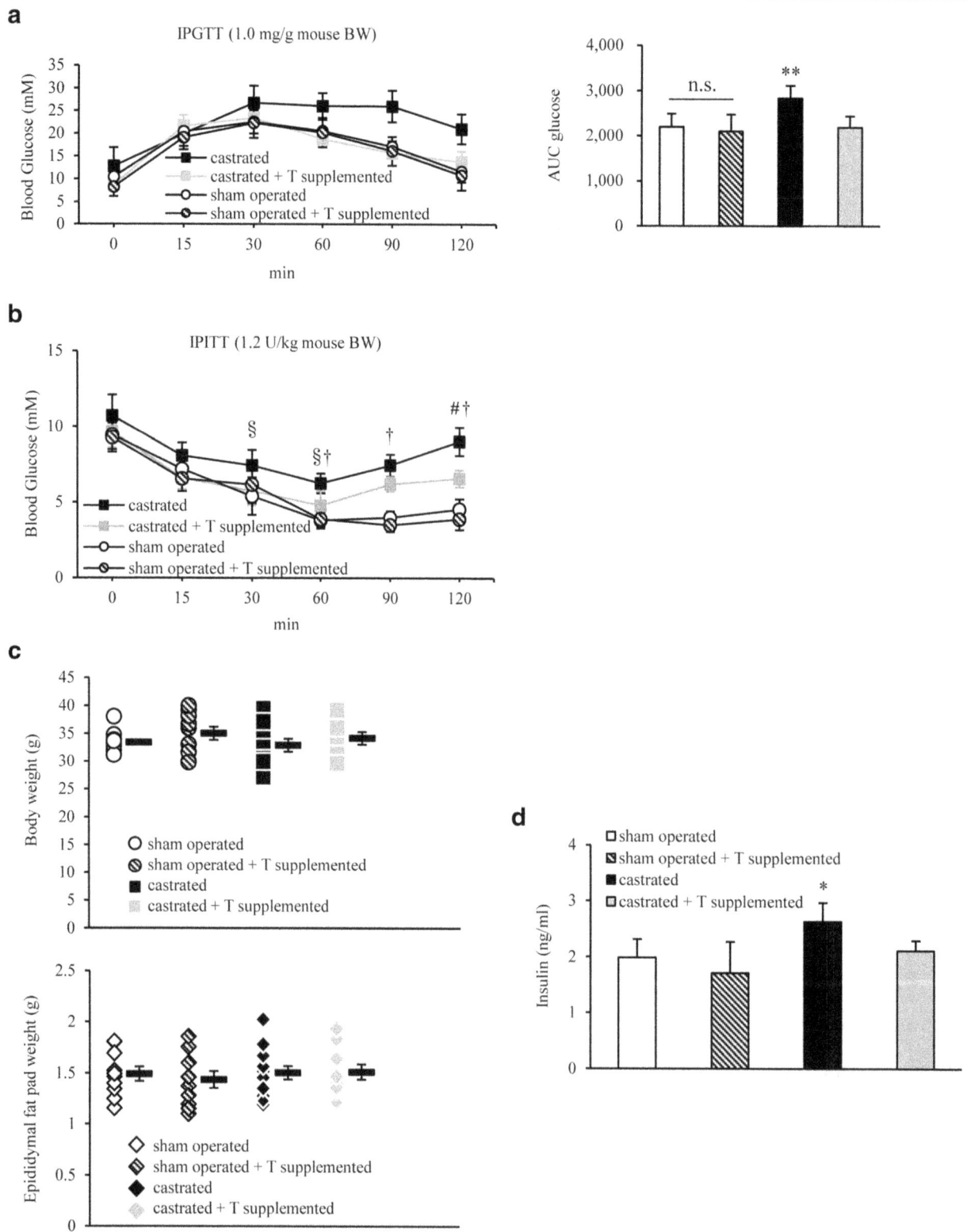

Fig. 2 (See legend on next page.)

in the sham+testosterone-supplemented group, 2839 ± 280 in the castrated group, and 2182 ± 252 in the castrated+testosterone replacement group; P < 0.01) (Fig. 2a). IpITT testing also showed that insulin sensitivity was lower in the castrated group than in the sham group, and tended to recover in the testosterone replacement group (Fig. 2b). Therefore, glucose intolerance mainly associated with insulin resistance was attributed to a decrease in endogenous testosterone levels in castrated mice. No significant differences were observed in the body weight or epididymal fat weight among these groups at 7 weeks of age (Fig. 2c). In addition, fasting blood insulin levels were slightly higher in the castrated group, and were significantly decreased upon testosterone replacement (Fig. 2d). Fat accumulation in and the TG content of liver and muscle were also evaluated. The percentage area of fat was higher in the castrated group, and was significantly lower in the testosterone replacement group (% area of fat: 36.5 ± 3.2 in the sham group, 30.7 ± 6.3 in the sham+testosterone replacement group, 42.4 ± 2.4 in the castrated group, and 29.4 ± 4.3 in the testosterone replacement group; sham vs. castrated group, P < 0.05; castrated vs. testosterone replacement group, P < 0.01) (Fig. 3a and b). The testosterone replacement group also lowered liver TG content (Fasting state: 20.9 ± 6.9 mg/g liver in the sham group, 22.5 ± 4.6 mg/g liver in the castrated group, and 15.8 ± 1.9 mg/g liver in the castrated+testosterone replacement group; castrated vs. testosterone replacement group, P < 0.05; Fed state: 32.1 ± 10.6 mg/g liver in the sham group, 52.0 ± 13.3 mg/g liver in the castrated group, and 37.7 ± 11.1 mg/g liver in the castrated+testosterone replacement group; sham vs. castrated group, P < 0.01; castrated vs. testosterone replacement group, P < 0.01) (Fig. 3c). No significant differences were observed in these parameters or in the weight of the soleus muscle at 7 weeks of age (data not shown). Insulin resistance in obesity was previously shown to manifest as a result of impaired suppression of hepatic glycogen synthesis and glucose output. Therefore, the hepatic glycogen contents were assessed, demonstrating no significant difference between the groups after 16 h of fasting. However, they

were significantly higher in the castrated mice than in the sham-operated mice in a fed state, and significantly reduced upon testosterone replacement (Fig. 3c). Pancreatic β cells were homogenously swollen in all groups, but no collapse (shrinkage of β cells) occurred, which indicated that a low testosterone level was unlikely to directly destroy pancreatic β cells (Fig. 3d).

Impact of testosterone replacement on castration-induced insulin resistance in the liver

Insulin-inducing Akt signals were investigated in the liver and soleus muscle by immunoblotting. Akt phosphorylation was significantly decreased in the liver of the castrated group, and recovered upon testosterone replacement (Fig. 4a). However, no significant difference was observed in Akt signals in the soleus muscle (Fig. 4b). A comparison of the relative *G6pc* and *Pck1* mRNA/*Gapdh* expression levels in the liver revealed that these levels were enhanced in the castrated group, and then the *Pck1* levels were mildly but significantly reduced upon testosterone replacement (Fig. 4c).

Based on the above findings, low blood testosterone levels appear to somewhat inhibit insulin signaling in the liver during the relatively young period in *db/db* mice.

Testosterone is almost not affected by circadian rhythms. To reduce subcutaneous testosterone injection-induced variations in blood testosterone levels (i.e., to prepare a steady state), a testosterone pellet was implanted under the cervical skin in castrated mice at 4 weeks of age (a placebo pellet was implanted in the control mice). In addition, to completely block the influence of aromatization, the aromatase inhibitor, anastrozole, was simultaneously and continuously infused using an osmotic pump (Fig. 4d). We found that aromatization was completely blocked by anastrozole administration (Additional file 1: Figure S1). When glucose metabolism were evaluated in 7-week-old mice, the results obtained were similar to those in animals treated with a subcutaneous testosterone injection alone (Fig. 4e and f), which suggests that the recovery of glucose metabolism with testosterone replacement involved at least the direct action of testosterone.

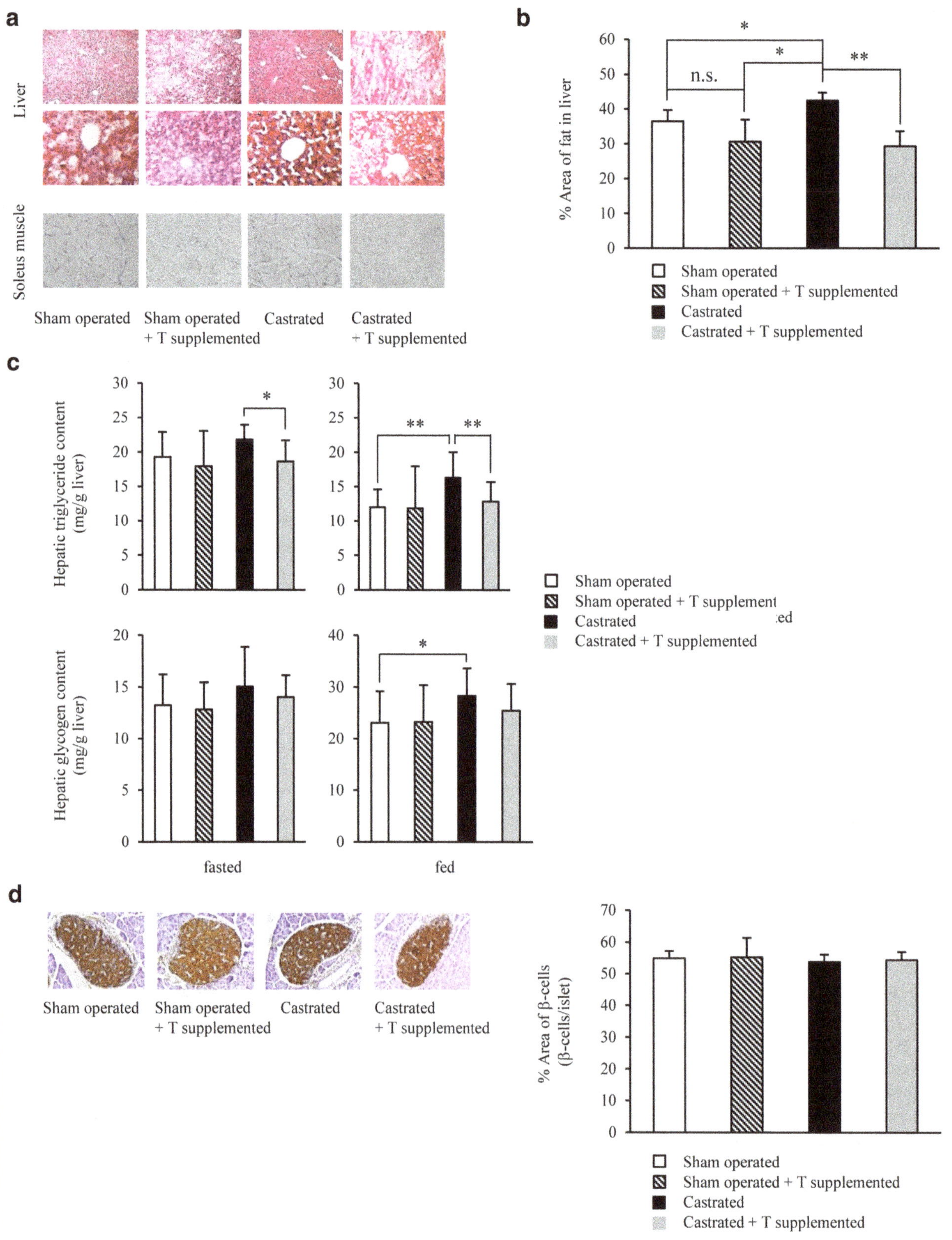

Fig. 3 (See legend on next page.)

(See figure on previous page.)
Fig. 3 Decreased blood testosterone levels exacerbated fatty liver in *db/db* mice, and exogenous testosterone replacement mildly reduced this exacerbation. **a** Microscopic views of the liver [upper (× 40 magnification) and middle (× 200 magnification)] and soleus muscle [bottom (× 200 magnification)] from 7-week-old *db/db* mice in each group [sham operated, sham operated + testosterone (T) supplemented, castrated, or castrated + T supplemented mice; $n = 9–12$/group]. Hepatic steatosis was most exacerbated in castrated mice and reduced with T supplementation as shown by Oil Red O staining. **b** Oil Red O-positive area. **c** Hepatic TG (upper) and glycogen (bottom) content in fasted and ad libitum-fed ($n = 11–13$/group). **d** Histological analyses of the pancreas ($n = 10–12$/group). Representative sections stained with anti-insulin antibodies [left (× 100 magnification)]. The proportion of β cells was calculated relative to islets (right). Results are expressed as means ± s.e.m. *P < 0.05, **P < 0.01 between the indicated groups, 2-way ANOVA. n.s., no significant

Aging- and dietary content-induced changes in blood testosterone levels and the influence of female mice in the reproductive period on blood testosterone levels in male mice

As shown in Fig. 5a, changes in blood testosterone levels with aging were compared between male *db/db* and *db/+* mice. Blood testosterone levels decreased with aging after reaching a peak during the reproductive period in male *db/+* mice. In contrast, these levels were already low from the juvenile period in male *db/db* mice, and remained low even during the reproductive period. Regarding the effect of the diet (NCD and HFD) on male *db/+* mice, blood testosterone levels were lower in the HFD- than in the NCD-fed group throughout the observation period (Fig. 5a). The levels of simultaneously measured LH and FSH gradually increased in male *db/+* mice at 32 weeks of age and older, but remained low in male *db/db* mice throughout the observation period from 4 weeks of age to the elderly period (Fig. 5b). In addition, the testis weight was lower in *db/db* mice than in age-matched *db/+* mice (Table 1).

To investigate the influence of mating on blood testosterone levels, on the assumption that mating elevates these levels, male and female mice were kept in the same cage for 2 weeks from 10 weeks of age (Fig. 5c). Blood testosterone levels significantly increased in 12-week-old male *db/+* mice regardless of whether the female mice in the same cage were *db/+* or *db/db*. In contrast, no significant increase was observed in blood testosterone levels in 12-week-old *db/db* mice in the presence of female mice of either genotype. hCG is known to stimulate the production of testosterone [39]. The hCG load test revealed that the increase in testosterone levels was significantly lower in male *db/+* HFD-fed mice than in *db/+* NCD-fed mice at 12 weeks of age. In contrast, although the hCG stimulating, testosterone levels were low in male *db/db* mice (Fig. 5d).

Discussion

In an obesity model, *db/db* mice, a decrease in blood testosterone levels significantly aggravated glucose intolerance even at a relatively young age. Previous reports have suggested that AR acts to reinforce the action of leptin [25–27]; however, our findings, obtained with the leptin

receptor knockout *db/db* mice, indicate the presence of a pathway not mediated by leptin signaling in the mechanism by which testosterone inhibited the exacerbation of glucose tolerance. To the best of our knowledge, no report has yet confirmed that fatty liver generally develops in men with hypogonadism, e.g., men with Klinefelter syndrome, Prader-Willi syndrome or Kallmann syndrome, or after castration. In this context, the actions of leptin and testosterone may complement each other, while their simultaneous reduction has been attributed to the aggravation of glucose tolerance observed in our model. Based on the results obtained from aromatization, we set the dose of exogenous testosterone replacement at 10 μg/g body weight/2 days (Fig. 1d and e). Variation of the blood testosterone level was marked in *db/+* mice supplemented with 10 μg/g body weight/2 days of testosterone, but the level was significantly higher than that in *db/db* mice, whereas no difference was noted in the blood estradiol level. Since exogenous supplementation with 10 μg/g body weight/2 days of testosterone did not reach the aromatization-inducing threshold in this mouse strain (both *db/+* and *db/db*), it was considered that sufficient conversion to estradiol by aromatization did not occur unless the dose of exogenous testosterone was increased to 100 μg/g body weight/2 days. Thus, we performed an additional experiment with 75 μg/g body weight/2 days of testosterone, and observed that the blood estradiol level was significantly higher in *db/+* than *db/db* mice (*db/+* mice vs. *db/db* mice; 10.5 vs. 7.6 pg/mL) (data graph not shown). However, a small amount of estradiol may still have been produced by aromatization because of variations in blood testosterone levels and the influence of glucose and lipid metabolism. To remove this possibility, a constant blood testosterone level was established by implanting a testosterone pellet under the cervical skin. Combined with the administration of anastrozole, the influence of aromatization was completely blocked and similar results were obtained (Fig. 4e and f, and Additional file 1: Figure S1). These findings indicate that testosterone directly alleviated the exacerbation of glucose tolerance, but not through leptin signaling. Although no significant difference was observed in the β cell rate relative to islets (Fig. 3d), testosterone

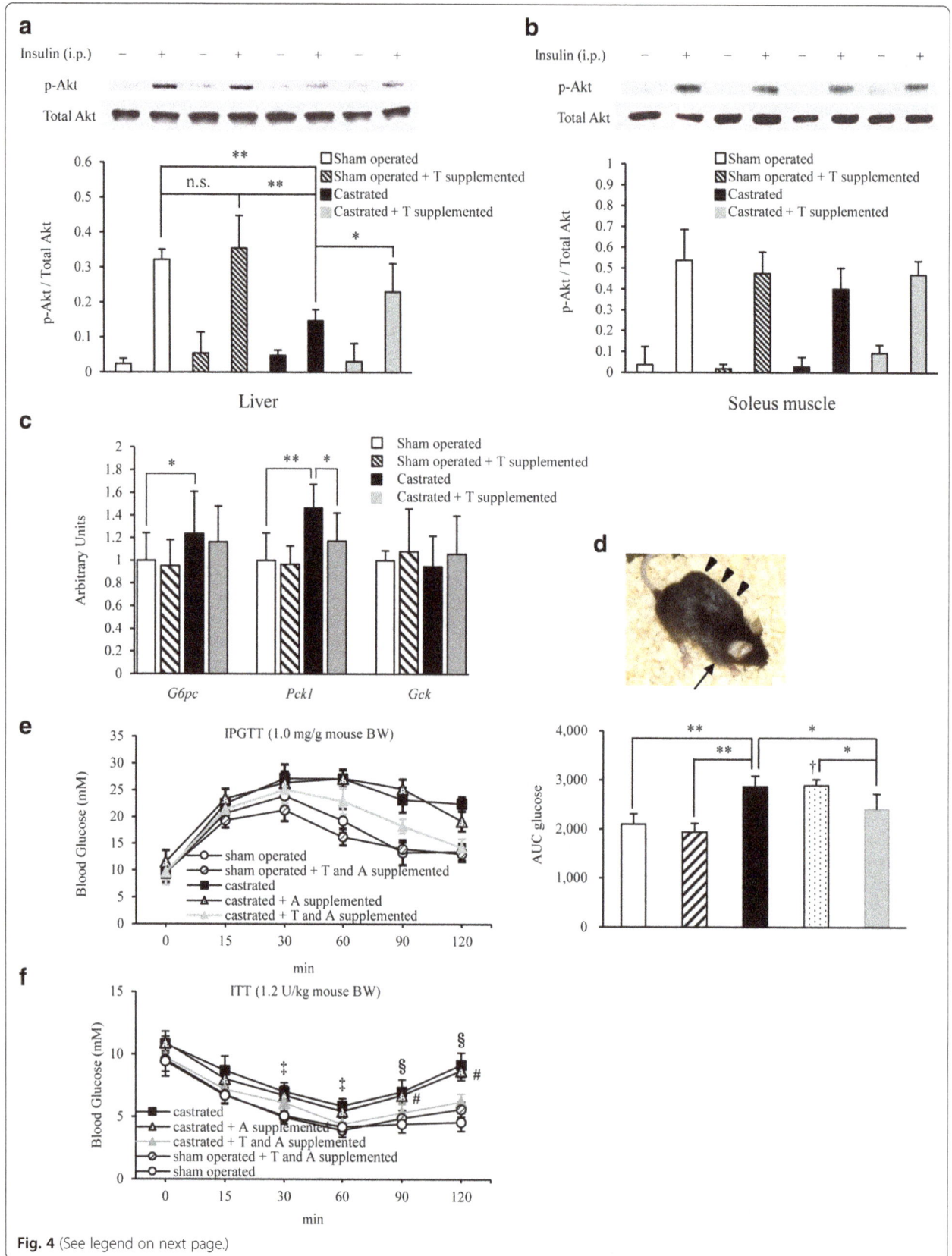

Fig. 4 (See legend on next page.)

(See figure on previous page.)
Fig. 4 Low testosterone-induced suppression of hepatic insulin signaling played a certain role in the development of insulin resistance in castrated *db/db* mice. **a** Representative immunoblots (top) and the ratio (bottom) of hepatic phosphorylated Akt (p-Akt) versus total Akt in sham operated, sham operated + testosterone (T) supplemented, castrated, or castrated + T supplemented mice (7 weeks of age) treated from 4 to 7 weeks of age (n = 10–13/group). **b** The ratio of muscular p-Akt versus total Akt, as assessed by immunoblotting, in the mice (7 weeks of age) in each group (n = 8–11/group). **c** Hepatic mRNA levels of *G6pc*, *Pck1*, and *Gck* as determined by quantitative real-time PCR (qRT-PCR) at 7 weeks of age (16 h-fasted) (n = 10–13/group). **d** A photograph of a mouse receiving the continuous anastrozole infusion from an osmotic pump (arrowhead). In addition, a T pellet was implanted under the cervical skin (arrow). **e** IpGTT analysis in 7-week-old *db/db* mice fed NCD in each group (n = 8–10/group) as indicated. The area under the curve (AUC glucose) is shown in the right panel. Glucose homeostasis was exacerbated by castration and ameliorated upon T supplementation. **f** IpITT analysis in 7-week-old mice in each group (n = 8–9/group) as indicated. The blood glucose levels 120 min after insulin loading were significantly higher in castrated than in sham operated mice, and were significantly lower in the T replacement after castration group than in the castrated group. Results are expressed as means ± s.e.m. *P < 0.05, **P < 0.01 between the indicated groups. [†]P < 0.01 versus sham operated or sham operated + T and A supplemented mice. [‡]P < 0.05 versus sham operated mice at each time, 2-way ANOVA. [§]P < 0.01, [#]P < 0.01 versus castrated + T and A supplemented, sham operated + T and A supplemented, or sham operated mice, respectively, at each time, 2-way ANOVA

replacement significantly improved insulin sensitivity (Fig. 2b) and decreased fasting insulin levels (Fig. 2d) accompanying mildly reduced hepatic fat accumulation and TG content (Fig. 3a–c) in castrated mice, suggesting that testosterone directly or indirectly decreases intrahepatic fat or may influence insulin-degrading enzyme (IDE). In each group, the power calculation values were low for fasting insulin levels, hepatic triglyceride contents, hepatic glycogen contents, and real-time PCR results (Additional file 2: Figure S2). However, they showed a tendency for significant differences, which could be simply explained by the small sample size.

We initially expected the recovery of insulin sensitivity in muscle to play an important role in glucose tolerance in this experimental system because testosterone increases muscle mass. However, no significant differences were observed in the fat content of, or Akt signals in, the soleus muscle between sham, castrated and testosterone-treated mice. Because no significant difference was noted in the soleus muscle weight among the groups at 7 weeks of age (data not shown), a 2-week testosterone replacement may have been too short to recover insulin sensitivity in muscle, and prolonging the replacement period may have led to different results.

Regarding the influence of aging, blood testosterone levels reached a peak in the reproductive period and then slowly decreased until 1 year of age in *db/+* mice (Fig. 5a), a pattern that is similar to that in healthy men. In contrast, blood testosterone levels in *db/db* mice were low throughout the period from 4 weeks to 1 year of age (Fig. 5a). Based on a comparison of the findings reported by Garris DR et al. [40], the decreased LH levels characteristic of *db/db* mice may have influenced these levels (Fig. 5b). This difference in gonadotropin levels was also implicated in the differences observed in the testis weight (Table 1). The decreased secretion of gonadotropin-releasing hormone (GnRH) from the hypothalamus may also have been attributed to the

decreased gonadotropin level measured in *db/db* mice; however, this needs to be investigated in more detail in future studies. Leptin gene knockout mice (*ob/ob* mice) are infertile. However, as reported by Chehab et al., female mice show restored fertility after receiving recombinant leptin [41]. Moreover, as reported by Mounzih et al., male *ob/ob* mice show restored fertility with estrus induction and testis weight gains as blood gonadotropins, especially LH, increase after administration of recombinant leptin [42].

In addition, as demonstrated by Wabitsch et al., young male patients with anorexia nervosa had lower gonadotropin (LH and FSH) and testosterone levels with decreasing blood leptin levels and, surprisingly, these parameters recovered along with weight gains (increases in body fat) [43].

The lower testosterone and gonadotropin levels with aging in the leptin receptor knockout mice (*db/db* mice) were comparable to those of *ob/ob* mice. However, the parameters were not recovered by the administration of recombinant leptin in *db/db* mice, unlike in *ob/ob* mice. Furthermore, although the infertility of *ob/ob* mice can be clearly explained by defects in the hypothalamic-pituitary axis, blood gonadotropin levels are elevated in castrated male *ob/ob* mice [44]. This finding suggests the existence of partial negative feedback in the hypothalamic-pituitary-gonadal axis. *db/db* mice showed non-significant negative feedback (slight elevations of gonadotropins) after castration, which disappeared after testosterone supplementation (data not shown). This result also has important implications in humans. Specifically, gonadal functions may decline after unnecessary testosterone supplementation in young men with low gonadotropin and testosterone levels due to decreased leptin.

Regarding dietary content, markedly lower blood testosterone levels were observed in male HFD-fed *db/+* mice than in NCD-fed mice (Fig. 5a). Although we did not investigate the dietary components in detail, obesity

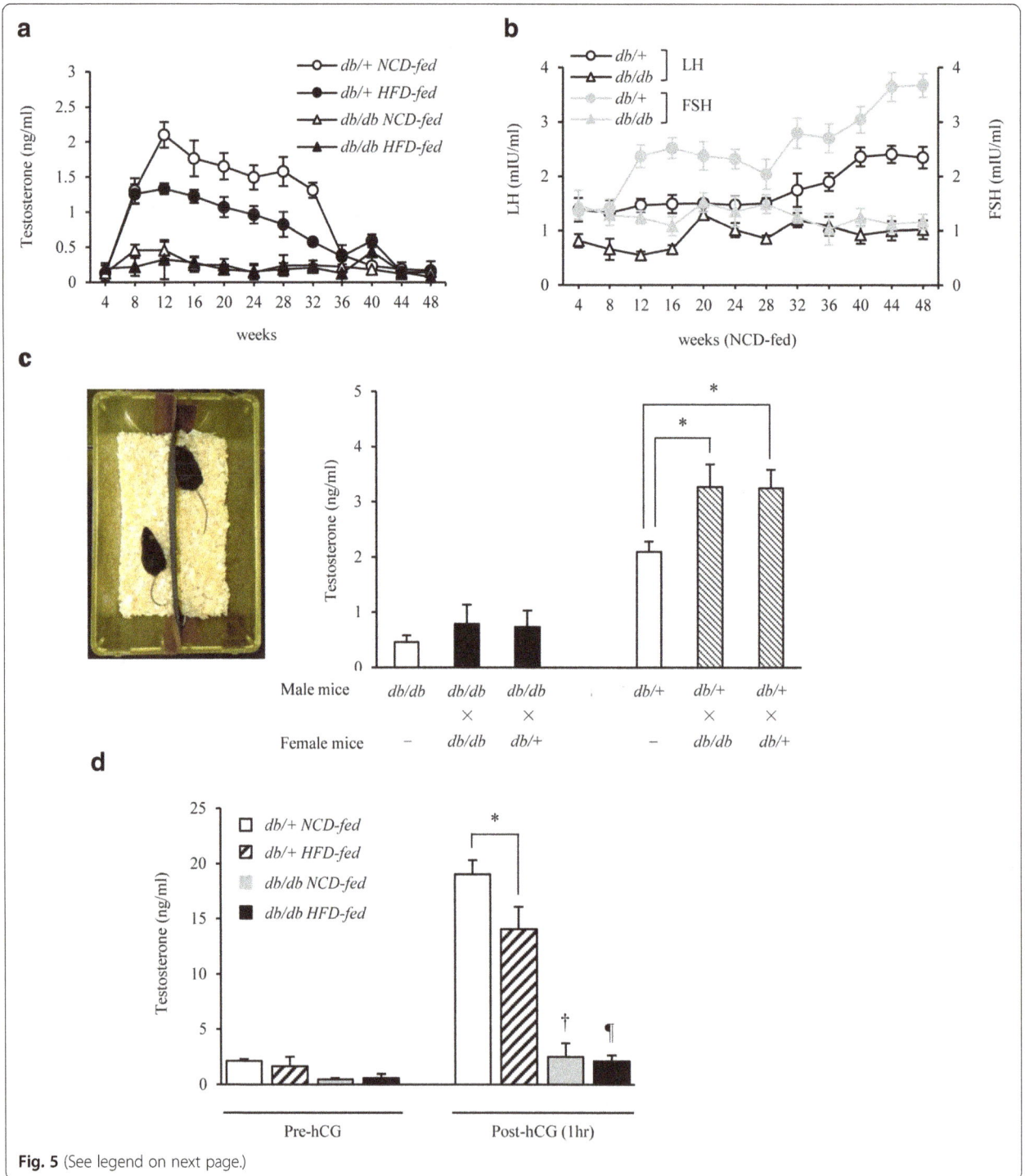

Fig. 5 (See legend on next page.)

(See figure on previous page.)

Fig. 5 Blood testosterone levels in male *db/db* mice were low throughout life from the juvenile period, and their reactions to female mice and hCG were weak. **a** Changes in blood testosterone levels from 4 to 48 weeks of age in each group are shown (*n* = 9–11/group). Blood testosterone levels rapidly decreased in NCD-fed male *db/+* mice at 36 weeks of age and older. These levels were lower in male *db/db* mice than in male *db/+* mice throughout life, and were also lower in male *db/+* mice in the HFD- than in NCD-fed group. **b** The changes in gonadotropin levels from 4 to 48 weeks of age in each group are shown (*n* = 9–11/group). The blood LH and FSH levels increased in male *db/+* mice after 32 weeks of age. In contrast, these levels were low in male *db/db* mice throughout life. **c** A pair of male and female mice were kept in the same cage for 2 weeks (from 10 to 12 weeks of age) in each group (left picture), and the blood testosterone levels were measured in male mice after 2 weeks (right) [*n* = 8–14 (7–8 males and 0–7 females)/group]. The presence of a female significantly increased blood testosterone levels in male *db/+* mice, whereas no significant change was noted in male *db/db* mice. **d** Increases in blood testosterone levels after hCG loading (0.5 IU/g body weight) in 12-week-old male *db/+* and *db/db* mice (*n* = 10/group). hCG increased blood testosterone levels by nearly 10 times in male *db/+* mice, but only by approximately 2 times in male *db/db* mice. Results are expressed as means ± s.e.m. *P < 0.01 between the indicated groups. †P < 0.01, ¶P < 0.01 versus pre-hCG in *db/db* mice on each diet

or the exacerbation of glucose and lipid metabolism induced low blood testosterone levels, which further promoted the aggravation of metabolic parameters, resulting in a vicious cycle. Decreased leptin signals may also have been strongly associated with this vicious cycle; however, further studies are needed to elucidate this mechanism in more detail.

When male and female mice were kept in the same cage during the reproductive period, blood testosterone levels were low in male *db/db* mice, possibly because of decreased LH levels (Fig. 5b and c). In addition, the hCG load test revealed that blood testosterone levels were nearly 10 times higher after hCG loading in *db/+* mice, while this increase was significantly lower in *db/db* mice (Fig. 5d). These findings indicate either that in addition to pituitary hypogonadism, functional Leydig cells are almost absent in *db/db* mice, or that the presence of leptin resistance or phenotypic obesity in males may suppress increases in blood testosterone levels. These findings support the hypothesis that testosterone inhibits the development and progression of lifestyle-related diseases, mainly diabetes [8, 17]. However, we did not investigate the influence of androgens produced by the adrenal gland. Moreover, elevation of the hematocrit value [45] and cardiovascular risk [46] resulting from an increase in

the blood testosterone level is of concern, but the increased risk of prostate cancer remains controversial [3, 47–49]. Furthermore, whether changes in blood testosterone levels are the cause or result of various diseases remains to be clarified. Because systemic disease may decrease testosterone levels, a reverse causal relationship should also be considered [50, 51]. Therefore, testosterone should not be administered to middle-aged to elderly men that do not have decreased testosterone levels (those that do not meet the diagnostic criteria of a general androgen deficiency). However, testosterone replacement was shown to be beneficial for men with decreased testosterone levels in several studies [52–54]. Therefore, the advantages and problems associated with testosterone replacement therapy need to be elucidated in more detail in future studies.

Conclusion

Our results strongly suggest that there are two pathways whereby testosterone affects glycometabolic functions: an indirect pathway via leptin signaling and a direct pathway that acts in a leptin-independent manner.

Additional files

Additional file 1: Figure S1. Aromatase inhibitor anastrozole blocks conversion of exogenous testosterone to estradiol (aromatization). The continuous anastrozole infusion rate was adjusted to 0, 20, or 200 μg/day (*n* = 8–10/group). A significant increase in blood estradiol levels was observed at an exogenous testosterone dose of 100 μg/g body weight/ 2 days, which were significantly decreased upon anastrozole infusion (20 or 200 μg/day) in castrated *db/db* mice. Results are expressed as means ± s.e.m. *P < 0.01 versus the other group of castrated *db/db* mice on the NCD. (ODP 17 kb)

Additional file 2: Figure S2. Power analysis of each experiment. After each experiment, we performed a post-hoc power analysis to assess the power of the experiment. Results are expressed as 1-β error probabilities. (ODP 20 kb)

Table 1 Mean body and testes weights of *db/+* and *db/db* mice at 12 and 40 weeks of age

	db/+ mice	*db/db* mice	*P* value
Body weight (g)			
12 wk	28.42 ± 0.82	48.14 ± 0.61	0.002
40 wk	35.06 ± 0.67	56.86 ± 0.91	0.004
Testes weight (g)			
12 wk	0.194 ± 0.009	0.131 ± 0.003	0.015
40 wk	0.186 ± 0.009	0.148 ± 0.011	0.031
Ratio of testes / body weight (%)			
12 wk	0.68 ± 0.02	0.30 ± 0.05	0.001
40 wk	0.53 ± 0.06	0.26 ± 0.08	0.001

Data are expressed as means ± SE, unless stated otherwise. Significance was considered as *P* < 0.05, calculated by an independent two-sample *t* test

Abbreviations

AR: Androgen receptor; AUC: Area under curve; DAB: Diaminobenzidine; DHT: Dihydrotestosterone; ECL: Enhanced chemiluminescence; ELISA: Enzyme-linked immunosorbent assay; FSH: Follicle stimulating hormone; GnRH: Gonadotropin-releasing hormone; hCG: Human chorionic gonadotropin; HDL: High-density lipoprotein; HFD: High-fat diet; IDE: Insulin-degrading enzyme; ipGTT: Intraperitoneal glucose tolerance test;

ipITT: Intraperitoneal insulin tolerance test; KO: Knockout; LH: Luteinizing hormone; MetS: Metabolic syndrome; NCD: Normal chow diet; PPARγ: Peroxisome proliferator-activated receptor gamma; QOL: Quality of life; SHR: Spontaneously hypertensive rat; STAT3: Signal transducer and activator of transcription 3; TG: Triglyceride

Acknowledgements
We thank N. Sensui for technical advice preparing castrated db/db mice; S. Nishijima for technical advice implanting osmotic mini-pumps into mice; and J. Bosma for editing the manuscript.

Funding
This research did not receive any specific grant from any funding agency in the public, commercial or not-for-profit sector.

Authors' contributions
"KY is the guarantor of this work and, as such, had full access to all the data in the study and takes responsibility for the integrity of the data and the accuracy of the data analysis. KN made conceptual contributions and assisted in conducting the experiments. AT assisted with power calculations. All authors read and approved the final manuscript.

Competing interests
The authors declare that they have no competing interests.

Author details
[1]Division of Endocrinology, Diabetes and Metabolism, Hematology, Rheumatology (Second Department of Internal Medicine), Graduate School of Medicine, University of the Ryukyus, 207 Uehara, Nishihara, Okinawa 903-0215, Japan. [2]GenomIdea Incorporated, Okinawa, Japan. [3]Clinical Pharmacology and Therapeutics University of the Ryukyus School of Medicine, Okinawa, Japan.

References
1. Wu FC. Commentary: Guideline for male testosterone therapy: a European perspective. J Clin Endocrinol Metab. 2007;92:418–9.
2. Bhasin S, Cunningham GR, Hayes FJ, Matsumoto AM, Snyder PJ, et al. Task force, Endocrine Society. Testosterone therapy in men with androgen deficiency syndromes: an Endocrine Society clinical practice guideline. J Clin Endocrinol Metab. 2010;95:2536–23.
3. Rhoden EL, Morgentaler A. Risks of testosterone-replacement therapy and recommendations for monitoring. N Engl J Med. 2004;350:482–92.
4. Snyder PJ. Might testosterone actually reduce mortality? J Clin Endocrinol Metab. 2008;93:32–3.
5. Muller M, Grobbee DE, den Tonkelaar I, Lamberts SW, van der Schouw YT. Endogenous sex hormones and metabolic syndrome in aging men. J Clin Endocrinol Metab. 2005;90:2618–23.
6. Kupelian V, Page ST, Araujo AB, Travison TG, Bremner WJ, et al. Low sex hormone-binding globulin, total testosterone, and symptomatic androgen deficiency are associated with development of the metabolic syndrome in nonobese men. J Clin Endocrinol Metab. 2006;91:843–50.
7. Laaksonen DE, Niskanen L, Punnonen K, Nyyssönen K, Tuomainen TP, et al.
8. Ding EL, Song Y, Malik VS, Liu S. Sex differences of endogenous sex hormones and risk of type 2 diabetes: a systematic review and meta-analysis. JAMA. 2006; 295:1288–99.
9. Oh JY, Barrett-Connor E, Wedick NM, Wingard DL, Rancho Bernardo Study. Endogenous sex hormones and the development of type 2 diabetes in older men and women: the rancho Bernardo study. Diabetes Care. 2002;25:55–60.
10. Tsai EC, Matsumoto AM, Fujimoto WY, Boyko EJ. Association of bioavailable, free, and total testosterone with insulin resistance: influence of sex hormone-binding globulin and body fat. Diabetes Care. 2004;27:861–8.
11. Meier C, Nguyen TV, Handelsman DJ, Schindler C, Kushnir MM, et al. Endogenous sex hormones and incident fracture risk in older men: the Dubbo osteoporosis epidemiology study. Arch Intern Med. 2008;168:47–54.
12. Araujo AB, Travison TG, Leder BZ, McKinlay JB. Correlations between serum testosterone, estradiol, and sex hormone-binding globulin and bone mineral density in a diverse sample of men. J Clin Endocrinol Metab. 2008; 93:2135–41.
13. Tracz MJ, Sideras K, Boloña ER, Haddad RM, Kennedy CC, et al. Testosterone use in men and its effects on bone health. A systematic review and meta-analysis of randomized placebo-controlled trials. J Clin Endocrinol Metab. 2006;91:2011–6.
14. Lorenz MW, Markus HS, Bots ML, Rosvall M, Sitzer M. Prediction of clinical cardiovascular events with carotid intima-media thickness: a systematic review and meta-analysis. Circulation. 2007;115:459–67.
15. Mäkinen J, Järvisalo MJ, Pöllänen P, Perheentupa A, Irjala K, et al. Increased carotid atherosclerosis in andropausal middle-aged men. J Am Coll Cardiol. 2005;45:1603–8.
16. Muller M, van den Beld AW, Bots ML, Grobbee DE, Lamberts SW, et al. Endogenous sex hormones and progression of carotid atherosclerosis in elderly men. Circulation. 2004;109:2074–9.
17. Liu PY, Death AK, Handelsman DJ. Androgens and cardiovascular disease. Endocr Rev. 2003;24:313–40.
18. Barrett-Connor E, Khaw KT. Endogenous sex hormones and cardiovascular disease in men. A prospective population-based study. Circulation. 1988;78:539–45.
19. Yarnell JW, Beswick AD, Sweetnam PM, Riad-Fahmy D. Endogenous sex hormones and ischemic heart disease in men. The Caerphilly prospective study. Arterioscler Thromb. 1993;13:517–20.
20. Reckelhoff JF, Zhang H, Granger JP. Testosterone exacerbates hypertension and reduces pressure-natriuresis in male spontaneously hypertensive rats. Hypertension. 1998;31:435–9.
21. Melis MR, Mauri A, Argiolas A. Apomorphine-and oxytocin-induced penile erection and yawning in intact and castrated male rats: effect of sexual steroids. Neuroendocrinology. 1994;59:349–54.
22. Chamness SL, Ricker DD, Crone JK, Dembeck CL, Maguire MP, et al. The effect of androgen on nitric oxide synthase in the male reproductive tract of the rat. Fertil Steril. 1995;63:1101–7.
23. Reilly CM, Zamorano P, Stopper VS, Mills TM. Androgenic regulation of NO availability in rat penile erection. J Androl. 1997;18:110–5.
24. Traish AM, Park K, Dhir V, Kim NN, Moreland RB, et al. Effects of castration and androgen replacement on erectile function in a rabbit model. Endocrinology. 1999;140:1861–8.
25. Satoh T, Matsumoto T, Yamada T, Watanabe T, Kawano H, et al. Late onset of obesity in male androgen receptor-deficient (AR KO) mice. Biochem Biophys Res Commun. 2003;300:167–71.
26. Lin HY, Xu Q, Yeh S, Wang RS, Sparks JD, et al. Insulin and leptin resistance with hyperleptinemia in mice lacking androgen receptor. Diabetes. 2005;54:1717–25.
27. Fan W, Yanase T, Nishi Y, Chiba S, Okabe T, et al. Functional potentiation of leptin-signal transducer and activator of transcription 3 signaling by the androgen receptor. Endocrinology. 2008;149:6028–36.
28. Longcope C, Kato T, Horton R. Conversion of blood androgens to estrogens in normal adult men and women. J Clin Invest. 1969;48:2191–201.
29. Longcope C, Pratt JH, Schneider SH, Fineberg SE. Aromatization of androgens by muscle and adipose tissue in vivo. J Clin Endocrinol Metab. 1978;46:146–52.
30. Qiu Y, Yanase T, Hu H, Tanaka T, Nishi Y, et al. Dihydrotestosterone suppresses foam cell formation and attenuates atherosclerosis development. Endocrinology. 2010;151:3307–16.

31. Misso ML, Murata Y, Boon WC, Jones ME, Britt KL, et al. Cellular and molecular characterization of the adipose phenotype of the aromatase-deficient mouse. Endocrinology. 2003;144:1474–80.

32. Brunham LR, Kruit JK, Pape TD, Timmins JM, Reuwer AQ, et al. Beta-cell ABCA1 influences insulin secretion, glucose homeostasis and response to thiazolidinedione treatment. Nat Med. 2007;13:340–7.

33. Le Bacquer O, Petroulakis E, Paglialunga S, Poulin F, Richard D, et al. Elevated sensitivity to diet-induced obesity and insulin resistance in mice lacking 4E-BP1 and 4E-BP2. J Clin Invest. 2007;117:387–96.

34. Hosooka T, Noguchi T, Kotani K, Nakamura T, Sakaue H, et al. Dok1 mediates high-fat diet-induced adipocyte hypertrophy and obesity through modulation of PPAR-gamma phosphorylation. Nat Med. 2008;14:188–93.

35. Higa M, Shimabukuro M, Shimajiri Y, Takasu N, Shinjyo T, et al. Protein kinase B/Akt signalling is required for palmitate-induced beta-cell lipotoxicity. Diabetes Obes Metab. 2006;8:228–33.

36. Ivashchenko Y, Kramer F, Schäfer S, Bucher A, Veit K, et al. Protein kinase C pathway is involved in transcriptional regulation of C-reactive protein synthesis in human hepatocytes. Arterioscler Thromb Vasc Biol. 2005;25:186–92.

37. Dahlman I, Forsgren M, Sjögren A, Nordström EA, Kaaman M, et al. Downregulation of electron transport chain genes in visceral adipose tissue in type 2 diabetes independent of obesity and possibly involving tumor necrosis factor-alpha. Diabetes. 2006;55:1792–9.

38. Singh J, O'Neill C, Handelsman DJ. Induction of spermatogenesis by androgens in gonadotropin-deficient (hpg) mice. Endocrinology. 1995;136:5311–21.

39. Larsen P, Kronenberg H, Melmed S, Polonsky K. Williams textbook of endocrinology. 10th ed. Philadelphia: Saunders; 2003.

40. Garris DR, Garris BL, Novikova L, Lau YS. Structural, metabolic and endocrine analysis of the diabetes (db/db) hypogonadal syndrome: relationship to hypophyseal hypercytolipidemia. Cell Tissue Res. 2005;319:501–12.

41. Chehab FF, Lim ME, Lu R. Correction of the sterility defect in homozygous obese female mice by treatment with the human recombinant leptin. Nat Genet. 1996;12:318–20.

42. Mounzih K, Lu R, Chehab FF. Leptin treatment rescues the sterility of genetically obese Ob/Ob males. Endocrinology. 1997;138:1190–3.

43. Wabitsch M, Ballauff A, Holl R, Blum WF, Heinze E, et al. Serum leptin, gonadotropin, and testosterone concentrations in male patients with anorexia nervosa during weight gain. J Clin Endocrinol Metab. 2001;86:2982–8.

44. Swerdloff RS, Batt RA, Bray GA. Reproductive hormonal function in the genetically obese (ob/ob) mouse. Endocrinology. 1976;98:1359–64.

45. Bhasin S, Cunningham GR, Hayes FJ, Matsumoto AM, Snyder PJ, et al. Testosterone therapy in adult men with androgen deficiency syndromes: an endocrine society clinical practice guideline. J Clin Endocrinol Metab. 2006; 91:1995–2010.

46. No authors listed. Testosterone for 'late-onset hypogonadism' in men? Drug Ther Bull 2010;48:69–72.

47. Huggins C, Hodges CV. Studies on prostatic cancer: I. The effect of castration, of estrogen and of androgen injection on serum phosphatases in metastatic carcinoma of the prostate. 1941. J Urol. 2002;168:9–12.

48. Shaneyfelt T, Husein R, Bubley G, Mantzoros CS. Hormonal predictors of prostate cancer: a meta-analysis. J Clin Oncol. 2000;18:847–53.

49. Stattin P, Lumme S, Tenkanen L, Alfthan H, Jellum E, et al. High levels of circulating testosterone are not associated with increased prostate cancer risk: a pooled prospective study. Int J Cancer. 2004;108:418–24.

50. Kaufman JM, Vermeulen A. The decline of androgen levels in elderly men and its clinical and therapeutic implications. Endocr Rev. 2005;26:833–76.

51. Karagiannis A, Harsoulis F. Gonadal dysfunction in systemic diseases. Eur J Endocrinol. 2005;152:501–13.

52. Allan CA, Strauss BJ, Burger HG, Forbes EA, McLachlan RI. Testosterone therapy prevents gain in visceral adipose tissue and loss of skeletal muscle in nonobese aging men. J Clin Endocrinol Metab. 2008;93:139–46.

53. Page ST, Amory JK, Bowman FD, Anawalt BD, Matsumoto AM, et al. Exogenous testosterone (T) alone or with finasteride increases physical performance, grip strength, and lean body mass in older men with low serum T. J Clin Endocrinol Metab. 2005;90:1502–10.

54. Isidori AM, Giannetta E, Greco EA, Gianfrilli D, Bonifacio V, et al. Effects of testosterone on body composition, bone metabolism and serum lipid profile in middle-aged men: a meta-analysis. Clin Endocrinol. 2005;63:280–93.

17

Glycaemic control for people with type 2 diabetes in Saudi Arabia – an urgent need for a review of management plan

Mohammed J. Alramadan[1], Dianna J. Magliano[1,2], Turky H. Almigbal[3], Mohammed Ali Batais[3], Afsana Afroz[1], Hesham J. Alramadhan[4], Waad Faozi Mahfoud[5], Adel Mehmas Alragas[6] and Baki Billah[1*]

Abstract

Background: The aim of this study was to assess inadequate glycaemic control and its associated factors among people with type 2 diabetes in Saudi Arabia.

Methods: A cross-sectional study design was used. Adults with type 2 diabetes attending diabetes centres in Riyadh, Hofuf and Jeddah cities were interviewed and their anthropometrics were measured. Their medical records were also reviewed to collect information related to recent lab tests, medications, and documented comorbidities. Multivariable logistic regression were used for data analysis.

Results: A total of 1111 participants were recruited in the study. Mean age was 57.6 (±11.1) years, 65.2% of the participants were females, and mean HbA1c was 8.5 ± 1.9%. About three-fourths of participants had inadequate glycaemic control (≥ 7%). Multivariable analysis showed that age ≤ 60 years, longer duration of diabetes, living in a remote location, low household income, low intake of fruits and vegetable, low level of physical activity, lack of knowledge about haemoglobin A1c, high waist-hip ratio, low adherence to medication, and using injectable medications were independent risk factors for inadequate glycaemic control.

Conclusions: Inadequate glycaemic control is prevalent among people with type 2 diabetes in Saudi Arabia. In order to improve glycaemic control diabetes management plan should aim at controlling the modifiable risk factors which include low intake of fruits and vegetable, low level of physical activity, lack of knowledge about haemoglobin A1c, high waist-hip ratio, and low adherence to medications.

Keywords: Saudi Arabia, Diabetes, Glycaemic control

Background

Diabetes mellitus is a major worldwide public health issue. A recent study showed that the prevalence of diabetes mellitus in Saudi Arabia was 13.4% [1], which is higher than the global prevalence of 8.8% and the prevalence in the Middle East of 10.7% [2]. In fact, Saudi Arabia is among the countries with the highest prevalence of diabetes regionally and globally [2], and the prevalence of diabetes in the country is on the rise [3].

The primary goal of the management of diabetes is to maintain blood glucose levels within or close to normal ranges [4]. It is well established that elevated blood glucose level increases the risk of diabetes complications and mortality [5, 6], while intensive glycaemic control substantially lower the risk [7, 8]. Unfortunately, studies from Saudi Arabia showed that half to two-thirds of people with type 2 diabetes mellitus (T2DM) have poor glycaemic control [9–13], and the prevalence of diabetes complications is higher than the global and regional prevalence [14–16].

A few studies have examined risk factors of poor glycaemic control among people with T2DM in Saudi Arabia [9, 10, 12, 13, 17]. Many of these studies were limited to a small geographical location and included a relatively small cohort of participants. In addition, some of these studies used random or fasting blood sugar test

* Correspondence: baki.billah@monash.edu
[1]Department of Epidemiology and Preventive Medicine, School of Public Health and Preventive Medicine, Monash University, Melbourne, Australia
Full list of author information is available at the end of the article

to assess glycaemic control which is not as accurate as the glycated haemoglobin A1c (HbA1c) level that measures the control over a number of weeks [4]. Moreover, not all potential risk factors of poor control were explored in the previous studies. A systematic review and meta-analysis showed that among other factors, diet and physical activity were significantly associated with glycaemic control [18]. Studies from Saudi Arabia, however, did not adequately explore the effect of physical activity and eating habits.

To achieve glycaemic control goals among people with T2DM, all possible associated risk factors of inadequate control must be identified and considered in the management. The aim of this study was to assess the current status of glycaemic control and to identify risk factors for inadequate control among people with T2DM in Saudi Arabia.

Methods

This study was conducted as a part of a research project that examined the status of glycaemic control, diabetes complications and quality of life for people with T2DM in Saudi Arabia. The study methodology has been described in detail in another article [19]. Ethical approval was obtained from the Monash University Human Research Ethics Committee in Australia and the Research Ethics Committee of the Ministry of Health in Saudi Arabia. All the study procedures were carried out in accordance with the principles of the Declaration of Helsinki as revised in 2013.

Participants

The study population were people with T2DM aged 18 years and over who were followed up at diabetes centres in three major cities (Hofuf, Riyadh, and Jeddah) in Saudi Arabia. The plan was to recruit 1082 participants based on a sample size calculation with 90% power, 5% significance level, a margin of error of 2.5%, and a prevalence of poor glycaemic control of 50% [9, 20]. Inclusion criteria include documented diagnosis of T2DM, aged 18 years and above, and duration of diabetes of at least 1 year. Pregnant women and participants who did not have a HbA1c test within 1 year were excluded.

Data collection

Participants were selected randomly from consecutive attendees of the diabetic centres between May 15 and November 30, 2017. After explaining the study and obtaining informed consent in writing, participants were interviewed using a pre-tested structured electronic questionnaire through Research Electronic Data Capture (REDCap) application [19, 21]. The questionnaire collects information related to socio-demographics, lifestyle, medical history, cognitive function, anxiety and depression. Socio-demographic data include gender, date of birth, marital status, education, and income. Lifestyle data include smoking status, physical activity (Global Physical Activity Questionnaire (GPAQ) [22]), and dietary habits. The dietary habit section included 10 questions selected from the UK diabetes and diet questionnaire (UKDDQ) [23] with some modifications to make some points more suitable for the eating habits of the Saudi population. The dietary questions include the frequency of consuming fruits, vegetables, red meat, desserts, date, sugary drinks, butter, bread, and rice and the fat content of consumed milk. The dietary habit variable was measured as a scale between zero and 48, where high score means the individual is following healthy eating habits. Medical history data include the duration of diabetes, modality of treatment, follow-up centre, other comorbidities, medication adherence (the 4 item Morisky Medication Adherence questionnaire) [24], family support in regards to diet and physical activity, and peripheral neuropathy (the Michigan Neuropathy Screening Instrument) [25]. Mental status data include anxiety (Generalized Anxiety Disorder Scale (GAD-2)) [26], depression (the Patient Health Questionnaire-2 (PHQ-2)) [27], and cognitive function (Rowland Universal Dementia Assessment Scale (RUDAS)) [28]. The establishers' permission to use the above-mentioned tools was obtained.

After interviewing participants, their anthropometrics were measured and recorded. Blood pressure was measured three times after sitting for at least 10 min using the Omron BP742N5 Series Upper Arm Blood Pressure Monitor with a cuff that fits standard and large arms. Weight was measured after instructing participants to remove their shoes and outer layers of clothing. Height, waist circumference, and hip circumference were measured twice and if the measurement varied by more than 2 cm, a third measurement was taken. Waist and hip circumference were measured against thin clothing. Participants' medical records were reviewed for most recent lab test results, namely HbA1c, creatinine, cholesterol, high density lipoprotein (HDL), low density lipoprotein (LDL), and triglycerides. Information regarding currently prescribed medication, and documented diagnosis of hypertension, coronary artery disease, retinopathy, and stroke was also collected from medical records.

Operational definitions

Glycaemic control was categorised into controlled (HbA1c < 53 mmol/mol (< 7%)), partially controlled (HbA1c 53–63 mmol/mol (7% to < 8%)), and poorly controlled (HbA1C ≥ 64 mmol/mol (≥ 8%)) [4]. A HbA1c cut-off value of > 68 mmol/mol (≥ 9%) was also used to represent very poor control [29]. Using the Global Physical Activity Questionnaire (GPAQ) [22], the total number of minutes of physical activity per week was categorised into ≥150 min and < 150 min [4]. Treatment modalities was categorized as oral tablets only, injectable medications (insulin and glucagon-like peptide-1 receptor agonists) only, and combined (oral tablets and injectable medications). Using the Morisky Medication Adherence questionnaire [24] medication adherence was categorized into adequate (a score of zero), and inadequate (a score of one or more). Hypoglycaemia was defined as episodes of mild or severe hypoglycaemia symptoms including hunger sweating, light headedness, headache, shaking, trembling, weakness, dizziness, confusion, loss of consciousness, and seizures. Family support in regards to healthy diet and physical activity was categorised as good support if healthy diet and physical activity were encouraged all the time, inadequate support if encouragement was sometimes, and poor support if family members rarely or never encouraged healthy diet or physical activity. Participants were considered unaware of HbA1c if they had not heard of HbA1c before or they did not know the recommended HbA1c target for people with diabetes. Body Mass Index (BMI) was categorised according to the current World Health Organization guidelines into normal (< 25.0 kg/m^2), pre-obesity (25.0–29.9 kg/m^2), and obesity (class I, II and II ≥ 30.0 kg/m^2). High waist-hip ratio was defined as a ratio of > 0.96 for men and > 0.98 for women [30]. Hypertension was defined as either a documented diagnosis of hypertension, taking antihypertension medications, or three previous high blood pressure readings (systolic ≥140 or diastolic ≥90) [4]. Dyslipidaemia was defined as any of the following: total cholesterol > 4.0 mmol/L (154.7 mg/dl), LDL > 2.0 mmol/L (77.3 mg/dl), triglycerides > 2.0 mmol/L (177.1 mg/dl), or HDL < 1.0 mmol/L (38.7 mg/dl) [31]. Impaired cognitive function was defined as a score of ≤22 in the Rowland Universal Dementia Assessment Scale (RUDAS) [28]. Depression was defined as a score of three and more using the Patient Health Questionnaire-2 (PHQ-2)) [27]. Anxiety was defined as a score of three and more using the Generalized Anxiety Disorder Scale (GAD-2)) [26]. Macrovascular complications were defined as having one of the following: documented diagnosis of stroke (irreversible cerebrovascular accident), documented diagnosis of coronary artery disease, taking medication for coronary artery disease, underwent a procedure for coronary artery disease, or self-reported lower extremity ulcers or amputations. Microvascular complication was defined as having one of the following: documented diagnosis of retinopathy, the participant had been told by an ophthalmologist that he or she had retinopathy, a score of seven or more using the Michigan Neuropathy Screening Instrument [25], or estimated glomerular filtration rate ≤ 60 ml/min/1.73m^2 calculated from serum creatinine using the Chronic Kidney Disease Epidemiology Collaboration (CKD-EPI) equation [32, 33].

Data analysis

Stata SE version 15.0 was used for data analysis. Data were summarised and presented as a mean (± standard deviation) for numerical data and frequency and percentage for categorical data. ANOVA and chi-square tests were used to examine univariate associations between risk factors and levels of glycaemic control. Potential risk factors with a p-value of 0.2 from univariate analysis were entered into multivariable logistic regression with step wise variable selection [34]. In the regression analysis, glycaemic control was categorised into controlled (HbA1c < 53 mmol/mol (< 7%)) and inadequately controlled (HbA1c ≥ 53 mmol/mol (≥ 7%)). The determinants were also examined for very poor glycaemic control (HbA1c > 68 mmol/mol (≥ 9%)). A p-value of 0.05 or less was considered as statistical significant.

Results

A total of 1111 participants were recruited in this study; 624 participants (56.2%) were from Riyadh, 239 (21.5%) were from Hofuf, and 248 (22.3%) were from Jeddah. Four hundred and-fifty participants (40.5%) were followed up at diabetes centres only, while 125 participants (11.3%) were followed up at both diabetes centres and hospitals and 535 participants (48.2%) were followed up at both diabetes centres and primary healthcare centres. Mean age was 57.6 (±11.1) years, mean duration of diabetes was 13.9 (±8.4) years, and 65.2% (724) of the participants were females, while 34.8% (387) were males. Mean body mass index was 32.9 (±8.1) kg/m^2. Mean HbA1c was 69.4 (±15.5) mmol/mol (8.5% (±1.9%)), and 24.1% of participants had good glycaemic control (HbA1c < 53 mmol/mol (< 7%)), 21.7% had partial control (HbA1c 53–63 mmol/mol (7–7.9%)), and 54.2% had poor control (HbA1C ≥ 64 mmol/mol (≥ 8%)). None of the study participants were on insulin pump or continuous glucose monitoring.

Table 1 summarises participants' demographic and lifestyle characteristics by different levels of glycaemic control. There was a higher prevalence of poor glycaemic control among those with lower levels of education (p-value: < 0.001), living in a remote place (p-value: 0.002), and not working including house-wives (p-value: 0.005). A higher proportion of those aged 60 years and younger had poor glycaemic control, however, the association was not statistically significant in univariate analysis. Similarly, gender, nationality, household income, and region were not significantly related to glycaemic control. Regarding lifestyle factors, there was no difference in the mean of healthy eating habit score among different categories of glycaemic control. However, higher proportions of those with less than daily intake of fruits and vegetables had poor glycaemic control (p-value: 0.011). Similarly, higher proportions of those with physical activity less than

Table 1 Demographic and lifestyle characteristics by level of glycaemic control

Variable	Glycaemic control			P-value
	Good (HbA1c < 7.0%) n = 263	Partial (HbA1c 7.0% - 7.9) n = 237	Poor (HbA1c ≥ 8%) n = 592	
Age % (n)				
> 60 years	28.4 (109)	22.4 (86)	49.2 (189)	0.106
46–60 years	21.4 (123)	21.6 (124)	57.0 (327)	
< 46 years	23.1 (31)	20.2 (27)	56.7 (76)	
Gender: female % (n)				
Female	22.9 (162)	20.9 (148)	56.3 (399)	0.173
Male	26.4 (101)	23.2 (89)	50.4 (193)	
Nationality % (n)				
Saudi	23.6 (246)	21.7 (226)	54.7 (570)	0.207
Non-Saudi	34.0 (17)	22.0 (11)	44.0 (22)	
Education level % (n)				
University/college	30.9 (60)	28.9 (56)	40.2 (78)	< 0.001
Lower education level	22.6 (203)	20.2 (181)	57.2 (514)	
Location of residency % (n)				
Urban	24.3 (229)	22.9 (216)	52.8 (497)	0.002
Rural	30.4 (28)	15.2 (14)	54.4 (50)	
Remote	10.3 (6)	12.1 (7)	77.6 (45)	
Working status % (n)				
Working	23.9 (55)	20.4 (47)	55.7 (128)	0.005
Not working / house-wife	21.6 (141)	21.0 (137)	57.4 (374)	
Retired	31.9 (67)	25.2 (53)	42.9 (90)	
Household income % (n)				
≥ 6001 SAR	25.2 (148)	23.7 (139)	51.1 (300)	0.074
< 6001 SAR	22.8 (115)	19.4 (98)	57.8 (292)	
Region % (n)				
Riyadh	26.4 (161)	22.5 (137)	51.1 (311)	0.125
Jeddah	22.7 (56)	21.5 (53)	55.9 (138)	
Hofuf	19.5 (46)	19.9 (47)	60.6 (143)	
Active smoking % (n)				
Never	24.6 (230)	21.9 (205)	53.5 (501)	0.563
In the past (> 1 year)	20.7 (19)	17.4 (16)	62.0 (57)	
Current smoker	22.2 (14)	25.4 (16)	52.4 (33)	
Eating habit score (mean ± SD)	30.2 ± 4.4	29.6 ± 5.1	29.8 ± 5.1	0.451
Fruits and vegetables % (n)				
Daily	31.3 (76)	20.2 (49)	48.6 (118)	0.011
Less frequent	21.9 (186)	22.2 (188)	55.9 (474)	
Physical Activity % (n)				
≥ 150 min/week	29.0 (94)	21.9 (71)	49.1 (159)	0.032
< 150 min/week	22.0 (169)	21.6 (166)	56.4 (433)	
Sitting hours (mean ± SD)	6.1 ± 3.6	5.8 ± 3.5	6.2 ± 3.8	0.380

150 min per week had poor control (p-value: 0.032). Mean number of sitting hours and smoking did not differ significantly among the categories of glycaemic control.

The association between various clinical characteristics and glycaemic control are presented in Table 2. Higher proportions of poor control were among people with longer duration of diabetes (p-value: < 0.001), and who were taking injectable medications (p-value: < 0.001), followed up mainly at primary health care or diabetes centres (p-value: 0.019), used glucometer twice or more a week (p-value: 0.017), and were not aware of HbA1c or the recommended HbA1c target for people with diabetes (p-value: 0.016). Similarly, higher proportions of poor control were among those who had less frequent hypoglycaemia events (p-value: 0.016), macrovascular complications (p-value: 0.019), microvascular complications (p-value < 0.001), and high waist-hip ratio (p-value: 0.001). Other clinical characteristics including family history of diabetes, family support, hypertension, adherence to medication, depression, anxiety, cognitive function, dyslipidaemia, and body mass index, did not appear to have an association with glycaemic control.

Figure 1 summarises the results of the multivariable logistic regression analysis. A total of 379 participants (34.1%) had very poor glycaemic control (HbA1c > 68 mmol/mol (> 9%)). Less than daily intake of fruits and vegetables increased the risk of inadequate and very poor control by 60% and 79% respectively. Low level of physical activity was associated with 48% and 62% higher risk of inadequate and very poor control respectively. Inadequate knowledge of HbA1c was associated with 1.9-fold and 2.5-fold higher risk of inadequate and very poor control respectively. High waist-hip ratio increased the risk of very poor control by 72%, while frequent episodes of hypoglycaemia is associated with lower risk of both inadequate and very poor control. Other risk factors that were associated with inadequate and very poor control include younger age, longer duration of diabetes, remote location of residence, and using injectable medications with or without oral tablets.

Figure 2 illustrates the adjusted association between risk factors and inadequate control (HbA1c ≥ 7%) for people who were on oral tablets only as well as for those on injectable medications (with or without oral tablets). Among people on oral tablets the risk of inadequate control was higher by: 56% for low intake of fruits and vegetables, 50% for high waist-hip ratio, and by 55% for inadequate adherence to medication. Inadequate knowledge of HbA1c was associated with 2.1-fold increased risk among those on oral tablets, while frequent hypoglycaemia reduced the risk by 58%. Other risk factors of inadequate control among those on oral tablets include younger age and longer diabetes duration. For

participants who were on injectable medications, low level of physical activity increased the risk of inadequate control by 2.1-folds, while high waist-hip ratio reduced the risk by 61%. Other risk factors of inadequate control among those on injectable medications were lower household income and followed up mainly at diabetes centres, while people from Jeddah appeared to have lower risk.

Discussion
In this current multi-centre study we have assessed the status of glycaemic control and its associated factors among people with T2DM attending diabetes centres in Saudi Arabia. One important finding was that only 24.1% of people with T2DM achieved the recommended HbA1c level of less than < 53 mmol/mol (< 7%), while the majority (75.9%) did not attained this target. Our findings, however, were comparable to the findings of recent studies from Saudi Arabia and other Arabian Gulf Countries [10–13, 35–39]. Despite quality health care services and various antidiabetic medications that are available for people with diabetes at no cost, the majority of people with T2DM in Saudi Arabia continue to have inadequate glycaemic control. A possible explanation could be the embracing of unhealthy lifestyle.

Sedentary lifestyle and the consumptions of processed, energy condensed, and fat-rich food have led to the increased prevalence of obesity and diabetes, and have made it difficult for people with diabetes to control their blood sugar. Recent studies showed that more than half of the Saudi population consumed less than one serving of fruits and vegetables per day [40], and 96.1% of them were physically inactive [41]. Furthermore, 51.0% of the adult Saudi population were either overweight or obese [42] and the prevalence of overweight and obesity among people with diabetes was significantly higher than the general population in the country [43, 44]. In addition, studies from Saudi Arabia found an association between low physical activity and poor glycaemic control [10, 13, 35], while a study from Bahrain [45], a country that shares boundaries and similar culture with Saudi Arabia, showed an association between unhealthy eating habits and higher HbA1c among people with T2DM.

Healthy eating habits and regular physical activity are key components in the management of T2DM. The current guidelines for people with diabetes recommend 8–10 servings of fruits and vegetables every day [4]. A serving of fruits is equal to a medium-size apple, orange, or banana, while a serving of vegetables is half a cup of corn, carrot or leafy vegetables. The guidelines also recommend at least 150 min of moderate to vigorous intensity physical activity per week [4]. The majority (77.5%) of participants in this study, however, did not eat fruits and vegetables daily, which has increased their risk of

Table 2 Clinical characteristics by level of glycaemic control

Variable	Glycaemic control			P-value
	Good (HbA1c < 7.0%) n = 263	Partial (HbA1c 7.0% - 7.9) n = 237	Poor (HbA1c ≥ 8%) n = 592	
Diabetes Duration % (n)				
≤ 10 years	34.7 (143)	25.5 (105)	39.8 (164)	< 0.001
> 10 years	17.5 (119)	19.4 (132)	63.0 (428)	
Family history of diabetes % (n)				
Yes	22.9 (187)	22.2 (181)	54.9 (447)	0.325
No	27.2 (75)	20.3 (56)	52.5 (145)	
Modality of treatment				
Oral tablets	36.4 (219)	25.8 (155)	37.9 (228)	< 0.001
Injectable	9.9 (22)	18.5 (41)	71.6 (159)	
Oral and injectable	7.9 (21)	15.4 (41)	76.8 (205)	
Main follow up centre % (n)				
Hospital	34.2 (42)	22.0 (27)	43.9 (54)	0.019
Primary care centre	24 (125)	23.0 (120)	53.0 (276)	
Diabetes centre	21.3 (95)	20.1 (90)	58.6 (262)	
Glucometer use % (n)				
Once or more a week	21.4 (145)	21.7 (147)	57.0 (387)	0.017
Less than once a week	28.6 (118)	21.8 (90)	49.6 (205)	
Hypoglycaemia events % (n)				
None	26.9 (170)	21.1 (133)	52.0 (328)	0.016
1–5 times	18.2 (71)	22.8 (89)	59.1 (231)	
6 times and more	30.4 (21)	21.7 (15)	47.8 (33)	
Medication adherence % (n)				
Adequate	26.0 (165)	22.4 (142)	51.7 (328)	0.110
Inadequate	21.4 (98)	20.8 (95)	57.8 (264)	
Family support with diet % (n)				
Good	23.5 (103)	22.2 (97)	54.3 (238)	0.621
Inadequate	23.0 (73)	23.9 (76)	53.1 (169)	
Poor	25.9 (87)	19.1 (64)	55.1 (185)	
Family support with physical activity % (n)				
Good	21.4 (66)	21.0 (65)	57.6 (178)	0.460
Inadequate	23.2 (74)	23.2 (74)	53.6 (171)	
Poor	26.5 (123)	21.1 (98)	52.4 (243)	
knowledge about HbA1c % (n)				
Aware	29.5 (103)	20.3 (71)	50.1 (175)	0.016
Not aware	21.5 (160)	22.3 (166)	56.1 (417)	
Body mass index % (n)				
Underweight/normal	22.7 (25)	20.9 (23)	56.4 (62)	0.075
Pre-obesity	26.4 (78)	26.4 (78)	47.1 (139)	
Obesity (class I – III)	23.3 (158)	20.0 (136)	56.7 (385)	
Waist-hip ratio % (n)				
Normal	26.4 (144)	24.8 (135)	48.8 (266)	0.001
High (male: > 0.96, female: > 0.98)	22.1 (96)	17.5 (76)	60.5 (263)	

Table 2 Clinical characteristics by level of glycaemic control *(Continued)*

Variable	Glycaemic control			P-value
	Good (HbA1c < 7.0%) n = 263	Partial (HbA1c 7.0% - 7.9) n = 237	Poor (HbA1c ≥ 8%) n = 592	
Depression % (n)				
No	24.1 (220)	22.3 (203)	53.6 (489)	0.563
Yes	23.9 (43)	18.9 (34)	57.2 (103)	
Anxiety % (n)				
No	24.2 (224)	22.4 (207)	53.4 (493)	0.328
Yes	23.2 (39)	17.9 (30)	58.9 (99)	
Cognitive function % (n)				
Intact	24.3 (169)	21.4 (149)	54.2 (377)	0.709
Impaired	22.1 (59)	23.2 (62)	54.7 (146)	
Dyslipidaemia % (n)				
No	29.6 (45)	23.0 (35)	47.4 (72)	0.142
Yes	23.2 (218)	21.5 (202)	55.3 (520)	
Hypertension % (n)				
No	22.8 (74)	20.3 (66)	56.9 (185)	0.503
Yes	24.6 (189)	22.3 (171)	53.1 (407)	
Macrovascular complications				
No	25.3 (199)	23.1 (182)	51.6 (406)	0.019
Yes	21.0 (64)	18.0 (55)	61.0 (186)	
Microvascular complication				
No	29.4 (146)	23.7 (118)	46.9 (233)	< 0.001
Yes	19.7 (117)	20.0 (119)	60.3 (359)	

inadequate and very poor glycaemic control. Similarly, more than two-thirds of participants (70.5%) did not achieve the recommended length of time of physical activity per week even though walking for transportation and physical activities at work were included in measuring it. Results of this current study also showed that a low level of physical activity was an independent risk factor for inadequate and very poor glycaemic control. Continuous education programs emphasising the role of lifestyle modification in controlling blood glucose level will be of great benefit for people with T2DM in Saudi Arabia.

Previous studies have shown that the more knowledge of diabetes a person has the more likely that he or she will have lower HbA1c level [17, 46]. Though the participants' knowledge of the disease was not evaluated in this study, their awareness of HbA1c and its recommended level for people with diabetes was assessed as a proxy for knowledge of the disease. Only 31.9% of participants were aware of HbA1c and knew the recommended target (< 53 mmol/mol (< 7%)). The remaining participants either have not heard of HbA1c before (32.0%) or did not know the recommended HbA1c target (36.1%), which was associated with increased risk of inadequate

and very poor control after adjustment for other risk factors. This finding is supported by the results of randomised control trials which showed that knowledge of actual and target HbA1c was associated with a significant reduction in HbA1c levels [47, 48]. In order to improve glycaemic control, physicians and health educators should ensure that people with diabetes are fully aware of their actual as well as the target HbA1c they should achieve.

Similar to studies conducted in the Arabian Gulf [49, 50] and other countries [18, 51] we found that younger age groups (≤60 years) were at higher risk of inadequate glycaemic control. Younger people are more likely to be affected by the change in lifestyle and less likely to be adherent to a management plan because of active occupational and social life [52]. Old people, in contrast, are less likely to be affected by the change in lifestyle and more likely to adhere to a management plan because they might be more concerned about their health, especially when they start to have comorbidities and complications [49]. Because of the beneficial effect of optimal glycaemic control on delaying complications, improving quality of life, and extending life expectancy among young

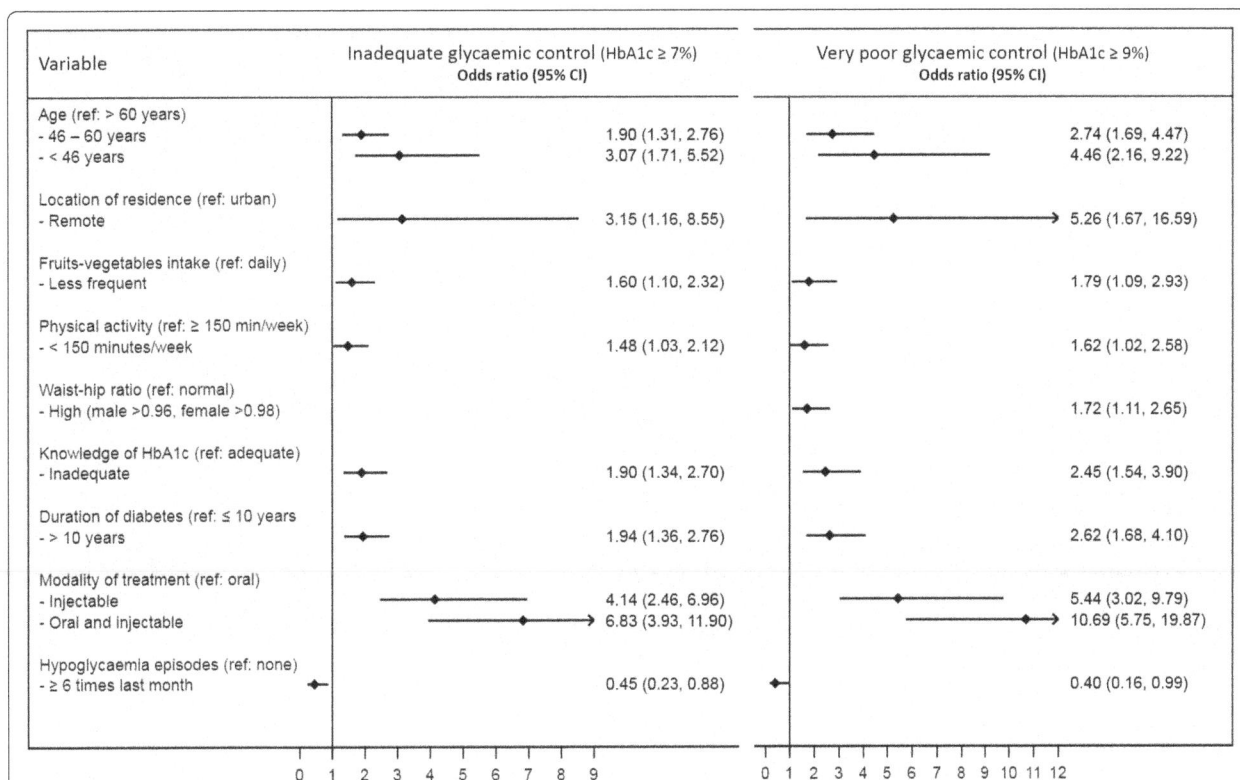

Variable	Inadequate glycaemic control (HbA1c ≥ 7%) Odds ratio (95% CI)	Very poor glycaemic control (HbA1c ≥ 9%) Odds ratio (95% CI)
Age (ref: > 60 years)		
- 46 – 60 years	1.90 (1.31, 2.76)	2.74 (1.69, 4.47)
- < 46 years	3.07 (1.71, 5.52)	4.46 (2.16, 9.22)
Location of residence (ref: urban)		
- Remote	3.15 (1.16, 8.55)	5.26 (1.67, 16.59)
Fruits-vegetables intake (ref: daily)		
- Less frequent	1.60 (1.10, 2.32)	1.79 (1.09, 2.93)
Physical activity (ref: ≥ 150 min/week)		
- < 150 minutes/week	1.48 (1.03, 2.12)	1.62 (1.02, 2.58)
Waist-hip ratio (ref: normal)		
- High (male >0.96, female >0.98)		1.72 (1.11, 2.65)
Knowledge of HbA1c (ref: adequate)		
- Inadequate	1.90 (1.34, 2.70)	2.45 (1.54, 3.90)
Duration of diabetes (ref: ≤ 10 years		
- > 10 years	1.94 (1.36, 2.76)	2.62 (1.68, 4.10)
Modality of treatment (ref: oral)		
- Injectable	4.14 (2.46, 6.96)	5.44 (3.02, 9.79)
- Oral and injectable	6.83 (3.93, 11.90)	10.69 (5.75, 19.87)
Hypoglycaemia episodes (ref: none)		
- ≥ 6 times last month	0.45 (0.23, 0.88)	0.40 (0.16, 0.99)

Fig. 1 Adjusted association between risk factors and inadequate (HbA1c ≥ 7%) and very poor (HbA1c ≥ 9%) glycaemic control. Variables introduced in the multivariable analysis were age, gender, education level, location of residence, work status, income, region, intake of fruits and vegetables, physical activity, duration of diabetes, treatment modality, glucometer use frequency, hypoglycaemia, follow-up location, adherence to medication, awareness of HbA1c, BMI, waist-hip ratio, macrovascular complications, microvascular complications and dyslipidaemia

people with diabetes [53], the management should aim at tight control once the diagnosis is made.

Another concerning finding of this study is that while the mean age of participants was 57.6 (±11.1) years (median: 57.8, 25th percentile: 51.8, 75th percentile: 63.9 years), they have a relatively long mean duration of diabetes of 13.9 (±8.4) years (median: 13.0, 25th percentile: 6.0, 75th percentile: 20 years). This indicates that the majority of people acquired diabetes in their early 40s. Early onset T2DM is associated with poor glycaemic control and a higher risk of comorbidities and complications [54]. With longer duration of T2DM, on the other hand, there is usually further deterioration of the function of the pancreas and the body's resistance to insulin increases, which makes it more difficult to control blood glucose level. The likelihood of acquiring diabetes complications also increases with longer duration, and complications can negatively affect the control either directly through inflammation and disturbance of the body's metabolism and indirectly through the effect of poly-pharmacy, anxiety, depression and stress. To prevent or delay diabetes and its complications, the healthcare system in Saudi Arabia should fully activate the screening programs and establish an intensive

management protocols to identify and treat people at risk of diabetes.

Though BMI did not appear to affect glycaemic control, we found that a high waist-hip ratio was an independent risk factor for inadequate and very poor control. Similar findings were also observed in studies from Japan and the United States [55, 56]. In addition, compared to BMI, a high waist-hip ratio was found to have stronger association with cardiovascular disease among people with type 2 diabetes [57]. Waist-hip ratio is a more accurate measure of central obesity which is strongly linked with T2DM, poor glycaemic control, and cardiovascular disease [58]. Therefore, similar to BMI, waist-hip ratio should be measured and recorded for people with diabetes with every follow up visit, and health care providers should raise the awareness of people with diabetes about high waist-hip ratio and the risk associated with it.

We found that living in a remote village was a strong predictor of inadequate and very poor glycaemic control. People living in remote villages are likely to have a low level of formal education and are likely to have less access to fresh healthy food options. Because of accessibility issues, they limit their follow-up to the local primary health care centre and may not visit a specialised diabetes clinic

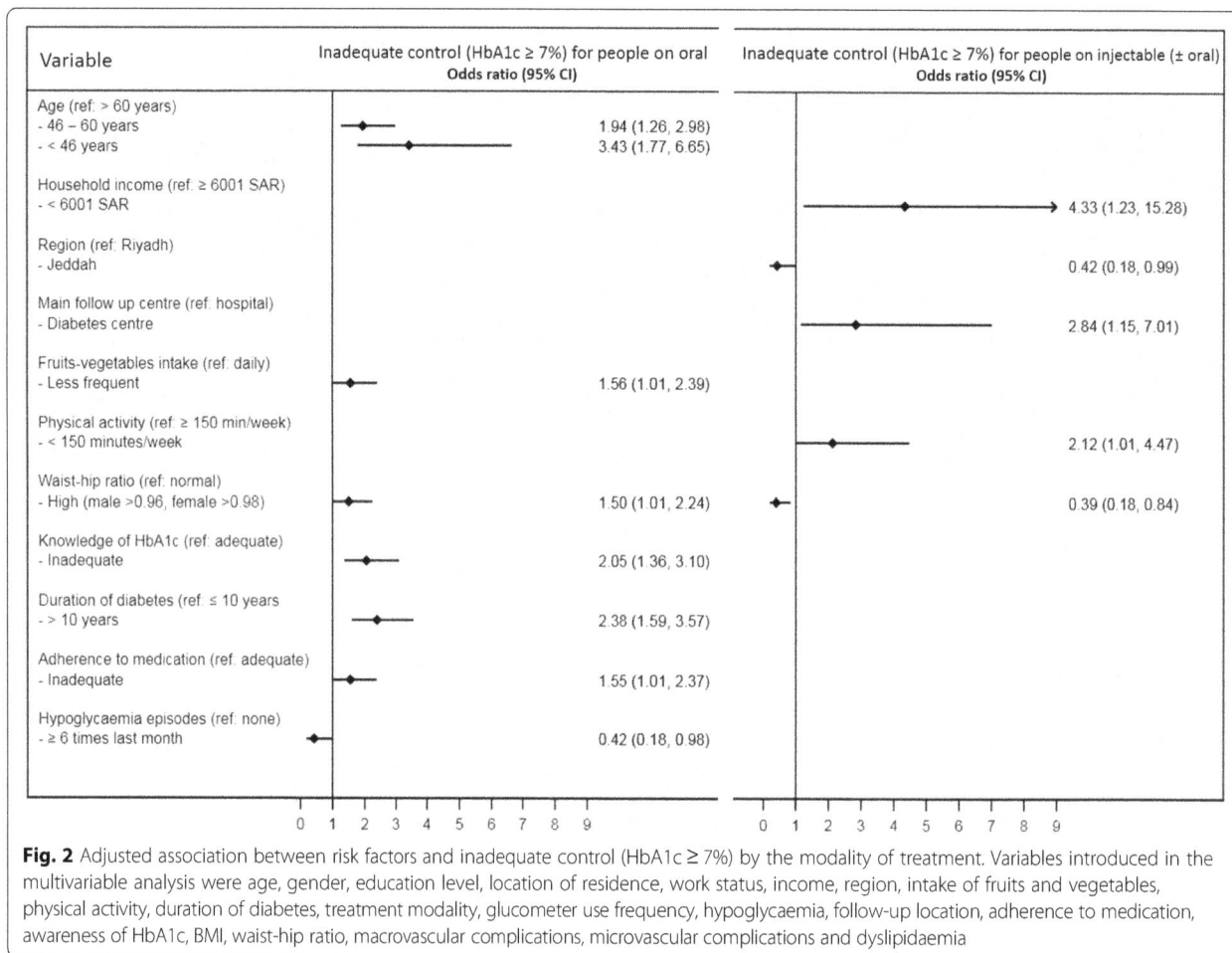

Variable	Inadequate control (HbA1c ≥ 7%) for people on oral Odds ratio (95% CI)	Inadequate control (HbA1c ≥ 7%) for people on injectable (± oral) Odds ratio (95% CI)
Age (ref: > 60 years)		
- 46 – 60 years	1.94 (1.26, 2.98)	
- < 46 years	3.43 (1.77, 6.65)	
Household income (ref: ≥ 6001 SAR)		
- < 6001 SAR		4.33 (1.23, 15.28)
Region (ref: Riyadh)		
- Jeddah		0.42 (0.18, 0.99)
Main follow up centre (ref: hospital)		
- Diabetes centre		2.84 (1.15, 7.01)
Fruits-vegetables intake (ref: daily)		
- Less frequent	1.56 (1.01, 2.39)	
Physical activity (ref: ≥ 150 min/week)		
- < 150 minutes/week		2.12 (1.01, 4.47)
Waist-hip ratio (ref: normal)		
- High (male >0.96, female >0.98)	1.50 (1.01, 2.24)	0.39 (0.18, 0.84)
Knowledge of HbA1c (ref: adequate)		
- Inadequate	2.05 (1.36, 3.10)	
Duration of diabetes (ref: ≤ 10 years		
- > 10 years	2.38 (1.59, 3.57)	
Adherence to medication (ref: adequate)		
- Inadequate	1.55 (1.01, 2.37)	
Hypoglycaemia episodes (ref: none)		
- ≥ 6 times last month	0.42 (0.18, 0.98)	

Fig. 2 Adjusted association between risk factors and inadequate control (HbA1c ≥ 7%) by the modality of treatment. Variables introduced in the multivariable analysis were age, gender, education level, location of residence, work status, income, region, intake of fruits and vegetables, physical activity, duration of diabetes, treatment modality, glucometer use frequency, hypoglycaemia, follow-up location, adherence to medication, awareness of HbA1c, BMI, waist-hip ratio, macrovascular complications, microvascular complications and dyslipidaemia

or centre until the disease has progressed and they acquire complications. To improve the control among this susceptible group, the healthcare system should provide special diabetes education programs for healthcare providers working at remote places, and motivate them to use the online continuous education programs that are currently available and accredited by the Saudi Health System. General physicians working on remote sittings should also be provided with timely hotline or email access to specialists including endocrinologists, ophthalmologist and podiatrist. Patients, on the other hand, should have frequent teleconference or phone calls by diabetes educators, dietitians and other allied health professionals if these healthcare professionals are not assigned to the remote place where patients live.

Similar to other previous studies [18, 49, 50], our results showed that the use of injectable medications was a strong predictor for inadequate control. It is of concern that even after management with insulin, which is highly effective modality of treatment [59], a large proportion of people continued to have high blood glucose level. Low adherence to injectable medication regimen because of social stigmata, interference with daily activity, and fear of hypoglycaemia, have been suggested to increase the risk of poor control among people using injectable medications [60]. In Addition, the progression of the disease, weight gain related to insulin use, and polypharmacy can also contribute to poor glycaemic control among people with T2DM who are on injectable medications [61].

Our findings support the previous study that showed an association between inadequate glycaemic control and low income as well as low adherence to medications [18, 52, 62]. Low income decreases the likelihood of adherence to lifestyle modifications and treatment regimen [62], and low adherence to management plan is a known risk factors for poor glycaemic control [18, 52].

The association between hypoglycaemia and glycaemic control is of interest. Our findings showed that people with infrequent symptoms of hypoglycaemia were at higher risk of poor glycaemic control compared to those who had frequent symptoms of hypoglycaemic. This may indicate that while an intensive treatment regimen improve glycaemic control, it may come at the cost of frequent hypoglycaemia symptoms. Severe hypoglycaemia is associated with lower productivity, reduced quality of life, and a higher risk of anxiety, depression and mortality [63, 64]. Therefore, hypoglycaemia should be prevented, and the treatment should aim at achieving the lowest HbA1c level without severe hypoglycaemia episodes and a minimum number of mild hypoglycaemia symptoms [65].

The strength of this study lays on the relatively large sample size that was recruited from multiple centres from different regions of Saudi Arabia. The consideration of several potential risk factors and the use of a validated electronic questionnaire, which reduce data errors, also add strength to this study. This study, however, has some limitations. Cross-sectional study design lack temporality and causality cannot be inferred. Another limitation is that information regarding individualised glycaemic control targets could not be collected because it was not documented in participants' medical records. Therefore, a HbA1c cut off point of 7% was selected to categorise adequate control which is too strict for old people with longer duration of the disease and those who have advanced cardiovascular disease [4]. In addition, we could not investigate the effect of new anti-hyperglycaemic agents such as the glucagon-like peptide-1 (GLP-1) receptor agonists on glycaemic control because only a very small number of participants in our database were using them. Nonetheless, this study clearly revealed the burden of inadequate glycaemic control among people with T2DM in Saudi Arabia and its associated risk factors.

Conclusion
Inadequate glycaemic control is a common and widespread problem among people with T2DM in Saudi Arabia. Healthcare providers should undertake a patient-centred approach and individualise management strategies with consideration to all identified risk factors for inadequate control. Continuous education programs should also be implemented to raise the awareness of the disease and the importance of lifestyle modification. The healthcare system should prioritise diabetes prevention strategies through active screening and intensive management of people at risk. The health system should also take special measures to improve glycaemic control for people with diabetes living at remote locations. Future research should investigate the effectiveness of education programs targeting people with diabetes and barriers to adhering to lifestyle modifications.

Abbreviations
BMI: Body Mass Index; eGFR: Estimated glomerular filtration rate; HbA1c: Glycated haemoglobin A1c; HDL: High density lipoprotein; LDL: Low density lipoprotein; T2DM: Type 2 diabetes mellitus

Acknowledgements
We would like to acknowledge the contribution of Fatema A. AlRamadan, Basmah J. Al Ramadhan, Ameera J. Alramadan, Ahmed J. Alramadhan, Talal A. Alzahrani, Hawra H. Alramadhan, Ayat S. Alabdullah, Noor A. Alabdullah, Husam M. Almaramhi, Nawaf F. Almukaibil, Nouf A. Alzaid, Nour A. Bayaseh, Sara M. Alameer, Wed A. Alkharras, Ghada M Amin, and Ahmad Alhammad in the data collection for this study.

Author contributions
All authors were involved in the conception and design of the study. MJA, HJA, WFM, and AMA contributed to the acquisition of data. MJA, DJM, AA, BB, THA and MAB contributed to data analysis and interpretation of results. MJA and BB drafted the manuscript. All authors critically reviewed the manuscript and approved the final version.

Funding
This research did not receive any specific grant from funding agencies in the public, commercial, or not-for-profit sectors.

Competing interests
The authors declare that they have no competing interests.

Author details
[1]Department of Epidemiology and Preventive Medicine, School of Public Health and Preventive Medicine, Monash University, Melbourne, Australia. [2]Baker Heart and Diabetes Institute, Melbourne, VIC, Australia. [3]College of Medicine, King Saud University, Riyadh, Saudi Arabia. [4]College of Medicine, King Faisal University, Al-Ahsa, Saudi Arabia. [5]Ibn Sina National College, Jeddah, Saudi Arabia. [6]Medical City - King Saud University, Riyadh, Saudi Arabia.

References
1. El Bcheraoui C, Basulaiman M, Tuffaha M, Daoud F, Robinson M, Jaber S, et al. Status of the diabetes epidemic in the Kingdom of Saudi Arabia, 2013. Int J Pub Health. 2014;59(6):1011–21.
2. Cho NH, Kirigia J, Mbanya JC, Ogurstova K, Guariguata L, Rathmann W, et al. IDF DIABETES ATLAS eighth edition 2017. Int Diabet Fed. 2017:1–147.
3. Al-Quwaidhi AJ, Pearce MS, Sobngwi E, Critchley JA, O'Flaherty M. Comparison of type 2 diabetes prevalence estimates in Saudi Arabia from a validated Markov model against the international diabetes federation and other modelling studies. Diabetes Res Clin Pract. 2014;103(3):496–503.
4. American Diabetes Association. American Diabetes Association Standards of Medical Care in Diabetes-2017. The Journal of Clinical and Applied Research and Education. 2017;40.
5. Collaboration ERF. Diabetes mellitus, fasting glucose, and risk of cause-specific death. N Engl J Med. 2011;2011(364):829–41.
6. Klein R, Klein BE, Moss SE. Relation of glycemic control to diabetic microvascular complications in diabetes mellitus. Ann Intern Med. 1996; 124(1_Part_2):90–6.
7. Ismail-Beigi F, Craven T, Banerji MA, Basile J, Calles J, Cohen RM, et al. Effect of intensive treatment of hyperglycaemia on microvascular outcomes in type 2 diabetes: an analysis of the ACCORD randomised trial. Lancet. 2010; 376(9739):419–30.
8. Duckworth W, Abraira C, Moritz T, Reda D, Emanuele N, Reaven PD, et al. Glucose control and vascular complications in veterans with type 2 diabetes. N Engl J Med. 2009;360(2):129–39.
9. Al-Nuaim AR, Mirdad S, Al-Rubeaan K, Al-Mazrou Y, Al-Attas O, Al-Daghari N. Pattern and factors associated with glycemic control of Saudi diabetic patients. Ann Saudi Med. 1998;18(2):109–12.

10. Al-Hayek AA, Robert AA, Alzaid AA, Nusair HM, Zbaidi NS, Al-Eithan MH, et al. Association between diabetes self-care, medication adherence, anxiety, depression, and glycemic control in type 2 diabetes. Saudi Med J. 2012; 33(6):681–3.

11. Alsulaiman TA, Al-Ajmi HA, Al-Qahtani SM, Fadlallah IM, Nawar NE, Shukerallah RE, et al. Control of type 2 diabetes in king Abdulaziz Housing City (Iskan) population, Saudi Arabia. J Family Community Med. 2016;23(1):1.

12. Almutairi MA, Said SM, Zainuddin H. Predictors of poor glycemic control among type two diabetic patients. Am J Med Medical Sci. 2013;3(2):17–21.

13. Alzaheb RA, Altemani AH. The prevalence and determinants of poor glycemic control among adults with type 2 diabetes mellitus in Saudi Arabia. Diabetes Metab Syndr Obes. 2018;11:15.

14. Alwakeel J, Sulimani R, Al-Asaad H, Al-Harbi A, Tarif N, Al-Suwaida A, et al. Diabetes complications in 1952 type 2 diabetes mellitus patients managed in a single institution. Ann Saudi Med. 2008;28(4):260.

15. Al Ghamdi AH, Rabiu M, Hajar S, Yorston D, Kuper H, Polack S. Rapid assessment of avoidable blindness and diabetic retinopathy in Taif, Saudi Arabia. Br J Ophthalmol. 2012;96(9):1168–72.

16. Halawa MR, Karawagh A, Zeidan A, Mahmoud A-E-DH, Sakr M, Hegazy A. Prevalence of painful diabetic peripheral neuropathy among patients suffering from diabetes mellitus in Saudi Arabia. Curr Med Res Opin. 2010; 26(2):337–43.

17. Binhemd TA. Diabetes mellitus: knowledge, attitude, practice and their relation to diabetes control in female diabetics. Ann Saudi Med. 1992; 12(3):247–51.

18. Sanal T, Nair N, Adhikari P. Factors associated with poor control of type 2 diabetes mellitus: a systematic review and meta-analysis. J Diabetol. 2011; 3(1):1–10.

19. Alramadan MJ, Afroz A, Batais MA, Almigbal TH, Alhamrani HA, Albaloshi A, et al. A study protocol to assess the determinants of Glycaemic control, complications and health related quality of life for people with type 2 diabetes in Saudi Arabia. J Health Edu Res Develop. 2017;5(2):1–6.

20. Al-Turki YA. Blood sugar control, ophthalmology referral and creatinine level among adult diabetic patients in primary health care, Riyadh, Saudi Arabia. Saudi Med J. 2002;23(11):1332–4.

21. Harris PA, Taylor R, Thielke R, Payne J, Gonzalez N, Conde JG. Research electronic data capture (REDCap)—a metadata-driven methodology and workflow process for providing translational research informatics support. J Biomed Inform. 2009;42(2):377–81.

22. Armstrong T, Bull F. Development of the world health organization global physical activity questionnaire (GPAQ). J Public Health. 2006;14(2):66–70.

23. England CY, Thompson JL, Jago R, Cooper AR, Andrews RC. Development of a brief, reliable and valid diet assessment tool for impaired glucose tolerance and diabetes: the UK diabetes and diet questionnaire. Public Health Nutr. 2017;20(2):191–9.

24. Morisky DE, Green LW, Levine DM. Concurrent and predictive validity of a self-reported measure of medication adherence. Med Care. 1986;24(1):67–74.

25. Moghtaderi A, Bakhshipour A, Rashidi H. Validation of Michigan neuropathy screening instrument for diabetic peripheral neuropathy. Clin Neurol Neurosurg. 2006;108(5):477–81.

26. Skapinakis P. The 2-item Generalized Anxiety Disorder scale had high sensitivity and specificity for detecting GAD in primary care. Evid Based Med. 2007;12(5):149.

27. Kroenke K, Spitzer RL, Williams JB. The patient health Questionnaire-2: validity of a two-item depression screener. Med Care. 2003;41(11):1284–92.

28. Storey JE, Rowland JT, Conforti DA, Dickson HG. The Rowland universal dementia assessment scale (RUDAS): a multicultural cognitive assessment scale. Int Psychogeriatr. 2004;16(01):13–31.

29. Oglesby AK, Secnik K, Barron J, Al-Zakwani I, Lage MJ. The association between diabetes related medical costs and glycemic control: a retrospective analysis. Cost Eff Resour Alloc. 2006;4(1):1.

30. Al-Lawati JA, Barakat NM, Al-Lawati AM, Mohammed AJ. Optimal cut-points for body mass index, waist circumference and waist-to-hip ratio using the Framingham coronary heart disease risk score in an Arab population of the Middle East. Diab Vasc Dis Res. 2008;5(4):304–9.

31. Deed G, Ackermann E, Newman R, Audehm R, Arthur I, Barlow J, et al. General Practice Management of Type 2 Diabetes: 2014–15: Royal Australian College of General Practitioners (RACGP); 2014.

32. Levey AS, Stevens LA, Schmid CH, Zhang YL, Castro AF, Feldman HI, et al. A new equation to estimate glomerular filtration rate. Ann Intern Med. 2009; 150(9):604–12.

33. Grams ME, Rebholz CM, McMahon B, Whelton S, Ballew SH, Selvin E, et al. Identification of incident CKD stage 3 in research studies. Am J Kidney Dis. 2014;64(2):214–21.

34. Billah B, Huq MM, Smith JA, Sufi F, Tran L, Shardey GC, et al. AusSCORE II in predicting 30-day mortality after isolated coronary artery bypass grafting in Australia and New Zealand. J Thorac Cardiovasc Surg. 2014;148(5):1850–5. e2

35. Al Baghli N, Al Turki K, Al Ghamdi A, El Zubaier A, Al Ameer M, Al Baghli F. Control of diabetes mellitus in the eastern province of Saudi Arabia: results of screening campaign. 2010.

36. Al-Rasheedi AAS. The role of educational level in glycemic control among patients with type II diabetes mellitus. Int J Health Sci. 2014;8(2):177.

37. Al Balushi KA, Al-Haddabi M, Al-Zakwani I, Al Z'a M. Glycemic control among patients with type 2 diabetes at a primary health care center in Oman. Prim Care Diabetes. 2014;8(3):239–43.

38. Al-Ibrahim AAH. Factors associated with compliance to diabetes self-care behaviors and glycemic control among Kuwaiti people with type 2 diabetes 2012.

39. Al-Kaabi J, Al-Maskari F, Saadi H, Afandi B, Parkar H, Nagelkerke N. Assessment of dietary practice among diabetic patients in the United Arab Emirates. Rev Diabet Stud. 2008;5(2):110–5.

40. Al-Hamdan N, Kutbi A, Choudhry A, Nooh R, Shoukri M, Mujib S. WHO stepwise approach to NCD surveillance country-specific standard report Saudi Arabia. In: Organization WH, editor. WHO Stepwise Approach. Geneva: WHO; 2005.

41. Al-Nozha MM, Al-Hazzaa HM, Arafah MR, Al-Khadra A, Al-Mazrou YY, Al-Maatouq MA, et al. Prevalence of physical activity and inactivity among Saudis aged 30-70 years. A population-based cross-sectional study. Saudi Med J. 2007;28(4):559–68.

42. Al Othaimeen A, Al Nozha M, Osman A. Obesity: an emerging problem in Saudi Arabia. Analysis of data from the National Nutrition Survey. East Mediterr Health J. 2007;13(2):441–8.

43. Al-Nozha MM, Al-Maatouq MA, Al-Mazrou YY, Al-Harthi SS, Arafah MR, Khalil MZ, et al. Diabetes mellitus in Saudi Arabia. Saudi Med J. 2004;25(11):1603–10.

44. Alqurashi K, Aljabri K, Bokhari S. Prevalence of diabetes mellitus in a Saudi community. Ann Saudi Med. 2011;31(1):19.

45. Shamsi N, Shehab Z, AlNahash Z, AlMuhanadi S, Al-Nasir F. Factors influencing dietary practice among type 2 diabetics. Bahrain Med Bull. 2013;35:3.

46. Tang YH, Pang S, Chan MF, Yeung GS, Yeung VT. Health literacy, complication awareness, and diabetic control in patients with type 2 diabetes mellitus. J Adv Nurs. 2008;62(1):74–83.

47. Cagliero E, Levina EV, Nathan DM. Immediate feedback of HbA1c levels improves glycemic control in type 1 and insulin-treated type 2 diabetic patients. Diabetes Care. 1999;22(11):1785–9.

48. Levetan CS, Dawn KR, Robbins DC, Ratner RE. Impact of computer-generated personalized goals on HbA1c. Diabetes Care. 2002;25(1):2–8.

49. Al-Lawati JA, Barakat MN, Al-Maskari M, Elsayed MK, Al-Lawati AM, Mohammed AJ. HbA1c levels among primary healthcare patients with type 2 diabetes mellitus in Oman. Oman Med J. 2012;27(6):465–70.

50. D'Souza MS, Karkada SN, Hanrahan NP, Venkatesaperumal R, Amirtharaj A. Do perceptions of empowerment affect glycemic control and self-care among adults with type 2 diabetes? Glob J Health Sci. 2015;7(5):80–90.

51. McBrien K, Manns B, Hemmelgarn B, Weaver R, Edwards A, Ivers N, et al. The association between sociodemographic and clinical characteristics and poor glycaemic control: a longitudinal cohort study. Diabet Med. 2016;33(11):1499–507.

52. Alramadan MJ, Afroz A, Hussain SM, Batais MA, Almigbal TH, Al-Humrani HA, et al. Patient-related determinants of Glycaemic control in people with type 2 diabetes in the Gulf cooperation council countries: a systematic review. J Diabet Res. 2018;2018:9389265.

53. Drewelow E, Wollny A, Pentzek M, Immecke J, Lambrecht S, Wilm S, et al. Improvement of primary health care of patients with poorly regulated diabetes mellitus type 2 using shared decision-making–the DEBATE trial. BMC Fam Pract. 2012;13(1):88.

54. Chuang L-M, Soegondo S, Soewondo P, Young-Seol K, Mohamed M, Dalisay E, et al. Comparisons of the outcomes on control, type of management and complications status in early onset and late onset type 2 diabetes in Asia. Diabetes Res Clin Pract. 2006;71(2):146–55.

55. Hsieh S, Yoshinaga H. Abdominal fat distribution and coronary heart disease risk factors in men-waist/height ratio as a simple and useful predictor. Int J Obes Relat Metab Disord. 1995;19(8):585–9.

56. Eberhardt MS, Lackland DT, Wheeler FC, German RR, Teutsch SM. Is race related to glycemic control? An assessment of glycosylated hemoglobin in two South Carolina communities. J Clin Epidemiol. 1994;47(10):1181–9.

57. Czernichow S, Kengne A-P, Huxley RR, Batty GD, De Galan B, Grobbee D, et al. Comparison of waist-to-hip ratio and other obesity indices as predictors of cardiovascular disease risk in people with type-2 diabetes: a prospective cohort study from ADVANCE. Eur J Cardiovasc Prev Rehabil. 2011;18(2):312–9.

58. Astrup A, Finer N. Redefining type 2 diabetes:'diabesity'or 'obesity dependent diabetes mellitus'? Obes Rev. 2000;1(2):57–9.

59. Nathan DM, Buse JB, Davidson MB, Ferrannini E, Holman RR, Sherwin R, et al. Medical management of hyperglycemia in type 2 diabetes: a consensus algorithm for the initiation and adjustment of therapy: a consensus statement of the American Diabetes Association and the European Association for the Study of diabetes. Diabetes Care. 2009; 32(1):193–203.

60. Peyrot M, Barnett A, Meneghini L, Schumm-Draeger PM. Insulin adherence behaviours and barriers in the multinational global attitudes of patients and physicians in insulin therapy study. Diabet Med. 2012;29(5):682–9.

61. Davies M. The reality of glycaemic control in insulin treated diabetes: defining the clinical challenges. Int J Obes. 2004;28:S14–22.

62. Brown AF, Ettner SL, Piette J, Weinberger M, Gregg E, Shapiro MF, et al. Socioeconomic position and health among persons with diabetes mellitus: a conceptual framework and review of the literature. Epidemiol Rev. 2004; 26(1):63–77.

63. Davis RE, Morrissey M, Peters JR, Wittrup-Jensen K, Kennedy-Martin T, Currie CJ. Impact of hypoglycaemia on quality of life and productivity in type 1 and type 2 diabetes. Curr Med Res Opin. 2005;21(9):1477–83.

64. Bonds DE, Miller ME, Bergenstal RM, Buse JB, Byington RP, Cutler JA, et al. The association between symptomatic, severe hypoglycaemia and mortality in type 2 diabetes: retrospective epidemiological analysis of the ACCORD study. BMJ. 2010;340:b4909.

65. Seaquist ER, Anderson J, Childs B, Cryer P, Dagogo-Jack S, Fish L, et al. Hypoglycemia and diabetes: a report of a workgroup of the American Diabetes Association and the Endocrine Society. J Clin Endocrinol Metabol. 2013;98(5):1845–59.

18

C-Peptide and cardiovascular risk factors among young adults in a southern Brazilian cohort

Romildo Luiz Monteiro Andrade[1,2,3*] (iD), Denise P. Gigante[2], Isabel Oliveira de Oliveira[2] and Bernardo Lessa Horta[2]

Abstract

Background: Proinsulin connecting peptide (C-Peptide) is a marker of the beta-cell function and has been considered a marker of insulin resistance whose evidence suggests were associated with cardiovascular mortality. Our study aims to evaluate the association of C-Peptide with metabolic cardiovascular risk factors among young adults followed since birth in southern Brazil.

Methods: In 1982, maternity hospital in Pelotas, a southern Brazilian city, were visited daily and all births were identified. Live births whose family lived in the urban area of the city were identified, their mothers interviewed, and these subjects have been prospectively followed. Casual hyperglycemia patients were excluded from analysis. C-Peptide was assessed at 23 years, when transversely analyzed its association with cardiometabolic and hemodynamic risk factors, and longitudinally 30 years of age.

Results: At age 23, 4297 individuals were evaluated, and C-Peptide was measured in 3.807. In a cross-sectional analysis at 23 years of age, C-Peptide was positively associated with waist circumference, body mass index, glycaemia, triglycerides, and C-reactive protein. The association with HDL cholesterol was negative. In the longitudinal analysis at 30 years, C-Peptide remained associated with BMI, waist circumference, glycated hemoglobin, triglycerides, and C-reactive protein, whereas the association was negative for HDL.

Conclusion: In the Pelotas birth cohort, the C-Peptide was associated with obesity indicators (waist circumference and BMI) cross-sectional (23 years) and longitudinal (30 years). We also observed cross-sectional and longitudinal associations of C-Peptide with cardiometabolic and inflammatory risk factors.

Keywords: C-Peptide, Cardiovascular disease, Risk, Young adults

Background

In 2012, cardiovascular diseases were the main cause of death, accounting for 17.5 million deaths [1]. And three quarters of these deaths, occurred in low and medium-income countries (70% of the global population) [2]. In face of population ageing and the increase in the prevalence of diabetes and obesity, cardiovascular mortality is estimated to rise over the next decades [3, 4].

Proinsulin connecting peptide-(C-Peptide) is considered a marker of insulin resistance, epidemiological studies suggest its performance as a cardiovascular risk factor [5–7]. Secreted by β cells in the pancreas at amounts equimolar to insulin [8], C-Peptide is also a marker of beta cell function, and studies have shown its association to overall cardiovascular risk and mortality [9]. Its pathophysiological activity would be linked to the stimulation of vascular permeability to monocytes, stimulating the differentiation in macrophages, promoting the phagocytosis of molecules of oxidized lipoproteins, such as low-density lipoprotein (LDL), and differentiating into foam cells, the classic cellular substrate of atherosclerotic lesions [10]. C-Peptide would also act in subsequent phases of the atherogenic process,

* Correspondence: rlmandrade@hotmail.com
[1]University Hospital Cassiano Antônio de Moraes (HUCAM) of the Federal, University of Espírito Santo (UFES), Vitória-ES, Brazil
[2]Post-Graduate Program in Epidemiology, Federal University of Pelotas (UFPel), Pelotas-RS, Brazil
Full list of author information is available at the end of the article

inducing the proliferation of smooth muscle cells and the cascade of release of pro-atherogenic components such as cytokines, metalloproteinases, and oxidative molecules, besides clotting factors such as the tissue plasminogen activator (tPA) [11, 12].

Population studies are in line with findings such as Cabrera et al. observed that individuals in the upper tercile of C-Peptide were at higher risk of coronary artery disease (RR 2.4; CI 95% 1.3–4.6) and myocardial infarction (RR 2.8; C I95% 1.1–6.9) [13]. Marx et al. reported that serum levels of C-Peptide in patients subjected to coronary angiography were associated with overall (HR 1.46 CI95% 1.15–1.85) and cardiovascular (HR 1.58 CI 95% 1.15–2.18) mortality [14]. Patel et al. evaluated individuals with fasting glycaemia ≥70 mg/dL and found that C-Peptide was associated with cardiovascular (HR 1.60, CI95% 1.07–2.39) and overall (HR 1.72, CI95% 1.34–2.21) mortality [15]. Min et al. also found an association with cardiovascular (HR 3.20 CI95% 2.07–4.93) and overall (HR 1.80 CI95% 1.33–2.43) mortality.

On the other hand, Bo et al. found no association between C-Peptide and cardiovascular mortality after adjusting for age, sex, body mass index, smoking, time on insulin therapy, glycated hemoglobin, systolic blood pressure, HDL cholesterol, triglycerides, and previous vascular complications [16]. However, the control for other metabolic cardiovascular risk factors may have blocked causal pathways between C-Peptide and mortality, underestimating the association.

Given the small number of studies assessing the association of C-Peptide with metabolic cardiovascular risk factors, and the possibility of analyzing their relation to the long period of follow-up we considered important to investigate such association. The present study aimed to evaluate the cardio-metabolic risk profiles in non-diabetic young stratified according to C-peptide quartiles in a southern Brazilian cohort [7].

Methods

In 1982, the maternity hospital in Pelotas, a southern Brazilian city, were visited daily and all births were identified. The neonates whose families lived in the urban area were examined and the mothers interviewed soon after birth (n 5914). These individuals have been prospectively followed at different moments of their life cycles.

In 2004, an attempt was made to locate all participants of the cohort, using multiple strategies. The subjects were interviewed at home and invited to visit the research laboratory to donate a blood sample [17]. At 30 ages, a new attempt was made to locate all cohort members, who were invited to visit the research clinic, where they were interviewed, examined, and blood samples were collected [18].

Anthropometric variables of weight, was measured at 23 years, using Seca (Uniscale®, Germany) portable electronic scales with 100 g precision. Aluminum anthropometers with 1 mm precision were used to measure height according to Lohman et al. [19]. At 30 years, weight was measured with a scale connected to Bod Pod (Cosmed®, USA) device and height with an aluminum vertical stadiometer with 1 mm precision. Waist circumference was measured while the subjects were standing upright with feet together and arms relaxed along the body. The measuring tape was extended on the horizontal plane at waist height (narrowest portion of the trunk) between the last rib and the iliac crest at the end of a regular exhaling and without compressing the skin, and the value was recorded with 0.1 cm precision. Body mass index (BMI) was calculated by dividing the weight in kilograms (kg) by the square of the height in meters (m).

Cardiometabolic variables were measured at 23 years: capillary glycaemia (mg/dL), total cholesterol (mg/dL), HDL cholesterol (mg/dL), triglycerides (mg/dL), C-reactive protein (mg/dL). At age 30, serum glycaemia (mg/dL), total cholesterol (mg/dL); HDL cholesterol (mg/dL); LDL cholesterol (mg/dL); triglycerides (mg/dL); C-reactive protein (mg/dL); glycated hemoglobin (%) were measured. At 23 years, glycaemia was measured using an Accu-Chek Advantage (Roche®) portable glucometer, total cholesterol, HDL, and triglycerides were measured using a Selectra 2 (Merck®, Darmstadt, Germany. C-Peptide was measured in the blood samples collected at 23 years, using the chemiluminescence technique (Immulite – Siemens) [20], because the analyses were performed on samples collected at random, the estimates were adjusted for fasting time.

At 30 years, serum glucose was measured using the colorimetric enzyme assay with K082 -Glicose Monoreagente kits (Bioclin®, Brazil), LDL cholesterol was measured with K088 (Bioclin®, Brazil) kits and glycated hemoglobin (HbA1c), with K09 -HbA1c Bi-reagent (Bio-Rad®, Berkeley, California, USA) kits. High-sensitivity C-reactive protein (Hs-CRP) was measured using the automated turbidimetry technique with a BS 380 (Shenzhen-Mindray Bio-Medical Electronics Co.; Ltd®, China) chemical analyzer. Those measures with values below the lower limit of detection of 0.1 mg/L were converted to 0.05 mg/L. Expressing acute inflammatory conditions, we excluded values above 10 mg / L [21]. We also excluded those subjects whose serum glucose level was > 200 mg / dL at 23 and 30 years due to diabetes mellitus [22].

Blood pressure was measured at 23 years, using an Omron® wrist monitor at the beginning and at the end of the interview, about 60 min apart, with the respondent sited with the arm on a support. At 30 years, blood pressure was measured twice with an HEM705 CPINT (Omron®) automated device coupled to an arm cuff, which was replaced by a proper model for obese subjects. The mean of two measurements was used in the analyses.

The following variables were considered as confounding factors: physical activity was measured at 23 and 30 years of age using the International Physical Activity Questionnaire (IPAQ) [23] maternal skin color (assessed by the interviewer in the perinatal study), monthly family income in minimum wage, tobacco use (those subjects who reported smoking at least one cigarette a day at 23 years were considered as smokers), alcohol consumption (daily intake in mg/L), family history of hypertension (father and/or mother), birthweight (grams), and rapid weight gain between 2 and 4 years (change in Z score above 0.67 standard deviation) [24] . Paternal and maternal history of dyslipidemia, hypertension, myocardial infarction, and/or stroke was also considered.

The means of the variables according to the quartiles of Pep-C were evaluated according to the trend tests of the ordered groups. Due to the asymmetric distribution, C-reactive protein and triglycerides were transformed into logarithm. Multiple linear regression was used to evaluate the association between C-Peptide and cardiovascular risk factors, estimates were adjusted for confounding variables like: fasting time (estimated as the time between the last meal and blood sample collection), physical activity practice per week (minutes), family

income, mother's skin color, birthweight, rapid growth between 2 and 4 years old, smoking at 23 years, alcohol consumption, family history of dyslipidemia, arterial hypertension and stroke, myocardial infarction [23].

The analyses were carried out using the software STATA version 13.1. The study was approved by the Research Ethics Committee of the Medical School of the Federal University of Pelotas under protocol OF. 16/12. All interviews and blood collections were performed after written consent was obtained from the participants.

Results

In 2004, 4297 individuals were interviewed, which – added to the 282 deaths identified in the cohort – represented a follow-up rate of 77.4%. In 2012, 3701 individuals were interviewed, which – given the 325 deaths identified in the cohort – represented a follow-up rate of 68.1%.

In ad-doc tests in the regression models, sex was not shown an interaction condition with the Pep-C values, because of these findings, the analyzes were not stratified between sex. The exclusion criteria used for Hs-CRP greater than 10 mg/L withdraw participants and the hyperglycemia in the casual glucose dosage (> 200 mg / dL), totaling the exclusion of 02 individuals at the 23[a] and 25 participants at 30[a]. Table 1 shows the distribution of the studied

Table 1 Participant characteristics at 23 and 30 years old

Variables	23 years		30 years	
	n	μ (CI95%)	n	μ (CI95%)
Anthropometric				
Weight (kg)	4263	67.0 (66.6; 67.46)	3525	75.6 (75.0; 76.2)
Height (cm)	4263	167.4 (167.1; 167.7)	3581	167.7 (167.4; 168.0)
Waist circumference (cm)	4260	78.2 (77.9; 78.5)	3540	84.7 (84.3; 85.1)
Body mass index	4136	23.6 (23.4; 23.7)	3508	26.8 (26.6; 27.0)
Metabolic				
Serum glycaemia (mg/dL)	3713	97.1 (96.6; 97.6)	3506	87.9 (87.4; 88.4)
Total cholesterol (mg/dL)	2417	155.9 (154.4; 157.3)	3506	190.6 (189.4; 191.8)
HDL cholesterol (mg/dL)	3801	55.5 (55.0; 55.9)	3506	58.7 (58.2; 59.1)
LDL cholesterol (mg/dL)			3506	109.4 (108.4; 118.1)
Triglycerides [a] (mg/dL)	3801	88.4 (86.9; 89.9)	3506	100.4 (98.5; 102.2)
C-reactive protein (mg/dL) #	3449	2.0 (2.0; 2.1)	3188	1.47 (1.4; 1.5)
Glycated hemoglobin (mg/dL)			3516	51.1 (5.0; 5.1)
C-Peptide [a] (ng/mL)	3807	1.6 (1.5; 1.6)		
Hemodynamic				
Systolic arterial pressure (mmHg)	4291	117.4 (116.9; 117.9)	3593	121.0 (120.6; 121.5)
Diastolic arterial pressure (mmHg)	4291	73.5 (73.2; 73.9)	3593	75,3 (75.0; 75.6)
Heart rate (bpm)	4291	74.5 (74.1; 74.8)	1565	70.7 (70.1; 71.3)
Behavioral				
Prevalence of sedentary lifestyle	4269	444.8 (428.3; 461.2)	3580	294.7 (282.5; 307.0)

μ: arithmetic mean;# [a]: Geometric mean

population according to the outcomes. C-Peptide was measured in 3807 subjects and the geometric mean was 1.6 ng/mL (CI 95% 1.5; 1.6). From 23 to 30 years, the mean total cholesterol increased from 155.9 to 190.6 mg/dL, HDL from 55.5 to 58.7 mg/dL, the geometric mean of triglycerides from 88.4 to 100.4 mg/dL, and Hs-CRP from 2.0 to 1.47 mg/dL. Concerning the anthropometric measures, mean waist circumference increased from 78.2 to 84.7 cm and BMI from 23.6 to 26.8 kg/m². Systolic blood pressure

increased from 117.4 to 121.0 mmHg and diastolic from 73.5 to 70.7 mmHg.

At 23 years, in transversal analysis, C-Peptide was positively associated with waist circumference, BMI, glycaemia, total cholesterol, triglycerides, and Hs-CRP, whereas a negative association was observed with HDL. Longitudinally at 30 years, C-Peptide remained associated with waist circumference and BMI at 30. Concerning the metabolic risk factors, only triglycerides and

Table 2 Cardiovascular risk factors according to C-Peptide quartiles at 23 and 30 years old

Cardiovascular risk factors	C-Peptide				[b]p Trend value
	1st quartile	2nd quartile	3rd quartile	4th quartile	
	23 years				
	$n = 968$	$n = 958$	$n = 1015$	$n = 865$	
Anthropometric					
Waist circumference (cm)	76.6 (75.9; 91.0)	77.3 (76.7; 77.9)	78.3 (77.6; 78.9)	80.8 (79.9; 81.6)	**< 0.001**
Body mass index	22.7 (22.5; 22.9)	23,4 (23.1; 23.6)	23.7 (23.4; 23.9)	24.7 (24.3; 25.1)	**< 0.001**
Metabolic					
Capillary glycaemia (mg/dL)	92.1 (91.4; 92.9)	94.4 (93.6; 95.2)	97, 9 (96.9; 98.8)	104.8 (103.7; 106.0)	**< 0.001**
Total cholesterol (mg/dL)	155.0 (152.2; 157.9)	154.5 (151.9; 157.2)	156.3 (153.4; 159.2)	157.9 (154.9; 161.0)	0.094
HDL cholesterol (mg/dL)	56,2 (55.3; 57.0)	55.6 (54.8; 56.4)	55.2 (54.4; 56.0)	54.9 (54.1; 55.8)	**0.032**
Triglycerides (mg/dL)[a]	76,5 (74,1; 78,9)	76,5 (74,1; 90,7)	96,3 (93,2; 99,5)	108,4 (104,4; 112,6)	**< 0.001**
C-reactive protein (mg/dL)[a]	1,0 (1,06; 1,08)	1,0 (1,06; 1,17)	1,3 (1,20; 1,39)	1,4 (1.3; 1.5)	**< 0.001**
Hemodynamic					
Systolic arterial pressure (mmHg)	118.2 (117.2; 119.2)	116.7 (115.8; 117.6)	116.7 (115.7; 117.6)	117.5 (116.6; 118.6)	0.356
Diastolic arterial pressure (mmHg)	73.9 (73.2; 74.7)	72.6 (71.9; 73.3)	72,9 (72.2; 73.6)	73.9 (73.1; 74.6)	0.765
Heart rate (bpm)	73.0 (72.2; 74.0)	73.3 (72.6; 74.0)	75.9 (75.2; 76.7)	76.30 (75.4; 77.0)	**< 0.001**
	30 years				
	$n = 966$	$n = 955$	$n = 1006$	$n = 857$	
Anthropometric					
Waist circumference (cm)	83.0 (82.1; 83.7)	84.2 (83.4; 85.1)	85.0 (84.1; 86.0)	87.7 (86.6; 88.8)	**< 0.001**
Body mass index	25.8 (25.4; 26.1)	26.6 (26.2; 27.0)	27.1 (26.7; 27.5)	28.3 (27.8; 28.8)	**< 0.001**
Metabolic					
Serum glycaemia (mg/dL)	88.3 (87.2; 89.4)	87.3 (86.2; 88.3)	87.9 (86.8; 88.9)	88.5 (87.2; 89.8)	0.702
Total cholesterol (mg/dL)	189.9 (187.3; 192.6)	190.7 (188.1; 193.3)	191.0 (188.4; 193.5)	192.1 (189.3; 194.9)	0.084
HDL cholesterol (mg/dL)	59.1 (58.1; 60.0)	58.8 (57.8; 59.7)	58.5 (57.5; 59.4)	58.6 (57.5; 59.7)	0.223
LDL cholesterol (mg/dL)	109.4 (107.3; 111.6)	109.3 (107.3; 111.4)	109.7 (107.6; 111.8)	110.3 (108.1; 112.4)	0.161
Triglycerides (mg/dL)[a]	94.5 (91.0; 98.1)	100.5 (96.6; 104.6)	101.9 (97.9; 105.9)	105.4 (101.0; 111.0)	**< 0.001**
C-reactive protein (mg/dL)[a]	1.17 (1.07; 1.29)	1.43 (1.31; 1.57)	1.64 (1.50; 1.79)	1.83 (1.66; 2.00)	**< 0.001**
Glycated hemoglobin (%)	5.06 (5.03; 5.09)	5.10 (5.07; 5.14)	5.11 (5.08; 5.15)	5.10 (5.06; 5.14)	0.087
Hemodynamic					
Systolic arterial pressure (mmHg)	122.0 (121.0; 122.8)	120.4 (119.5; 121.4)	121.7 (120.0; 121.6)	121.1 (120.0; 122.2)	0.215
Diastolic arterial pressure (mmHg)	75.1 (74.17; 75.8)	74.8 (74.2; 76.1)	75.4 (74.8; 76.0)	76.4 (75.6; 77.14)	**0.003**
Heart rate (bpm)	69.7 (68.5; 70.9)	70.5 (69.3; 71.7)	72.1 (69.8; 72.5)	71.2 (70.0; 72.5)	**0.014**

[a]μ Geometric mean (CI95%)
[b]Test for trend across ordered groups
Values presented in bold present statistical significance

Hs-CRP at 30 years were associated with C-Peptide. At 23 and 30 years, only diastolic blood pressure was associated with C-Peptide, but this association did not show a linear pattern (Table 2).

Considering that the independent variable of positive family history for myocardial infarction was not significant in any of the multivariate stages used in the analysis (p = 0.56), it was thus excluded from participation in subsequent level adjustments. Table 3 shows that, even after adjusting for confounding factors, C-Peptide remained associated with waist circumference and BMI at 23 and 30 years of age. Among the metabolic variables at 23 years, C-Peptide was positively associated with glycaemia, triglycerides, and Hs-CRP and negatively with HDL cholesterol.

In the longitudinal analysis at 30 years, C-Peptide was positively associated with glycated hemoglobin, triglycerides, and HS-CRP, and negatively with HDL cholesterol. Regarding hemodynamic variables, C-Peptide was not associated with systolic blood pressure, whereas diastolic blood pressure at 30 years was higher among those subjects in the upper quartile of C-Peptide.

Discussion

In the present study, the cross-sectional analysis at 23 years showed that C-Peptide was positively associated with waist circumference, BMI, glycaemia, triglycerides, and Creactive protein, whereas the association with

Table 3 Multivariate regression of cardiovascular risk factors and C-Peptide at 23 and 30 years old[a]

Cardiovascular risk factors	1st quartile μ (CI95%)	2nd quartile β (CI95%)	3rd quartile β (CI95%)	4th quartile β (CI95%)
	23 years			
Anthropometric				
Waist circumference (cm)	Reference	0.88 (− 0.46; 2.22)	**1.78 (0.41; 3.15)**	**4.90 (3.45; 6.36)**
	Reference	0.49 (−0.38; 1.02)	**0.97 (0.44; 1.52)**	**2.15 (1.57; 2.72)**
Metabolic				
Serum glycaemia (mg/dL)	Reference	**2.58 (0.67; 4.50)**	**5.55 (3.60; 7.49)**	**11.19 (9.80; 13.94)**
Total cholesterol (mg/dL)	Reference	−0.38 (−5.04; 4.28)	0.95 (−3.79; 5.70)	1.76 (− 3.28; 6.80)
HDL cholesterol (mg/dL)	Reference	**−2.12 (−3.80; − 0.44)**	**− 2.33 (− 4.04; − 0.61)**	**− 2.10 (− 3.93; − 0.29)**
Triglycerides (mg/dL)	Reference	**1.12 (1.05; 1.20)**	**1.19 (1.05; 1.20)**	**1.28 (1.19; 1.38)**
C-reactive protein (mg/dL)	Reference	**0.94 (0.81; 1.10)**	**1.26 (1.08; 1.47)**	**1.42 (1.20; 1.67)**
Hemodynamic				
Systolic pressure (mmHg)	Reference	−1.32 (−3.39; 0.75)	− 1.93 (−4.05; 0.18)	−0.25 (−2.48; 2.01)
Diastolic pressure (mmHg)	Reference	**−1.88 (− 3.43; − 0.32)**	**−1.93 (− 3.52; − 0.35)**	−0.20 (− 1.88; 1.47)
	30 years			
Anthropometric				
Waist circumference (cm)	Reference	1.0 (−0.39; 2.41)	**1,74 (0.30; 3.17)**	**4.18 (2.65; 5.70)**
Body mass index	Reference	**0.75 (0.15; 1.34)**	**1.26 (0.65; 1.88)**	**2.26 (1.61; 2.91)**
Metabolic				
Serum glycaemia (mg/dL)	Reference	−1.28 (−3.18; 0.62)	−0.39 (−2.33; 1.55)	−0.66 (− 2.72; 1.40)
Glycated hemoglobin (%)	Reference	**0.06 (0.01; 0.12)**	**0.07 (0.02; 0.13)**	**0.07 (0.01; 0.14)**
Total cholesterol (mg/dL)	Reference	−0.62 (−4.93; 3.68)	−0.69 (−5.11; 3.71)	−2.20 (−6.88; 2.47)
HDL cholesterol (mg/dL)	Reference	−0.79 (−2.42; 0.84)	−1.30 (− 2.97; 0.36)	**−1.82 (− 3.59; − 0.05)**
LDL cholesterol (mg/dL)	Reference	−0.76 (− 4.23; 2.70)	−0.68 (− 4.23; 2.86)	−0.98 (− 4.75; 2.78)
Triglycerides (mg/dL)	Reference	**1,06 (0,99; 1,13)**	**1,07 (1,0; 1,14)**	**1,06 (0,99; 1,14)**
C-reactive protein (mg/dL)	Reference	**1,23 (1,06; 1,42)**	**1,51 (1,30; 1,75)**	**1,54 (1,32; 1,80)**
Hemodynamic				
Systolic pressure (mmHg)	Reference	−0.96 (−2.54; 1.62)	−0.25 (−1.87; 1.36)	−0.03 (− 1.75; 1.68)
Diastolic pressure (mmHg)	Reference	−0.44 (−1.53; 0.65)	0.45 (− 0.66; 1.56)	1.12 (− 0.06; 2.30)

μ geometric mean
[a]adjusted for: time of fasting, physical activity practice per week (minutes), family income, mother's skin color, birthweight, rapid growth between 2 and 4 years old, smoking at 23 years, alcohol consumption, family history of dyslipidemia, arterial hypertension and stroke, myocardial infarction
Values presented in bold present statistical significance

HDL cholesterol was in the opposite direction. In the longitudinal analysis, C-Peptide remained positively associated with waist circumference, BMI, glycated hemoglobin, triglycerides, and C-reactive protein and negatively with HDL cholesterol. The direction of the association with diastolic blood pressure changed, i.e., at 23 years' diastolic blood pressure was higher among those in the first quartile of C-Peptide whereas the opposite was observed at 30 years.

Studies on the effect of C-Peptide on glycaemia have yielded conflicting evidence. Whereas Hoogwerf et al. found no association [24], Oskarsson et al. reported that C-Peptide enhances insulin-induced hypoglycemia among diabetic patients [25]. Nordquist et al. showed that C-Peptide infusion in patients with type-I diabetes improves glucose use by about 25% [26]. In the present study, C-Peptide was positively associated with glycaemia at 23 years, but no association was observed in the longitudinal analysis at 30 years. That may be due to the increase in insulin resistance, which would be the result of the rise in the prevalence of overweight – from 28.3 to 57.6% – from 23 to 30 years [27], increasing the peripheral resistance to insulin, which, along with hyperinsulinemia, would result in a temporary reduction in glycemic status.

On the other hand, the findings of the associations with abdominal circumference and body mass index are based on the understanding that increased visceral fat contributes to insulin resistance and pro-inflammatory adipokine production by means of monocyte attraction protein (MCP-1) in addition to its greater performance on catecholaminergic receptors and lower performance on insulin receptors, which favors a greater release of free fatty acids and hypertriglyceridemia, which in turn favors the lipotoxicity phenomenon, which was

transversely identified and remained associated longitudinally at 30 years [28, 29].

C-Peptide was associated with triglycerides at 23 and 30 years. Although they cannot be considered a marker of atherogenic risk by themselves, triglycerides in association with other components such as obesity, diabetes, or hypertension are a marker of cardiovascular risk [30]. In addition to this condition, the negative relation with HDL cholesterol at 23 and 30 years old stands out. Suggesting that C-Peptide is associated with metabolic factors related to cardiovascular risk. C-reactive protein, a marker of systemic inflammatory process, was considered a cardiovascular risk factor [31–34]. Danesh (2004), in a meta-analysis of observational studies, observed that those in the highest tercile of C-reactive protein were at higher risk of cardiovascular events (OR 1.45; CI95% 1.25–1.68) [35]. However, a Mendelian randomization study showed that Hs-CRP was not independently associated with cardiovascular risk and that it could be a marker of risk [36]. In the present study, C-Peptide remained associated with Hs-CRP at 23 and 30 years old, which suggests that C-Peptide is associated with the systemic inflammatory process.

Diastolic blood pressure was positively associated with C-Peptide at 23 years, but, unlike Chen and Every [37, 38] systolic blood pressure was not associated with C-Peptide. Although it accepts the association between insulin resistance and the condition of hypertension due to favoring the conditions of vasoconstriction, greater renal resorption of sodium and increased production of angiotensin II at the level of visceral fat. Which in turn, leads to less production of oxide nitric acid and hypertrophy in the mucosal mean of vessels by the action of hyperinsulinemia, our findings did not observe association with the

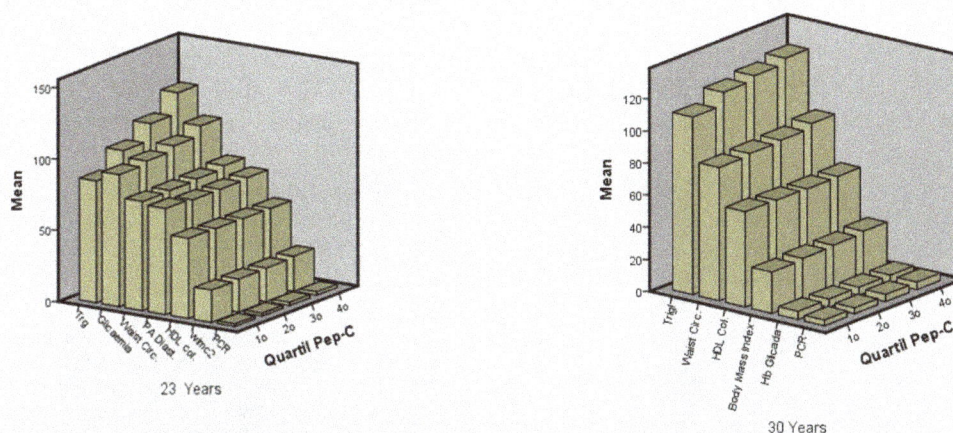

Fig. 1 Cardiovascular risk components associated with Pep-C at 23 and 30 years

tensional state and the levels of the pep-C quartiles at 23 or 30 years.

The majority prevalence of diabetes in developing countries, stay in the 45 to 64 -year age range, in contrast, with developed countries (> 64 years of age) [39]. Our findings are in line with the epidemiological profile indicated, since the associates found to be pre-findings point to a condition of insulin resistance associated with conditions of cardiometabolic risk already present at 23[a] and is maintained longitudinally at the end of the 3[a] decade of life. A strength of this study is its population-based design and the large proportion of the sample successfully followed, which minimized the likelihood of selection bias. Among the limitations, it could be pointed that the biochemical tests were carried out in non-fasting samples. On the other hand, more recent evidence indicates that casual exams allow better risk estimate [40] and, furthermore, the analyses were adjusted for time of fasting.

Conclusion

In a population that has been prospectively followed since birth, we observed a positive relationship between C-Peptide and obesity indicators such as waist circumference and BMI at 23 years and 30 years of age (as shown in Fig. 1). C-Peptide was also associated with the systemic inflammatory process and the higher level of metabolic cardiovascular risk factors.

Abbreviations

23[a]: Twenty-three years; 30[a]: Thirty years; BMI: Body mass index; cm: Centimeters; C-Peptide: Insulin-binding peptide; HbA$_{1c}$: Glycated hemoglobin; HDL: High-density lipoprotein – HDL cholesterol; HR: Hazard ratio; HS-CRP: High-sensitivity C-reactive protein; IPAQ: International physical activity questionnaire; kg: Kilograms; LDL: Low-density lipoprotein – LDL cholesterol; MCP-1: Monocyte attraction protein; mg/dL: Milligrams per deciliter; mm: Millimeters; mmHg: Millimeters of mercury; ng/mL: Nanogram per milliliter; RR: Relative risk; tPA: Tissue plasminogen activator; μ: Geometric mean

Acknowledgements
The Wellcame Trust and ABRASCO for the collaboration and support of the creation of the Pelotas Cohort and publication assistance.

Funding
Institutional PhD Program of the Coordination of Improvement of Higher Education Personnel- CAPES/MEC; Brasil, through technical cooperation between UFPel / UFES, developed by the Graduate Program in Epidemiology of UFPel.

Authors' contributions
RLMA - designed the study, performed the statistical analysis and prepared the initial manuscript. DPG - Interpreted the analyzed results and revised the manuscript. IOO - Interpreted the results and revised and revised the manuscript. BLH - Contributed to the design of the study, supervised the statistical analysis, interpreted the results analyzed and revised the manuscript. All authors have approved the final version to be submitted and agree to be responsible authors for the aspects of the work in order to ensure that issues related to the accuracy or completeness of any part of the work are properly investigated and resolved.

Competing interests
The authors declare that they have no competing interests.

Author details
[1]University Hospital Cassiano Antônio de Moraes (HUCAM) of the Federal, University of Espírito Santo (UFES), Vitória-ES, Brazil. [2]Post-Graduate Program in Epidemiology, Federal University of Pelotas (UFPel), Pelotas-RS, Brazil. [3]Vitória, Brazil.

References
1. Mendis S, Puska P, Norrving B, editors. Global Atlas on Cardiovascular Disease Prevention and Control. Geneva: World Health Organization; 2011. ISBN 978 92 4 156437 3. http://www.who.int/cardiovascular_diseases/publications/atlas_cvd/en/
2. Global action plan for the prevention and control of noncommunicable diseases 2013–2020. 1. Chronic diseases. 2. Cardiovascular diseases. 3. Neoplasms. 4. Respiratory tract diseases. 5. Diabetes mellitus. 6. Health planning. 7. International cooperation. I.World Health Organization. ISBN 978 92 4 1506236. http://apps.who.int/iris/bitstream/10665/94384/1/9789241506236_eng.pdf. Accessed 25 Oct 2018.
3. Piepoli MF, Hoes AW, Agewall S, Albus C, Brotons C, Catapano AL, et al. 2016 European Guidelines on cardiovascular disease prevention in clinical practice. Eur Heart J. 2016;37(29):2315. https://doi.org/10.1093/eurheartj/ehw106.
4. Ordunez P, Prieto-Lara E, Pinheiro Gawryszewski V, Hennis AJM, Cooper RS. Premature Mortality from Cardiovascular Disease in the Americas – Will the Goal of a Decline of "25% by 2025" be Met? PLoS One. 2015;10(10): e0141685. https://doi.org/10.1371/journal.pone.0141685.
5. Younk LM, Lamos EM, Davis SN. The cardiovascular effects of insulin. Expert Opin Drug Saf. 2014;13(7):955–66. https://doi.org/10.1517/14740338.2014.919256 Epub 2014 Jun 5. Review. PubMed PMID: 24899093. http://www.tandfonline.com/doi/abs/10.1517/14740338.2014.919256?journalCode=ieds20.
6. Li Y, Li Y, Meng L, Zheng L. Association between serum C-Peptide as a risk factor for cardiovascular disease and high-density lipoprotein cholesterol levels in nondiabetic individuals. PLoS One. 2015;10(1):e112281. https://doi.org/10.1371/journal.pone.0112281 eCollection 2015. PubMed PMID: 25559358; PubMed Central PMCID: PMC4283961. http://journals.plos.org/plosone/article?id=10.1371/journal.pone.0112281.
7. Min JY, Min KB. Serum C-Peptide levels and risk of death among adults without diabetes mellitus. CMAJ. 2013;185(9):E402–8. https://doi.org/10.1503/cmaj.121950 Epub 2013 Apr 15. PubMed PMID: 23589428; PubMed Central PMCID: PMC3680586. http://www.cmaj.ca/content/185/9/E402.long.
8. Steiner DF, Cunningham D, Spigelman L, et al. Insulin biosynthesis: evidence for a precursor. Science. 1967;157(3789):697–700 http://science.sciencemag.org/content/157/3789/697.long.

9. Hirai FE, Moss SE, Klein BE, Klein R. Relationship of glycemic control, exogenous insulin, and C-Peptide levels to ischemic heart disease mortality over a 16-year period in people with older-onset diabetes: the Wisconsin Epidemiologic Study of Diabetic Retinopathy (WESDR). Diabetes Care. 2008; 31(3):493–7 https://www.ncbi.nlm.nih.gov/pmc/articles/PMC2773445/.

10. Wahren J, Shafqat J, Johansson J, Chibalin A, Ekberg K, Jornvall H. Molecular and cellular effects of C-Peptide- new perspectives on an old peptide. Exp Diabesity Res. 2004;5(1):15–23 https://www.ncbi.nlm.nih.gov/pmc/articles/PMC2892072/pdf/125_2010_Article1736.pdf.

11. Walcher D, Babiak C, Poletek P, Rosenkranz S, Bach H, Betz S, Durst R, Grüb M, Hombach V, Strong J, Marx N. C-Peptide induces vascular smooth muscle cell proliferation: involvement of SRC-kinase, phosphatidylinositol 3-kinase, and extracellular signal-regulated kinase 1/2. Circ Res. 2006;99(11): 1181–7 PubMed PMID: 17068290 http://circres.ahajournals.org/content/99/11/1181.long.

12. Marx N, Walcher D. C-Peptide and Atherogenesis: C-Peptide as a Mediator of Lesion Development in Patients with Type 2 Diabetes Mellitus? Exp Diabesity Res. 2008;2008:385108. https://doi.org/10.1155/2008/385108 5 pages. https://www.hindawi.com/journals/jdr/2008/385108/.

13. Cabrera de Leon A, Oliva Garcia JG, Marcelino Rodriguez I, Almeida Gonzalez D, Aleman Sanchez JJ, Brito Diaz B, et al. C-Peptide as a risk factor of coronary artery disease in the general population. Diab Vasc Dis Res. 2015;12(3):199–207 http://dvr.sagepub.com/content/12/3/199.long.

14. Marx N, Silbernagel G, Brandenburg V, Burgmaier M, Kleber ME, Grammer TB, et al. C-Peptide levels are associated with mortality and cardiovascular mortality in patients undergoing angiography: the LURIC study. Diabetes Care. 2013;36(3):708–14 http://care.diabetesjournals.org/content/36/3/708.

15. Patel N, Taveira TH, Choudhary G, Whitlatch H, Wu WC. Fasting serum C-Peptide levels predict cardiovascular and overall death in nondiabetic adults. J Am Heart Assoc. 2012;1(6):e003152. https://doi.org/10.1161/JAHA.112.003152 PubMed PMID: 23316320; PubMed Central PMCID: PMC3540682 https://www.ncbi.nlm.nih.gov/pmc/articles/PMC3540682/.

16. Bo S, Gentile L, Castiglione A, Prandi V, Canil S, Ghigo E, et al. C-Peptide and the risk for incident complications and mortality in type 2 diabetic patients: a retrospective cohort study after a 14-year follow-up. Eur J Endocrinol. 2012;167(2):173–80 https://eje.bioscientifica.com/view/journals/eje/167/2/173.xml.

17. Victora CG, Barros FC. Cohort Profile: The 1982 Pelotas (Brazil) Birth Cohort Study. Int J Epidemiol. 2006;35(2):237–42. https://doi.org/10.1093/ije/dyi290 First published online December 22, 2005. https://academic.oup.com/ije/article/35/2/237/694731.

18. Horta BL, Gigante DP, Goncalves H, dos Santos Motta J, Loret de Mola C, Oliveira IO, et al. Cohort Profile Update: https://academic.oup.com/ije/article/44/2/441/753028. Accessed 25 Oct 2018.

19. Lohman TG, Roche AF, Martorell R, editors. Anthropometric Standardization Reference Manual. Champaign: Human Kinetics Books; 1988. p. 5570.

20. C-Peptide Assay Specifications. The 1982 Pelotas (Brazil) Birth Cohort Study. Int J Epidemiol. 2015;44(2):441 Siemens Healthcare Diagnostics Products Ltd. Llanberis, Gwynedd LL 55 4EL United Kingdom. https://www.healthcare.siemens.com/clinical-specialities/diabetes/diabetes-related-assays/clinicalsignificance.

21. Nazmi A, Oliveira IO, Horta BL, Gigante DP, Victora CG. Lifecourse socioeconomic trajectories and C-reactive protein levels in young adults: findings from a Brazilian birth cohort. Soc Sci Med. 2010;70(8):1229–36. https://doi.org/10.1016/j.socscimed.2009.12.014 PubMed PMID: 20137842; PubMed Central PMCID: PMC2877874. https://www.ncbi.nlm.nih.gov/pmc/articles/PMC2877874/.

22. American Diabetes Association. (2) Classification and diagnosis of diabetes. Diabetes Care. 2015;38(Suppl):S8–S16. https://doi.org/10.2337/dc15-S005 Review. PubMed PMID: 25537714. http://care.diabetesjournals.org/content/diacare/38/Supplement_1/S8.full.pdf.

23. Brasil. Ministério da Saúde. Secretaria de Atenção à Saúde. Departamento de Atenção Básica. Atenção ao pré-natal de baixo risco / Ministério da Saúde. Secretaria de Atenção à Saúde. Departamento de Atenção Básica. – Brasília: Editora do Ministério da Saúde, 2012. 318 p.: il. – (Série A. Normas e Manuais Técnicos) (Cadernos de Atenção Básica, n° 32) ISBN978–85–334-1936-0. http://bvsms.saude.gov.br/bvs/publicacoes/cadernos_atencao_basica_32_prenatal.pdf

24. Andrade RLM, Gigante DP, de Oliveira IO, Horta BL. Conditions of gestation, childbirth and childhood associated with C-peptide in young adults in the 1982 Birth Cohort in Pelotas-RS; Brazil. BMC Cardiovasc Disord. 2017;17(1):

181. https://doi.org/10.1186/s12872-017-0613-3 PubMed PMID: 28693499; PubMed Central PMCID: PMC5504841.

25. Hoogwerf BJ, Bantle JP, Gaenslen HE, Greenberg BZ, Senske BJ, Francis R, Goetz FC. Infusion of synthetic human C-Peptide does not affect plasma glucose, sérum insulin, or plasma glucagon in healthy subjects. Metabolism. 1986;35(2):122–5 PubMed PMID: 3511350 http://www.sciencedirect.com/science/article/pii/0026049586901113?via%3Dihub.

26. Oskarsson P, Johansson BL, Adamson U, Lins PE. Effects of C-Peptide on insulin-induced hypoglycaemia and its counterregulatory responses in IDDM patients. Diabet Med. 1997;14(8):655–9 PubMed PMID: 9272591. https://onlinelibrary.wiley.com/doi/pdf/10.1002/%28SICI%291096-9136%28199708%2914%3A8%3C655%3A%3AAID-DIA435%3E3.0.CO%3B2-G.

27. Nordquist L, Johansson M. Proinsulin C-Peptide: friend or foe in thedevelopment of diabetes-associated complications? Vasc Health Risk Manag. 2008;4(6):1283–8 Review. PubMed PMID: 19337542; PubMed Central PMCID: https://www.ncbi.nlm.nih.gov/pmc/articles/PMC2663462/pdf/VHRM-4-1283.pdf.

28. Schaffer JE. Lipotoxicity: when tissues overeat. Curr Opin Lipidol. 2003;14(3): 281–7. Review. PubMed PMID: 12840659. https://doi.org/10.1097/01.mol.0000073508.41685.7f.

29. Ertunc ME, Hotamisligil GS. Sinalização lipídica e lipotoxicidade em metaflammation: indicações para patogênese e tratamento da doença metabólica. J Lipid Res. 2016 dez; 57 (12): 2099-2114. Epub 2016 Jun 21. Review. PubMed PMID: 27330055; PubMed Central PMCID: PMC5321214.

30. Lima NP, Horta BL, Motta JV d S, Valença MS, Oliveira V, dos Santos TV, Gigante DP, Barros FC. Evolução do excesso de peso e obesidade até a idade adulta, Pelotas, Rio Grande do Sul, Brasil, 1982-2012. Cad Saude Publica. 2015;31(9):2017–25. https://doi.org/10.1590/0102-311X00173814.

31. Miller M, Stone NJ, Ballantyne C, Bittner V, Criqui MH, Ginsberg HN, Goldberg AC, Howard WJ, Jacobson MS, Kris-Etherton PM, Lennie TA, Levi M, Mazzone T, Pennathur S. American Heart Association Clinical Lipidology, Thrombosis, and Prevention Committee of the Council on Nutrition, Physical Activity, and Metabolism.; Council on Arteriosclerosis, Thrombosis and Vascular Biology.; Council on Cardiovascular Nursing.; Council on the Kidney in Cardiovascular Disease. Triglycerides and cardiovascular disease: a scientific statement from the American Heart Association. Circulation. 2011; 123(20):2292–333. https://doi.org/10.1161/CIR.0b013e3182160726 PubMed PMID: 21502576. http://circ.ahajournals.org/content/123/20/2292.

32. Harchaoui KE, Visser M, Kastelein JJ, Stroes E, Dallinga-Thie G. Triglycerides and Cardiovascular Risk. Curr Cardiol Rev. 2009;5(3):216–22. https://doi.org/10.2174/157340309788970315 https://www.ncbi.nlm.nih.gov/pmc/articles/PMC2822144/pdf/CCR-5-216.pdf.

33. Galper BZ, Wang YC, Einstein AJ. Strategies for Primary Prevention of Coronary Heart Disease Based on Risk Stratification by the ACC/AHA Lipid Guidelines, ATPIII Guidelines, Coronary Calcium Scoring, and C-Reactive Protein, and a Global Treat-All Strategy: A Comparative--Effectiveness Modeling Study. PLoS One. 2015;10(9):e0138092. https://doi.org/10.1371/journal.pone.0138092 PubMed PMID: 26422204; PubMed Central PMCID: PMC4589241. https://www.ncbi.nlm.nih.gov/pmc/articles/PMC4589241/pdf/pone.0138092.pdf.

34. Kearney PM, Whelton M, Reynolds K, Muntner P, Whelton PK, He J. Global burden of hypertension: analysis of worldwide data. Lancet. 2005;365(9455): 217–23 https://www.sciencedirect.com/science/article/pii/0033062074900346.

35. Ridker PM, Cook N. Clinical usefulness of very high and very low levels of C-reactive protein across the full range of Framingham Risk Scores. Circulation. 2004;109(16):1955–9 PubMed PMID: 15051634 http://circ.ahajournals.org/content/109/16/1955.long.

36. Blaha MJ, Budoff MJ, DeFilippis AP, Blankstein R, Rivera JJ, Agatston A, et al. Associations between C-reactive protein, coronary artery calcium, and cardiovascular events: implications for the JUPITER population from MESA, a population-based cohort study. Lancet. 2011;378:684–92. https://doi.org/10.1016/S0140-6736(11)60784-8.

37. Danesh J, Wheeler JG, Hirschfield GM, Eda S, Eiriksdottir G, Rumley A, Lowe GD, Pepys MB, Gudnason V. C-reactive protein and other circulating markers of inflammation in the prediction of coronary heart disease. N Engl J Med. 2004;350(14):1387–97 PubMed PMID: 15070788. http://www.nejm.org/doi/full/10.1056/NEJMoa032804.

38. C Reactive Protein Coronary Heart Disease Genetics Collaboration (CCGC), Wensley F, Gao P, Burgess S, Kaptoge S, Di Angelantonio E, Shah T, Engert JC, Clarke R, Davey-Smith G, Nordestgaard BG, Saleheen D, Samani NJ, Sandhu M, Anand S, Pepys MB, Smeeth L, Whittaker J, Casas JP, Thompson

SG, Hingorani AD, Danesh J. Association between C reactive protein and coronary heart disease: mendelian randomisation analysis based on individual participant data. BMJ. 2011;342:d548. https://doi.org/10.1136/bmj.d548 https://www.ncbi.nlm.nih.gov/pmc/articles/PMC3039696/.

39. Wild S, Roglic G, Green A, Sicree R, King H. Global prevalence of diabetes: estimates for the year 2000 and projections for 2030. Diabetes Care. 2004; 27(5):1047–53 PubMed PMID: 15111519. http://care.diabetesjournals.org/content/27/5/1047.full-text.pdf.

40. Chen CH, Tsai ST, Chuang JH, Chang MS, Wang SP, Chou P. Population-based study of insulin, C-Peptide, and blood pressure in Chinese with normal glucose tolerance. Am J Cardiol. 1995;76(8):585–8 http://www.sciencedirect.com/science/article/pii/S000291499980160X?via%3Dihub.

19

Glycemic control with a basal-bolus insulin protocol in hospitalized diabetic patients treated with glucocorticoids: a retrospective cohort study

Elena Chertok Shacham[1*], Hila Kfir[1], Naama Schwartz[2] and Avraham Ishay[1]

Abstract

Background: Improved glycemic control is the desired outcome after the discharge of patients with diabetes. We aimed to determine the efficacy of a basal-bolus insulin protocol in hospitalized patients with diabetes treated with glucocorticoids.

Methods: A retrospective cohort study compared the glycemic control of 150 hospitalized patients with diabetes and elevated inflammatory markers who were either treated with ($n = 61$) or without glucocorticoids ($n = 89$). All patients were treated with a basal-bolus regimen.

Results: Glycosylated hemoglobin A1C (HbA1C) levels, mode of diabetes treatment before admission, length of hospitalization and inflammatory markers were similar in both groups of patients (treated and untreated with glucocorticoid). There was a trend toward female predominance in the glucocorticoid-treated group. Mean daily glucose levels were higher in patients taking glucocorticoids when compared with untreated patients (12.5 ± 2.7 mmol/l vs. 10.9 ± 2.4 mmol/l, $p < .0001$), and significantly higher at 5:00 PM (13.1 ± 3.4 vs. 10.2 ± 3 mmol/l, $p < .0001$), and 8:00 P.M. (13.9 ± 4.1 mmol/l vs. 11 ± 3.1 mmol/l, $p < 0.001$) . No difference was detected between the two groups in prandial and basal insulin doses during hospitalization. Overall, 64% of patients in the glucocorticoid-treated group versus 39% in the untreated group had inadequate glycemic control during hospitalization ($p = 0.003$).

Conclusion: A significantly higher percentage of patients with diabetes who were treated with glucocorticoids during hospitalization did not achieve glycemic control with a basal-bolus insulin protocol. These patients had significantly higher mean blood glucose levels due to elevated levels in the afternoon and evening. New basal-bolus protocols with appropriate adjustments of short acting insulin are needed to treat patients with diabetes on glucocorticoid therapy.

Keywords: Type 2 diabetes mellitus, Basal-bolus insulin protocol, Glucocorticoid treatment, Glycemic control

Background

The deleterious effects of hyperglycemia on the length of hospitalization, rate of infection, in-hospital mortality, and disability after hospitalization are well known from previous studies [1–3], so enhancing glycemic control during the hospital stay is a reasonable and logical target for improving patient outcomes [4, 5]. The management of

patients with diabetes in noncritical care settings is based on basal-bolus insulin protocols according to contemporary guidelines [6, 7]. The recommended pre-meal target glucose levels for the majority of inpatients are 100–140 mg/dl (5.6–7.8 mmol/l), and random blood glucose levels should be less than 180 mg/dl (10.0 mmol/l) [7].

Glucocorticoids are widely used for treating inflammatory, autoimmune and malignant diseases [8]. New-onset hyperglycemia and difficulties in controlling existing diabetes are known to accompany glucocorticoid treatment [8, 9]. Indeed, a number of studies have reported elevated

* Correspondence: elena_ch@clalit.org.il; elenachertok12@gmail.com
[1]Endocrinology Unit, Haemek Medical Center, Rabin Ave 21, Afula, Israel, 18134 Afula, Israel
Full list of author information is available at the end of the article

blood glucose levels in more than 50% of patients without diabetes who were treated with glucocorticoids during hospitalization [10–12].

Although a growing body of studies have examined various glycemic control protocols for glucocorticoid-treated patients with diabetes [13–15], there are still no uniform guidelines, as previous studies failed to demonstrate benefits of one regimen over another, and there is a paucity of randomized clinical trials. The aim of this study was to examine the efficacy of the currently implemented basal bolus insulin protocol in our institution among patients with diabetes who were hospitalized with an acute inflammatory state, and to examine whether there is a difference in glycemic control between those receiving glucocorticoids and those who were not.

Methods

This retrospective study was approved by HaEmek Medical Center Research Ethics Committee (Afula, Israel). We reviewed the electronic charts of patients diagnosed with type 2 diabetes mellitus (T2DM) admitted to the

internal medicine department of the Medical Center from 2013 to 2015 and treated with a basal-bolus insulin protocol during their stay. Patients were included in the analysis if they were hospitalized for a minimum of 4 days, were 18 years of age or older, and had elevated inflammatory markers (C-reactive protein [CRP] ≥20) on admission. Exclusion criteria were pregnancy, type 1 diabetes and the presence of diabetic ketoacidosis. A total of 150 patients met the inclusion criteria: 61 who received glucocorticoid treatment during hospitalization (with prednisone ≥10 mg/day or an equivalent dose of glucocorticoid) and 89 who did not (Fig. 1).

The amounts of long- and short-acting insulin were recorded in units/day. The baseline characteristics collected at admission were recorded for each group. The most recent glycosylated hemoglobin A1C (HbA1C) for each patient (in the preceding 3 months) was retrieved.

Both patient groups were treated according to the hospital's standard protocol for treating of patients with hyperglycemia. The protocol was written by an endocrinologist, a clinical pharmacologist and a nurse responsible for

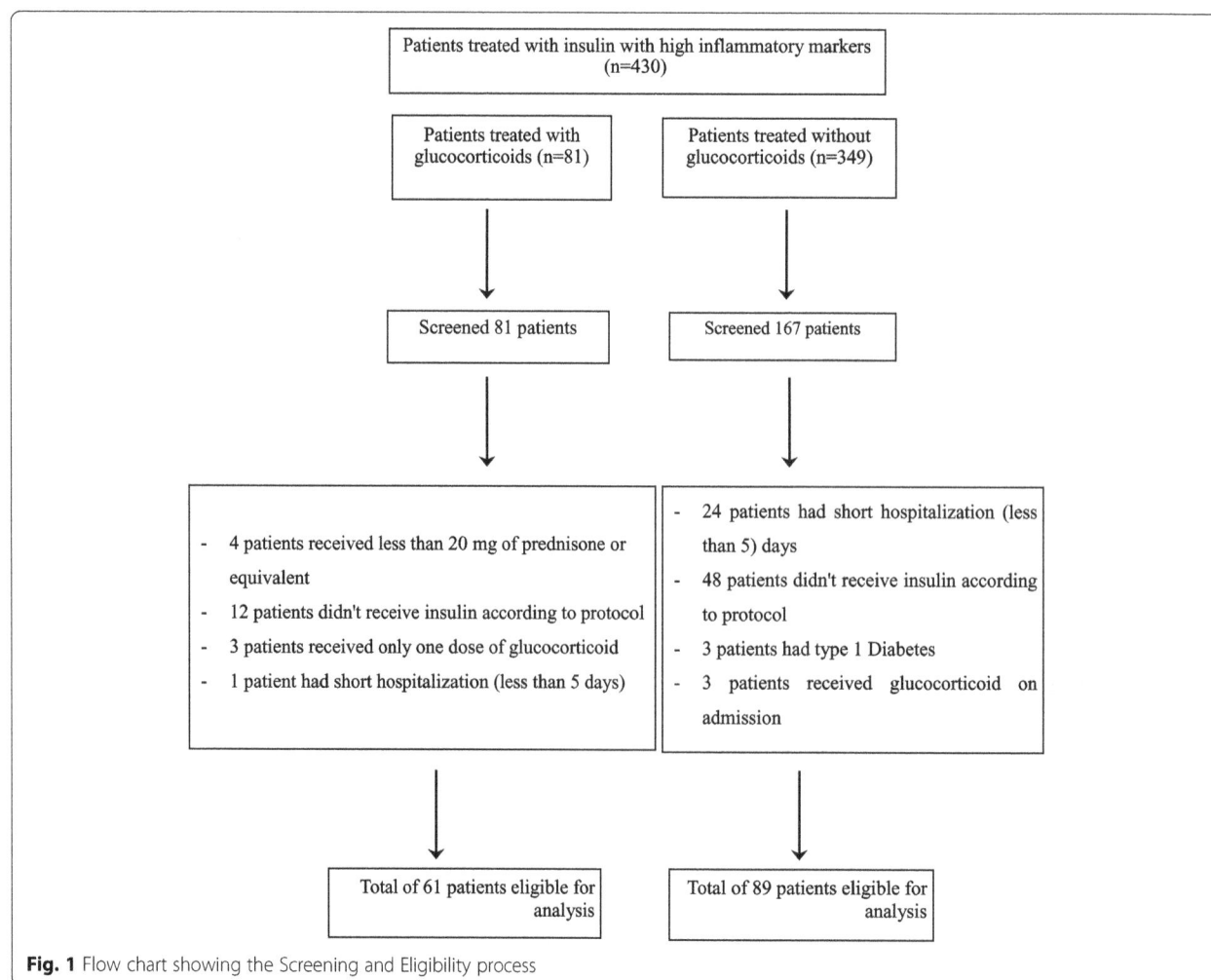

Fig. 1 Flow chart showing the Screening and Eligibility process

diabetes treatment in our hospital. The treatment protocol was first implemented in July 2011 and has been used since then as the standard recommended care for diabetes in the hospital's internal medicine departments (Fig. 2).

In accordance with our standard practice, patients with two consecutive glucose measurements above 180 mg/dl (10 mmol/l) were started on a basal–bolus insulin regimen. All oral hypoglycemic and non-insulin injectable diabetes medications were discontinued in patients eligible for insulin treatment. A total daily dose (TDD) of insulin was estimated as 0.5 units /kg/day for glucose levels of 180–400 mg/dl (10–22.2 mmol/l) on admission. Patients treated with glucocorticoids or having a glucose level > 400 mg/dl (22.2 mmol/l) were treated with 0.7 units/kg/day of insulin. The TDD was distributed as follows: 50% long-acting, defined as basal insulin, and 50% prandial fast, defined as bolus insulin. The long-acting insulins used in the study were insulin glargine (Lantus) and insulin detemir (Levemir) given in the evening. The short-acting insulins were glulisine (Apidra) and aspart (NovoRapid). We analyzed blood glucose levels by type of long-acting insulin in both patient groups (steroid-treated and control). If pre-meal glucose levels were > 180 mg/dl(10 mmol/l), a correction factor insulin was given (Fig. 2). Patients treated with insulin before admission continued their insulin regimen if blood glucose levels on admission were < 180 mg/dl (10 mmol/l). If more than two subsequent glucose measurements were > 180 mg/dl (10 mmol/l), correction doses of insulin were added at meal times. After the first 24 h of treatment, the insulin doses (including the additional insulin given at meal-time during the previous day) were calculated. Basal insulin doses were adjusted if the 08.00 AM blood glucose level was outside the target range (110–180 mg/dl; 6.1–10 mmol/l) for hyperglycemia as well as hypoglycemia (Fig. 3). Attending physicians were provided with the titration schedule as written in the standard protocol of care in an attempt to achieve glucose readings within the target range.

The primary endpoint of the study was to determine the differences in glycemic control between the treatment groups as measured by the mean daily blood glucose concentration. Mean blood glucose during hospitalization, daily blood glucose according to hours of point-of-care capillary blood glucose, and the number of hypoglycemic and hyperglycemic episodes were also analyzed. Additional endpoints were the number of consecutive blood glucose readings > 200 mg/dl (11.1 mmol/l) during hospitalization: patients with three or more such readings were considered not controlled and the percentage of such patients in each group was recorded.

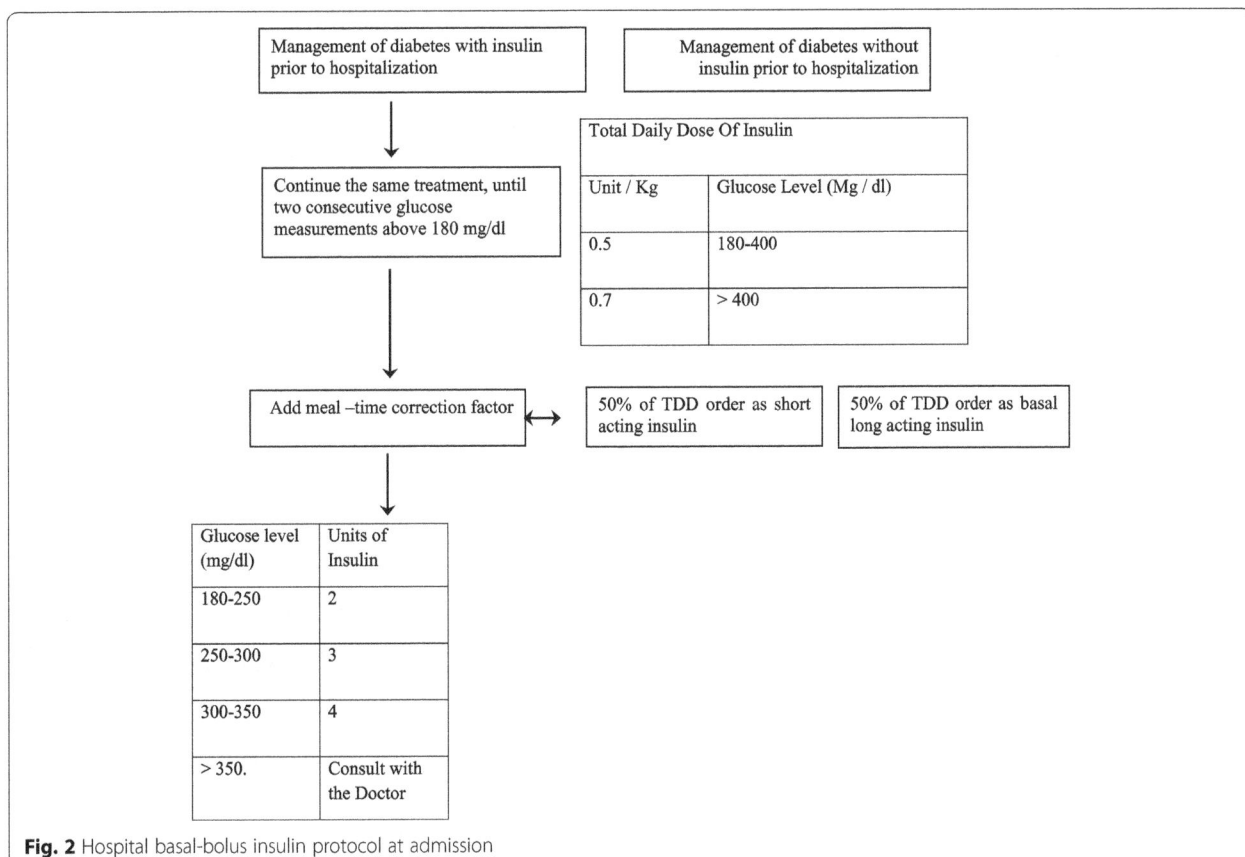

Fig. 2 Hospital basal-bolus insulin protocol at admission

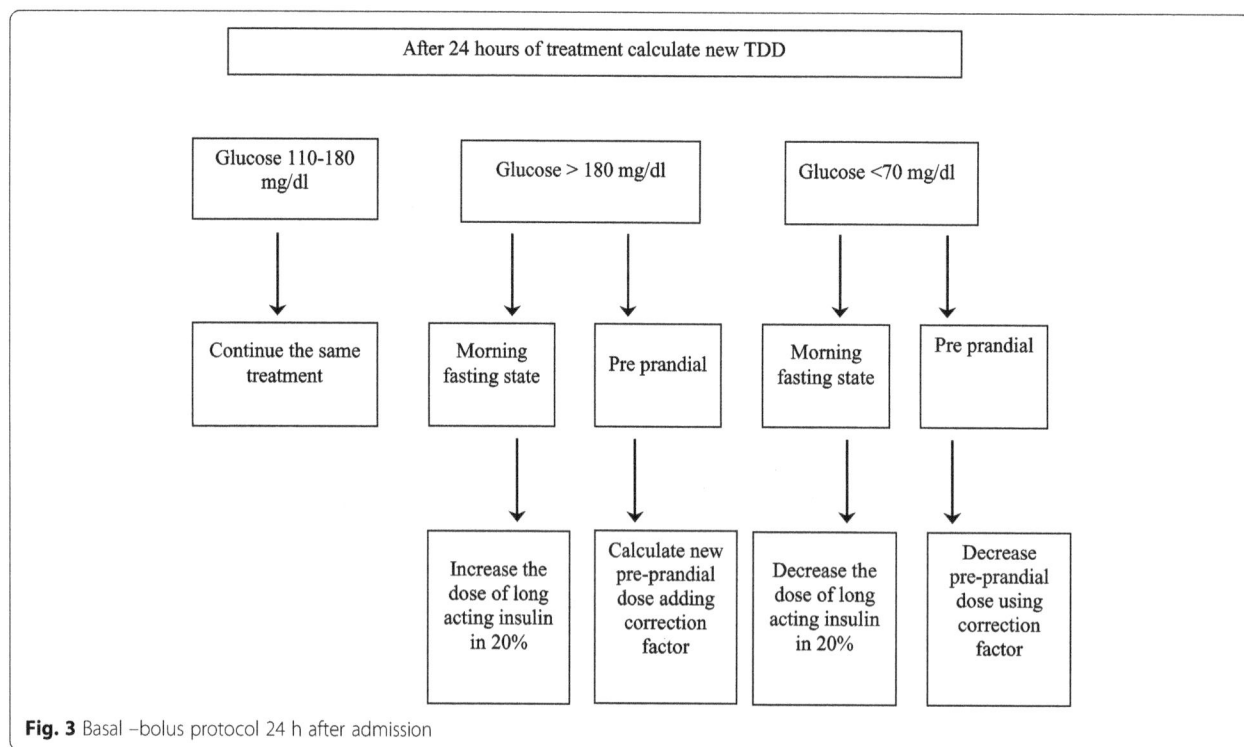

Fig. 3 Basal –bolus protocol 24 h after admission

We compared blood glucose levels of patients treated with glucocorticoids before their hospitalization to those of patients who were not treated with glucocorticoids and performed additional analysis of these two groups of patients. In the group of patients treated with glucocorticoids, we also compared blood glucose levels of patients treated with prednisone with those of patients treated with other steroids.

Statistical analysis

We hypothesized that the difference in mean blood glucose between patients treated with steroids and those in the control group (patient with diabetes who were not treated with glucocorticoids) would be at least 20 mg/dl (1.1 mmol/l) (SD 40). A sample size of 64 patients in each study group was required for a power of 80% and alpha 5% (two sided test). The final sample included 61 patients treated with steroids and 89 patients in the control group. As a result the study power increased to 85%. Categorical variables were presented with frequencies and percent, and continuous variables were presented with a mean ± standard deviation (SD) and median. The association between the glucocorticoid-treated and the control groups and categorical variables was examined by the Chi-square test or Fisher's exact test. Continuous variables were analyzed by T-test or Wilcoxon two sample tests. The difference in insulin dosage between the first and last day of hospitalization was calculated in each group and analyzed by the Wilcoxon signed-rank test.

The statistical analyses were performed with the SAS 9.4 software. A p value < 0.05 was considered significant.

Results

The demographic characteristics of the treated and untreated groups were similar, but a trend towards female sex predominance was found in the glucocorticoid group (Table 1). The mean length of hospitalization, inflammatory markers, diabetes treatment prior to admission and HbA1C levels (8.5 ± 1.9% vs. 8.6 ± 1.8%, $p = 0.5$), were the same in both groups. Treated patients received either prednisone (81%), methylprednisolone (5.9%), hydrocortisone (11%) or dexamethasone (2.2%).

The mean daily glucocorticoid dose was 42.0 ± 29.4 mg of prednisone or its equivalent. The main reason for glucocorticoid treatment was pulmonary diseases. (Table 2).

The mean blood glucose level was significantly higher in patients treated with glucocorticoids compared with those untreated: 225 ± 48.0 mg/dl (12.5 ± 2.7 mmol/l) vs. 196.5 ± 43.1 mg/dl (10.9 mmol/l ± 2.4 mmol/l), respectively, $p < 0.001$. The mean blood glucose level at 5 PM in the glucocorticoid-treated group was significantly higher than in the untreated group: 235.8 ± 61.9 mg/dl (13.1 ± 3.4 mmol/l) vs. 183.5 ± 54.2 mg/dl (10.2 ± 3.0 mmol/l), respectively, $p < 0.001$. Similarly, the mean blood glucose level at 8 PM was also significantly higher in the glucocorticoid-treated group compared with the untreated group: 251.2 ± 74.6 mg/dl (13.9 ± 4.1 mmol/l) vs. 198.3 ± 55 (11 ± 3.1), respectively, $p < 0.001$ (Table 3).

Table 1 Clinical characteristics at admission in the glucocorticoid treated and control groups

	Glucocorticoids treated group ($n = 61$) mean ± SD	Control group ($n = 89$) mean ± SD	p-value
HbA1C (%)	8.6 ± 1.8	8.5 ± 1.9	0.7
Male sex (n (%))	27 (40.3%)	54 (60.8%)	0.05
Age (yrs.)	70.1 ± 11.9	68.3 ± 12.1	0.4
BMI (kg/m²)	29.5 ± 5.2	29.6 ± 7.1	0.9
CRP[1] (mg/L)	139.2 ± 94	136.4 ± 99.2	0.7
Prior treatment			
-Oral hypoglycemic only (n (%))	46 (51.7%)	32 (52.4%)	0.9
-Oral hypoglycemic and/or insulin (n (%))	68 (76.4%)	43 (70.5%)	0.4
Hospitalization length (Days)	16.8 ± 15.9	15.34 ± 16	0.99

Fasting blood glucose levels and blood glucose levels measured at 12:00 noon did not differ between the two groups. Low blood glucose levels were rare during the study. Five clinically significant events of hypoglycemia (glucose values < 54 mg/dl, [< 3 mmol/l]) occurred in the study population: two in the glucocorticoid treated group and three in the untreated group. Basal and prandial insulin dosages were not significantly different between the two groups during hospitalization ($p > 0.1$). Comparing the daily insulin dose between the first and last day of hospitalization, a significantly higher daily insulin dose was recorded at the end of hospitalization only in the steroid treated group (Table 4). Nineteen patients in the steroid treated group were treated with glucocorticoids before hospitalization. Mean pre-admission steroid dose was $10 ± 7.5$ mg prednisone. Mean blood glucose levels during hospitalization in these 19 patients did not differ significantly compared with the remaining patients in the group who did not receive glucocorticoids before admission: $228 ± 48$ mg/dl ($12.7 ± 2.7$ mmol/l) vs. $212 ± 50.7$ ($11.8 ± 2.8$), $p = 0.3$. There was no difference in mean blood glucose levels among patients in the glucocorticoid-treated group, regardless of the type of steroid they received during hospitalization. Similarly, in both study groups, the type of long-acting insulin used did not affect mean blood glucose levels.

A significantly lower proportion of patients in the steroid treatment group were controlled with the basal-bolus treatment protocol, i.e. had less than three consecutive measurements of blood glucose > 200 mg/dl (11.1 mmol/l) (36% of patients in the steroid group vs. 61% in the control group, $p = 0.003$).

Discussion

We conducted a real-life study to assess the efficacy of glycemic control achieved with a basal-bolus insulin protocol in hospitalized patients with T2DM treated with glucocorticoids compared with patients who were not treated with glucocorticoids.

Many of the patients hospitalized in internal medicine wards have inflammatory or infectious diseases and elevated markers of tissue injury such as CRP. Previous studies have suggested that serum high sensitivity (hs)-CRP levels are higher in patients with T2DM with macrovascular complications [16]. A recent study has shown that patients with higher level of hs-CRP and high HbA1c levels have higher glycemic excursion [17]. Considering that patients treated with glucocorticoids have higher levels of inflammation and thus elevated CRP levels compared to patients who are not treated with glucocorticoids, we used elevated CRP levels as an inclusion criterion for patient analysis in this study as it allowed us to maintain patient homogeneity between two groups.

Approximately two-thirds of steroid-treated patients had inadequate glycemic control compared with only one-third of the control group patients, according to the

Table 2 Underlying conditions in the glucocorticoid group

Pulmonary	Rheumatology	Gastro	Other
COPD (14)	Still's disease (2)	IBD (4)	Acute pericarditis (1)
Pneumonia (18)	Polymyalgia rheumatica (1)		West- Nile Encephalitis (1)
Interstitial lung (2)	Giant cell arteritis (2)		Multiple sclerosis (2)
Lung carcinoma (2)	Behcet's disease (1)		Demyelinating disease (1)
	Gout (1)		Ig-a Nephropathy (1)
			Severe sepsis (8)

In parentheses () is the number of patients

Table 3 Blood glucose levels and insulin doses at 8 A.M., 12 noon, 5 P.M. and 8 P.M.

Hours	8 A.M.		12:00		5 P.M.		8 P.M.	
	Glucocorticoids	Control	Glucocorticoids	Control	Glucocorticoids	Control	Glucocorticoids	Control
BGL(mg/dl) mean ± SD	197.1 ± 52.8	184.8 ± 53.9	220.1 ± 61.1	212.9 ± 54.7	235.8 ± 61.9	183.5 ± 54.2	251.2 ± 74.6	198.3 ± 55.7
BGL mmol/l ± SD	10.9 ± 2.4	10.3 ± 3	12.2 ± 3.4	11.8 ± 3	13.1 ± 3.4	10.2 ± 3	13.9 ± 4.1	11 ± 3.1
p-value	0.16		0.45		<.0001		<.0001	
Insulin (units) mean ± SD	9.7 ± 3.9	9.86 ± 4.08	10.1 ± 4.3	10.2 ± 4.0	10.48 ± 3.9	9.9 ± 3.9	10.8 ± 5.4	18.7 ± 8.4
p-value	0.8		0.85		0.41		<.0001	

criteria arbitrarily defined for the present study. Specifically, the glucocorticoid-treated patients had higher blood glucose measurements in the afternoon and evening compared with the untreated patients. Insulin prandial doses were similar in the two groups. These findings are in agreement with those of Donihi et al. [12] who reported that excessive blood glucose levels occurred in two-thirds of hospitalized patients treated with steroids, and with those of Burt et al. [10] who found that patients treated with high-dose glucocorticoids had higher postprandial, afternoon and evening blood glucose levels and relatively mild elevations of morning glucose levels. Our findings are also in accordance with a recent study which found that the current basal-bolus insulin regimens were inadequate for controlling hyperglycemia in inpatients receiving prednisolone ≥10 mg/d [11].

Comparing the results obtained using the basal-bolus regimen with those of other reported treatment modalities suggest that the basal-bolus regimen is more effective for glycemic control. The regimen demonstrated better glycemic control and lower frequency of hospital complications compared to the sliding scale insulin regimen (SSI) for treatment of inpatients with diabetes, without increasing the number of severe hypoglycemic events [18, 19]. Gosmanov et al. [13] also found that the basal-bolus regimen is more effective than the SSI regimen for treating steroid-induced hyperglycemia, although the difference in insulin doses between the two groups (49 ± 29 units/day in the SSI group and 122 ± 39 units/day in the basal-bolus group) may have affected the results of their study. Two other studies [14, 20] compared the neutral protamine Hagedorn (NPH) insulin to glargine, both in a basal-bolus protocol, for treatment of steroid-induced hyperglycemia in hospitalized patients. Both agents were equally as effective as basal insulin for the management of these patients, and both groups experienced a similar number of hypoglycemic

episodes. Ruiz de Adana et al. [14] reported that patients in the glargine group spent 42% of their hospital stay within a glucose level target range compared to 38% in the NPH group.

In a recent randomized parallel-arm study comparing two different protocols for glucocorticoid-treated patients, only 54% of patients in the basal-bolus group had blood glucose levels within the target range compared to 62% of patients in the NPH group [15]. In our study 61% of patients in the control group versus 36% in glucocorticoid treated group were adequately controlled during hospitalization. It's clear that in the control group the main reason for insufficient control was inappropriate dose adjustment, but in the steroid treatment group more adjustments were performed during hospitalization however fewer patients achieved appropriate blood glucose control .

Considering that prednisone induced hyperglycemia takes place in the afternoon and evening, it seems reasonable to switch basal insulin glargine to insulin NPH and perform appropriate adjustments to short acting insulins. Nonetheless, several previous studies [14, 15, 20] failed to show significant improvement in glucose control using insulin NPH.

Although a significant proportion of patients hospitalized in internal medicine department are treated with steroids other than from prednisone, with different glycemic profiles, our results showed that glycemic control was not influenced by the type of steroid administered. Therefore, we think it wiser to treat all of these patients with a uniform protocol. In addition, we need to take into account that a significant proportion of patients with diabetes are treated with basal insulin on a permanent basis. In Israel insulin NPH is not used as basal insulin, so it seemed unwise to change their home insulin to insulin NPH without achieving a clear benefit in diabetes control. Patients treated with glucocorticoids have a

Table 4 Difference in dosage of insulin in first and last day of hospitalization in each the groups

	Insulin dose(units) mean ± SD in first day of hospitalization	Insulin dose(units) mean ± SD in last day of hospitalization	P-value
Steroid treated patients	39.3 ± 19.8 [36]	46.8 ± 21.7 [44]	0.0098
Untreated patients	42.5 ± 18.1 [40]	43.9 ± 18.9 [40]	0.13

distinct pattern of blood glucose distribution during the day (with elevation of blood glucose in the latter part of the day). This is in accordance with Burt's study [11] which found that blood glucose control was inadequate despite of higher insulin doses in glucocorticoid treated patients. Although we were not able to address this issue in this study we speculate that a different insulin protocol would be more effective in controlling glucocorticoid treated patients during hospitalization. The protocol we suggest includes less basal insulin and a higher ratio of prandial insulin at lunch and at supper (Fig. 4).

Study limitations

We conducted a retrospective real data study in order to evaluate the existing basal-bolus protocol in our institution and to assess its implementation. In addition to the inherent limitations due to its retrospective design, the main limitation of our study is in the failure of our

patients with diabetes on glucocorticoid treatment to achieve adequate glycemic control on the basal-bolus insulin protocol. A high proportion of patients in both groups were undertreated, according to the existing protocol. We attribute this to the inadequate insulin dosing adjustments done by junior doctors and nurses responsible for the treatment of each specific patient; thus, a substantial proportion of patients did not receive an appropriate insulin dose, essentially due to excessive caution taken to avoid hypoglycemia and inability to make appropriate fine tuning, especially of prandial dosing of insulin. On the other hand, the strength of our study lies in the collecting of data about real-world patient experience thus assisting in filling the knowledge gap between clinical trials and actual clinical practice, by adding to the understanding of how best to incorporate new therapies into everyday clinical practice. We hope that our study will help to guide changes in protocols to

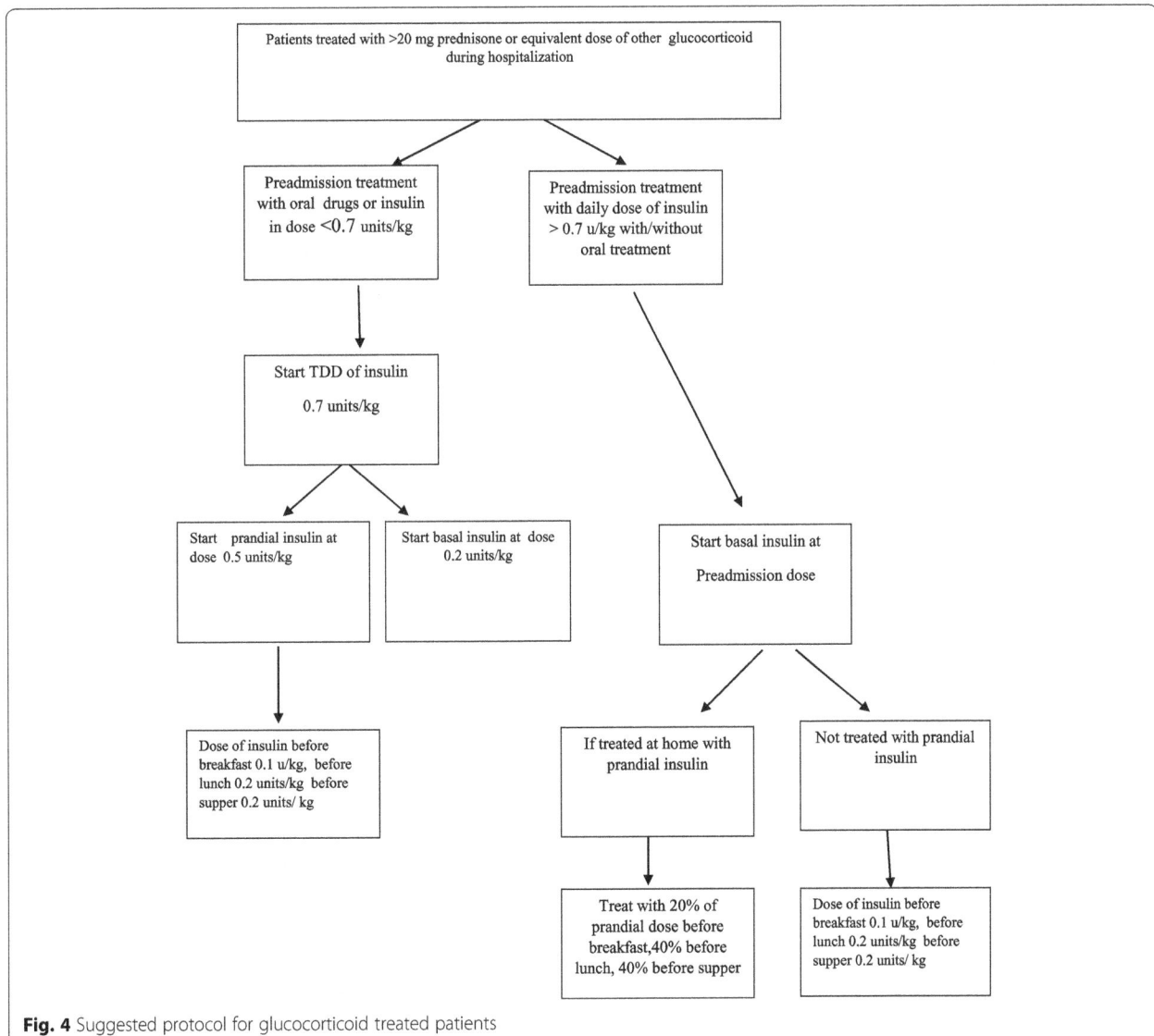

Fig. 4 Suggested protocol for glucocorticoid treated patients

achieve better glycemic control for inpatients receiving glucocorticoid treatment. Moreover, that this has the potential to improve the quality and delivery of medical care, reduce overall costs and improve outcomes.

Conclusion

Treatment of hyperglycemia in inpatients with T2DM receiving glucocorticoids remains challenging. Raising the awareness of medical staff about the appropriate use of insulin protocols during hospitalization and increasing the doses of short acting insulin in the afternoon and evening in glucocorticoid-treated patients with diabetes could optimize the inherent benefits of the basal-bolus protocol.

Abbreviations

CRP: C-reactive protein; HbA1C: Glycosylated hemoglobin A1C; NPH: Neutral protamine Hagedorn; SSI: Sliding scale insulin therapy; T2DM: Type 2 diabetes mellitus; TDD: Total daily dose

Acknowledgements

The authors wish to acknowledge Mrs. Snait Ayalon for helping to collect data from electronic charts. The authors express their gratitude to Ms. Dalia Dawn Orkin for her important English language contributions and professional editing services.

Authors' contributions

ECS designed and conceived the study and drafted the manuscript, HK participated in the study design and data collection, NS performed the statistical analysis, AI drafted and critically revised the manuscript. All authors read and approved the final manuscript.

Authors' information

All the authors are from the Emek Medical Center, a community 500-bed teaching hospital in Northern Israel, serving a population of 500,000 inhabitants. ECS, the corresponding author, is an Internal Medicine and Endocrinology Consultant physician, HK is a research assistant, NS is a biostatistician, AI is an Endocrinology Consultant physician and the Director of the Endocrinology Clinic.

Competing interests

The authors declare that they have no competing interests.

Author details

[1]Endocrinology Unit, Haemek Medical Center, Rabin Ave 21, Afula, Israel, 18134 Afula, Israel. [2]Statistics Department, Haemek Medical Center, Afula, Israel.

References

1. Umpierrez GE, Isaacs SD, Bazargan N, You X, Thaler LM, Kitabchi AE. Hyperglycemia: an independent marker of in hospital mortality in patients with undiagnosed diabetes. JCEM. 2002;87:978–82.
2. McAlister FA, Majumdar SR, Blitz S, Rowe BH, Romney J, Marrie TJ. The relation between hyperglycemia and outcomes in 2471 patients admitted to the hospital with community-acquired pneumonia. Diabetes Care. 2005; 28:810–5.
3. Saxena A, Anderson CS, Wang X, Sato S, Arima H, Chan E, et al. Prognostic significance of hyperglycemia in acute intracerebral hemorrhage: the INTERACT2 study. Stroke. 2016;47(3):682–8.
4. Van den Berghe G, Wouters PJ, Bouillon R, Weekers F, Verwaest C, Schetz M, et al. Outcome benefit of intensive insulin therapy in the critically ill: insulin dose versus glycemic control. Critical Care Med. 2003;31:359–66.
5. Frisch A, Chandra P, Smiley D, Peng L, Rizzo M, Gatcliffe C, et al. Prevalence and clinical outcome of hyperglycemia in the perioperative period in noncardiac surgery. Diabetes Care. 2010;33:1783–8.
6. American Diabetes Association. Standards of medical care in diabetes-2017. Diabetes Care. 2017;40(suppl. 1):S121.
7. Umpierrez GE, Hellman R, Korytkowski MT, Kosiborod M, Maynard GA, Montori VM, et al. Management of hyperglycemia in hospitalized patients in non -critical care setting. JCEM. 2012;97:16–38.
8. Clore JN, Thurby-Hay L. Glucocorticoid- induced hyperglycemia. Endocr Pract. 2009;15:469–71.
9. Kwon S, Hermayer KL. Glucocorticoid- induced hyperglycemia. Am J Med Sci. 2013;345:274–7.
10. Burt MG, Roberts GW, Aguilar-Loza NR, Frith P, Stranks SN. Continuous monitoring of circadian glycemic patterns in patients receiving prednisolone for COPD. J Endocr Metab. 2011;96:1789–96.
11. Burt MG, Drake SM, Aguilar-Loza NR, Esterman A, Stranks SN, Roberts GW. Efficacy of a basal bolus insulin protocol to treat prednisolone-inducedhyperglycaemia in hospitalised patients. J Intern Med. 2015;45:261–6.
12. Donihi AC, Raval D, Saul M, Korytkowski MT, DeVita MA. Prevalence andpredictors of corticosteroid-related hyperglycemia in hospitalized patients. Endocr Pract. 2006;12:358–62.
13. Gosmanov AR, Goorha S, Stelts S, Peng L, Umpierrez GE. Management of hyperglycemia in diabetic patients with hematologic malignancies during dexamethasone therapy. Endocr Pract. 2013;19:231–5.
14. Ruiz de Adana MS, Colomo N, Maldonado-Araque C, Fontalba MI, Linares F, García-Torres F, et al. Randomized clinical trial of the efficacy and safety of insulin glargine vs. NPH insulin as basal insulin for the treatment of glucocorticoid induced hyperglycemia using continuous glucose monitoring in hospitalized patients with type 2 diabetes and respiratory disease. Diabet Res Clin Practice. 2015;110:158–65.
15. Grommesh B, Lausch MJ, Vannelli AJ. Hospital insulin protocol aims for glucose control in glucocorticoid–induced hyperglycemia. Endocr Pract. 2016;22:180–9.
16. Misra DP, Das S, Sahu PK. Prevalence of inflammatory markers (high-sensitivity C-reactive protein, nuclear factor-κB and adiponectin) in Indian patients with type 2 diabetes mellitus with and without macrovascular complications. Metab Syndr Relat Disord. 2012;10:209–13.
17. Shi CH, Wang C, Bai R, Zhang XY, Men LL, Du JL. Associations among glycemic excursions, glycated hemoglobin and high-sensitivity C-reactive protein in patients with poorly controlled type 2 diabetes mellitus. Exp Ther Med. 2015;10:1937–42.
18. Umpierrez GE, Smiley D, Zisman A, Prieto LM, Palacio A, Ceron M, et al. Randomized study of basal-bolus insulin therapy in the inpatient management of patients with type 2 diabetes (RABBIT 2 trial). Diabetes Care. 2007;30:2181–6.
19. Umpierrez GE, Smiley D, Jacobs S, Peng L, Temponi A, Mulligan P, et al. Randomized study of basal-bolus insulin therapy in the inpatient management of patients with type 2 diabetes undergoing general surgery (RABBIT 2 surgery). Diabetes Care. 2011;34:256–61.
20. Dhital SM, Shenker Y, Meredith M, Davis DB. A retrospective study comparing neutral protamine hagedorn insulin with glargine as basal therapy in prednisone-associated diabetes mellitus in hospitalized patients. Endocr Pract. 2012;18:712–9.

20

Effect of imatinib on plasma glucose concentration in subjects with chronic myeloid leukemia and gastrointestinal stromal tumor

Miguel Ángel Gómez-Sámano[1], Jorge Enrique Baquerizo-Burgos[2], Melissa Fabiola Coronel Coronel[2], Buileng Daniela Wong-Campoverde[2], Fernando Villanueva-Martinez[3], Diego Molina-Botello[4], Jose Alonso Avila-Rojo[5], Lucía Palacios-Báez[1], Daniel Cuevas-Ramos[1], Francisco Javier Gomez-Perez[1], Alejandro Zentella-Dehesa[6], Álvaro Aguayo-González[7] and Alfonso Gulias-Herrero[8*]

Abstract

Background: Type 2 diabetes mellitus has become one of the most important public health concerns worldwide. Due to its high prevalence and morbidity, there is an avid necessity to find new therapies that slow the progression and promote the regression of the disease. Imatinib mesylate is a tyrosine kinase inhibitor that binds to the Abelson tyrosine kinase and related proteins. It enhances β-cell survival in response to toxins and pro-inflammatory cytokine. The aim of this study is to evaluate the effect of imatinib on fasting plasma glucose in subjects with normal fasting glucose, subjects with impaired fasting glucose and in subjects with type 2 diabetes mellitus.

Methods: We identified 284 subjects diagnosed with chronic myeloid leukemia or gastrointestinal stromal tumors from the Instituto Nacional de Ciencias Medicas y Nutricion Salvador Zubiran database. 106/284 subjects were treated with imatinib. We compared the effect of imatinib on fasting plasma glucose after 1 and 6 months of treatment. We used ANOVA test of repeated samples to determine statistical significance in fasting plasma glucose before imatinib treatment and the follow-up. Statistical analysis was performed with Statistical Package for the Social Sciences v22.

Results: We included a total of 106 subjects: 76 with fasting plasma glucose concentrations < 100 mg/dL (normal FG), 19 subjects with fasting plasma glucose concentrations ≥100 mg/dL (impaired fasting glucose), and 11 subjects with ≥126 mg/dL (type 2 diabetes mellitus). We found a significant increase in fasting plasma glucose concentration in the normal fasting glucose group ($p = 0.048$), and a significant decrease in fasting plasma glucose concentration in the type 2 diabetes mellitus group ($p = 0.042$). In the impaired fasting glucose group, we also found a tendency towards a decrease in fasting plasma glucose ($p = 0.076$). We identified 11 subjects with type 2 diabetes mellitus, of whom, 7 (64%) had a reduction in their fasting plasma glucose concentrations after 6 months. A significant glycosylated hemoglobin reduction ($p = 0.04$) was observed.

Conclusion: Subjects with chronic myeloid leukemia or gastrointestinal stromal tumor with type 2 diabetes mellitus had a significant reduction in fasting plasma glucose and glycosylated hemoglobin at 1 and 6 months while using imatinib.

Keywords: Imatinib, Fasting plasma glucose concentrations, Chronic myeloid leukemia, Gastrointestinal stromal tumor, Type 2 diabetes mellitus

* Correspondence: alfonso.tiranicida@gmail.com
[8]Department of Internal Medicine, Instituto Nacional de Ciencias Medicas y Nutricion Salvador Zubiran, Vasco de Quiroga #15, Sección XVI Tlalpan, 14000 Mexico City, Mexico
Full list of author information is available at the end of the article

Background

Type 2 diabetes mellitus (T2DM) has become one of the most important public health concerns worldwide, reaching epidemic proportions. Currently, T2DM affects over 425 million people and is estimated that the number of cases will reach 629 million by 2045 [1]. Due to its high prevalence and morbidity, there is a necessity to find new therapies that slow the progression and promote the regression of the disease. Previous publications have shown an improvement of glucose metabolism with the use of imatinib in diabetic subjects with chronic myeloid leukemia (CML) and gastrointestinal stromal tumors (GIST) [2, 3].

Imatinib mesylate is a tyrosine kinase inhibitor (TKI) that binds to the Abelson tyrosine kinase (c-Abl) and related proteins. It became the very first molecular inhibitor drug to be clinically approved [4]. Also, it inhibits the platelet-derived growth factor receptor (PDGFR) and transmembrane stem-cell factor receptor (c-Kit) [5, 6], as well as it enhances β-cell survival in response to toxins and pro-inflammatory cytokines [7, 8].

The aim of this study is to evaluate the effect of imatinib on fasting plasma glucose (FPG) concentrations in subjects with CML and GIST, classified by their FPG status: normal fasting glucose (normal FG) compared to subjects with impaired fasting glucose (IFG) and subjects with T2DM. Our hypothesis is that subjects with IFG or T2DM will show an improvement in fasting glucose concentrations.

Methods

This is a retrospective cohort study that included subjects with a diagnosis of CML or GIST that received treatment with imatinib from January 2000 to October 2016. The study was submitted and approved by the Instituto Nacional de Ciencias Medicas y Nutricion Salvador Zubiran Comite de etica en Investigacion/Comite de investigacion on July 11th, 2016.

Study population

We identified 284 Hispanic subjects diagnosed with CML and GIST from the Instituto Nacional de Ciencias Medicas y Nutricion Salvador Zubiran (INCMNSZ) database. Of these, 106 were treated with imatinib. We selected subjects aged 18 years and older. We excluded subjects who did not have enough data, such as 1-month follow-up, FPG, triglycerides (Tg), low-density lipoprotein (LDL), high-density lipoprotein (HDL), and subjects treated with imatinib in another hospital (Fig. 1).

Three study groups were formed depending on their FPG concentrations: subjects with FPG < 100 mg/dL, subjects with FPG ≥100 to < 126 mg/dL (IFG), and FPG ≥ 126 mg/dL (T2DM). Data were collected following the next criteria:

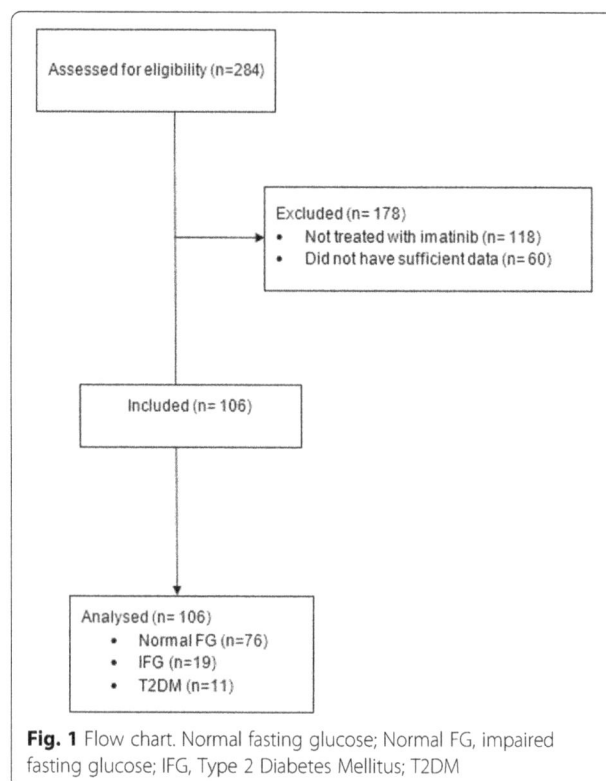

Fig. 1 Flow chart. Normal fasting glucose; Normal FG, impaired fasting glucose; IFG, Type 2 Diabetes Mellitus; T2DM

- Basal information was collected with a maximum period of 3 months prior to the treatment with imatinib.
- 1-month follow-up: information was collected with a period of ±2 weeks of completing 1 month of treatment with imatinib.
- 6-month follow-up: information was collected with a period of ±1 month of completing 6 months of treatment with imatinib.

Biochemical and anthropometric measurements

We reviewed subject charts to retrieve laboratory data from the central laboratory of INCMNSZ, including fasting glucose, HbA1c, total cholesterol, LDL, HDL, triglycerides (Tg), alanine aminotransferase (ALT), magnesium (Mg), and creatinine. The measurements were carried out with commercially available standardized methods. In addition, other variables obtained from the subjects were age, sex, weight, and treatment for diabetes or other conditions.

Statistical analysis

Normally distributed data are expressed as the mean and standard deviation (±SD), whereas variables with a skewed distribution are reported as median (interquartile range). In addition, we used the Kruskal-Wallis test to determine the statistical significance between the FPG concentrations before treatment and at 1 and 6 months follow-up among the three study groups. Mauchly's sphericity test was used to evaluate equality and homogeneity of the studied population, and Greenhouse-Geisser test to obtain the p-value to determine if the changes of FPG were statistically and clinically significant. Data were analyzed with Statistical Package for the Social Sciences (SPSS) v22.

Results

We included a total of 106 subjects that received imatinib for 6 months: 76 with normal fasting glucose concentrations < 100 mg/dL (normal FG), 19 subjects with glucose concentrations ≥100 to < 126 mg/dL (IFG), and 11 subjects with glucose concentrations ≥126 mg/dL (T2DM). Baseline characteristics of the studied subjects are shown in Table 1. Characteristics of subjects according to their FPG concentrations are shown in Table 2, there were significant differences in age ($p = 0.023$) and ALT concentration after 1 month of treatment with Imatinib ($p = 0.008$). The comparison of mean FPG concentration variations through time in each group are presented in Table 3. We analyzed the sphericity of the mean FPG within each group with the Mauchly's sphericity test and found a $p = 0.960$ in the normal FG group, a $p = 0.184$ in the IFG group, and a $p = 0.702$ in the T2DM group. Due to these values, we corrected the significance with the Greenhouse-Geisser test. We found a significant increase in FPG concentration in the normal FG group, before (87.6 ± 8.3), after 1 month (93.6 ± 7.6), and after 6 months (93.4 ± 10.5), $p = 0.048$; and a statistically significant decrease in FPG concentration in the T2DM group, before (241 ± 120.7), after 1 month (152.7 ± 74.5), and after 6 months (128.6 ± 33.9), $p = 0.042$. In the IFG group, there is also a decrease in FPG concentration, at baseline (121 ± 28.7), after 1 month (97.3 ± 12.8), and after 6 months (96.1 ± 7.3), $p = 0.076$. The latter result

Table 1 Baseline characteristics of the studied subjects ($n = 106$)

Variable	Value
Sex (male: %)	52.5
CML (%)	81.8
GIST (%)	18.2
Age (years)	40.2 ± 16.7
Weight (kg)	68.3 ± 14.4
Overweight (%)	47.7
IFG (%)	17.9
DM2 (%)	10.4
Creatinine (mg/dL)	0.93 (0.68–1.0)
ALT (U/L)	28.3 (14.2–31.0)
Mg (mg/dL)	2.1 ± 0.26
Glucose (mg/dL)	109 (86–104.5)

Variables with normal distribution are expressed as mean ± s.d. Variables with non-parametric distribution are expressed as median (interquartile range). *CML* chronic myeloid leukemia, *GIST* gastrointestinal stromal tumor, *IFG* impaired fasting glucose, *ALT* alanine aminotransferase, *Mg* magnesium

shows imatinib's tendency to decrease FPG concentration, even though is not statistically significant. These results are represented in Fig. 2, where we can observe an important reduction of FPG concentration in the group with T2DM and IFG; having a decrease in concentrations at one-month follow-up, and 6-month follow-up. On the other hand, we can observe that the normal FG group had a small, yet significant increase in the FPG concentrations. Also, we decided to compare all patients with normal fasting glucose against IFG plus T2DM, in the first group we obtained a $p = 0.059$ and in the second group a significant p value = 0.034. These results are shown in Additional file 1: Table S1 and Additional file 2: Figure S1.

We identified 11 subjects with T2DM, which are represented in Table 4, from the INCMNSZ database. As shown in the table, two subjects (18.2%) had an increase in FPG concentration after 1 month of treatment with imatinib, one did not have sufficient follow-up data, and the remaining (72.7%) decreased their FPG concentration. According to the FPG concentration after 6 months of treatment, one subject (9.1%) had an elevation, seven decreased their glucose concentrations (63.6%), and three did not have sufficient data. HbA1c decreased from 7.48 (±1.82) to 6.2 (±0.57), with a significant reduction at 6 months after imatinib treatment ($p = 0.04$). Finally, according to the hypoglycemic treatment, four subjects (36.4%) stayed with the same treatment, two (18.2%) reduced the doses, one (9.1%) stopped taking metformin, one (9.1%) increased doses, another one (9.1%) started using insulin, and the last two subjects did not have sufficient follow-up data after 6 months of imatinib administration. With these results, we can observe that most subjects did have a reduction in the FPG concentration at 1-month follow-up (72.7%) and 6-month follow-up (63.6%), indicating a benefit of imatinib on glucose metabolism. In Table 5 we depict the studies assessing the effect of imatinib on glucose metabolism in subjects with T2DM.

Discussion

We observed that imatinib reduced the FPG and HbA1c concentration in subjects with T2DM. However, due to the design of our study, we cannot establish a real therapeutic effect of imatinib in subjects with T2DM. As described previously, only three of the eleven subjects with T2DM reduced their hypoglycemic therapy, but four remained with the same anti-diabetic treatment. HbA1c reduction indicates that FG was reduced, especially in subjects with high-starting HbA1c values; as in most diabetes clinical trials the magnitude of improvement in HbA1c is related to baseline A1c, the higher the A1c the greater the drop, so when A1c is normal you cannot expect a lot of improvement.

Table 2 Characteristics of subjects according to fasting glucose

Variable	Subjects with fasting glucose < 100 mg/dL (n = 76)	Subjects with fasting glucose ≥100 mg/dL and < 126 mg/dL (n = 19)	Subjects with T2DM (n = 11)	p
Sex (male: n, %)	41, 53.9	9, 47.4	5, 45.5	0.721
Cigarette (yes: n, %)	22, 28.9	4, 26.7	3, 30	0.663
CML (n, %)	59, 80.8	13, 72.2	10, 90.9	0.747
GIST (n, %)	14, 18.4	5, 27.8	1, 9.1	
Age (years)	38.6 ± 15.7	41.8 ± 16.8	53 ± 14.2	0.023
Weight (kg)	70.5 ± 15.1	64.2 ± 14.4	65.3 ± 10.7	0.486
Weight (after 1 month, kg)	69.6 ± 14.9	63.7 ± 12.6	74.4 ± 27.5	0.645
Weight (after 6 months, kg)	74.9 ± 16.6	78.5 ± 10	61.6 ± 7.5	0.127
Mg (mg/dL)	2.2 ± 0.25	2 ± 0.20	2.1 ± 0.38	0.098
Mg (after 1 month, mg/dL)	2 ± 0.6	1.9 ± 0.18	2.25 ± 0.21	0.343
Creatinine (before, mg/dL)	0.90 (0.68–1)	1.02 (0.62–1.13)	1.02 (0.75–1.12)	0.260
Creatinine (after 1 month, mg/dL)	0.81 (0.70–0.90)	0.94 (0.68–1.05)	0.90 (0.60–1.10)	0.549
Creatinine (after 6 months, mg/dL)	0.86 (0.73–0.99)	0.84 (0.58–1.06)	0.84 (0.73–0.98)	0.239
ALT (before, U/L)	23.6 (14–26.5)	45.8 (14.2–48.2)	31 (17–48.5)	0.293
ALT (after 1 month, U/L)	24.9 (15–30)	51.3 (19–54.7)	17.8 (13–23.5)	0.008
ALT (after 6 months, U/L)	22.3 (17–26)	23.4 (20–27.5)	16. 5 (15.2–17.7)	0.106

p value was obtained with Kruskal-Wallis or chi-square test

CML chronic myeloid leukemia, GIST gastrointestinal stromal tumor, IFG impaired fasting glucose, Mg magnesium, ALT alanine aminotransferase

Imatinib inhibits the phosphorylation of proteins which may result in better signaling, better function of effectors, or both, with improvement in insulin sensitivity; thus, decreasing HbA1c levels in patients with high-starting values. Therefore, we can assume there is a therapeutic benefit in patients with T2DM. We cannot attribute this effect entirely to the imatinib treatment, but data in our study suggests there is a relationship between its administration and the lowering of FPG concentration.

Due to our study population, formed by Hispanic subjects with cancer, many confounding factors can alter the results. Nausea, vomiting, weight loss, hydroxyurea, and redistribution of adipose tissue [9] could influence glucose metabolism and insulin resistance. Even though there are animal trials that confirm the effect of imatinib on insulin resistance and glucose metabolism, these confounding variables need to be evaluated in prospective studies. We could not assess the effect after discontinuing therapy as Agostino et al. [2].

Ethnicity could affect imatinib's treatment response. Several studies compared the difference of imatinib therapy response between different ethnic groups, but few studies have enough Hispanic subjects to compare against other ethnic groups. Lee et al. performed a study with more Hispanic subjects with CML compared to non-Hispanics [60.9% vs 39.1%, respectively], and concluded that Hispanic subjects achieved better treatment responses to imatinib when compared to non-Hispanic subjects [10].

We reviewed the pathophysiology of T2DM and several animal and human studies that aimed to establish the mechanism by which imatinib lowers FPG concentration. T2DM derives from the abnormal metabolism of carbohydrates, fats, and proteins which leads to hyperglycemia and hyperlipidemia. Within time, high levels of glucose and lipids induce changes in the metabolic pathways of insulin causing impaired insulin secretion from the β-cells of pancreatic islets, insulin resistance and decreased glucose use in peripheral

Table 3 Repeated measures ANOVA

	Glucose before	Glucose after 1 month	Glucose after 6 months	Mauchly's sphericity test	Greenhouse-Geisser p value
Subjects with fasting glucose < 100 mg/dL (n = 76)	87.6 ± 8.3	93.6 ± 7.6	93.4 ± 10.5	0.960	0.048
Subjects with fasting glucose ≥100 mg/dL (n = 19)	121 ± 28.7	97. 3 ± 12.8	96. 1 ± 7.3	0.184	0.076
Subjects with T2DM (n = 11)	241 ± 120.7	152.5 ± 74.5	128.6 ± 33.9	0.702	0.042

Database was analyzed through the ANOVA test of repeated samples to determine the statistical significance between normal FG, IFG and T2DM subjects before treatment and at 1 and 6 months follow-up. The Mauchly's sphericity test was used to evaluate equality and homogeneity of the studied population, and the p value was obtained through the Greenhouse-Geisser test

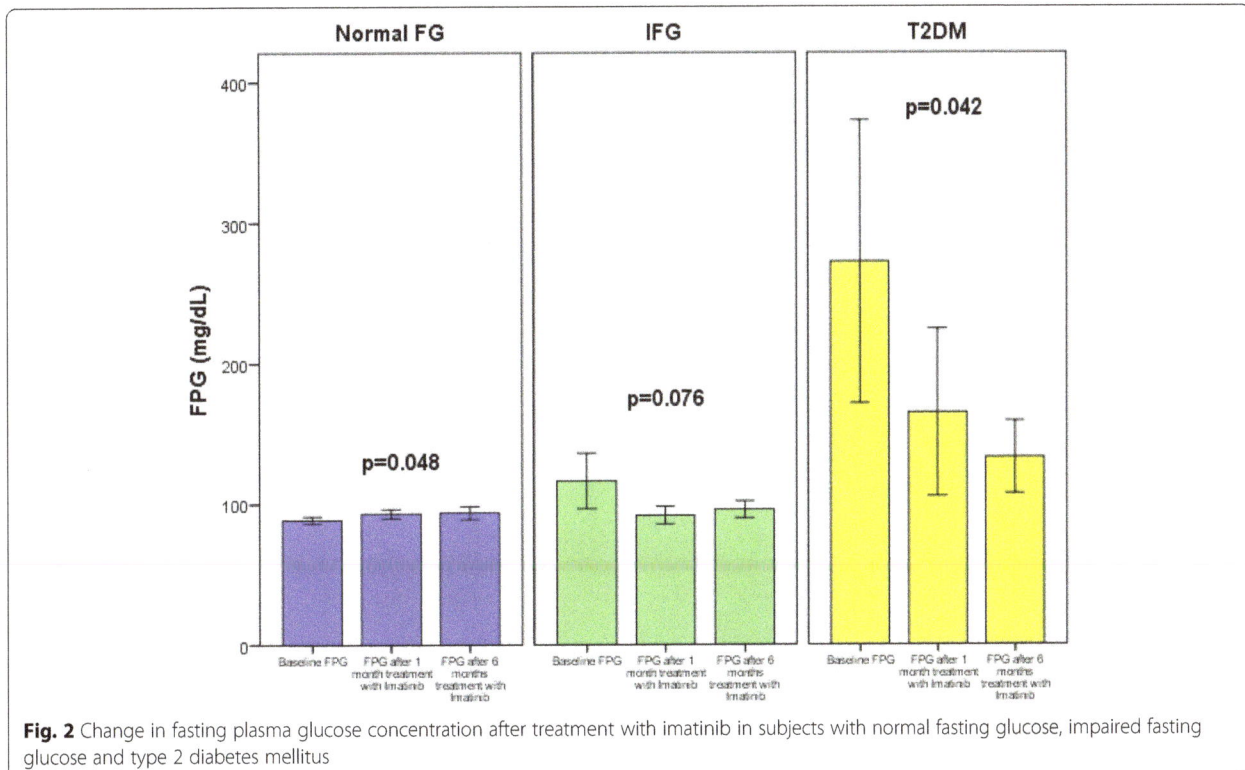

Fig. 2 Change in fasting plasma glucose concentration after treatment with imatinib in subjects with normal fasting glucose, impaired fasting glucose and type 2 diabetes mellitus

tissues, and abnormal hepatic glucose production. Imatinib has shown to interfere in these pathways [11].

Mice models with type 1 diabetes mellitus (T1DM) and T2DM treated with TKIs have shown beneficial effects, improving several aspects of the disease. A study by Louvet et al. reported non-obese diabetic mice with new-onset T1DM experienced the regression of the disease when treated with imatinib [7]. Additionally, Chang Qing et al. established that there is an increase in the production of insulin in residual β-cells, with or without glucose stimulation, through an indirect control of the genetic expression of insulin in response to glucose, and through the promotion of the expression of glucose transporter-2 (GLUT-2) in β-cells [12]. Furthermore, it has been proven that TKIs prevent β-cell apoptosis via activation of antiapoptotic nuclear factor kappa-light-chain-enhancer of activated B cells (NF-Kb) and/or inhibition of the proapoptotic mitogen-activated protein kinase/c-jun N-terminal kinase (MAPK/JNK) [13, 14]. Moreover, Wijesekara et al. found that adiponectin promotes the phosphorylation of the protein kinase B (Akt/pkB) and the extracellular signal-regulated kinase (ERK) which leads to protection against apoptosis and stimulation of gene expression and secretion in pancreatic beta cells [15]. It has been proven that adiponectin concentration rises three times in plasma after three months of treatment with imatinib [16].

The hypoglycemic effect of this drug might be due to the inhibition of the multiple tyrosine kinases, such as c-Abl [12], PDGFR, Akt/pkB [4], and the extracellular regulatory kinases ERK1 and ERK2 which are crucial to the control and signaling activity of cellular effectors in the insulin pathway [17]. Phosphorylation of ERK by imatinib could result in better signaling, better functioning of the effectors or both [18], and it could also have an antiapoptotic effect [17]. In addition, inhibition of vascular endothelial growth factor receptor 2 (VEGFR2) reduces the degree of islet cell inflammation (insulitis) [19]. Likewise, the tyrosine phosphorylation of insulin receptor and phosphorylation of Akt/pkB after insulin administration was dose-dependent [20]. It is noteworthy that c-kit inhibition is not required for the reversal of hyperglycemia [5]. Markers of endoplasmic reticulum (ER) stress, protein kinase RNA-like endoplasmic reticulum kinase (PERK), eukaryotic initiation factor 2α (eIF2α), phosphorylated tribbles homolog 3 protein (TRB3), C/EBP homologous protein (CHOP), and phosphorylated JNK, decreased with imatinib [21].

Several case reports and retrospective human studies have been published assessing the effect of imatinib on glucose metabolism. Salalori et al. reported a subject with T1DM with the translocation-ets-leukemia/platelet-derived growth factor receptor β (TEL/PDGFRβ) rearrangement mutation and symptomatic hypoglycemia that had a reduction in the insulin dosage after treatment with imatinib

Table 4 Subjects with type 2 diabetes

Subjects	1	2	3	4	5	6	7	8	9	10	11
Baseline Glucose	117	173	323	321	113	110	254	261	137	386	457
Glucose after 1 month	51	187	137	135	133	106	–	186	118	334	138
Glucose after 6 months	–	164	167	158	–	107	97	–	143	116	77
HbA1c before	8.6	10	8.8	14.6	6	6.5	12.1	–	6.3	8.6	–
HbA1c after 1 month	–	–	5.2	7.5	–	–	–	11	6	6.7	–
HbA1c after 6 months	–	7.1	6.2	7.6	–	6.3	6	–	5.7	7.6	5.7
Treatment before	Glyburide 5 mg TID Metformin 500 mg TID	Metformin 500 mg TID Glyburide 5 – 2.5	Metformin / glyburide 500 mg/5 mg TID	Glyburide 5 mg BID Metformin 850 mg QD	Metformin 500 mg QD	Metformin 500 mg QD	Glyburide 5 mg TID Metformin 850 TID	Insulin Glargine 30 U QD Metformin 850 mg QD	Metformin / glyburide 500 mg/5 mg half dose TID	NPH 45–0–20 Lispro 10–10–2	Glyburide 5 mg TID Metformin 850 mg TID
Treatment after 6 months	Stayed the same	Metformin 500 mg TID Glyburide 5 mg TID	Metformin /glyburide 500 mg/5 mg BID	Stayed the same	–	Stayed the same	NPH insulin 25 U QD Metformin 850 mg TID	–	Stayed the same	NPH 25–0–20 Lispro 10–10–3	Suspended Metformin Glyburide 5 mg TID

HbA1c Glycated hemoglobin, TID three times a day, BID two times a day, QD once a day, NPH neutral protamine Hagedom

Table 5 Studies assessing effect of imatinib on glucose metabolism of subjects with T2DM

Author	Year	N	Effect	Reference
Agostino et al.	2011	17	47% of the subjects could discontinue their medications. All the subjects had a reduction in FPG.	[2]
Breccia et al.	2004	7	85.7% of the subjects reduced FPG concentration allowing dose decrease of oral hypoglycemic agents.	[3]
Iurlo et al.[a]	2015	27	Improve FPG levels and reduction of the dosage of antihyperglycemic drugs.	[22]
Dingli et al. [b]	2007	7	There was no reduction of FG, HbA1c or antidiabetic treatment in any of the patients.	[9]

FPG fasting plasma glucose
[a]In this study, the authors did not separate subjects with IFG and T2DM
[b]Two patients of the group with normal fasting glucose developed diabetes during the treatment with imatinib

[22]. Breccia et al. performed a study of 7 diabetic subjects with CML treated with imatinib, 6 showed improvements in fasting glucose concentrations, allowing a dose decrease of oral hypoglycemic agents and insulin. Before starting imatinib, they had a mean glucose of 220 mg/dL, after 3 months of treatment the mean FPG concentration was 110 mg/dL and after 12 months 108 mg/dL. The subject who was resistant to imatinib had also a decrease in FPG concentrations [3]. A similar study by Agostino et al. analyzed the effect of multiple TKIs in glucose metabolism, and a subgroup of diabetic subjects (8 of 17, 47%) could discontinue their medications, including insulin in some of them. The mean FPG decreased in all individuals associated with treatment with TKI [2]. Additionally, other case series not only found beneficial effects of imatinib on FPG concentrations, but also in the lipid profile, lowering total, high-density lipoprotein (HDL), and low-density lipoprotein (LDL) cholesterol concentrations [16, 23]. It has been proven that imatinib's effect on glucose concentrations is stable after the end of treatment in comparison with dasatinib, which also lowered glucose concentrations [23, 24]. It is important to recall that this study has the biggest number of subjects, compared with others with the same topic.

For future studies in this topic, it would be very important to adjust the effect of imatinib on glucose metabolism for important confounders such as weight changes.

Conclusion

We conclude that subjects with CML or GIST with T2DM had a statistically and clinically reduction in mean FPG and HbA1c at 1 and 6 months of imatinib therapy. Clinicians should consider the hypoglycemic effect of this drug when treating CML or GIST subjects with T2DM, and investigations on this drug need to continue to discover its potential use in diabetes therapy.

Acknowledgements
MAGS would like to acknowledge Luz del Carmen Abascal-Olascoaga for her support.

Funding
This research received no specific grant from any funding agency in the public, commercial, or not-for-profit sectors.

Authors' contribution
MAGS, JEBB, MCC, BDWC, FVM, DMB, JAAR, LPB, DCR, FJGP, AZD, AAG, and AGH recollected the patients' information from the hospital database. MAGS and DCR made the statistical analysis, MAGS, JEBB, MCC, BDWC, FVM, DMB, JAAR, LPB, DCR, FJGP, AZD, AAG, and AGH interpreted the results obtained from the statistical analysis. All authors read and approved the final manuscript.

Competing interest
The authors declare that they have no competing interests.

Author details
[1]Department of Endocrinology and Metabolism, Instituto Nacional de Ciencias Medicas y Nutricion Salvador Zubiran, Vasco de Quiroga #15, Sección XVI Tlalpan, 14000 Mexico City, Mexico. [2]Universidad Catolica de Santiago de Guayaquil, Av. Carlos Julio Arosemena Km. 1½ vía Daule, Guayaquil, Ecuador. [3]Department of Internal Medicine, Hospital San Angel Inn, Av Chapultepec 489, Juárez, 06600 Mexico City, Mexico. [4]Universidad Anahuac Mexico Sur, Av. de las Torres No. 131, Alvaro Obregon, Olivar de los padres, 01780 Mexico City, Mexico. [5]Universidad Autonoma de Baja California, Campus Mexicali, Av. Alvaro Obregon y Julian Carrillo S/N, Colonia Nueva, 21100 Mexicali, B.C, Mexico. [6]Department of Biochemistry, Instituto Nacional de Ciencias Medicas y Nutricion Salvador Zubiran, Vasco de Quiroga #15, Sección XVI Tlalpan, 14000 Mexico City, Mexico. [7]Department of Hematology, Instituto Nacional de Ciencias Medicas y Nutricion Salvador Zubiran, Vasco de Quiroga #15, Sección XVI Tlalpan, 14000 Mexico City, Mexico. [8]Department of Internal Medicine, Instituto Nacional de Ciencias Medicas y Nutricion Salvador Zubiran, Vasco de Quiroga #15, Sección XVI Tlalpan, 14000 Mexico City, Mexico.

References
1. International Diabetes Federation. IDF Diabetes Atlas. 8th ed. Brussels: International Diabetes Federation; 2017. http://www.diabetesatlas.org
2. Agostino NM, Chinchilli VM, Lynch CJ, Koszyk-Szewczyk A, Gingrich R, Sivik J, et al. Effect of the tyrosine kinase inhibitors (sunitinib, sorafenib, dasatinib, and imatinib) on blood glucose levels in diabetic and nondiabetic patients in general clinical practice. J Oncol Pharm Pract. 2011;17:197–202. https://doi.org/10.1177/1078155210378913.
3. Breccia M, Muscaritoli M, Aversa Z, Mandelli F, Alimena G. Imatinib mesylate may improve fasting blood glucose in diabetic Ph+ chronic myelogenous leukemia patients responsive to treatment. J Clin Oncol. 2004;22:4653–5. https://doi.org/10.1200/JCO.2004.04.217.
4. Mokhtari D, Welsh N. Potential utility of small tyrosine kinase inhibitors in the treatment of diabetes. Clin Sci (Lond). 2010;118:241–7.
5. Lau J, Zhou Q, Sutton SE, Herman AE, Schmedt C, Glynne R. Inhibition of c-kit is not required for reversal of hyperglycemia by imatinib in NOD mice. PLoS One. 2014;9:1–5.
6. Tuveson DA, Willis NA, Jacks T, Griffin JD, Singer S, Fletcher CD, et al. STI571 inactivation of the gastrointestinal stromal tumor c-KIT oncoprotein: biological and clinical implications. Oncogene. 2001;20: 5054–8. https://doi.org/10.1038/sj.onc.1204704.
7. Louvet C, Szot GL, Lang J, Lee MR, Martinier N, Bollag G, et al. Tyrosine kinase inhibitors reverse type 1 diabetes in nonobese diabetic mice. Proc Natl Acad Sci U S A. 2008;105:18895–900. https://doi.org/10.1073/pnas.0810246105.

8. Hägerkvist R, Sandler S, Mokhtari D, Welsh N. Amelioration of diabetes by imatinib mesylate (Gleevec): role of beta-cell NF-kappaB activation and anti-apoptotic preconditioning. FASEB J. 2007;21:618–28. https://doi.org/10.1096/fj.06-6910com.

9. Dingli D, Wolf RC, Vella A. Imatinib and type 2 diabetes. Endocr Pract. 2007; 13:126–30.

10. Lee JP, Birnstein E, Masiello D, Yang D, Yang AS. Gender and ethnic differences in chronic myelogenous leukemia prognosis and treatment response: a single-institution retrospective study. J Hematol Oncol. 2009;2:30.

11. Akash MSH, Rehman K, Chen S. Role of inflammatory mechanisms in pathogenesis of type 2 diabetes mellitus. J Cell Biochem. 2013;114:525–31.

12. Xia CQ, Zhang P, Li S, Yuan L, Xia T, Xie C, et al. C-Abl inhibitor imatinib enhances insulin production by β cells: C-Abl negatively regulates insulin production via interfering with the expression of NKx2.2 and GLUT-2. PLoS One. 2014;9:1–11.

13. Wolf AM, Wolf D, Rumpold H, Ludwiczek S, Enrich B, Gastl G, et al. The kinase inhibitor imatinib mesylate inhibits TNF-α production in vitro and prevents TNF-dependent acute hepatic inflammation. Proc Natl Acad Sci U S A. 2005;102:13622–7.

14. Hägerkvist R, Makeeva N, Elliman S, Welsh N. Imatinib mesylate (Gleevec) protects against streptozotocin-induced diabetes and islet cell death in vitro. Cell Biol Int. 2006;30:1013–7. https://doi.org/10.1016/j.cellbi.2006.08.006.

15. Wijesekara N, Krishnamurthy M, Bhattacharjee A, Suhail A, Sweeney J, Wheeler MB. Adiponectin-induced ERK and Akt phosphorylation protects against pancreatic beta cell apoptosis and increases insulin gene expression and secretion. J Biol Chem. 2010;285:33623–31. https://doi.org/10.1074/jbc.M109.085084.

16. Fitter S, Vandyke K, Schultz CG, White D, Hughes TP, Zannettino ACW. Plasma adiponectin levels are markedly elevated in imatinib-treated chronic myeloid leukemia (CML) patients: a mechanism for improved insulin sensitivity in type 2 diabetic CML patients? J Clin Endocrinol Metab. 2010;95: 3763–7. https://doi.org/10.1210/jc.2010-0086.

17. Fred RG, Boddeti SK, Lundberg M, Welsh N. Imatinib mesylate stimulates low-density lipoprotein receptor-related protein 1-mediated ERK phosphorylation in insulin-producing cells. Clin Sci (Lond). 2015;128:17–28. https://doi.org/10.1042/CS20130560.

18. Mokhtari D, Al-Amin A, Turpaev K, Li T, Idevall-Hagren O, Li J, et al. Imatinib mesilate-induced phosphatidylinositol 3-kinase signalling and improved survival in insulin-producing cells: role of Src homology 2-containing inositol 5'-phosphatase interaction with c-Abl. Diabetologia. 2013;56:1327–38.

19. Fountas A, Diamantopoulos LN, Tsatsoulis A. Tyrosine kinase inhibitors and diabetes: a novel treatment paradigm? Trends Endocrinol Metab. 2015;26: 643–56. https://doi.org/10.1016/j.tem.2015.09.003.

20. Prada PO, Ropelle ER, Moura RH, de Souza CT, Pauli JR, Rocco SA, et al. EGFR tyrosine kinase inhibitor (PD153035) improves glucose tolerance and insulin action in high-fat diet-fed mice. Diabetes. 2009;58:2910–9. https://doi.org/10.2337/db08-0506.P.O.P.

21. Han MS, Chung KW, Cheon HG, Rhee SD, Yoon C-H, Lee M-K, et al. Imatinib mesylate reduces endoplasmic reticulum stress and induces remission of diabetes in db/db mice. Diabetes. 2009;58:329–36. https://doi.org/10.2337/db08-0080.

22. Salaroli A, Loglisci G, Serrao A, Alimena G, Breccia M. Fasting glucose level reduction induced by imatinib in chronic myeloproliferative disease with TEL-PDGFRβ rearrangement and type 1 diabetes. Ann Hematol. 2012;91:1823–4.

23. Iurlo A, Orsi E, Cattaneo D, Resi V, Orofino N, Sciumè M, et al. Effects of first- and second-generation tyrosine kinase inhibitor therapy on glucose and lipid metabolism in chronic myeloid leukemia patients : a real clinical problem ? Oncotarget. 2015;6:33944–51.

24. Breccia M, Muscaritoli M, Cannella L, Stefanizzi C, Frustaci A, Alimena G. Fasting glucose improvement under dasatinib treatment in an accelerated phase chronic myeloid leukemia patient unresponsive to imatinib and nilotinib. Leuk Res. 2008;32:1626–8.

21

Long-term follow-up in a Chinese child with congenital lipoid adrenal hyperplasia due to a *StAR* gene mutation

Xiu Zhao[1], Zhe Su[1]* ⓘ, Xia Liu[1], Jianming Song[2], Yungen Gan[3], Pengqiang Wen[4], Shoulin Li[5], Li Wang[1] and Lili Pan[1]

Abstract

Background: Congenital lipoid adrenal hyperplasia (CLAH) is an extremely rare and the most severe form of congenital adrenal hyperplasia. Typical features include disorder of sex development, early-onset adrenal crisis and enlarged adrenal glands with fatty accumulation.

Case presentation: We report a case of CLAH caused by mutations in the steroidogenic acute regulatory protein (*StAR*) gene. The patient had typical early-onset adrenal crisis at 2 months of age. She had normal-appearing female genitalia and a karyotype of 46, XY. The serum cortisol and adrenal steroids levels were always nearly undetectable, but the adrenocorticotropic hormone levels were extremely high. Genetic analysis revealed compound heterozygous mutations at c. 229C > T (p.Q77X) in exon 3 and c. 722C > T (p.Q258X) in exon 7 of the *StAR* gene. The former mutation was previously detected in only two other Chinese CLAH patients. Both mutations cause truncation of the StAR protein. The case reported here appears to be a classic example of CLAH with very small adrenal glands and is the second reported CLAH case with small adrenal glands thus far. In a 15-year follow-up, the patient's height was approximately average for females before age 4 and fell to − 1 SDS at 10 years of age. Her bone age was similar to her chronological age from age 4 to age 15 years.

Conclusions: In conclusion, this is a classic case of CLAH with exceptionally small adrenal glands. Q77X mutation seems to be more common in Chinese CLAH patients. Additionally, this is the first report of the growth pattern associated with CLAH after a 15-year follow-up.

Keywords: Congenital lipoid adrenal hyperplasia, Steroidogenic acute regulatory protein, Mutation, Growth

Background

Congenital lipoid adrenal hyperplasia (CLAH, OMIM 201710) is the most severe form of congenital adrenal hyperplasia (CAH) and may cause 46, XY disorders of sex development (DSD). CLAH is an autosomal recessive inherited disorder caused by mutations of the steroidogenic acute regulatory protein (*StAR*; OMIM 600617) gene [1]. Currently, more than 83 different mutations of the *StAR* gene have been reported in approximately 190 patients [2]. However, only 17 cases of CLAH have been reported in Chinese patients [3–9]. The clinical features include severe adrenal and gonadal steroidogenesis defects due to disorder of the conversion of cholesterol to pregnenolone (P). All affected individuals with classic CLAH are phenotypically female regardless of their gonadal sex [1]. Hormone replacement enables long-term survival for these patients, but the literature regarding their long-term outcomes is limited.

Here, we report a 15-year follow-up of a Chinese patient with typical clinical manifestations of CLAH except for small adrenal glands.

Case presentation

The patient was Chinese individual who was raised as a female. She was born full-term by vaginal delivery. She was the fourth child of nonconsanguineous parents. She was admitted to our hospital at 2 months of age with recurrent vomiting, diarrhea and dehydration. She was found to have hyperpigmentation, hyponatremia

* Correspondence: su_zhe@126.com
[1]Department of Endocrinology, Shenzhen Children's Hospital, 7019# Yitian Road, Futian District, Shenzhen 518038, Guangdong Province, China
Full list of author information is available at the end of the article

(sodium 114 mmol/L) and hyperkalemia (potassium 6.98 mmol/L). The serum adrenocorticotropic hormone (ACTH) level was greater than 1250 pg/ml accompanied by very low levels of cortisol (0.17 µg/dl) and aldosterone (4.21 pg/ml). The levels of all adrenal steroids, including testosterone (T), P, dehydroepiandrosterone sulfate, androstenedione and 17-hydroxyprogesterone, were always nearly undetectable. She was diagnosed with primary adrenal insufficiency and was prescribed hydrocortisone and 9α-fludrocortisone orally [10]. However, her treatment compliance was poor. She often did not take the medications on time or at the recommended dose. She was followed up irregularly. Several episodes of adrenal crisis occurred, and she was admitted again at the age of 13.2 years. On admission, her blood pressure was 90/60 mmHg, and her height, weight and body mass index (BMI) were 148.7 cm (− 1.3 SDS), 35.3 kg (− 1.5 SDS) and 15.96 kg/m^2 (− 1.0 SDS), respectively. Hyperpigmentation was found on her tongue, gums, face, trunk, elbows, knees, palms, and soles. The patient was in Tanner stage 1. External female genitalia were observed, including a normal-sized clitoris and a normal urethral orifice and vaginal orifice. No palpable gonads were identified in the inguinal or labial regions. No pubic or axillary hair was observed. She had a high ACTH level and lower levels of cortisol, adrenal steroids and aldosterone. She exhibited gonadal dysgenesis, including: 1) high baseline levels of luteinizing hormone (38.2 mIU/ml) and follicle-stimulating hormone (68.3 mIU/ml); 2) very low levels of baseline T (< 0.35 nmol/L) and T after administration of the human chorionic gonadotropin stimulation test (0.47 nmol/L); and 3) low levels of anti-Müllerian

hormone and Inhibin b. The patient's karyotype was 46, XY (big Y). Ultrasonography revealed the presence of testes-like masses in the pelvic cavity (1.4 cm × 0.8 cm × 1.0 cm on the left and 1.5 cm × 0.6 cm × 1.0 cm on the right). Neither ovaries nor a uterus was identified. After 13 years of steroid replacement therapy, the patient underwent an adrenal computed tomography (CT) scan at the age of 13.2 years. Adrenal CT scans revealed that the adrenal glands on both sides were much smaller than normal (Fig. 1). Magnetic resonance imaging of the abdominal and pelvic cavities showed no uterus or ovaries. The patient's bone age (BA) was 13.5 years old (Fig. 2).

The patient was given hydrocortisone (17.3 mg/m^2 of body surface area per day) and 9α-fludrocortisone (0.1 mg/day) regularly. Her hyperpigmentation was slightly alleviated, and she had no adrenal crisis episodes thereafter. At the age of 15.2 years, the patient began estrogen replacement therapy. After 4 months of estrogen treatment, her breasts began developing. Photos of the patient are shown in Fig. 3. Laboratory and treatment data were collected during the 15-year follow-up and are shown in Table 1. Growth data are shown in Table 2. Compared to healthy Chinese girls [11], the patient's growth charts were drawn and are shown in Fig. 4. At 15.5 years old, she nearly reached her final adult height (154 cm), which was similar to her midparent height (152.5 cm) but shorter than the heights of her two sisters (156 cm, 160 cm).

The patient had no other diseases and exhibited normal intelligence. One of her elder sisters died during infancy from an unknown cause. Her parents and her other two sisters were healthy and underwent normal

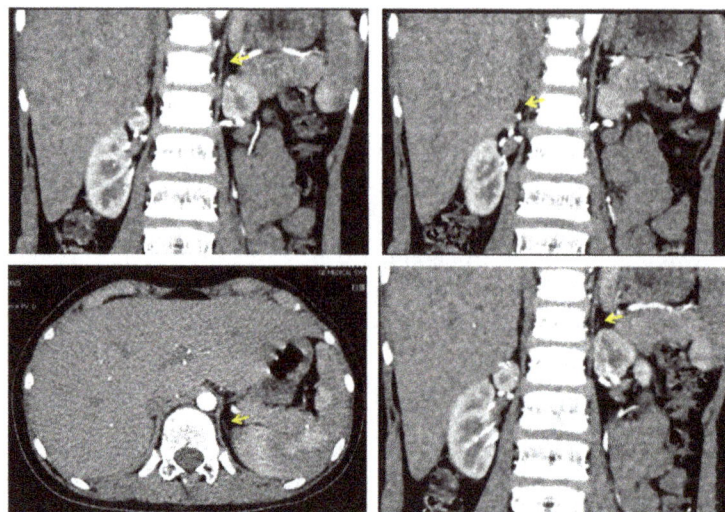

Fig. 1 At the age of 13.2-year adrenal computed tomography (CT) scans revealed that the adrenal glands on both sides were much smaller than normal. The yellow arrows indicate the adrenal gland

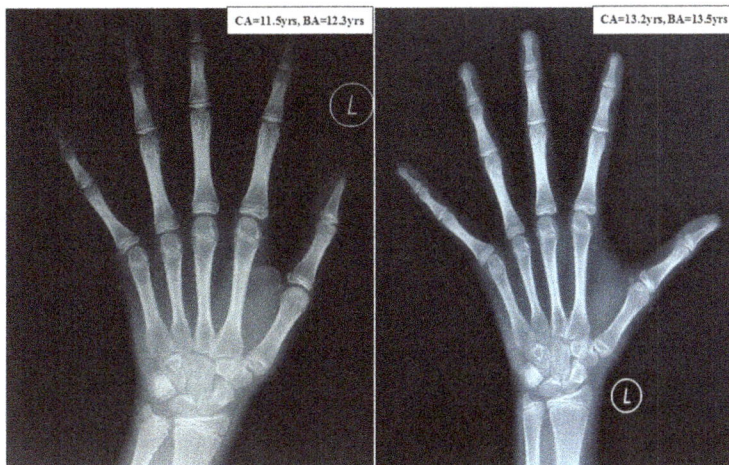

Fig. 2 Bone age of the patient. *CA* chronological age, *BA* bone age, yrs. = years old

puberty. Her mother died in a traffic accident when she was 10 years old. No family history of DSD was noted.

Considering the above clinical picture, an initial diagnosis of 46, XY DSD caused by severe deficiency of adrenal and gonadal steroids was established. The most plausible causes of the patient's condition include some specific types of CAH (3β-hydroxysteroid dehydrogenase deficiency, 17 hydroxysteroid dehydrogenase deficiency, CLAH) and congenital adrenal hypoplasia caused by mutations of the *NR0B1* or *NR5A1* genes [12]. Medical exome sequencing was the method of choice for a clear diagnosis.

Gene analysis

The sex-determining region on the Y chromosome gene was positive. Gene sequencing was performed with medical exome sequencing. The interpretation of the sequence variants and pathogenicity was conducted according to guidelines set by the American College of Medical Genetics and Genomics [13]. The Human Gene Mutation Database (HGMD), db SNP database, and 1000 database were used to identify whether the observed mutations have been reported previously. Compound heterozygous mutations were found in the *StAR* gene, with c. 229C > T (p. Q77X) in exon 3 and c.

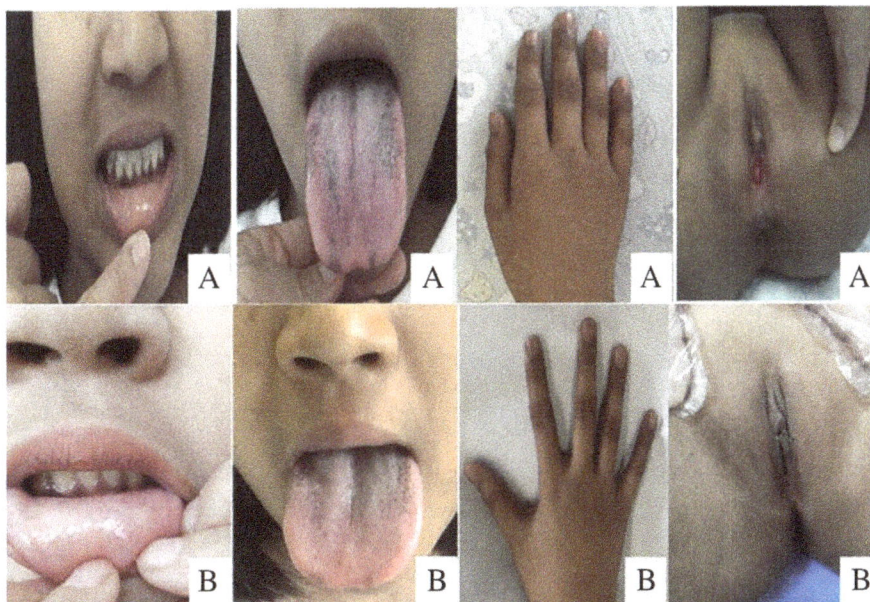

Fig. 3 Photos of the patient with CLAH. (**a**) Photos at age 13.2 years, (**b**) Photos at age 15.5 years

Table 1 Laboratory test results and treatment of the patient during the 15-year follow-up

Age (year)	Cor	ACTH	17OHP	DHEAS	P	AD	LH	FSH	E2	T	PRL	Sodium	Chloride	Potassium	FBG	TC	TG	LDL	HDL	ATII	Renin	ALD	INH-b	AMH	HC	FC
Variable unit	μg/dl	pg/ml	ng/ml	μg/dl	ng/ml	ng/ml	mIU/ml	mIU/ml	pg/ml	nmol/L	ng/ml	mmol/L	mmol/L	mmol/L	mmol/L	mmol/L	mmol/L	mmol/L	mmol/L	pg/ml	ng/ml/hr	pg/ml	pg/ml	ng/ml	mg/m²/d	μg/d
Normal range	4.5–23	0–53	0.16–1.85	45–139	0.1–8.45	0.3–1.97	0.3–15	0.6–25	20–85	0.35–2.1	5–35	135–145	96–105	3.5–5.5	3–5.6	3.1–5.18	0.23–1.7	2.07–3.37	0.9–1.04	23–75	0.15–2.33	10–160	92–147	5.6–18.8		
0.2	0.17	>1250	0.1	0.11	1.4	<0.3			<20	<0.35		114	82.2	6.98											18.7	100
0.3	0.51	1229		<0.1						<0.35		134.6	102.4	5.58								4.21			14.6	100
0.5	3.45	1229		<0.1	0.57				<20	<0.35															17.2	100
0.9	0.92	>1250		<0.1	<0.15				<20	<0.35															15.5	100
11.3	0.8	>1250	0.03	0.1	<0.15	<0.3	40.8	58	<20	<0.35	16.4	128	93.2	5.2	4.5										17.5	100
13.2	0.67	723	0.04	0.8	<0.15	<0.3	38.2	68.3	<20	<0.35	21.15	130	97.6	4.79	4.7	5.39	1.03	3.54	0.85	48.97	1.73	114.87	79.28	4.03	17.3	100
14.2	0.11	804	0.07	0.9	0.3	<0.3	35.1	49	<20	<0.35	22.71	138	103	4.4	4.5	5.51	1.25	3.68	0.81	57.91	0.5	113.4			16.2	100

Cor Cortisol, ACTH Adrenocorticotropic hormone, P Pregnenolone, DHEAS Dehydroepiandrosterone sulfate, AD Androstenedione, 17OHP 17-hydroxyprogesterone, E2 Estradiol, PRL Prolactin, FBG Fasting blood glucose, AT Angiotensin, ALD Aldosterone, TC Cholesterol, LDL Low density lipoprotein, HDL High density lipoprotein, TG Triglyceride, LH Luteinizing hormone, FSH Follicle stimulating hormone, INH-b Inhibin b, AMH Anti-Müllerian hormone, HC Hydrocortisone, T Testosterone, FC Fludrocortisone

Table 2 Physical assessments of the patient during the 15-year follow-up

Age (year)	BA (year)	Height (cm)	HtSDS	Weight (kg)	WtSDS	BMI (kg/m²)
Newborn		–		3.0	−0.6	–
0.2		50.0	0.2	3.7	1.1	14.80
0.9		72.5	−0.5	8.6	−0.1	15.27
1.5		80.0	−0.5	11.0	0.3	17.19
1.9		84.0	−0.1	12.0	0.5	17.01
3.7		99.0	−0.1	15.5	0.2	15.81
4.2	5	102.0	−0.3	18.0	0.9	17.30
10.2		134.0	−1.0	30.5	−0.2	16.99
11.3		138.8	−1.2	35.2	−0.1	18.27
11.5	12.3	139.5	−1.5	36.0	−0.4	18.50
13.2	13.5	148.7	−1.3	35.3	−1.5	15.96
14.2		153.3	−0.9	45.6	− 0.3	19.40
15.2	15	154.0	−1.1	52.4	0.3	22.09
15.5		154.0	−1.2	53.0	0.4	22.35

HtSDS Height standard deviation score, *WtSDS* Weight standard deviation score, *BMI* Body mass index, *BA* Bone age

722C > T (p. Q258X) in exon 7. The patient's father had the same heterozygous mutation at c. 229C > T (p. Q77X) (Fig. 5). Unfortunately, the samples from her mother and her two sisters could not be obtained. No other variants were observed in the *CYP11A1, CYP17A1, HSD3β2, StAR, P450scc, MC2R, NR0B1* and *NR5A1* genes.

Surgery and gonadal histology

After discussion with the DSD multidisciplinary team and consent from the patient and her father, the patient underwent surgery at 14.2 years old. Surgical exploration showed no Müllerian structures. Both gonads were removed, and the pathological results indicated hypogenesis of both testes. Hyalinization of the seminiferous tubules, the presence of spermatogonia and spermatocytes, and no sperm or sperm cells in the gonads were noted during the procedure. Immunohistochemical staining of the gonadal tissue was partly positive for CD117 and OCT 3/4 and positive for TSPY1 and Inhibin A (Fig. 6).

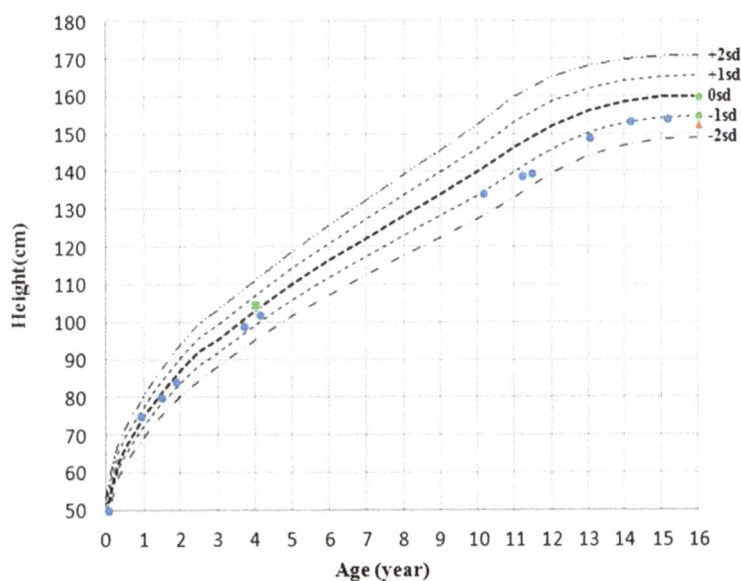

Fig. 4 Chart showing the progression of the patient's height during the 15-year follow-up. Blue dots indicate the patient's height. Green dots indicate the height of the patient's sisters. The red triangle represents the midparent height. The green square represents the height of the patient reported in Fu's paper

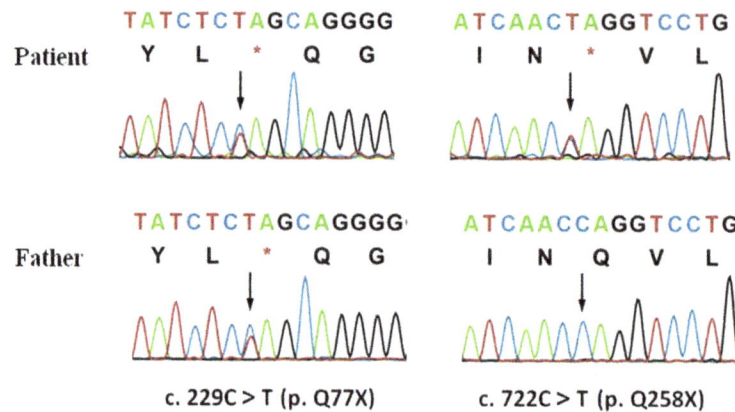

Fig. 5 Sequence electropherograms showing the StAR gene mutations in the patient and her father. Sequence analysis of the StAR gene revealed two hemizygous nonsense mutations at c. 229C > T (p. Q77X) and c. 722C > T (p. Q258X). The heterozygous mutation of c. 229C > T (p. Q77X) was found in the patient's father. Because the patient's mother had died due to a traffic accident, the mother's sequences could not be tested. The black arrows indicate the hemizygous nucleotides of c. 229C > T (p. Q77X) and c. 722C > T (p. Q258X) from the patient and the heterozygous mutation from the patient's father

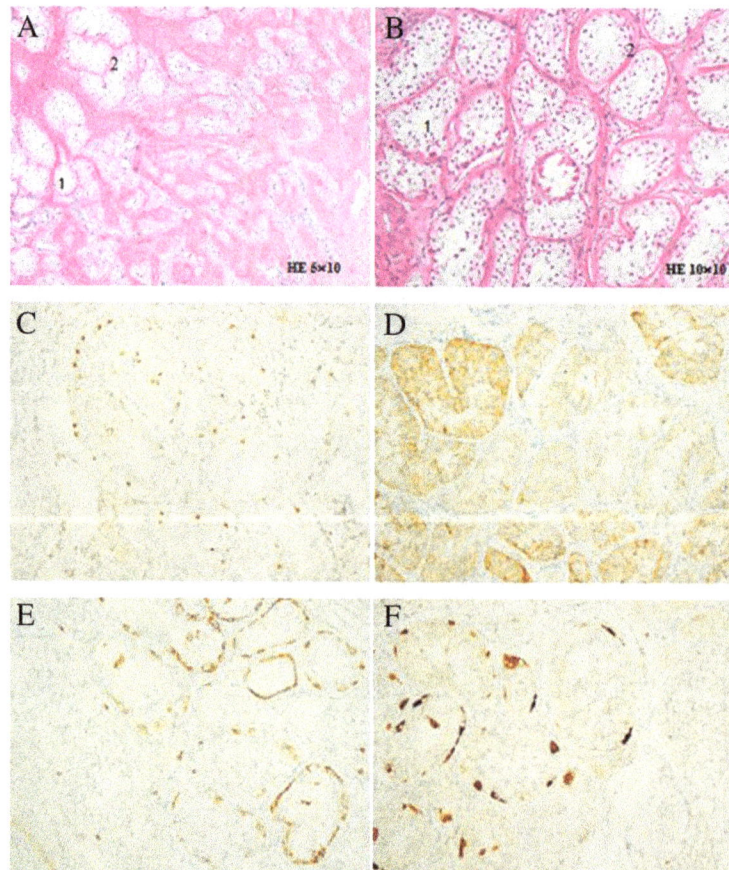

Fig. 6 Histology of the removed gonads. **a** Testis at low magnification: Seminiferous tubules (1). Hyaline thickening of the basal membranes (2). **b** Testis at higher magnification: Seminiferous tubules (1). Hyaline thickening of the basal membranes (2). **c** Testis stained for OCT 3/4. **d** Testis stained for Inhibin A. **e** Testis stained for CD117. **f** Testis stained for TSPY1

Discussion and conclusion

CLAH is an autosomal recessive inherited disorder caused by to mutations in the *StAR* gene. The human *StAR* gene is located on chromosome 8p11.2 and consists of 7 exons that translate into a protein of 285 amino acids in length. *StAR* is required for translocation of cholesterol from the outer to the inner mitochondrial membranes to synthesize P [14] and is involved in the first step of adrenal and gonadal steroidogenesis. Individuals with mutations in this gene may have severe deficiency of adrenal and/or gonadal steroids accompanied by fatty accumulation in enlarged adrenal glands in most cases. The amino acid sequence of the StAR protein is highly conserved from 67 to 280 [4]. The full length of the protein consists of a mitochondrial target sequence on its N-terminus and a cholesterol-binding site on its C terminus [15]. In vitro studies have revealed that the StAR protein without the C-terminal region had severe defects in function, while deletion of the N-terminus resulted in less loss-of-function [16].

We presented a case of CLAH caused by mutations in the *StAR* gene with a 15-year follow-up. This patient exhibited typical features of primary adrenal insufficiency shortly after birth. She was raised as a female and had visibly normal external female genitalia despite the presence of the male sex chromosome. The patient carried compound heterozygous mutations c. 229C > T (p. Q77X) and c. 722C > T (p. Q258X) in the *StAR* gene, both of which are nonsense mutations. Q258X is a known pathogenic hotspot mutation in Japanese, Korean and Chinese individuals with CLAH [5, 17]. Deleting 10 amino acids from the C-terminus has been shown to decrease StAR activity by approximately 50% [18]. With the nonsense mutation p. Q258X, StAR protein activity decreases to 16% of that of wild-type activity due to truncation of 27 amino acids in the C-terminal region [19].

The other mutation in our patient is c. 229C > T (p. Q77X) in exon 3. Q77 is a highly conserved residue from zebrafish (Fig. 7). The nonsense mutation c. 229C > T (p. Q77X) changes glutamine 77 to a terminal codon. Therefore, the StAR protein became truncated to a length much shorter than that of the Q258X mutant

and may have exhibited less than 16% activity. Therefore, the Q77X mutation was predicted to be pathogenic. The Q77X mutation has been previously reported in only two other Chinese patients with CLAH [7, 9]. Therefore, this mutation may be more common in the Chinese population.

The typical features of CLAH are enlarged adrenal glands with lipid deposits [20]. However, a suspected diagnosis of CLAH in the absence of adrenal enlargement cannot be ruled out [21, 22]. Huang et al. [5] studied images of the adrenal glands from CLAH patients and found that 7 of 9 cases had enlarged adrenal glands, one had normal-sized adrenal glands with fatty deposits, and one had normal adrenal glands. Only one CLAH case with small-sized adrenal glands, as observed in our patient, has been reported previously [20] (Table 3); however, the paper provided no corresponding speculation. The physiological mechanism for small adrenal glands remains unclear.

Data regarding the growth patterns of CLAH patients are limited (Table 4). The heights of CLAH patients from 1.2 years to 4 years of age were reported to be between the 10th and 50th percentiles of that among the normal population [4, 23]. The final heights in patients with CLAH were reported to be shorter or similar to the calculated midparent height [9, 24, 25]. Here, we constructed the first growth curve of a CLAH patient before and after sex hormone replacement. Birth length and heights before age 4 were similar to the average value of the general population. However, her height decreased to approximately − 1 SDS at 10 years old. At 15.5 years old, the patient's height was near her final adult height, which was similar to her midparent height but shorter than her two sisters' heights. The patient's BA was similar to her chronological age from age 4 to age 15.2 (Fig. 2), which is different from the retarded BA reported in other cases [24].

Limitations: Growth data in children with CLAH have rarely been analyzed. Our study plotted the patient's anthological measurement data from infancy to adolescence. However, accurate descriptions of growth patterns in children with CLAH require more cases and longer follow-ups.

In conclusion, we identified a CLAH patient with a 15-year follow-up. Small-sized adrenal glands were the

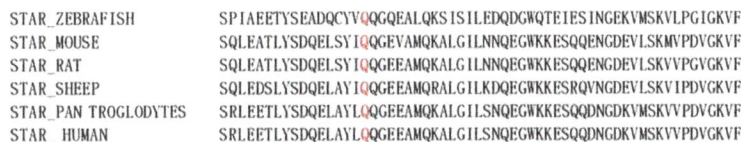

STAR_ZEBRAFISH	SPIAEETYSEADQCYVQQGQEALQKSISILEDQDGWQTEIESINGEKVMSKVLPGIGKVF
STAR_MOUSE	SQLEATLYSDQELSYIQQGEVAMQKALGILNNQEGWKKESQQENGDEVLSKMVPDVGKVF
STAR_RAT	SQLEATLYSDQELSYIQQGEEAMQKALGILNNQEGWKKESQQENGDEVLSKVVPGVGKVF
STAR_SHEEP	SQLEDSLYSDQELAYIQQGEEAMQRALGILKDQEGWKKESRQVNGDEVLSKVIPDVGKVF
STAR_PAN TROGLODYTES	SRLEETLYSDQELAYLQQGEEAMQKALGILSNQEGWKKESQQDNGDKVMSKVVPDVGKVF
STAR_ HUMAN	SRLEETLYSDQELAYLQQGEEAMQKALGILSNQEGWKKESQQDNGDKVMSKVVPDVGKVF

Fig. 7 Sequence alignment of the StAR protein from seven species. Q77 is a highly conserved amino acid (highlighted in red)

Table 3 Data of two CLAH cases with small-size adrenals due to *StAR* gene mutation

Author	Ethnicity	Rearing gender	Consanguineous parents	Age at onset (month)	Manifestations	Adrenal imaging by CT	Treatment	Karyotype	Alleles	Mutation area	Gene mutation	Type of mutation
Bose et al. [20]	Guatemalan/Amerindian	Female	Yes	2	typical	The left adrenal gland was not seen, the right one was small	HC, FC	46, XY	H	Exon 6	c.InsA677	Frameshift
Our case	Chinese/Asian	Female	No	2	typical	Both were small	HC, FC	46, XY (big Y)	C	Exon 3 Exon 5	c. 229C>T c. 722C>T	Nonsense

HC Hydrocortisone, *FC* Fludrocortisone, *CT* Computed tomography, *H* Homozygote, *C* Compound heterozygote

Table 4 Available growth data of CLAH cases due to *StAR* gene mutations

Author	Ethnicity	Relation	Age at onset (month)	Manifestations	Ht (percentile)	FAH (cm)	FAH vs MP	BA	Treatment	Karyotype	Alleles	Mutation
Khoury et al. [24]	French Canadian	siblings	11	typical	NM	NM	similar	significantly delayed	HC, FC, SH	46, XY	H	p.L275P
	French Canadian	siblings	1.5	typical	NM	NM	similar	slightly delayed	HC, FC, SH	46, XX	H	p.L275P
Fluck et al. [25]	Caucasian	siblings	10	typical	NM	143	low	NM	HC, FC	46, XX	C	p.T44HfsX3 p.G221S
	Caucasian	siblings	14	typical	NM	159.5	similar	NM	HC, FC	46, XY	C	p.T44HfsX3 p.G221S
Qiu et al. [9]	Chinese		1.3	typical	NM	152	low	NM	HC, FC, SH	46, XY	C	p.Q77X c.838delA
Fu et al. [4]	Chinese		11	typical	P50th (4 years)	NM	NM	NM	HC, FC	46, XY	H	p.K236Tfs∗47
Park et al. [23]	Korean	twins	1.3	typical	P3-10th (14 months)	NM	NM	NM	HC, FC	46, XX	C	p.R182C p.Q258X
	Korean	twins	< 1	typical	P10-25th (14 months)	NM	NM	NM	HC, FC	46, XX	C	p.R182C p.Q258X
Our case	Chinese		2	typical	P25-50th (18 months) P25th (4.2 years)	154	similar	NM	HC, FC, SH	46, XY	C	p.Q77X p.Q258X

HC Hydrocortisone, *FC* Fludrocortisone, *SH* Sex hormone, *CT* Computed tomography, *AI* Adrenal insufficiency, *GD* Gonadal dysplasia, *BA* Bone age, *NM* No mention, *H* Homozygote, *C* Compound heterozygote, *E* Estradiol

primary characteristic in our patient. Based on her long-term follow-up, her growth profile is the first reported growth pattern of CLAH. Our patient is the third reported case with the Q77X mutation in the *StAR* gene, which seems to be more common in the Chinese population.

Abbreviations
ACTH: Adrenocorticotropic hormone; AHC: Adrenal hypoplasia, congenital; BA: Bone age; BMI: Body mass index; CLAH: Congenital lipoid adrenal hyperplasia; CT: Computed tomography; DSD: Disorders of sex development; P: Pregnenolone; SDS: Standard deviation score; SF-1: Steroidogenic factor-1; StAR: Steroidogenic acute regulatory protein; T: Testosterone

Acknowledgments
The authors thank the patient and her father for their participation in this study and their consent to report these findings and pictures.

Funding
This research did not receive any specific grant from any funding agency in the public, commercial or not-for-profit sector.

Authors' contributions
XZ contributed to the data collection, data interpretation and writing of the report. ZS contributed to the study design and reviewed the report. JMS contributed to the histology data collection and data interpretation. YGG contributed to the imaging data collection and data interpretation. PQW contributed to the gene mutation interpretation. SLL contributed to the surgical data collection. XL contributed to the data collection and study conception and design. LW contributed to the growth data collection, data interpretation and revision of the report. LLP contributed to the photo data collection, image processing of the report and revision of the report. All authors read and approved the final manuscript.

Competing interests
The authors declare that they have no competing interests.

Author details
[1]Department of Endocrinology, Shenzhen Children's Hospital, 7019# Yitian Road, Futian District, Shenzhen 518038, Guangdong Province, China. [2]Pathology Department, Shenzhen Children's Hospital, Shenzhen 518038, China. [3]Radiology Department, Shenzhen Children's Hospital, Shenzhen 518038, China. [4]Pediatrics Research Institute, Shenzhen Children's Hospital, Shenzhen 518038, China. [5]Department of Urology, Shenzhen Children's Hospital, Shenzhen 518038, China.

References
1. Hauffa BP, Miller WL, Grumbach MM, Conte FA, Kaplan SL. Congenital adrenal hyperplasia due to deficient cholesterol side-chain cleavage activity (20, 22-desmolase) in a patient treated for 18 years. Clin Endocrinol. 1985;23:481–93.
2. Kaur J, Casas L, Bose HS. Lipoid congenital adrenal hyperplasia due to STAR mutations in a Caucasian patient. Endocrinol Diabetes Metab Case Rep. 2016;2016:150119.
3. Lihong W, Lei W, Yanhua S, Qinfang W, Mei F, Gaixiu Z, et al. A case report of congenital lipoid adrenal hyperplasia and literature review. Chin J Med. 2017;52:92–6.
4. Fu R, Lu L, Jiang J, Nie M, Wang X, Lu Z. A case report of pedigree of a homozygous mutation of the steroidogenic acute regulatory protein causing lipoid congenital adrenal hyperplasia. Medicine (Baltimore). 2017;96:e6994.
5. Huang Z, Ye J, Han L, Qiu W, Zhang H, Yu Y, et al. Identification of five novel STAR variants in ten Chinese patients with congenital lipoid adrenal hyperplasia. Steroids. 2016;108:85–91.

6. Xie T, Zheng JP, Huang YL, Fan C, Wu DY, Tan MY, et al. Clinical features and StAR gene mutations in children with congenital lipoid adrenal hyperplasia. Zhongguo Dang Dai Er Ke Za Zhi. 2015;17:472–6.

7. Ruimin C, Xin Y, Ying Z, Xiaohong Y, Xiangquan L. Mutation analysis of steroid acute regulatory protein gene in a patient affected with congenital lipoid adrenal hyperplasia. Chinese J Endocrinol Metab. 2014; 30:980–4.

8. Shiqin L, Huicui Y, Linqi C, Wenxiang W, Haiying W, Fengyun WY, et al. case report of lipoid congenital adrenal hyperplasia. J Appl Clin Pediatr. 2010;25:263–4.

9. Qiu WJ, Ye J, Han B, Han LS, Gu XF. Molecular genetic analysis of congenital lipoid adrenal hyperplasia. Zhonghua Er Ke Za Zhi. 2004;42:585–8.

10. Oelkers W. Adrenal insufficiency. N Engl J Med. 1996;335:1206–12.

11. Li H, Ji CY, Zong XN, Zhang YQ. Height and weight standardized growth charts for Chinese children and adolescents aged 0 to 18 years. Zhonghua Er Ke Za Zhi. 2009;47:487–92.

12. Houk CP, Lee PA. Consensus statement on terminology and management: disorders of sex development. Sex Dev. 2008;2:172–80.

13. Boehm U, Bouloux PM, Dattani MT, de Roux N, Dode C, Dunkel L, et al. Expert consensus document: European consensus statement on congenital hypogonadotropic hypogonadism--pathogenesis, diagnosis and treatment. Nat Rev Endocrinol. 2015;11:547–64.

14. Lin D, Sugawara T, Strauss JR, Clark BJ, Stocco DM, Saenger P, et al. Role of steroidogenic acute regulatory protein in adrenal and gonadal steroidogenesis. Science. 1995;267:1828–31.

15. Sugawara T, Lin D, Holt JA, Martin KO, Javitt NB, Miller WL, et al. structure of the human steroidogenic acute regulatory protein (StAR) gene: StAR stimulates mitochondrial cholesterol 27-hydroxylase activity. Biochemistry-Us. 1995;34:12506–12.

16. Miller WL. Androgen biosynthesis from cholesterol to DHEA. Mol Cell Endocrinol. 2002;198:7–14.

17. Kim JM, Choi JH, Lee JH, Kim GH, Lee BH, Kim HS, et al. High allele frequency of the p.Q258X mutation and identification of a novel mis-splicing mutation in the STAR gene in Korean patients with congenital lipoid adrenal hyperplasia. Eur J Endocrinol. 2011;165:771–8.

18. Arakane F, Sugawara T, Nishino H, Liu Z, Holt JA, Pain D, et al. Steroidogenic acute regulatory protein (StAR) retains activity in the absence of its mitochondrial import sequence: implications for the mechanism of StAR action. Proc Natl Acad Sci U S A. 1996;93:13731–6.

19. Kang E, Kim YM, Kim GH, Lee BH, Yoo HW, Choi JH. Mutation spectrum of STAR and a founder effect of the p.Q258* in Korean patients with congenital lipoid adrenal hyperplasia. Mol Med. 2017;23:149–54.

20. Bose HS, Sato S, Aisenberg J, Shalev SA, Matsuo N, Miller WL. Mutations in the steroidogenic acute regulatory protein (StAR) in six patients with congenital lipoid adrenal hyperplasia. J Clin Endocrinol Metab. 2000;85: 3636–9.

21. Hashemipour M, Ghasemi M, Hovsepian S. a case of congenital lipoid adrenal hyperplasia. Int J Prev Med. 2012;3:510–4.

22. Sahakitrungruang T, Soccio RE, Lang-Muritano M, Walker JM, Achermann JC, Miller WL. Clinical, genetic, and functional characterization of four patients carrying partial loss-of-function mutations in the steroidogenic acute regulatory protein (StAR). J Clin Endocrinol Metab. 2010;95:3352–9.

23. Park HW, Kwak BO, Kim GH, Yoo HW, Chung S. P.R182C mutation in Korean twin with congenital lipoid adrenal hyperplasia. Ann Pediatr Endocrinol Metab. 2013;18:40–3.

24. Khoury K, Barbar E, Ainmelk Y, Ouellet A, Lavigne P, LeHoux JG. Thirty-eight-year follow-up of two sibling lipoid congenital adrenal hyperplasia patients due to homozygous steroidogenic acute regulatory (STARD1) protein mutation. Molecular structure and modeling of the STARD1 L275P mutation. Front Neurosci. 2016;10:527.

25. Fluck CE, Pandey AV, Dick B, Camats N, Fernandez-Cancio M, Clemente M, et al. Characterization of novel StAR (steroidogenic acute regulatory protein) mutations causing non-classic lipoid adrenal hyperplasia. PLoS One. 2011;6:e20178.

22

Switching from glargine+insulin aspart to glargine+insulin aspart 30 before breakfast combined with exercise after dinner and dividing meals for the treatment of type 2 diabetes patients with poor glucose control – a prospective cohort study

Jing Li*, Liming Wang, Fen Chen, Dongxia Xia and Lingling Miao

Abstract

Background: This study aimed to examine the switch from glargine+once daily insulin aspart (1 + 1 regimen) to glargine+insulin aspart 30 before breakfast combined with exercise and in patients with type 2 diabetes mellitus (T2DM) with poorly controlled blood glucose levels.

Methods: Consecutive patients with poorly controlled T2DM ($n = 182$) were switched from the 1 + 1 regimen to glargine+insulin aspart 30 before breakfast in combination with exercise after dinner and dividing meals in two (same final calories intake). The insulin doses were adjusted according to blood glucose levels within 4 weeks after the switch and maintained for 12 weeks. Fasting blood glucose (FBG), 2-hpostprandial glucose (2hPG), glycosylated hemoglobin (HbA1c), body mass index (BMI), daily insulin dose, and hypoglycemia events were assessed.

Results: Sixteen weeks after the switch, 2 h PG levels and HbA1c levels (from 8.5 to 7.4%, $P = 0.001$) were improved. The proportions of patients reaching the HbA1c targets of 7.5% were improved (from 22.5 to 58.7%, $P = 0.001$). Among the 182 patients, 24 (13.2%) divided one meal into two meals, and 23 (12.6%) divided two meals into four meals. Among all patients, 8.5% had to reuse insulin aspart before dinner after the study. One patient with diarrhea and poor appetite experienced severe hypoglycemia. The rate of hypoglycemia was 3.76 events/patient-year. The daily insulin Aspart 30 dose was higher than the original insulin aspart dose ($P = 0.001$).

Conclusions: For patients with poorly controlled T2DM under the 1 + 1 regimen, switching to glargine+insulin aspart 30 before breakfast combined with exercise after dinner and dividing meals showed promising benefits.

Keywords: Glargine, Insulin aspart 30, Type 2 diabetes, Glycemic control

* Correspondence: 627168316@qq.com
Department of Endocrinology, The Affiliated Hospital of Medical School of
Ningbo University, Zhejiang, China

Background

Type 2 diabetes (T2DM) is an endocrine disorder characterized by hyperglycemia that results from variable degrees of insulin resistance and deficiency [1]. Chronic hyperglycemia associated with T2DM eventually leads to renal, neurologic, and cardiovascular complications [1]. In 2014, the worldwide prevalence of T2DM was 9% in men and 7.9% in women [2]. In China, a cross-sectional study carried out in 2010 showed an estimated prevalence of T2DM of 12.1% in men and 11% in women, and a 50.1% prevalence of prediabetes [3]. Therefore, T2DM represents a serious threat to the health of the Chinese population and this state should become worse because of the Westernization of the nutritional patterns in China [4].

For patients with a long course of T2DM that is still uncontrolled despite glargine combined with oral drugs, a regimen of glargine+prandial insulin is usually proposed [5–7]. The "1 + 1 regimen" (glargline+ 1-time prandial insulin) is usually started first, but it often has to be changed to the "1 + 3 regimen" (glargine+ 3-times prandial insulin) to achieve glycemic control [5–8]. With time, β-cell function progressively declines and secretagogues gradually lose their effectiveness, ultimately leading to the progression from the 1 + 1 to the 1 + 3 regimen [5–7]. The 1 + 3 regimen is associated with better glycemic control than the 1 + 1 regimen [8–10].

The 1 + 3 regimen requires injections before meals every day, resulting in low compliance. Shifting from the 1 + 1 regimen to the 1 + 3 regimen is associated with significantly decreased quality of life and treatment adherence [11]. The APOLLO trial showed that a single daily injection of insulin glargine resulted in better quality of life and compliance than injections thrice daily [10].

We hypothesized that optimizing treatment approaches based on a single daily injection could achieve appropriate glycemic control, possibly because of better compliance, compared with three injections each day. Therefore, this study aimed to examine the switch from glargine+once daily insulin aspart 30 (1 + 1 regimen) to glargine+insulin aspart 30 before breakfast combined with exercise after dinner and reduced servings in patients with type 2 diabetes mellitus (T2DM) with poorly controlled blood glucose levels, and to assess whether targets of the blood glucose and HbA1c were achieved.

Methods

Study design and subjects

This was an observational prospective single-arm cohort study (registration number: ChiCTR-OOC-17011177). Consecutive patients with T2DM treated at the Endocrinology Department of the Affiliated Hospital of Medical School of Ningbo University during June 2014 and February 2015 were consecutively enrolled and followed.

This study was approved by the ethics committee of the Affiliated Hospital of School of Medicine of Ningbo University. Informed consent was obtained from all patients.

The inclusion criteria were: 1) Chinese patients with type 2 diabetes according to the 1999 criteria of the World Health Organization [12]; 2) 50–82 years of age; 3) T2DM course of 10–30 years; 4) had constantly received the 1 + 1 regimen (combined with at least two kinds of oral antidiabetic drugs including secretagogues, α-glycosidase inhibitor, metformin, TZD, and DPP-IV inhibitors) for at least 3 months; 5) HbA1c > 6.5% but < 11.0%; 6) fasting blood glucose (FBG) of 5–7 mmol/l and at least one postprandial blood glucose (PG) > 11.0 mmol/l; and 7) patients were willing and able to use a blood glucose meter, and to provide informed consent. The exclusion criteria were: 1) non-type 2 diabetes patients (such as type 1 diabetes, diabetes secondary to pancreatic diseases, or diabetes due to drugs or chemicals); 2) pregnant or lactating women, or women willing to be pregnant; 3) patients accompanied with acute diabetic complications such as diabetic ketoacidosis and hyperosmolar coma; 4) patients with liver and renal failure (alanine transaminase > 2 times the upper limit of normal or patients with obvious kidney diseases or serum creatinine ≥ 133 μmol/L); 5) other endocrine and metabolic diseases, newly discovered tumors, or autoimmune diseases; 6) diseases in the thyroid, pituitary, or adrenal gland, or any other endocrine disease; 7) participating or had participated in another study within 3 months; or 8) received steroids within 3 months. In addition, the patients showing one of the following criteria were ruled out of the study: 1) allergic reactions, severe adverse reactions, or intolerance after receiving insulin aspart 30, acarbose, or metformin; 2) any protocol deviation; or 3) could not continue this study due to any factors, for which the reasons would be recorded.

Intervention

Prior to the study, all patients received guidelines on diet and exercise [13, 14], as well as on the use of blood glucose meters, on self-monitoring knowledge, and on hypoglycemia symptoms and appropriate countermeasures.

Each patient visited the outpatient 10 times during the 16-week study treatment period. During the first 4 weeks (adjustment period), each patient was seen each week, and then every 2 weeks for weeks 5–16.

Adjustment period (1–4 weeks)

The patients were required to perform moderate-intensity exercise for ≥ 30 min after dinner each day (e.g., walking, jogging, square dancing, ball games). Moderate-intensity exercise was defined as keeping the exercise workload at 65% of maximum heart rate (HR max = 220 - age). This method was used because it can be easily self-monitored.

During this period, patients were asked to monitor fasting blood glucose and 2-h postprandial glucose (2hPG) after each meal, every 3 days. Then, they adjusted their antidiabetic drugs according to the results.

The original 1 + 1 regimen was discontinued and breakfast insulin aspart 30 was added to glargine. In addition, an individualized treatment approach was developed according to the patients' body mass index (BMI). The adjustment procedures were: 1) the initial dose of insulin aspart 30 analogues was set at 1.5 times the dose of breakfast insulin aspart in the original "1 + 1" regimen or as 6 U. Then, the insulin aspart 30 was gradually adjusted by 2–8 U until at least one of the 2 h PG level readings after breakfast or lunch met the targets; 2) dividing one meal into two meals was required in the following situations: a) 2 h PG failing to meet the target after one or two meals (except for patients with 2 h PG failing to meet the requirement at both breakfast and lunch); or b) hypoglycemia between meals. 3) If the 2 h PG levels still failed to meet the standard after dividing meals, then the patients were switched to glargine+multiple prandial insulin doses after the study (Fig. 1). In terms of dividing meals, the patients were asked to reduce by 1/4–1/3 (about 25–50 g) their carbohydrate-rich food amount (rice, dried pasta, or bread) for the meal which was supplemented with equal amounts of low-fat crackers, bread, or other carbohydrates at 2 h after the meal. If their BMI failed to fall below 25 kg/m^2, the snack at 2 h after meal was withdrawn in order to control the weight and to improve insulin sensitivity of overweight patients.

In addition, patients were given oral administration of acarbose at dinner (minimum and maximum doses of 50 mg qd and 100 mg tid) and metformin (minimum and maximum doses of 0.5 g bid and 1.0 g bid). At the same time, they stopped taking secretagogues, TZDs, and DPP-IV inhibitors. The doses of insulin and oral drugs were adjusted according to the blood profiles. Patients were asked to have regular meal times. The purpose of the treatment was to achieve 2 h PG < 11.0 mmol/L and the target HbA1c level was set to 7.5%.

Stable period (5–16 weeks)

Once adjusted, the treatment protocol was maintained for 12 weeks, and had to remain unchanged. Nevertheless, if fine adjustments were needed due to disease

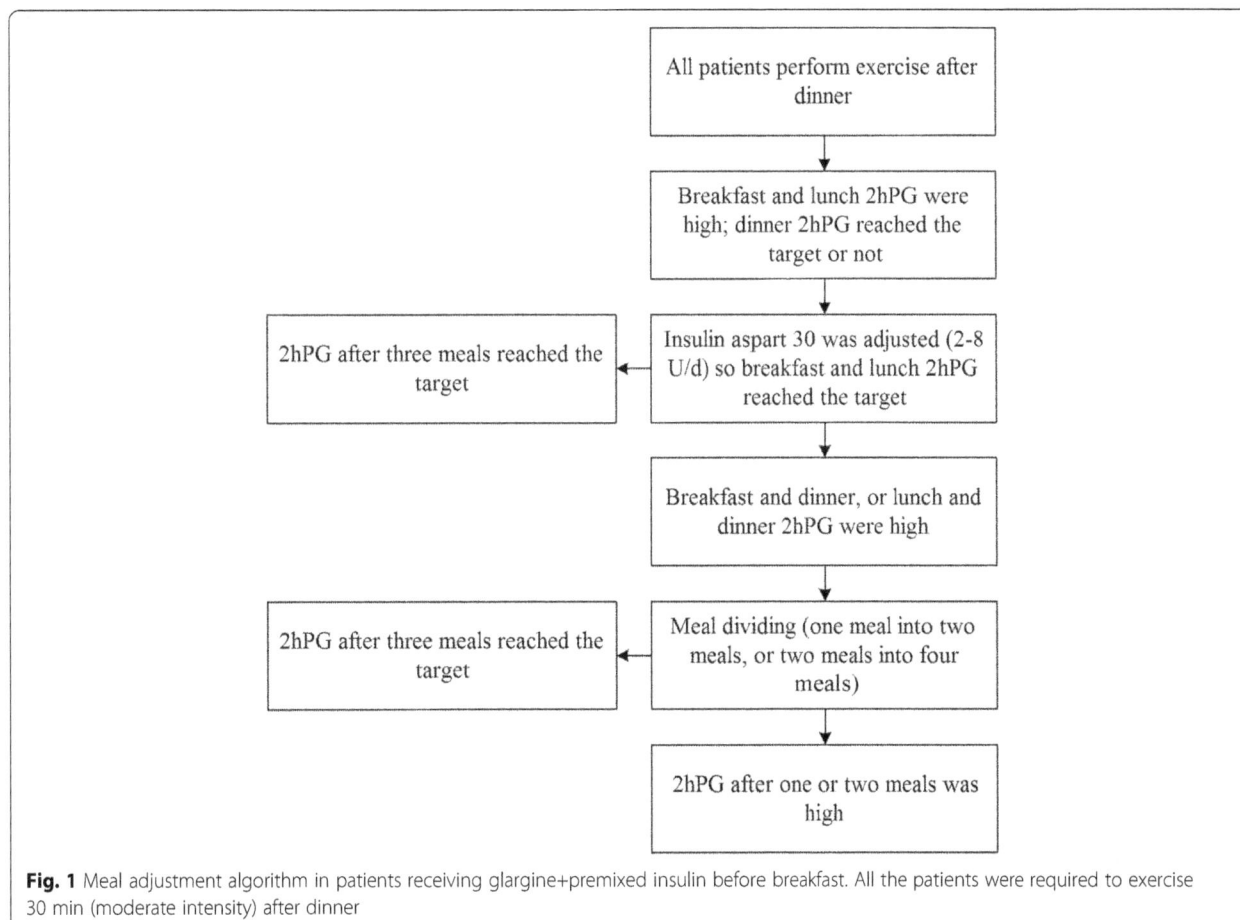

Fig. 1 Meal adjustment algorithm in patients receiving glargine+premixed insulin before breakfast. All the patients were required to exercise 30 min (moderate intensity) after dinner

conditions, the dose of glargine and variety of oral hypoglycemic agents (metformin tablet and acarbose tablet) could only be reduced rather than increased, while the doses of insulin aspart 30 could be increased or decreased.

Data collection

The following baseline data were recorded: age, gender, course of disease, insulin dose, BMI, HbA1c, fasting glucose, glucose before and 2 h after meals, glucose before sleep and insulin injection time-point before main meal (breakfast, lunch, or dinner). At the 16th weekend, HbA1c was measured.

Study drugs

In this study, insulin glargine (Lantus) (Sanofi Aventis, Paris, France) and insulin aspart 30 (NovoMix 30 Flexpen) (Novo Nordisk, Bagsvaerd, Denmark) were selected, both of which were injected simultaneously and separately on both sides around the umbilicus before breakfast. Other drugs included metformin tablet (Glucophage) (Bristol-Meyer Squibb, New York, NY, USA) and 100 mg Glucobay (acarbose tablet) (Bayer Health-Care Pharmaceuticals, Montville, NJ, USA).

Laboratory parameters

All blood glucose measurements were performed using fingertip blood using a steady blood glucose meter (Johnson & Johnson, New Brunswick, NJ, USA). The average blood profiles 1 week prior to participation and at the 16th week of treatment (average value within 1 week was taken) were monitored. HbA1c was monitored using high-pressure liquid chromatography (Bio-Rad, Hercules, CA, USA).

Outcomes

The primary outcomes were changes in HbA1c and 2 h PG at the end of the study compared to the baseline levels. The secondary outcomes were: 1) achieving HbA1c < 7.5%; and 2) changes of insulin dose and BMI.

Adverse effects

The number of hypoglycemia events and their duration and severity throughout the study period were analyzed. Hypoglycemia was defined as the patient feeling or were found to have symptoms and signs of hypoglycemia, and blood glucose ≤ 3.9 mmol/l at any time point. Severe hypoglycemia referred to the occurrence of coma, psychotic symptoms, or necessity of injection of glucose, the remaining cases were considered as general hypoglycemia. If patients showed recurrent general hypoglycemia within a few days, they were asked to inform their doctors by telephone. If non-drug factors (such as excessively less or late ingress, or excessive exercise, etc.) were excluded from

causing hypoglycemia in the patients, the insulin dose had to be adjusted promptly. Patients suffering from severe hypoglycemia had to visit the hospital for treatment immediately. All other adverse reactions were recorded.

Statistical analysis

Categorical variables were expressed as frequency and percentage, while continuous variables were expressed as mean, standard deviation, median, maximum and minimum, as appropriate. Changes between data before and after treatment were compared using analysis of covariance (ANCOVA). Categorical variables were described using frequency, and changes between data before and after treatment were analyzed using the chi-square test or non-parametric tests. Changes of HbA1c levels were assessed using the hybrid model. Statistical analyses were performed using SAS 6.12 software (SAS Institute, Cary, NY, USA). Two-sided P-values ≤ 0.05 were considered statistically significant.

Results

Characteristics of the patients

Two hundred and two patients were screened. Five patients were reluctant to participate since they could not adhere to the exercise program. Three patients were lost to follow-up. Twelve patients withdrew during treatment: three because they were unable to meet the requirements of the exercise program and nine because of adverse reaction to the oral hypoglycemic drugs. Ultimately, 182 patients were analyzed. Table 1 presents the baseline characteristics of the patients. The BMI of 87 (47.8%) patients was below 25 kg/m^2.

Glucose and HbA1c levels

Table 2 present the FBG and PG profiles before and after switching to glargine+insulin aspart 30 before breakfast. Switching to glargine+insulin aspart 30 before breakfast resulted in lower breakfast, lunch, and dinner 2 h PG and HbA1c, (all $P = 0.001$).

Table 1 Baseline characteristics of the patients

Variables	$n = 182$
Gender	
Male (n, %)	90 (49.5)
Female (n, %)	92 (50.5)
Age (years)	62.0 ± 10.9
BMI (kg/m^2)	24.9 ± 2.7
Course of disease (years) (min, max)	14.6 ± 4.5 (10, 21)
Insulin glargine dose (U)	25.5 ± 8.2
Daily insulin dose (U)	32.2 ± 8.5

BMI body mass index

Table 2 Comparisons of blood glucose profile before and after glargine+ Insulin Aspart 30 before breakfast

Variables	Glargine+once daily insulin aspart	Glargine+insulin aspart 30 before breakfast	P
FPG (mmol/L)	6.3 ± 0.6	6.2 ± 0.5	0.085
Breakfast 2 h PG (mmol/L)	13.9 ± 2.8	9.8 ± 2.6	0.001
Before lunch	9.1 ± 2.2	6.3 ± 1.9	0.001
Lunch 2 h PG (mmol/L)	13.8 ± 2.8	9.5 ± 2.5	0.001
Before dinner	8.7 ± 2.6	6.5 ± 2.1	0.001
Dinner 2 h PG (mmol/L)	12.3 ± 2.9	9.6 ± 2.5	0.001
Before sleep	8.5 ± 2.0	7.3 ± 1.8	0.001
HbA1c (n, %)	8.5 ± 1.6	7.4 ± 1.2	0.001
Rate of reaching HbA1c < 7.5% (n, %)	41 (22.5)	107 (58.7)	0.001

FPG fasting plasma glucose, *2 h PG* 2-h postprandial glucose
$n = 182$
Changes between data before and after treatment were compared using analysis of covariance (ANCOVA)
Frequencies were analyzed using the chi-square test

Tables 2 show the HbA1c levels before and after switching to glargine+insulin aspart 30 before breakfast. In addition, the HbA1c targets < 7.5% were examined. Sixteen weeks after the switch, 2 h PG levels at each meal and HbA1c levels were improved (all P = 0.001). The proportions of patients reaching the HbA1c targets of 7.5% were improved (7.5%: from 22.5 to 58.7%, P = 0.001); Table 3 and Fig. 2 present the hypoglycemia events, BMI, and insulin doses. The daily insulin dose was higher after the switch (P = 0.001). Patients had lost weight 16 weeks after the switch (P = 0.002). One patient suffered from severe hypoglycemia. The rate of hypoglycemia was 3.76 events/patient-year. The daily insulin aspart 30 dose was higher than the original insulin aspart dose (P = 0.001).

Insulin dose
Table 4 presents the proportions of patients receiving or needing prandial insulin at different meals before the switch and patients still needing prandial insulin at the end of study, The proportions of patients receiving prandial insulin at meals were 60.4% at

breakfast, 23.1% at lunch, and 16.9% at dinner. Before the switch. The proportions of patients needing prandial insulin at meals were, 96.1% at breakfast, 86.8% at lunch, and 30.2% at dinner. Sixteen weeks after the switch, the proportion of patients needing prandial insulin at dinner was decreased to 8.5% by dividing out dinner into two meals and exercise after dinner.

Meal adjustment
Meal adjustments are shown in Fig. 3. At the end of study, the ratio of patients dividing meal(s) at the 16th week after switching was 16.9% for breakfast, 8.3% for lunch, and 20.6% for dinner. Dividing at least one meal into two meals was conducted by 47 (25.8%) patients, among whom 23 (12.6%) patients finally needed dividing two meals into four meals, and the remaining 24 (13.2%) patients needed dividing one meal into two meals.

Discussion
This study aimed to examine the switch from glargine +once daily insulin aspart (1 + 1 regimen) to glargine+insulin aspart 30 before breakfast combined with exercise after dinner and dividing meals in patients with type 2

Table 3 Incidence of hypoglycemia (times/patient-year), insulin dose (U), and BMI (kg/m^2) after switching to glargine+ insulin aspart 30 before breakfast

Item	Glargine+once daily insulin aspart	Glargine+insulin aspart 30 before breakfast	P
Insulin glargine dose	25.5 ± 8.2	24.8 ± 8.0	0.410
Daily insulin dose	32.2 ± 8.5	40.7 ± 8.1	0.001
BMI	24.9 ± 2.7	24.1 ± 2.2	0.002
Patients with hypoglycemia event	N/A	159/182 (87.3%)	N/A
Hypoglycemia (times/patient-year)	N/A	3.76	N/A

BMI body mass index, *N/A* not available
Results are presented as mean ± SD
$n = 182$
Changes between data before and after treatment were compared using analysis of covariance (ANCOVA)

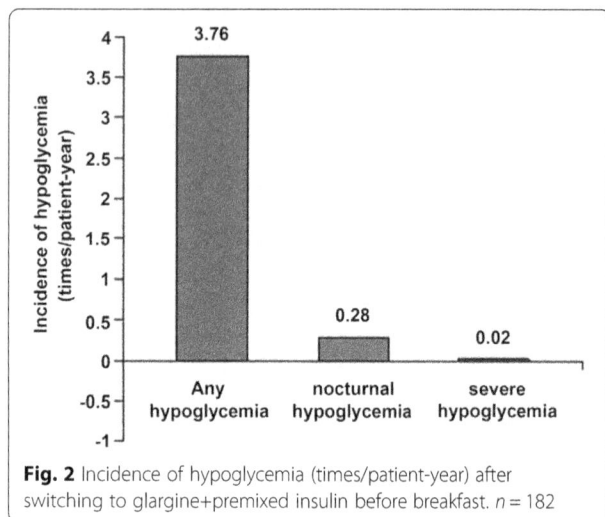

Fig. 2 Incidence of hypoglycemia (times/patient-year) after switching to glargine+premixed insulin before breakfast. $n = 182$

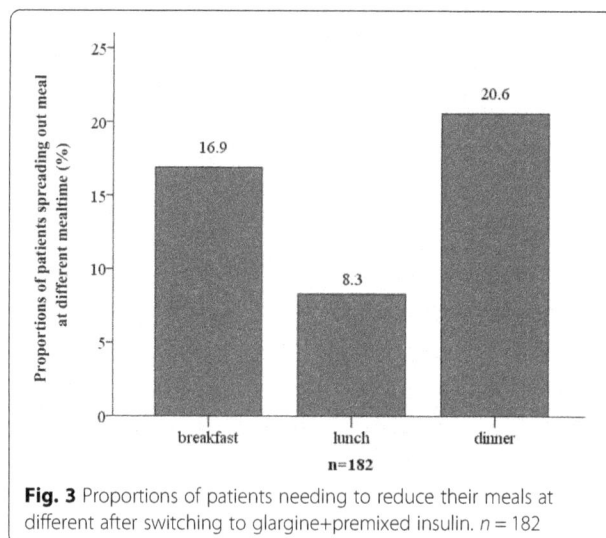

Fig. 3 Proportions of patients needing to reduce their meals at different after switching to glargine+premixed insulin. $n = 182$

diabetes mellitus (T2DM) with poorly controlled blood glucose levels, and to assess whether the blood glucose targets were achieved after dinner. The results suggest that for patients with poorly controlled T2DM under the 1 + 1 regimen, switching to glargine+insulin aspart 30 after breakfast could have promising benefits.

In this study, we adopted a new regimen of glargine +insulin aspart 30 before breakfast, which meant to separately inject glargine and insulin aspart 30 before breakfast, hereby to make the 30% of insulin aspart to play the action of insulin before breakfast. At lunch, the remaining 70% of protamine insulin aspart started to peak, and played the role of lunch insulin. Therefore, the principle of this regimen is probably similar to that of the 1 + 2 regimen. Nevertheless, since insulin aspart 30 has a fixed proportion, its regulatory effects on blood glucose after breakfast and lunch may not be as flexible as that of the 1 + 2 and 1 + 3 regimens. Thus, to compensate this disadvantage, patients were asked to divide one or two meals to improve the blood glucose fluctuations after meal. Therefore, 47 (25.8%) of the 182 patients had to divide their at least one meal,into two meals, of which it was respectively adopted in 16.9% and 8.3% of the 182 patients at breakfast and lunch.

The glargine+insulin aspart 30 before breakfast regimen did not affect 2 h PG after dinner. Indeed, the proportion of patients who needed insulin injection before dinner was not high before switch (30.2%). Patients from western countries often consume most of their energy of the day at dinner, while older Chinese patients often have a lower calorie intake at dinner. Thus, the need for insulin injection before dinner was not high. This phenomenon was also confirmed in a study by Feng et al. [15], in which the 1 + 1 regimen showed the highest proportion of injections before breakfast (55.9%) and the lowest proportion of injections before dinner (20.3%). This suggests that the need for insulin before dinner could be less in Chinese elderly patients with T2DM. Secondly, acarbose, an α-glucosidase inhibitor, played a synergistic hypoglycemic effect with glargine at dinner, which could have reduced prandial insulin. Thirdly, 30 min of exercise after dinner and/or dividing dinner into two meals were adopted. Compared to baseline, the exercise and/or dividing dinner could lower the proportion of patients who needed insulin at dinner from 30.2 to 8.5%.

Exercise efficiently improves the postprandial blood glucose levels of patients with T2DM [1–3, 14]. The

Table 4 Proportions of patients receiving or needing additional prandial insulin at different meal time before and after switching to glargine+insulin aspart 30 before breakfast

	Receiving prandial insulin before switching to glargine+insulin aspart 30	Needing prandial insulin before switching to glargine+insulin aspart 30	Needing prandial insulin at dinner after switching to glargine+insulin aspart 30
Breakfast insulin aspart (n, %)	110 (60.4)	175 (96.1)	48 (26.3)
Lunch insulin aspart (n, %)	42 (23.1)	158 (86.8)	38 (20.8)
Diner insulin aspart (n, %)	30 (16.9)	55 (30.2)	16 (8.5)[a]

[a]Proportions of patients needing insulin at dinner 16 weeks after switching to glargine + insulin aspart 30
$n = 182$
Frequencies were analyzed using the chi-square test

insulin-like effect generated by exercise can significantly decrease the blood glucose levels, especially for patients with seriously impaired glucose metabolism [13]. According to the present study, the increased area under the glucose curve among the patients who performed postprandial exercises declined more obviously than that of patients who just walked once a day, especially for the patients who performed exercise after dinner. In addition, this effect on postprandial blood glucose was more obvious for patients who consumed a large amount of carbohydrates [16]. Chinese patients with T2DM have both these features, i.e. using carbohydrates as main calorie source and exercising after dinner.

It is worth mentioning that the long disease course in the present study may have resulted in a poor effect of secretagogues. Nevertheless, because of the high proportion of carbohydrates in the Chinese diet compared to the Western diet [17], the therapeutic effect of α-glucosidase inhibitor is significantly superior to that in European diabetic population [18, 19]. Meanwhile, acarbose plays a significant "peak shaving" effect through delaying the absorption of carbohydrates, thereby saving the prandial insulin dose to some extent. Therefore, patients were asked to stop secretagogues. Instead, they took at least 50 mg of acarbose at dinner or, if possible, at the three meals.

In this study, for patients with poorly controlled T2DM under the 1 + 1 regimen, switching to glargine+insulin aspart 30 before breakfast showed promising benefits. A previous study showed that basal-bolus insulin detemir/insulin aspart could be more effective than biphasic insulin aspart in reducing HbA1c [20]. Another study showed that a flexible glargine dosing regimen achieved better outcomes than a fixed one [21]. A systematic review showed that regimens based on prandial premixed insulin analogues (thus providing both basal and prandial insulin coverage) could result in better overall, preprandial, and postprandial glycemic control compared to basal insulin alone regimens [22]. Nevertheless, direct comparisons among studies are difficult because of the variety of regimens.

In this study, the overall hypoglycemia and nocturnal hypoglycemia rates were not very high, suggesting that this approach could be acceptable. Compared to conventional multiple preprandial insulin regimens, injecting premixed fixed proportion of insulin before breakfast may increase the risk of hypoglycemia between meals, but this shortcoming can be solved using dividing one meal into two meals. The included patients were mainly elderly patients with a long T2DM course. These patients often display poor self-regulation ability of blood glucose levels and higher risk of hypoglycemia [23, 24]. Therefore, the safety of treatments is particularly important in this population,since hypoglycemia often leads

to even more serious consequences in these patients, such as aggravating cardiovascular diseases and neurological disorders, fall fracture, coma, and even death [23, 24]. Based on these risks, the target HbA1c level was set to 7.5% in this study.

According to previous studies, the proportion of Chinese elderly T2DM patients doing exercise is continuously rising [25, 26]. In this study, patients were provided with health guidance and individualized exercise programs according to their living habits and hobbies, which resulted in good exercise compliance in the majority of patients. It is noteworthy that the subjects in this study were middle-aged and elderly patients (50–82 years old) and most of them had regular daytime activities (housework, grocery shopping, taking care of the third generation of children, etc.). Thus, it could be difficult for them to improve blood glucose after breakfast and lunch by performing additional exercise. Meanwhile, nowadays in China, nocturnal exercise like night "square dance", night walking, cycling, jogging or boxing, etc., are increasingly popular. Therefore, postprandial exercise after dinner was conform to the life habits of most middle-age and elderly patients with T2DM.

In this study, the overweight patients were asked to reduce carbohydrate-rich food intake by about 25–50 g in the meal for which 2hPG levels failed to meet the targets. Therefore, the weight of the overweight patient could be decreased by properly reducing their food intake and increasing their exercise (regular moderate-intensity exercise for 30 min after supper).

Our success in terminating insulin before dinner without effect on postprandial blood glucose is possibly based on the following factors. First, we and the Tianjin '1 + 1' regimen study [15] both found that the proportion of patients using insulin at dinner was low (30.2% and 20.3%, respectively). Therefore, dinnertime insulin was not widely used in these patients. Secondly, 2 h PG levels can be further improved through regular moderate-intensity exercise for 30 min after dinner and dividing dinner into two meals [27, 28]. Thirdly, acarbose has a synergistic effect on insulin glargine. In the present study, only 8.5% of the patients with T2DM needed dinnertime insulin injection to control 2 h PG by using glargine+insulin aspart 30 in combination with exercise after dinner and dividing dinner.

The present study is not without limitations. The sample size was small and from a single center. No control group was neither included, nor other types of insulin regimens or dosages were tried. Only Chinese middle-aged and elderly subjects were recruited, limiting the generalizability of the results. We selected patients of ≥ 50 years of age because they were retired or nearly retired and they could more easily keep up with the 30-min of exercise compared with younger working people, probably with children at home, and with less available time. Since it was an observational study, a run-in period was not included and we could not reliably record the hypoglycemic events before switching. Additional studies are necessary to compare the efficacy and safety of this new insulin regimen with other regimens.

Conclusions

In conclusion, for patients with poorly controlled T2DM under the 1 + 1 regimen, switching to glargine+ insulin aspart 30 before breakfast combined with exercise after dinner and dividing meals showed promising benefits. Interventional study was needed to evaluate efficacy and safety.

Abbreviations
2hPG: 2-hpostprandial glucose; ANCOVA: Analysis of covariance; FBG: Fasting blood glucose; HbA1c: Glycosylated hemoglobin; T2DM: Type 2 diabetes mellitus

Authors' contributions
JL carried out the studies, participated in collecting data, and drafted the manuscript. LMW, FC and DXX performed the statistical analysis and participated in its design. LLM helped to draft the manuscript. All authors read and approved the final manuscript.

Competing interests
All authors declare that they have no competing interests.

References
1. American Diabetes A. Diagnosis and classification of diabetes mellitus. Diabetes Care. 2014;37(Suppl 1):S81–90.
2. Collaboration NCDRF. Worldwide trends in diabetes since 1980: a pooled analysis of 751 population-based studies with 4.4 million participants. Lancet. 2016;387(10027):1513–30.
3. Xu Y, Wang L, He J, Bi Y, Li M, Wang T, Wang L, Jiang Y, Dai M, Lu J, et al. Prevalence and control of diabetes in Chinese adults. Jama. 2013; 310(9):948–59.
4. Pan A, Malik VS, Hu FB. Exporting diabetes mellitus to Asia: the impact of Western-style fast food. Circulation. 2012;126(2):163–5.
5. American Diabetes Association. Standards of Medical Care in Diabetes-2016: Summary of Revisions. Diabetes Care 2016, 39 Suppl 1:S4–5.
6. American Diabetes Association. Professional Practice Committee for the Standards of Medical Care in Diabetes-2016. Diabetes Care 2016, 39 Suppl 1: S107–108.
7. American Diabetes A. Standards of medical Care in Diabetes-2016 abridged for primary care providers. Clin Diab. 2016;34(1):3–21.
8. Weng J, Ji L, Jia W, Lu J, Zhou Z, Zou D, Zhu D, Chen L, Chen L, Guo L, et al. Standards of care for type 2 diabetes in China. Diabetes Metab Res Rev. 2016; 32(5):442–58.
9. Jia W, Xiao X, Ji Q, Ahn KJ, Chuang LM, Bao Y, Pang C, Chen L, Gao F, Tu Y, et al. Comparison of thrice-daily premixed insulin (insulin lispro premix) with basal-bolus (insulin glargine once-daily plus thrice-daily prandial insulin lispro) therapy in east Asian patients with type 2 diabetes insufficiently controlled with twice-daily premixed insulin: an open-label, randomised, controlled trial. Lancet Diabetes Endocrinol. 2015;3(4):254–62.
10. Bretzel RG, Nuber U, Landgraf W, Owens DR, Bradley C, Linn T. Once-daily basal insulin glargine versus thrice-daily prandial insulin lispro in people with type 2 diabetes on oral hypoglycaemic agents (APOLLO): an open randomised controlled trial. Lancet. 2008;371(9618):1073–84.
11. Hartman I. Insulin analogs: impact on treatment success, satisfaction, quality of life, and adherence. Clin Med Res. 2008;6(2):54–67.
12. World Health Organization. Definition, Diagnosis and Classification of Diabetes Mellitus and its Complications. Report of a WHO Consultation. In: Part 1: Diagnosis and classification of diabetes mellitus. Geneva: World health Organization; 1999.
13. Duclos M, Virally ML, Dejager S. Exercise in the management of type 2 diabetes mellitus: what are the benefits and how does it work? Phys Sportsmed. 2011;39(2):98–106.
14. MacLeod SF, Terada T, Chahal BS, Boule NG. Exercise lowers postprandial glucose but not fasting glucose in type 2 diabetes: a meta-analysis of studies using continuous glucose monitoring. Diabetes Metab Res Rev. 2013;29(8):593–603.
15. Efficacy of the addition of a single bolus of insulin glulisine in combination with basal insulin glargine and oral antidiabetic drugs. Int J Endocrinol Metab 2011, 31(1).
16. Reynolds AN, Mann JI, Williams S, Venn BJ. Advice to walk after meals is more effective for lowering postprandial glycaemia in type 2 diabetes mellitus than advice that does not specify timing: a randomised crossover study. Diabetologia. 2016;59(12):2572–8.
17. Cui Z, Dibley MJ. Trends in dietary energy, fat, carbohydrate and protein intake in Chinese children and adolescents from 1991 to 2009. Br J Nutr. 2012;108(7):1292–9.
18. Weng J, Soegondo S, Schnell O, Sheu WH, Grzeszczak W, Watada H, Yamamoto N, Kalra S. Efficacy of acarbose in different geographical regions of the world: analysis of a real-life database. Diabetes Metab Res Rev. 2015;31(2): 155–67.
19. Ma RC, Chan JC. Type 2 diabetes in east Asians: similarities and differences with populations in Europe and the United States. Ann N Y Acad Sci. 2013;1281:64–91.
20. Liebl A, Prager R, Binz K, Kaiser M, Bergenstal R, Gallwitz B, Group PS. Comparison of insulin analogue regimens in people with type 2 diabetes mellitus in the PREFER study: a randomized controlled trial. Diabetes Obes Metab. 2009;11(1):45–52.
21. Riddle MC, Bolli GB, Home PD, Bergenstal RM, Ziemen M, Muehlen-Bartmer I, Wardecki M, Vinet L, Jeandidier N, Yki-Jarvinen H. Efficacy and safety of flexible versus fixed dosing intervals of insulin glargine 300 U/mL in people with type 2 diabetes. Diabetes Technol Ther. 2016;18(4):252–7.
22. Umpierre D, Ribeiro PA, Kramer CK, Leitao CB, Zucatti AT, et al. Physical activity advice only or structured exercise training and association with HbA1c levels in type 2 diabetes: a systematic review and meta-analysis. JAMA. 2011;305:1790–9.
23. Abdelhafiz AH, Rodriguez-Manas L, Morley JE, Sinclair AJ. Hypoglycemia in older people - a less well recognized risk factor for frailty. Aging Dis. 2015;6(2): 156–67.
24. Chelliah A, Burge MR. Hypoglycaemia in elderly patients with diabetes mellitus: causes and strategies for prevention. Drugs Aging. 2004;21(8):511–30.
25. Sun F, Norman IJ, While AE. Physical activity in older people: a systematic review. BMC Public Health. 2013;13:449.
26. Muntner P, Gu D, Wildman RP, Chen J, Qan W, Whelton PK, He J. Prevalence of physical activity among Chinese adults: results from the international collaborative study of cardiovascular disease in Asia. Am J Public Health. 2005;95(9):1631–6.
27. Hirshman MF, Wallberg-Henriksson H, Wardzala LJ, Horton ED, Horton ES. Acute exercise increases the number of plasma membrane glucose transporters in rat skeletal muscle. FEBS Lett. 1988;238(2):235–9.
28. Chen Y, Yuan X. The effect of exercise intensity,duration and postprandial exercise initial time on postprandial glucose metabolism in patients with type 2 diabetes mellitus. Chin J Sports Med. 2007;26(1):29–33.

23

Exploring how patients understand and assess their diabetes control

Anjali Gopalan[1,2]* ⓘ, Katherine Kellom[3], Kevin McDonough[4] and Marilyn M. Schapira[2,4]

Abstract

Background: Poor understanding of diabetes management targets is associated with worse disease outcomes. Patients may use different information than providers to assess their diabetes control. In this study, we identify the information patients use to gauge their current level of diabetes control and explore patient-perceived barriers to understanding the hemoglobin A1c value (HbA1c).

Methods: Adults who self-reported a diagnosis of diabetes were recruited from outpatient, academically-affiliated, Internal Medicine clinics. Semi-structured interviews were conducted with participants and collected data were analyzed using thematic analysis.

Results: The mean age of the 25 participants was 56.8 years. HbA1c was one of several types of information participants used to assess diabetes control. Other information included perceived self-efficacy and adherence to self-care, the type and amount of medications taken, the presence or absence of symptoms attributed to diabetes, and feedback from self-monitoring of blood glucose. Most participants reported familiarity with the HbA1c (22 of 25), though understanding of the value's meaning varied significantly. Inadequate diabetes education and challenges with patient-provider communication were cited as common barriers to understanding the HbA1c.

Conclusions: In addition to the HbA1c, several categories of information influenced participants' assessments of their diabetes control. Increased provider awareness of the factors that influence patients' perceptions of diabetes control can inform effective, patient-centered approaches for communicating vital diabetes-related information, facilitating behavior change towards improved patient outcomes.

Keywords: Diabetes, Qualitative research, Hemoglobin A1c, Glycemic targets, Doctor-patient relationships

Background

Correct knowledge of diabetes management targets is associated with better glycemic control and improved diabetes self-care [1–4]. However, past studies estimate that as few as 25% of people with diabetes can accurately describe the meaning of the hemoglobin A1c value (HbA1c) or recall their most recent value [2, 5]. While this may not seem surprising given the conceptual complexity of the HbA1c value (e.g., expressed as a percentage, non-intuitive goal range), even simpler assessments of diabetes control appear difficult [6–8]. In two prior studies, individuals with poor glycemic control were asked to more generally describe their current diabetes control using Likert scales with qualitative descriptors. Many of these individuals, particularly those with low health literacy, erroneously described their diabetes as well-controlled in spite of average HbA1c values over 9% (11.7 mmol/L) [7, 8]. While these findings may simply indicate a lack of patient understanding of the HbA1c, they may also reflect differences in the ways patients and providers conceptualize and gauge diabetes control. Though providers may expect patients to also use the HbA1c value, the rubric used by patients to assess control may be different and remains incompletely understood.

In several established models of health behaviors and outcomes, individuals' awareness and assessment of their current disease status are important predictors of behavior change or outcomes. Examples include perceived "disease severity," cited in the Health Belief Model, the

* Correspondence: Anjali.Gopalan@kp.org
[1]Division of Research, Kaiser Permanente Northern California, 2000 Broadway, Oakland, CA 94612, USA
[2]Michael J. Crescenz VA Medical Center, 3900 Woodland Ave, Philadelphia, PA 19104, USA
Full list of author information is available at the end of the article

role of "consciousness raising" in the Transtheoretical Model of Health Behavior Change, where knowledge or information can contribute to a shift from the pre-contemplation stage to the contemplation stage, and the "informed, activated patient" in Wagner's Chronic Care Model [9, 10]. Still, little remains known about the factors that contribute to these disease-related assessments for patients with diabetes. Better knowledge of the factors influencing patients' evaluations of their diabetes may enable providers to communicate more effectively regarding diabetes management targets and current levels of diabetes control.

We conducted semi-structured interviews with patients with diabetes to address the following research questions: 1) *What information do patients use to assess their current level of diabetes control?* and 2) *What are patient-perceived barriers to understanding the HbA1c value?*

Methods

Study design and oversight
The study was approved by the University of Pennsylvania's Institutional Review Board. Oral informed consent, including approval for audio-recording, was obtained prior to the start of each interview.

Setting and participants
We recruited patients from the waiting rooms of two academically-affiliated Internal Medicine practices located in West Philadelphia. The individuals approached regarding participation were those that happened to have an appointment with a provider on a day we were recruiting (i.e., a convenience sample). Eligible individuals were at least 18 years of age and self-reported a diagnosis of diabetes. Pregnant women, non-English speakers, and individuals unable to verbalize understanding of the provided study information sheet were excluded. Participants received a $30 gift card to CVS (a common drugstore) for their participation.

Data collection
Interviews, 30–60 min in length, were conducted by a research assistant (KM) and then transcribed verbatim. AG directly observed the initial interviews and regularly reviewed interview transcripts to provide feedback to KM on interview techniques. KM also took field notes. Sociodemographic information and diabetes history was collected from participants. The interview first focused on what information participants use to decide if their diabetes control is "good" or "bad" from day-to-day, month-to-month, and year-to-year. Participants were then asked if they were familiar with the HbA1c value. If they reported familiarity, they were asked what the value meant and about their most recent value. All participants, regardless of stated familiarity, were then read a short

description: "*The hemoglobin A1c is a blood test that doctors use to measure how well a person is managing their diabetes. The test measures a person's average blood sugar over the past 2-3 months. For most people with diabetes, the goal for the hemoglobin A1c is 7% or less.*" Participants were then asked how this description changed their previous understanding of their level of diabetes control. Next, participants were asked to perform an assessment of comprehension, referred to as the *Sharon* vs. *John HbA1c Comprehension Test*. They were presented with two written scenarios: 1) "*John is a 56-year-old man with a history of diabetes. His most recent hemoglobin A1c value was 9%*" and 2) "*Sharon is a 65-year-old woman with a history of diabetes. Her most recent hemoglobin A1c value was 6.8%.*" Participants were asked to select the individual (Sharon or John) that they believed had better diabetes control. The *Sharon* vs. *John HbA1c Comprehension Test* was done after, rather than before, the above description of HbA1c as it was intended to test participants' comprehension and application of this provided information (i.e., not intended to test baseline HbA1c understanding). Finally, participants were told that many patients with diabetes have trouble understanding the HbA1c value and were asked for their thoughts on plausible reasons for this difficulty. The interview guide is included in the Additional file 1: Appendix.

Analysis
Descriptive statistics were performed on the collected demographic and diabetes history data, as well as on participant accuracy on the *Sharon* vs. *John HbA1c Comprehension Test*. Participants' interview responses (identified by study ID only) were analyzed using a thematic analysis approach as described by Braun and Clarke and summarized in Fig. 1 [11]. Two independent reviewers, KK (a qualitative methods consultant) and AG (a health services researcher with qualitative methods training), read and re-read the transcripts to familiarize themselves with the data. With input from the entire research team, units of meaning, or "codes," within the data were then systematically defined. As additional transcripts were reviewed, these codes were organized into larger themes. The thematic definitions were refined and revised as the analysis proceeded, and variations and connections within the themes were noted and explored. The entire research team worked to determine the most salient themes pertaining to the research questions and to select the relevant data elements (participant [P] quotes) to synthesize a narrative addressing these questions. The reviewers independently coded transcripts until thematic saturation (no new themes emerging) was achieved ($N = 20$). The five remaining transcripts were then coded by AG only. KK and AG met to review coding comparison query results and

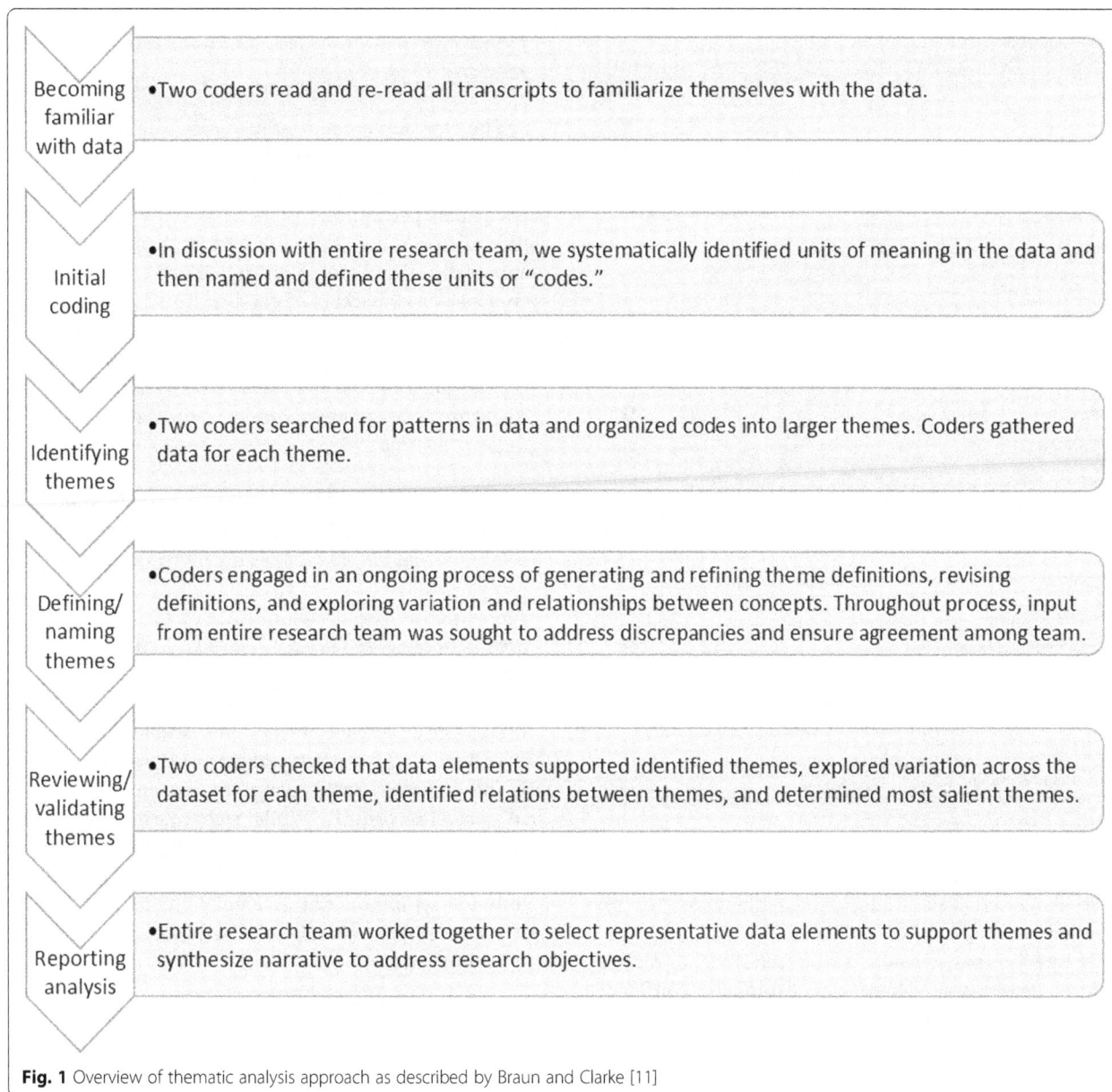

Fig. 1 Overview of thematic analysis approach as described by Braun and Clarke [11]

Becoming familiar with data
•Two coders read and re-read all transcripts to familiarize themselves with the data.

Initial coding
•In discussion with entire research team, we systematically identified units of meaning in the data and then named and defined these units or "codes."

Identifying themes
•Two coders searched for patterns in data and organized codes into larger themes. Coders gathered data for each theme.

Defining/ naming themes
•Coders engaged in an ongoing process of generating and refining theme definitions, revising definitions, and exploring variation and relationships between concepts. Throughout process, input from entire research team was sought to address discrepancies and ensure agreement among team.

Reviewing/ validating themes
•Two coders checked that data elements supported identified themes, explored variation across the dataset for each theme, identified relations between themes, and determined most salient themes.

Reporting analysis
•Entire research team worked together to select representative data elements to support themes and synthesize narrative to address research objectives.

discrepancies were resolved through study team discussion leading to consensus, with the coding scheme and definitions updated as needed. This process resulted in an average final inter-reviewer agreement of 97.6% (high inter-rater reliability was defined a priori as ≥90% agreement). NVivo Qualitative Analysis Software (QSR International Pty. Ltd., Version 10, 2014) was used to facilitate data management, coding, inter-rater reliability review, and analysis.

Results

Between June 2013 and December 2013, approximately 240 individuals were approached regarding participation. Of those approached, 83 reported having diabetes, and 25 individuals agreed to participate. Of this 25, 68% were women and 84% were Black. There was a wide range of educational attainment, the mean duration of diabetes was 11 years, 36% of participants self-reported a diabetes-related health complication, and 40% reported current treatment with insulin (Table 1).

Factors influencing participants' assessments of diabetes control

Participants' assessments of current control fell into the following thematic domains: 1) perceived self-efficacy and adherence to self-management; 2) the types and amount of medications taken; 3) the presence or absence of symptoms attributed to diabetes; 4) numerical data, both the HbA1c and self-monitoring of blood glucose (SMBG); and 5) connections between these domains.

Table 1 Participant characteristics and diabetes history

Characteristic	N = 25	%
Age (mean years ± SD[a])		57 ± 13
Gender		
Female	17	68
Ethnicity		
Hispanic	1	4
Race		
Black	21	84
White	1	4
Multiple[b]	3	12
Education		
Less than High School	3	12
High School or GED[c]	13	52
Some College/Technical School	6	24
College or beyond	3	12
Years since diabetes diagnosis (mean ± SD)		11 ± 7
Experienced a diabetes-related complication (Yes)	9	36
Diabetes Treatment		
Oral medications only	12	48
Insulin	6	24
Oral medications & Insulin	4	16
Diet only	3	12

[a]SD Standard deviation
[b]Multiple = Individual 1: Black, White, and Asian, Individual 2: Black and Native American, Individual 3: Black and White
[c]GED General equivalency diploma

1) Perceived self-efficacy and adherence to self-management

Of the 25 participants, seven referred to diabetes control in terms of self-efficacy, expressing confidence in their abilities to complete self-care and prioritize their health. For 17 participants, diabetes control was intrinsically linked with their perceived adherence to diabetes self-management behaviors. For the majority of participants (*n* = 17), self-care activities used in assessing diabetes control centered on maintaining a healthy diet, exercising, and weight management. In addition, four participants cited routine contact with providers as part of self-care used to assess their current diabetes control.

I'm on top of my job…I'm on top of doing what I'm supposed to do to maintain this thing here. (P4)

[Referring to poor control] *Not being disciplined, not setting my priorities and my priority is my body. (P9)*

If I keep this excess weight off me. That's how I'll know [about level of diabetes control]. *(P25)*

I go to the doctor. Make sure that I get examinations for my eyes and for my feet, and come into my doctor regularly. (P18)

2) The type and amount of medication taken

Perceived medication adherence, as well as the number and type of medications taken, affected ten of the participants' perceptions of their current control. The ability to stop a medication (based on a physician's recommendation) and not requiring insulin therapy were both considered markers of good control.

When you're not taking your medicine or doing what the doctors told you, you could tell by your health digressing. Like, more and more complications could arise or whatnot. (P13)

It's well under control because I got a letter from my doctor telling me that my diabetes is well under control and if I wanted to stop the medication, I could. (P5)

I took insulin three times a day. And my doctor told me I'm doing good because I haven't been back on insulin in ten years. (P8)

3) Presence or absence of symptoms attributed to diabetes

Over half of the participants (*n* = 14) cited the presence of diabetes-related symptoms as an indicator of "bad" diabetes control. While eight participants mentioned specific symptoms often ascribed to hyperglycemia (e.g., polyuria, polydipsia, blurry vision), others mentioned symptoms not as readily attributable to diabetes, such as pain (*n* = 3) or general feeling of low energy and malaise (*n* = 9).

Because, of course because you feel better, for one thing. And like I said, some of the things like I was doing, running to the bathroom frequently. (P15)

Because sometimes it be real high cause you get headaches and a lot of pain. Your bones ache and stuff and you're in pain. (P21)

Things in your body that say, hey, it's not right. (P18)

How do I tell if I'm in good control? When I don't feel tired. (P7)

4) Numerical data

Of the 25 participants, 16 referred to the HbA1c without prompting (i.e., prior to any mention of the HbA1c by the interviewer) as information used to assess diabetes control. However, seven patients did not refer to the value correctly by name (e.g., A1, AC1 U).

Besides the current HbA1c, eight participants stated that improvements in the HbA1c over time were an indicator of good diabetes control. Nearly all participants ($n = 21$) also mentioned the use of SMBG as a means of assessing current diabetes control.

Numbers—like when you take your sugar, hopefully all your numbers are where they're supposed to be. (P1)

I have to do finger pricks. I take my—got machine where I take my diabetes, and that tells me what amount the diabetes is. (P16)

5) Connections between domains

There were several commonly made connections between domains. Adherence to diabetes self-management or medications, together with numerical data (SMBG or HbA1c), was a combination that 11 participants used to assess their diabetes control. Another combination used by 13 participants to assess current control was numerical data (SMBG or HbA1c) along with the presence or absence of diabetes-attributed symptoms.

I try to keep my weight down, but I'm picking up weight now. So I'll be looking any day when I come to the doctor that she tells me that the count [referring to the HbA1c] is up again because I'm gaining weight. And I know that. (P8)

Doing well, yeah, by my finger sticks. And even when I go to the doctor, they check the blood through the arm. That's when they told me my A1c was up. But now it's down because I've been taking the medicine twice. (P7)

It's mainly the hemoglobin A1c and just how I feel. (P22)

Exploring understanding of the HbA1c value

Although nearly all participants ($n = 22$) had at least heard of the HbA1c in the past, and the majority mentioned the HbA1c without prompting ($n = 16$), understanding of the value varied greatly. When asked what the value meant, six participants described what the test measured (e.g., an average over a period of time), ten participants described their general interpretation (both accurately and inaccurately) of the value (i.e., goal to be lower, target range), three participants described a more personal importance of the value, and three participants had just heard of the test before but could not provide further description. After being given the basic description of the HbA1c, seven participants reported

that this information changed their previous understanding in some way.

How much sugar was in my body for the last three months. The HbA1c measures for the last three months. And it's supposed to be seven or below. But I keep mine at 6.2, once in a while at 6.4. Once it goes 6.4, I get back on my strict diet to knock it down to 6.2. I don't like for it to pass 6.2. (P24)

No, I don't know the meaning. All I know is it's got to be low instead of high. (P21)

Like you could do your sugars every day and you could see it, but that's the main number that shows that all of them numbers. (P3)

It means lot, it means that this is something that can affect my health if I don't stay on top of it. (P10)

I know it is life saving for me and like it helps like it's a super guideline. If it is off course, then my doctor can correct it through the medication. (P11)

Several participants ($n = 3$) thought of the HbA1c as a sort of detector of non-adherence to diabetes self-management.

And so, that level [referring to the HbA1c] let me know I was cheating, and I have to just get back on track. (P20)

Because that's the only way that you can really find out if a person is really doing what they supposed to be doing as far as diabetes is concerned. (P4)

John vs. Sharon HbA1c Comprehension Test After hearing our description of the HbA1c, most participants ($n = 22$) accurately stated that Sharon (HbA1c = 6.8%) had better diabetes control than John (HbA1c = 9%). Most of the participants who answered Sharon stated that their choice was based on Sharon's lower HbA1c value ($n = 19$), however, three participants explained their choice differently (based on Sharon's age, based on decimal point) or doubted their choice (needed more information).

Given she's 65, I'm going with 6.8%. Because she's 10 years older than John. And I don't know, that was my analogy of it. (P15)

I want to say the 6.8, but you don't know all of the factors that relate to why John's is 9. He could be doing everything he's supposed to be doing. He could have his weight under control and he could be one of those folks whose insulin levels is high. (P2)

Of note, the three individuals who answered incorrectly were not the same three who reported no prior familiarity with the HbA1c. The reasoning provided by these individuals exposed general misunderstanding of the HbA1c and its interpretation.

Because of the levels of it [referring to the HbA1c]. They're supposed to be like I think seven, eight and nine. So I think his is in more control because I think nine is the top number or something, I think. (P5)

Participant Perceived Barriers to Understanding the HbA1c Value Participants' thoughts on why the HbA1c might cause confusion for some patients fell into two main categories: 1) need for more diabetes-related education ($n = 6$) and 2) need for better provider communication of this information ($n = 8$).

I think people need to be a little more education...just don't give them the class and after they're done, they go about their business. They really need a follow-up. (P2)

So I think education, if a diabetic is educated from the door [referring to the time of diabetes diagnosis], it would be more beneficial. (P20)

I think people psych their selves out listening to medicalese. Like to me, the best doctors are doctors that can make it plain. (P12)

They're [referring to patients] scared of the doctors. They think they [referring to doctors] went to school all this time, they know what they're talking about. (P8)

Discussion

While the HbA1c was an important contributor to participants' evaluations of their diabetes control, participants also considered other information, including perceived self-efficacy and adherence to self-care activities, the types and amounts of medications used, the presence or absence of symptoms attributed to diabetes, and SMBG.

The importance participants placed on diabetes self-efficacy and self-care activities is well-founded and supported by existing literature [12, 13]. Provider awareness of the roles that self-efficacy and self-care activities play in patients' model of diabetes control is vital. By focusing on building self-efficacy, and supporting and reinforcing self-care in their communications with patients,

providers' recommendations and feedback can be more in line with patients' perspectives and priorities, hopefully increasing the effectiveness of these communications [14].

Medications, particularly the use of insulin, were linked to many participants' perceived diabetes control. The belief that more medications or insulin use is an indicator of worse or "end-stage" disease is established in the current literature and is a common barrier to medication intensification, particularly insulin initiation [15, 16]. Dispelling the idea that insulin use is an indicator of current diabetes control and addressing beliefs regarding the number of medications taken could shift patients' perceptions regarding diabetes control. Re-framing the types of pharmacologic treatments prescribed not as failures of management, but rather as results of individual physiologic differences, could have a beneficial impact on patient-provider communication, patient self-efficacy, and adherence to these prescribed medications.

Associations of patient-reported symptoms and symptom severity with diabetes outcomes, including patients' self-rated health status and measured glycemic control, have been noted in past work [17, 18]. Although symptoms can be an indicator of poor glycemic control, two potential issues complicate patients' use of this metric to gauge their current diabetes control. First, patients and providers may differentially attribute certain symptoms to diabetes. Patients may attribute symptoms such as general malaise and fatigue to poorly controlled diabetes, even though these are symptoms providers may not immediately associate with this disease [19, 20]. Notably, malaise and fatigue may actually be symptoms of depression, a condition that disproportionately affects patients with diabetes, remains underdiagnosed in this population, and may contribute to worse diabetes outcomes [21]. Second, the absence of symptoms may provide false reassurance to patients regarding their current diabetes control. Many patients with blood glucose levels well above goal do not experience any symptoms in spite of their increased risk for future diabetes-related complications. Providers should emphasize this point to patients in their communications about diabetes control.

Numerical information, either SMBG or the HbA1c, was part of many participants' assessment of diabetes control. The frequent mention of SMBG as an important source of information is noteworthy given mixed evidence regarding the reported clinical value of ongoing SMBG in patients not on insulin (only 40% of interviewed participants reported insulin use) [22]. The importance given to the HbA1c in assessing control and management was somewhat surprising given the varying levels of actual understanding of the value's meaning. Given past evidence supporting the value of an accurate understanding of disease management targets, like the HbA1c, further efforts are needed to improve the way care providers present this information to patients with diabetes [2–4]. Improving providers' communication of this value could address the current barriers to HbA1c understanding and, hopefully, increase the HbA1c's informational value for patients with diabetes. Further work is needed to identify optimal approaches for communicating information on glycemic control to patients. Towards this goal, in an in-progress mixed-methods study, we elicited input from participants with diabetes on a variety of visual formats for presenting the HbA1c value (e.g., color-based scales, depictions of distance from goal). Based on qualitative analysis of participants' input, two formats were chosen for testing against standard presentation of the HbA1c in a three-arm randomized, controlled trial of patients with diabetes to assess their impact on patients' assessments of their current diabetes control.

The study has several key limitations. First, the population is small and demographically homogenous, limiting the generalizability of the findings to other populations. Of note, the race/ethnic demographics of the participants do reflect that of West Philadelphia, a predominantly Black neighborhood. Because demographic information was not collected from eligible individuals who declined participation, differential participation by race or educational attainment cannot be assessed. Second, while the investigator AG's supervision and coding of the initial interviews may have introduced potential bias, it was necessary for the interviewer's (KM) training and unavoidable given limited study staff. We feel that the use of a structured interview script, coding by two independent individuals, and input from the broader study team during the analysis process, helped to mitigate this potential bias. Third, participants willing to take part in this type of interview may be more engaged and activated than the typical patient with diabetes. Finally, we did not ask participants to specify whether they had Type 1 or Type 2 diabetes. In our clinical experience, many patients are not sure of their diabetes type and, in the absence of blood tests (i.e., insulin autoantibodies, c-peptide), providers cannot always be entirely certain of diabetes type among patients treated only with insulin. However, the age of participants and use of oral medications or diet for management suggest most participants would be classified as having type 2 diabetes.

Conclusions

In this qualitative exploration of how patients with diabetes gauge their level of diabetes control we identified several types of information used by participants to assess their diabetes control. Most participants correctly emphasized the role of medication adherence and a healthy lifestyle in diabetes management and accurately equated lower HbA1c and blood glucose values with good diabetes control. However, many participants inaccurately believed that the type and amount of medication taken was an indicator of diabetes control and felt falsely reassured by the absence of diabetes-related symptoms. Provider awareness of the factors influencing patients' assessments of their diabetes control may help providers communicate more effectively with patients about their diabetes management status and targets, towards the goal of improved outcomes.

Abbreviations
Hemoglobin A1c: HbA1c; P: Participant; SD: Standard deviation; SMBG: Self-monitoring of blood glucoses

Acknowledgements
Not applicable.

Funding
This study was funded by a pilot grant from the University of Pennsylvania Department of Medical Ethics and Health Policy. The funder had no role in conducting the study, analysis and interpretation of the results, the construction of this manuscript, or the decision to submit the article for publication.

Authors' contributions
All listed authors have met the necessary criteria for authorship. AG was involved in the conception and design of the study, data analysis and interpretation, and construction of the manuscript. KK was involved in data analysis and interpretation, and review of the manuscript. KM was involved in study design, data acquisition and interpretation, and review of the manuscript. MS was involved in the conception and design of the study, data interpretation, and review of the manuscript. All authors have approved the final version of this manuscript.

Author's information
No additional information.

Competing interests
The authors declare that they have no competing interests.

Author details
[1]Division of Research, Kaiser Permanente Northern California, 2000 Broadway, Oakland, CA 94612, USA. [2]Michael J. Crescenz VA Medical Center, 3900 Woodland Ave, Philadelphia, PA 19104, USA. [3]Policy Lab, The Children's Hospital of Philadelphia, 3401 Civic Center Blvd, Philadelphia, PA 19104, USA. [4]Division of General Internal Medicine, The Perelman School of Medicine at the University of Pennsylvania, 3400 Civic Center Blvd, Philadelphia, PA 19104, USA.

References

1. Trivedi H, et al. Self-knowledge of HbA1c in people with type 2 diabetes mellitus and its association with glycaemic control. Prim Care Diabetes. 2017;11:414–20.

2. Beard E, Clark M, Hurel S, Cooke D. Do people with diabetes understand their clinical marker of long-term glycemic control (HbA1c levels) and does this predict diabetes self-care behaviours and HbA1c? Patient Educ Couns. 2010;80:227–32.

3. Berikai P, et al. Gain in patients' knowledge of diabetes management targets is associated with better glycemic control. Diabetes Care. 2007;30:1587–9.

4. Yang S, et al. Knowledge of A1c predicts diabetes self-management and A1c level among Chinese patients with type 2 diabetes. PLoS One. 2016;11:e0150753.

5. Heisler M, et al. The relationship between knowledge of recent HbA1c values and diabetes care understanding and self-management. Diabetes Care. 2005;28:816–22.

6. Zikmund-Fisher BJ, Exe NL, Witteman HO. Numeracy and literacy independently predict patients' ability to identify out-of-range test results. J Med Internet Res. 2014;16:e187.

7. Ferguson MO, et al. Low health literacy predicts misperceptions of diabetes control in patients with persistently elevated A1C. Diabetes Educ. 2015;41: 309–19.

8. Gopalan A, et al. Translating the hemoglobin A1C with more easily understood feedback: a randomized controlled trial. J Gen Intern Med. 2014; 29:996–1003.

9. K. Glanz, B.K. Rimer, K. Viswanath, Health behavior : theory, research, and practice, Fifth edition. ed., 2015.

10. Wagner EH. Chronic disease management: what will it take to improve care for chronic illness? Eff Clin Pract. 1998;1:2–4.

11. Braun V, Clarke V. Using thematic analysis in psychology. Qual Res Psychol. 2006;3:77–101.

12. Jones H, et al. Changes in diabetes self-care behaviors make a difference in glycemic control: the diabetes stages of change (DiSC) study. Diabetes Care. 2003;26:732–7.

13. Gao J, et al. Effects of self-care, self-efficacy, social support on glycemic control in adults with type 2 diabetes. BMC Fam Pract. 2013;14:66.

14. Lee YY, Lin JL. The effects of trust in physician on self-efficacy, adherence and diabetes outcomes. Soc Sci Med. 2009;68:1060–8.

15. Grant RW, et al. Diabetes oral medication initiation and intensification: patient views compared with current treatment guidelines. Diabetes Educ. 2011;37:78–84.

16. Ng CJ, et al. Barriers and facilitators to starting insulin in patients with type 2 diabetes: a systematic review. Int J Clin Pract. 2015;69:1050–70.

17. Nielsen AB, Gannik D, Siersma V, Olivarius Nde F. The relationship between HbA1c level, symptoms and self-rated health in type 2 diabetic patients. Scand J Prim Health Care. 2011;29:157–64.

18. Bulpitt CJ, Palmer AJ, Battersby C, Fletcher AE. Association of symptoms of type 2 diabetic patients with severity of disease, obesity, and blood pressure. Diabetes Care. 1998;21:111–5.

19. Fritschi C, Quinn L. Fatigue in patients with diabetes: a review. J Psychosom Res. 2010;69:33–41.

20. Fritschi C, et al. Fatigue in women with type 2 diabetes. Diabetes Educ. 2012;38:662–72.

21. Holt RI, de Groot M, Golden SH. Diabetes and depression. Curr Diab Rep. 2014;14:491.

22. Professional Practice Committee. Standards of Medical Care in Diabetes-2016. Diabetes Care. 2016;39(Suppl 1):S107–8.

24

The ratio of AGE to sRAGE independently associated with albuminuria in hypertensive patients

Kuang-Hsing Chiang[1,2], Jaw-Wen Chen[3,4,5,6], Shao-Sung Huang[3,5,7,8], Hsin-Bang Leu[3,5,7,8], Shing-Jong Lin[3,4,5,8,9] and Po-Hsun Huang[3,5,8*] (iD)

Abstract

Background: Soluble receptor for advanced glycation end-products (sRAGE) and advanced glycation end-products (AGE) have been associated with risks of cardiovascular disease. Because sRAGE is regarded as a scavenger to AGE, we hypothesized that the ratio of AGE to sRAGE (AGE/sRAGE) is associated with albuminuria in hypertensive patients.

Methods: In this cross-sectional study, a total of 104 patients with essential hypertension were recruited. Hypertension was defined as a systolic blood pressure ≥ 140 mmHg, a diastolic blood pressure ≥ 90 mmHg, or use of antihypertensive treatment. Albuminuria was defined as albumin excretion rate ≥ 20 μg/min. Multivariate logistic regression analyses were performed to evaluate the association between AGE/sRAGE and albuminuria.

Results: Among the 104 patients, 30 (28.8%) patients had albuminuria and 74 (71.2%) patients did not. Patients with albuminuria had higher AGE (2.15 vs. 1.71 μg/mL), lower sRAGE (424.5 vs. 492.5 pg/ml) and higher AGE/sRAGE (3.79 vs. 3.29 μg/pg) than those without albuminuria. Multivariate logistic regression model revealed that AGE/sRAGE (OR = 1.131, 95% CI = 1.001–1.278, P = 0.048) was independently associated with albuminuria. There was no significant relationship between AGE and sRAGE alone with albuminuria.

Conclusion: This study suggests that the ratio of AGE to sRAGE may be a surrogate biomarker for microvascular injury. Further prospective studies of the prognostic value of the ratio in relation to microvasular injury are needed.

Keywords: Advanced glycosylation end products, Advanced glycosylation end product-specific receptor, Hypertension, Albuminuria

Background

In hypertensive patients, the association between albuminuria and several cardiovascular risk factors has been widely demonstrated [1]. The existence of albuminuria is associated with signs of subclinical end-organ damage [2, 3] and is a strong indicator of microvascular damage in patients with essential hypertension [4]. Additionally, microalbuminuria is associated with an increased risk of all-cause mortality and cardiovascular mortality and is an early surrogate marker for cardiovascular events in hypertensive patients [5, 6]. Reduction of

albuminuria was also associated with cardiovascular protection [7]. Combing conventional Framingham score for cardiovascular risks with albuminuria may exert higher efficiency to determine a primary prevention strategy [8].

Advanced glycation end-products (AGE) is a group of modified proteins or lipids which become glycated and oxidized after exposure to sugars. The interaction of AGE and receptor for advanced glycation end-products (RAGE) on the membrane of endothelial cells can activate intracellular signal cascade, elicit reactive oxygen species production, activate nuclear factor-κB, and increase gene expression and release of inflammatory cytokines, resulting in the progression of atherosclerosis [9]. Soluble RAGE (sRAGE), either cleaved proteolitically from the membranous receptor via matrix metalloproteinases or

* Correspondence: huangbs@vghtpe.gov.tw
[3]Division of Cardiology, Department of Internal Medicine, Taipei Veterans General Hospital, Taipei, Taiwan
[5]Cardiovascular Research Center, National Yang-Ming University, Taipei, Taiwan
Full list of author information is available at the end of the article

secreted endogenously, can bind with AGE as a decoy receptor and therefore may play a protective role by avoiding the AGE-RAGE interaction [10]. Animal models have showed that inhibiting AGE-RAGE axis by sRAGE could attenuate the development and progression of cerebrovascular and cardiovascular disease [11, 12].

Both AGE and sRAGE play a critical role in the process of atherosclerosis; however, a number of studies revealed controversial results for either AGE or sRAGE alone. Fujisawa et al. reported that sRAGE was positively associated with the risk of cardiovascular disease in type 2 diabetes patients [13]. But Falcone et al. reported an inversely association of sRAGE with the presence of coronary artery disease in non-diabetes patients [14]. Similar controversy was also noted for AGE. The association of AGE with cardiovascular events was significant in some situations [15, 16], but insignificant in others [17]. As commented by Prasad et al., a potential solution to the above mentioned controversy is to consider the AGE and sRAGE simultaneously because AGE-RAGE axis involves AGEs, cellular receptor RAGE, sRAGE, and endogenous secretory RAGE. In humans, cellular receptor RAGE cannot be measured and the serum concentration of sRAGE are five times higher than endogenous secretory RAGE in healthy subjects. Therefore, the ratio of AGE to sRAGE (AGE/sRAGE) might be the most appropriate biomarker for AGE-RAGE axis [18].

To date, numerous studies have investigated the association of AGE/sRAGE with various conditions, for example, adiponectin [19], log trimethylamine-N-oxide [20], vascular function [21] end-stage renal disease [22], and idiopathic pulmonary fibrosis [23]. However, there is a lack of studies on the role of AGE/sRAGE in early-stage of atherosclerosis. Because current evidence implied that identifying novel biomarkers which is associated with albuminuria is possibly a way to find a surrogate for early evaluation of future cardiovascular risk, this study aimed to test the hypothesis that increased AGE/sRAGE may associate with the existence of albuminuria in patients with essential hypertension.

Methods
Study subjects
In this cross-sectional study, a total of 104 patients with essential hypertension were recruited from the outpatient clinic at Taipei Veterans General Hospital. Hypertension was defined as a systolic blood pressure (SBP) ≥ 140 mmHg, a diastolic blood pressure (DBP) ≥ 90 mmHg, or use of antihypertensive treatment. None of the patients had a history or clinical evidence of diabetic nephropathy, chronic nephritis, renal failure, liver cirrhosis, inflammatory disease, or hematological disease. Patients with diabetes or taking anti-diabetes drugs were excluded. Secondary hypertension was also

excluded by appropriate investigations, including measurement of plasma renin activity and aldosterone, Doppler studies of the renal arteries, renal scintigraphy or renal angiography. Medical history, including cardiovascular risk factors, previous and present cardiovascular events, and current drug treatment, was obtained during a personal interview and from medical records.

All patients gave written informed consent, and the study was approved by the Institute of Review Board in Taipei Veterans General Hospital (VGHIRB No: 96–12-42A).The protocols of this study were consistent with ethical guidelines provided in the 1975 Helsinki Declaration.

Data collection
For the study, a detailed review of each patient's chart and an interview was conducted to collect information on the patient's symptoms, medications, coronary risk factors, smoking status, family history of coronary artery disease, and other systemic diseases. All participants underwent a standard clinical examination. The Framingham risk score was determined for each participant to estimate the 10-year incidence of cardiovascular events (angina, myocardial infarction, or death). This score was based on age, sex, total cholesterol, high density lipoproteins (HDL), diabetes, history of smoking, left ventricular hypertrophy, and SBP. Hyperlipidemia was defined as total cholesterol concentration of 200 mg/dl. The body mass index (BMI) was calculated by dividing the weight of the patient in kilograms by the square of the height in meters. Concentration of fasting blood glucose, uric acid, blood urea nitrogen, creatinine, triglycerides, total cholesterol, HDL cholesterol and low-density lipoprotein (LDL) cholesterol, serum total bilirubin, aspartate aminotransferase (AST), and alanine aminotransferase in blood samples drawn after a 12-h fasting were measured using a Hitachi 7600 autoanalyzer (Hitachi Ltd., Tokyo, Japan).

Laboratory investigations
After a 12-h overnight fasting, blood samples were also collected to measure sRAGE, AGE, and high-sensitive C-reactive protein (hsCRP) concentrations. The blood samples were centrifuged at 3000 rpm for 10 min immediately after collection to obtain plasma and the plasma samples were kept frozen at -70 °C until analysis. Concentration of sRAGE was determined using a commercially available enzyme-linked immunosorbent assay (ELISA) kit (Quantikine, R&D systems, Minneapolis, Minnesota, USA). Another commercial enzyme immunoassay (ELISA) kit (OxiSelect, Cell Biolabs, San Diego, California, USA) was used to detect a variety of AGE structures, including N-epsilon-(Carboxymethyl) lysine and pentosidine but not N-epsilon-(Carboxyethyl) lysine or methylglyoxal. Determination of hsCRP concentration

was performed using a latex-enhanced immunophelo-metric assay (Dade Behring, Marburg, Germany) [19]. All procedures were carried out according to the instructions of the manufacturers and all measurements were performed by technicians who were blinded to all clinical data. Each standard and plasma sample was analyzed twice and the mean value was used in all subsequent analyses. The intra-assay and interassay variation coefficients were less than 10%.

Estimated creatinine clearance rate (eCCr) was calculated by the Cockcroft–Gault formula [20]. Morning urine samples were obtained for the creatinine to albumin ratio to determine the albumin excretion rate. Normoalbuminuria was defined as albumin excretion rate of < 20 μg/min, microalbuminuria was defined as albumin excretion rate of 20–200 μg/min, and macroalbuminuria was defined as albumin excretion rate > 200 μg/min.

Statistical analysis

This study aimed to analyze the association of AGE/sRAGE with the presence of albuminuria in hypertensive patients. Patients with microalbuminuria or macroalbuminuria were grouped as 'with albuminuria' group and patients with normoalbuminuria as 'without albuminuria' group. Continuous data are presented as mean with standard deviation, and categorical data presented as count with percentage. The differences between patients with and without albuminuria for continuous and categorical data were tested using Mann-Whitney U test and Chi-square test, respectively. Multivariate logistic regression analyses with backward stepwise method were performed to evaluate the association between AGE/sRAGE and albuminuria with a P-value of less than 0.1 in the univariable analysis. A two-tailed P-value of < 0.05 indicated statistical significance. All statistical analyses were performed using IBM SPSS Statistics for Windows, Version 19.0 (Armonk, NY, USA).

Results

Sample characteristics

Among the 104 patients, 30 (28.8%) patients had micro-albuminuria or macroalbuminuria, and 74 (71.2%) patients had normoalbuminuria. Demographic and clinical characteristics of the 104 hypertensive patients were provided in Table 1. Patients with albuminuria were older (58 vs. 56 years, $P < 0.001$), had significant higher SBP (150 mmHg vs. 137 mmHg, $P = 0.002$), higher DBP (83 vs. 78 mmHg, $P = 0.039$), higher pulse pressure (65 mmHg vs. 58 mmHg, $P = 0.047$), and more number of drugs ($P = 0.027$). Regarding the laboratory data, patients with albuminuria had significant higher AST (8 U/L vs. 6 U/L, $P = 0.008$). Patients with albuminuria had higher AGE (2.15 μg/mL vs. 1.71 μg/mL), lower

sRAGE (424.5 pg/ml vs. 492.5 pg/ml) and higher AGE/sRAGE (3.79 μg/pg vs. 3.29 μg/pg) than those without albuminuria (Table 1).

Association of AGE/sRAGE with albuminuria

The results of univariate and multivariate analysis were presented in Table 2. Variables with P-value < 0.1 in univariate analysis included SBP, DBP, pulse pressure, number of drugs, AST, N-terminal prohormone of brain natriuretic peptide (NT-proBNP), and AGE/sRAGE. Due to the collinearity among pulse pressure, systolic blood pressure and diastolic blood pressure, only pulse pressure was included into the multivariate analysis. The results of multivariate logistic regression models revealed that number of drugs (odds ratio [OR] = 1.986, 95% confident interval [CI] = 1.082–3.645, $P = 0.027$), NT-proBNP (OR = 1.015, 95% CI = 1.001–1.030, $P = 0.030$), and AGE/sRAGE (OR = 1.131, 95% CI = 1.001–1.278, $P = 0.048$) were independently associated with albuminuria (Table 2).

Discussion

To the best of our knowledge, this is the first study to investigate relationship of the ratio of AGE to sRAGE with micro- and macroalbuminuria in hypertensive patients. As our results showed a positive and independent association of AGE/sRAGE with albuminuria, the ratio may be a potentially surrogate biomarker for microvascular injury.

There is growing evidence that the AGE-RAGE axis plays a critical role in the development of atherosclerosis. In a cross-sectional study, Tahara et al. evaluated the correlation among adiponectin, AGE, sRAGE and AGE/sRAGE in 316 patients. The results showed that AGE/sRAGE was inversely related with adiponectin ($\beta = -0.126$, $P = 0.006$), independent of the metabolic and clinical variables such as insulin resistance, triglycerides, HbA1c, HDL, age and sex. The significance correlation of AGE and sRAGE with adiponectin did not exist after adjusting for AGE/sRAGE in multiple regression analysis [19]. As adiponectin is an anti-inflammatory and vascular protective adipocytokine with insulin-sensitizing properties, the following study by Kajikawa et al. extended the observation by evaluating the association of AGE, sRAGE, and AGE/sRAGE with endothelial function measured by flow-mediated vasodilation. The results of multivariate regression analysis showed that AGE/sRAGE independently predicted flow-mediated vasodilation ($\beta = -0.23$, $P = 0.02$) after adjusting several confounders, including age, sex, BMI, presence of hypertension, dyslipidemia, fasting glucose, and smoking status. Meanwhile, the association was not observed in either AGE or sRAGE alone [21]. Another study by Prasad et al. compared the AGE, sRAGE, endogenous secretory RAGE, cleaved RAGE

Table 1 Demographic and clinical characteristics of study population

		Without albuminuria (n = 74)	With albuminuria (n = 30)	P
Age (year)		56 (51–66)	58 (46–71)	< 0.001
Gender[a]	Male	48 (64.9)	19 (63.3)	0.882
	Female	26 (35.1)	11 (36.7)	
Smoking[a]	Not smoker	45 (60.8)	19 (63.3)	0.839
	Past smoker	16 (21.6)	5 (16.7)	
	Current smoker	13 (17.6)	6 (20.0)	
Body mass index (kg/m^2)		25.4 (23.9–27.3)	25.2 (23.7–27.0)	0.925
Heart rate (/min)		76 (68–86)	75 (72–84)	0.854
Systolic blood pressure (mmHg)		137 (126–147)	150 (132–158)	0.002
Diastolic blood pressure (mmHg)		78 (73–88)	83 (77–92)	0.039
Pulse pressure (mmHg)		58 (51–66)	65 (52–71)	0.047
Impaired fasting glucose[a]		36 (48.6)	16 (53.3)	0.829
Current medication				
ARB[a]		46 (62.2)	21 (70.0)	0.449
ACEI[a]		14 (18.9)	5 (16.7)	0.788
Calcium-channel blocker[a]		46 (62.2)	24 (80.0)	0.079
Diuretics[a]		17 (23.0)	8 (26.7)	0.690
Beta-blocker[a]		13 (17.6)	10 (33.3)	0.079
Statin[a]		9 (12.2)	3 (10.0)	1.000
Number of drugs		2 (1–3)	2 (2–3)	0.027
Laboratory				
Total cholesterol (mg/dl)		191.5 (170.0–214.0)	195.5 (182.0–214.0)	0.487
Triglycerides (mg/dL)		119.0 (76.0–184.0)	129.5 (102.0–197.0)	0.262
HDL (mg/dL)		42 (37–50)	43.5 (39–51)	0.586
LDL (mg/dL)		118.0 (95.6–140.0)	118.6 (101.0–133.4)	0.933
Fasting glucose (mg/dL)		99 (94–105)	100 (93–108)	0.950
ALT (U/L)		10 (8–13)	8 (7–11)	0.386
AST (U/L)		6 (5–9.5)	8 (7–11)	0.008
Uric acid (mg/dL)		6.05 (5.2–6.8)	6.5 (5.4–7.3)	0.264
eCCr (mL/min)		88.2 (72.9–104.6)	70.4 (55.0–103.0)	0.061
hs-CRP (mg/dL)		0.20 (0.16–0.36)	0.27 (0.16–0.55)	0.246
Adiponectin (µg/mL)		17.8 (11.0–27.6)	15.4 (11.2–25.1)	0.840
ADMA (µmol /L)		0.36 (0.33–0.40)	0.36 (0.32–0.41)	0.970
NT-proBNP (pg/mL)		84.1 (54.6–102.0)	93.7 (71.5–124.0)	0.077
AGE (µg/mL)		1.71 (0.82–2.45)	2.15 (0.87–2.65.00)	0.394
sRAGE (pg/ml)		492.5 (375.0–682.0)	424.5 (310.0–583.0)	0.200
AGE / sRAGE (µg/pg)		3.29 (1.78–5.18)	3.79 (1.77–7.59)	0.212

Data were presented as median (interquartile range) or count (percentage)[a]

Abbreviation: *ARB* angiotensin II receptor blocker; *ACEI* angiotensin-converting enzyme inhibitor, *HDL* high-density lipoprotein, *LDL* low-density lipoprotein, *ALT* alanine aminotransferase, *AST* aspartate aminotransferase, *eCCr* estimated creatinine clearance rate, *hs-CRP* high-sensitivity C-reactive protein, *ADMA* asymmetric dimethylarginine, *NT-proBNP* N-terminal pro-brain natriuretic peptide, *AGE* advanced glycation end product, *sRAGE* soluble form of receptor for AGE, *AGE/sRAGE* ratio of levels of AGE to soluble form of RAGE

between 88 patients with end-stage renal disease and 20 healthy people. Regarding the performance of identifying patients with end-stage renal disease, the results of receiver operating characteristic revealed that AGE/sRAGE had higher area under the curve of 0.918 than the ratio of AGE to endogenous secretory RAGE and the ratio

Table 2 Univariate and multivariate analysis for associated factors of albuminuria by logistic regression model with forward stepwise method

		Univariate		Multivariate	
		OR (95% CI)	P	OR (95% CI)	P
Age (year)		1.002 (0.97–1.035)	0.191		
Gender	Male	–	–		
	Female	0.936 (0.387–2.262)	0.883		
Smoking	Not smoker	–	–		
	Past smoker	0.915 (0.303–2.765)	0.875		
	Current smoker	0.677 (0.168–2.730)	0.584		
Body mass index		1.046 (0.909–1.202)	0.531		
Heart rate (/min)		1.001 (0.970–1.034)	0.928		
Systolic blood pressure (mmHg)		1.034 (1.010–1.059)	0.006		
Diastolic blood pressure (mmHg)		1.040 (1.006–1.076)	0.022		
Pulse pressure (mmHg)		1.040 (1.002–1.079)	0.038	1.020 (0.979–1.062)	0.350
Number of drugs		1.775 (1.074–2.934)	0.025	1.986 (1.082–3.645)	0.027
Impaired fasting glucose		1.206 (0.516–2.822)	0.665		
Laboratory					
Total cholesterol (mg/dl)		1.003 (0.991–1.016)	0.607		
Triglycerides (mg/dL)		1.001 (0.998–1.005)	0.541		
HDL (mg/dL)		1.002 (0.958–1.048)	0.927		
LDL (mg/dL)		1.001 (0.988–1.014)	0.933		
Fasting glucose (mg/dL)		1.002 (0.966–1.039)	0.931		
ALT (U/L)		0.979 (0.913–1.048)	0.538		
AST (U/L)		1.113 (0.998–1.241)	0.055	1.095 (0.962–1.246)	0.169
Uric acid (mg/dL)		1.220 (0.921–1.616)	0.166		
eCCr (mL/min)		0.989 (0.973–1.004)	0.149		
hs-CRP (mg/dL)		1.227 (0.501–3.002)	0.654		
Adiponectin (µg/mL)		0.994 (0.973–1.017)	0.622		
ADMA (µmol/L)		1.575 (0.003–732.211)	0.885		
NT-proBNP (pg/mL)		1.011 (1.000–1.022)	0.049	1.015 (1.001–1.030)	0.030
AGE (µg/mL)		1.208 (0.838–1.741)	0.311		
sRAGE (pg/ml)		0.999 (0.996–1.001)	0.189		
AGE/sRAGE (µg/pg)		1.109 (1.005–1.224)	0.039	1.131 (1.001–1.278)	0.048

Abbreviation: *ARB* angiotensin II receptor blocker, *ACEI* angiotensin-converting enzyme inhibitor, *HDL* high-density lipoprotein; *LDL* low-density lipoprotein; alanine aminotransferase, *eCCr* estimated creatinine clearance rate, *hs-CRP* high-sensitivity C-reactive protein, *ADMA* asymmetric dimethylarginine, *NT-proBNP* N-terminal pro-brain natriuretic peptide, *AGE* advanced glycation end product, *sRAGE* soluble form of receptor for AGE, *AGE/sRAGE* ratio of levels of AGE to soluble form of RAGE

of AGE to cleaved RAGE. The findings suggested that AGE/sRAGE is a better risk biomarker for end-stage renal disease [22]. Our study examined the role of AGE/sRAGE in relation to albuminuria, a strong clinical surrogate for cardiovascular diseases, in patients with essential hypertension. We observed that AGE/sRAGE was independently associated with presence of albuminuria (OR = 1.131, P = 0.048), but either AGE or sRAGE alone did not. Our results provide further support to the above evidence that AGE/sRAGE is a better biomarker for AGE-RAGE axis. Additionally,

our results were also consistent with the above studies that AGE/sRAGE was positively associated with early-stage of atherosclerosis. However, the causal relationship between AGE/sRAGE and albuminuria as well as the prognostic performance of AGE/sRAGE deserve more investigations in the future longitudinal cohort study.

Many pharmaceutical studies have already applied AGE, RAGE, or sRAGE as a beneficial endpoint. Simvastatin stabilized plaque in type 2 diabetes by suppression of RAGE [24]. Enalapril/lercanidipine combination and nifedipine/telmisartan increased sRAGE [25, 26]. AGE were decreased after 6 and 12 months valsartan therapy [27]. But another study showed that irbesartan does not influence AGE in patients with type 2 diabetes and microalbuminuria [28]. Those findings triggered us to clarify the interactions between sRAGE and AGE and the clinical role of AGE/sRAGE as a biomarker, whereas the investigation of either AGE or sRAGE alone may result in insignificance [28]. In this way, we may understand more deeply the pharmaceutical benefits, which may decrease AGE formation and increase sRAGE effects to reduce cardiovascular risks [25, 26, 29–31]. Our study also found that the number of antihypertensive agents was also one of the associated factor of albuminuria. As the number of antihypertensive agents reflected the severity of hypertension and medication could influence the concentration of AGE and sRAGE, further studies are warranted to explore the causal relationship among AGE/sRAGE, medications, and clinical outcomes.

Some limitations should be considered in this study. First, the study population was composed of participants with hypertension merely; therefore, the results cannot be generalized to normal individuals. The results also may not applied in patients with previous or present cardiovascular events because this study did not include this group of patients. The observed association can only provide information for clinical judgment and risk stratification. Second, concentration of total sRAGE were measured; therefore, specific sRAGE variants could not be discriminated. Third, this is a cross-sectional study. Further studies will be necessary for the biomarker's prognostic value.

Conclusion

This study found that the ratio of AGE to sRAGE was independently associated with the existence of albuminuria in hypertensive patients. The results suggest that the ratio of AGE to sRAGE may be a surrogate biomarker for microvascular injury. Further prospective studies of the prognostic value of the ratio in relation to microvasular injury are needed.

Abbreviations

AGE: Advanced glycation end-products; AST: Aspartate aminotransferase; BMI: Body mass index; DBP: Diastolic blood pressure; eCCr: Estimated creatinine clearance rate; ELISA: Enzyme-linked immunosorbent assay; HDL: High density lipoproteins; hsCRP: High-sensitive C-reactive protein; LDL: Low-density lipoprotein; NT-proBNP: N-terminal prohormone of brain natriuretic peptide; RAGE: Receptor for advanced glycation end-products; SBP: Systolic blood pressure; sRAGE: Soluble receptor for advanced glycation end-products

Acknowledgements

None.

Funding

This research did not receive any specific grant from funding agencies in the public, commercial, or not-for-profit sectors.

Authors' contributions

CKH, CJW, LHB interpreted the results, drafted the manuscript, and approved the final submission. CKH, CJW, LHB coordinated the data collection process, reviewed the manuscript. CKH, HSS, LSJ carried out the initial analyses. CJW, HSS interpreted the pathology and gave description. HSS, LSJ conceptualized the study and supervised the lab operation. HPH designed the data collection process, supervised data collection, and critically reviewed the manuscript. All authors read and approved the final manuscript.

Competing interests

The authors declare that they have no competing interests.

Author details

[1]Division of Cardiology and Cardiovascular Research Center, Department of Internal Medicine, Taipei Medical University Hospital, Taipei, Taiwan. [2]Graduate Institute of Biomedical Electronics and Bioinformatics, National Taiwan University, Taipei, Taiwan. [3]Division of Cardiology, Department of Internal Medicine, Taipei Veterans General Hospital, Taipei, Taiwan. [4]Department of Medical Research and Education, Taipei Veterans General Hospital, Taipei, Taiwan. [5]Cardiovascular Research Center, National Yang-Ming University, Taipei, Taiwan. [6]Institute of Pharmacology, National Yang-Ming University, Taipei, Taiwan. [7]Healthcare and Service Center, Taipei Veterans General Hospital, Taipei, Taiwan. [8]Institute of Clinical Medicine, National Yang-Ming University, Taipei, Taiwan. [9]Department of Internal Medicine, School of Medicine, College of Medicine, Taipei Medical University, Taipei, Taiwan.

References

1. Pontremoli R. Microalbuminuria in essential hypertension--its relation to cardiovascular risk factors. Nephrol Dial Transplant. 1996;11(11):2113–5.
2. Pontremoli R, Ravera M, Bezante GP, Viazzi F, Nicolella C, Berruti V, Leoncini G, Del Sette M, Brunelli C, Tomolillo C, et al. Left ventricular geometry and function in patients with essential hypertension and microalbuminuria. J Hypertens. 1999;17(7):993–1000.
3. Leoncini G, Sacchi G, Ravera M, Viazzi F, Ratto E, Vettoretti S, Parodi D, Bezante GP, Del Sette M, Deferrari G, et al. Microalbuminuria is an integrated marker of subclinical organ damage in primary hypertension. J Hum Hypertens. 2002;16(6):399–404.
4. Viazzi F, Leoncini G, Ratto E, Vaccaro V, Tomolillo C, Falqui V, Parodi A, Conti N, Deferrari G, Pontremoli R. Microalbuminuria, blood pressure load, and systemic vascular permeability in primary hypertension. Am J Hypertens. 2006;19(11):1183–9.
5. Jensen JS, Feldt-Rasmussen B, Strandgaard S, Schroll M, Borch-Johnsen K. Arterial hypertension, microalbuminuria, and risk of ischemic heart disease. Hypertension. 2000;35(4):898–903.
6. Asselbergs FW, de Boer RA, Diercks GF, Langeveld B, Tio RA, de Jong PE, van Veldhuisen DJ, van Gilst WH. Vascular endothelial growth factor: the link between cardiovascular risk factors and microalbuminuria? Int J Cardiol. 2004;93(2–3):211–5.
7. Heerspink HJ, Ninomiya T, Persson F, Brenner BM, Brunel P, Chaturvedi N, Desai AS, Haffner SM, McMurray JJ, Solomon SD, Pfeffer MA, Parving HH, de Zeeuw D. Is a reduction in albuminuria associated with renal and cardiovascular protection? A post hoc analysis of the ALTITUDE trial. Diabetes Obes Metab. 2016;18(2):169–77.
8. Asselbergs FW, Hillege HL, van Gilst WH. Framingham score and microalbuminuria: combined future targets for primary prevention? Kidney Int Suppl. 2004;92:S111–4.
9. Stirban A, Gawlowski T, Roden M. Vascular effects of advanced glycation endproducts: clinical effects and molecular mechanisms. Mol Metab. 2014;3(2):94–108.

10. Yamagishi S, Matsui T. Soluble form of a receptor for advanced glycation end products (sRAGE) as a biomarker. Front Biosci (Elite Ed). 2010;2:1184–95.

11. Park L, Raman KG, Lee KJ, Lu Y, Ferran LJ Jr, Chow WS, Stern D, Schmidt AM. Suppression of accelerated diabetic atherosclerosis by the soluble receptor for advanced glycation endproducts. Nat Med. 1998;4(9):1025–31.

12. Schmidt AM, Yan SD, Wautier JL, Stern D. Activation of receptor for advanced glycation end products: a mechanism for chronic vascular dysfunction in diabetic vasculopathy and atherosclerosis. Circ Res. 1999; 84(5):489–97.

13. Fujisawa K, Katakami N, Kaneto H, Naka T, Takahara M, Sakamoto F, Irie Y, Miyashita K, Kubo F, Yasuda T, et al. Circulating soluble RAGE as a predictive biomarker of cardiovascular event risk in patients with type 2 diabetes. Atherosclerosis. 2013;227(2):425–8.

14. Falcone C, Emanuele E, D'Angelo A, Buzzi MP, Belvito C, Cuccia M, Geroldi D. Plasma levels of soluble receptor for advanced glycation end products and coronary artery disease in nondiabetic men. Arterioscler Thromb Vasc Biol. 2005;25(5):1032–7.

15. Hanssen NM, Beulens JW, van Dieren S, Scheijen JL, van der AD, Spijkerman AM, van der Schouw YT, Stehouwer CD, Schalkwijk CG. Plasma advanced glycation end products are associated with incident cardiovascular events in individuals with type 2 diabetes: a case-cohort study with a median follow-up of 10 years (EPIC-NL). Diabetes. 2015;64(1):257–65.

16. Kizer JR, Benkeser D, Arnold AM, Ix JH, Mukamal KJ, Djousse L, Tracy RP, Siscovick DS, Psaty BM, Zieman SJ. Advanced glycation/glycoxidation endproduct carboxymethyl-lysine and incidence of coronary heart disease and stroke in older adults. Atherosclerosis. 2014;235(1):116–21.

17. Busch M, Franke S, Wolf G, Brandstadt A, Ott U, Gerth J, Hunsicker LG, Stein G. The advanced glycation end product N(epsilon)-carboxymethyllysine is not a predictor of cardiovascular events and renal outcomes in patients with type 2 diabetic kidney disease and hypertension. Am J Kidney Dis. 2006;48(4):571–9.

18. Prasad K. Low levels of serum soluble receptors for advanced glycation end products, biomarkers for disease state: myth or reality. Int J Angiol. 2014;23(1):11–6.

19. Tahara N, Yamagishi S, Tahara A, Ishibashi M, Hayabuchi N, Takeuchi M, Imaizumi T. Adiponectin is inversely associated with ratio of serum levels of AGEs to sRAGE and vascular inflammation. Int J Cardiol. 2012;158(3):461–2.

20. Tahara A, Tahara N, Yamagishi SI, Honda A, Igata S, Nitta Y, Bekki M, Nakamura T, Sugiyama Y, Sun J, et al. Ratio of serum levels of AGEs to soluble RAGE is correlated with trimethylamine-N-oxide in non-diabetic subjects. Int J Food Sci Nutr. 2017;68(8):1013–20.

21. Kajikawa M, Nakashima A, Fujimura N, Maruhashi T, Iwamoto Y, Iwamoto A, Matsumoto T, Oda N, Hidaka T, Kihara Y, et al. Ratio of serum levels of AGEs to soluble form of RAGE is a predictor of endothelial function. Diabetes Care. 2015;38(1):119–25.

22. Prasad K, Dhar I, Zhou Q, Elmoselhi H, Shoker M, Shoker A. AGEs/sRAGE, a novel risk factor in the pathogenesis of end-stage renal disease. Mol Cell Biochem. 2016;423(1–2):105–14.

23. Machahua C, Montes-Worboys A, Llatjos R, Escobar I, Dorca J, Molina-Molina M, Vicens-Zygmunt V. Increased AGE-RAGE ratio in idiopathic pulmonary fibrosis. Respir Res. 2016;17(1):144.

24. Cuccurullo C, Iezzi A, Fazia ML, De Cesare D, Di Francesco A, Muraro R, Bei R, Ucchino S, Spigonardo F, Chiarelli F, et al. Suppression of RAGE as a basis of simvastatin-dependent plaque stabilization in type 2 diabetes. Arterioscler Thromb Vasc Biol. 2006;26(12):2716–23.

25. Derosa G, Bonaventura A, Romano D, Bianchi L, Fogari E, D'Angelo A, Maffioli P. Effects of enalapril/lercanidipine combination on some emerging biomarkers in cardiovascular risk stratification in hypertensive patients. J Clin Pharm Ther. 2014;39(3):277–85.

26. Falcone C, Buzzi MP, Bozzini S, Boiocchi C, D'Angelo A, Schirinzi S, Esposito C, Torreggiani M, Choi J, Ochan Kilama M, et al. Microalbuminuria and sRAGE in high-risk hypertensive patients treated with nifedipine/telmisartan combination treatment: a substudy of TALENT. Mediat Inflamm. 2012;2012:874149.

27. Komiya N, Hirose H, Saisho Y, Saito I, Itoh H. Effects of 12-month valsartan therapy on glycation and oxidative stress markers in type 2 diabetic subjects with hypertension. Int Heart J. 2008;49(6):681–9.

28. Engelen L, Persson F, Ferreira I, Rossing P, Hovind P, Teerlink T, Stehouwer CD, Parving HH, Schalkwijk CG. Irbesartan treatment does not influence plasma levels of the advanced glycation end products N(epsilon)(1-carboxymethyl)lysine and N(epsilon)(1-carboxyethyl)lysine in patients with type 2 diabetes and microalbuminuria. A randomized controlled trial. Nephrol Dial Transplant. 2011;26(11):3573–7.

29. Gugliucci A, Menini T. The axis AGE-RAGE-soluble RAGE and oxidative stress in chronic kidney disease. Adv Exp Med Biol. 2014;824:191–208.

30. Quade-Lyssy P, Kanarek AM, Baiersdorfer M, Postina R, Kojro E. Statins stimulate the production of a soluble form of the receptor for advanced glycation end products. J Lipid Res. 2013;54(11):3052–61.

31. Rabbani N, Adaikalakoteswari A, Rossing K, Rossing P, Tarnow L, Parving HH, Thornalley PJ. Effect of Irbesartan treatment on plasma and urinary markers of protein damage in patients with type 2 diabetes and microalbuminuria. Amino Acids. 2012;42(5):1627–39.

25

Bisphenol A exposure and type 2 diabetes mellitus risk: a meta-analysis

Semi Hwang[1], Jung-eun Lim[1], Yoonjeong Choi[2] and Sun Ha Jee[1]*

Abstract

Background: This meta-analytic study explored the relationship between the risk of type 2 diabetes mellitus (T2DM) and bisphenol A concentrations.

Methods: The Embase and Medline (PubMed) databases were searched, using relevant keywords, for studies published between 1980 and 2018. A total of 16 studies, twelve cross-sectional, two case-control and one prospective, were included in the meta-analysis. The odds ratio (OR) and its 95% confidence interval (CI) were determined across the sixteen studies. The OR and its 95% CI of diabetes associated with bisphenol A were estimated using both fixed-effects and random-effects models.

Results: A total of 41,320 subjects were included. Fourteen of the sixteen studies included in the analysis provided measurements of urine bisphenol A levels and two study provided serum bisphenol A levels. Bisphenol A concentrations in human bio-specimens showed positive associations with T2DM risk (OR 1.28, 95% CI 1.14, 1.44). A sensitivity analysis indicated that urine bisphenol A concentrations were positively associated with T2DM risk (OR 1.20, 95% CI 1.09, 1.31).

Conclusions: This meta-analysis indicated that Bisphenol A exposure is positively associated with T2DM risk in humans.

Keywords: Bisphenol a (BPA), Endocrine disrupting chemicals (EDCs), Diabetes mellitus (DM), Type 2 diabetes mellitus (T2DM), Hemoglobin A1c (HbA1c), Fasting plasma glucose, Obesity, Meta-analysis

Background

Type 2 diabetes mellitus (T2DM) is a metabolic disease that presents with symptoms of insulin resistance and lack of insulin [1]. The global prevalence of T2DM among adults is about 415million, but based on projections by the International Federation of Diabetes is expected to reach 642 million in 2040 [2, 3].

Bisphenol A (BPA) is a role for endocrine disrupting chemicals (EDCs) and especially used in epoxy resin and polycarbonate plastic products such as food packaging, drink containers, and dental sealants [4–7]. Once the EDCs is deposited in the body, they can interfere with the physiological effects of estrogen, androgen and thyroid hormones by functioning as a hormone agonists and antagonists. Especially, BPA or EDCs interfere with cell signal pathways related to weight and glucose homeostasis. A number of previous experimental and epidemiological studies have found that EDCs can penetrate the body in several ways, including dietary intake, inhalation, skin contact, and other pathways. Thus, EDCs may have been associated with mainly the occurrence of hormone-like effects disorders and even cancers [7].

Competitive with 17- beta estradiol (E2), BPA is a type of endocrine disrupting chemical (EDCs) that disrupts estrogenic response by binding to estrogen receptors. BPA binds to androgen receptors and thyroid receptors. Unfortunately, humans are exposed to BPA through the daily exposure to BPA containing products such as canned food, plastic products, dental sealants, and household dust [7, 8].

In recent studies, research findings suggest that low levels of BPA can cause significant health problems. A number of scientists hypothesized that adverse health effects might be associated with high urinary BPA concentrations. Epidemiological studies have been carried out to evaluate the possible association between BPA exposure and the risk of T2DM, but the results were not consistent [9–24].

* Correspondence: jsunha@yuhs.ac
[1]Department of Epidemiology and Health Promotion, Institute for Health Promotion, Graduate School of Public Health, Yonsei University, 50-1 Yonsei-ro, Seodaemun-gu, Seoul 03722, Republic of Korea
Full list of author information is available at the end of the article

In this study, a meta-analysis focusing on the association between BPA concentrations (measured in urine or serum) and the risk of T2DM was performed. In addition, subgroup analyses were performed according to the sample type (urine or serum) and the study design.

Methods

Study selection

Figure 1 shows a PRISMA flow diagram that describes the selection process of this meta-analysis (Additional file 1: Table S1). As shown in the figure, the Embase and Medline (PubMed) databases were searched between 1980 and 2018 using Medical Subject Headings (MeSH) terms related to BPA and diabetes.

The keywords used in the Embase and Medline (PubMed) database searches were: Bisphenol A, BPA, 4, 4 isopropylidenediphenol or Bisphenol A bis (2 hydroxypropyl) ether dimethacrylate and Noninsulin dependent diabetes mellitus or Type 2 diabetes or Diabetes Mellitus, Type 2 or Diabetes Mellitus, Noninsulin-Dependent or Diabetes Mellitus, Ketosis-Resistant or Diabetes Mellitus, Fasting blood sugar or Fasting plasma glucose or Blood glucose, HbA1c or Glycosylated hemoglobin or Hemoglobin A1cor Glycated Hemoglobin A or Hemoglobin A, Glycated. A total of 420 articles were found: 246 were from Embase and 174 were from Medline (PubMed). First, 139 duplicated articles were

removed., After, an initial review, 148 studies were excluded; 85 studies were not human research such as animal and invitro experiment, 43 studies had irrelevant exposures or outcomes and 20 studies were reviews or meta-analyses papers. Next, 133 studies were selected for full-text article review. From these studies, 117 studies, including 44 studies were not human research, 38 with irrelevant exposures or outcomes, 10 studies were reviews or meta-analyses, 22 were letter or book or comment papers, and 3 had not find full text from the same database were excluded. Finally, a total of 16 articles were included in this meta-analysis (Fig. 1).

Data extraction

Data extraction was completed twice by two reviewers, Hwang, S. and Lim, J.E. independently, with no disagreement in the selection of the final sixteen articles [9–24]. The reviewers selected the variables while considering authors, year of publication, country, type of study, type of sample, unit of measurement, population, comparison categories, and adjusted odds ratios (OR) with corresponding confidence intervals, and model adjustments. To be included in the meta-analysis, a published study had to be the original article published between 1980 and 2018. A total of 16 studies published between September, 2008 and January, 2018 were selected for final inclusion. We conducted quality assessment using the

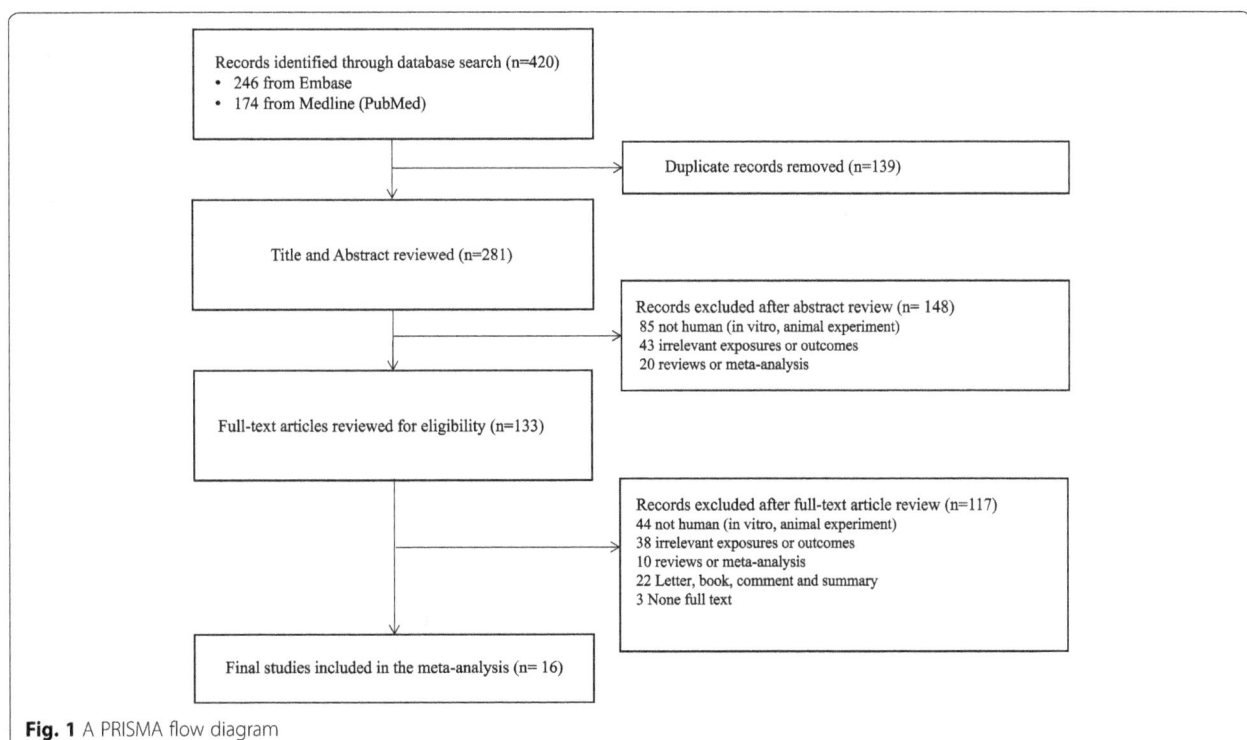

Fig. 1 A PRISMA flow diagram

Downs and Black score [25]. The average quality score was 16 with scores ranging from 13 to 18.

Statistical analyses

Odds ratios (OR) and 95% confidence intervals (95% CI) were obtained from the selected articles using the standard guidelines for meta-analysis [26]. Fixed-effects model and random-effects model were implemented. Heterogeneity was tested using the Cochrane Q-test and I^2 statistic, considering an I^2 value > 50% as indicative of substantial heterogeneity. A study with a significantly high OR was omitted from the meta-analysis to avoid overrepresentation. Analyses were performed by sub-groups: type of sample (serum or urine), and type of study (cross-sectional, case-control and prospective) as possible sources of heterogeneity. A Begg's Funnel Plot and an Egger's Regression Test were conducted to minimize publication bias and asymmetry of the studies. When publication bias exists, the Begg's Funnel Plot is asymmetric, or the Egger's Test P-value < 0.05 [27].

To adjust for the cross-study differences between the BPA concentration units and the range of measured values, a dose-response meta-analysis (DRMA) was implemented. The dose-response meta-analyses (DRMA) was implemented by using the STATA GLST command [28] on a sample off our studies (Additional file 2: Figure S2).

Statistical analyses were performed using STATA version 13.0 software (Stata Corp, College Station, Texas).

Results

The 420 studies were searched using a systematic search strategy, referring to the PRISMA flow chart that describes the selection process of the meta-analysis [29]. After the duplicate records were removed, each article was reviewed by title, abstract, and full-text. Sixteen studies, 12 cross-sectional, 3 case-control and 1 prospective studies remained. A total of 6855 diabetic patients from among 141,320 subjects were included in the study.

Table 1 represents the characteristics of the studies included in the meta-analysis. The selected studies were performed in the USA, Korea, Iran, China and Thailand. While using funnel plot asymmetry to detect publication bias and applying Egger's regression test to measure for asymmetry, a very low publication bias was confirmed .

BPA exposure was positively associated with the risk of T2DM (Fig. 2). The pooled OR of the random-effects model was 1.28 (95% CI, 1.14–1.44). Figure 3 presents the forest plot of sensitivity analysis after three studies were excluded, one for exhibiting highly heterogeneous results (OR 57.60; 95% CI 21.10–157.05) [20] and two for using serum BPA concentrations [22, 24].

In Fig. 4 and Additional file 2: Figure S2, the funnel plot shows publication bias in the meta-analysis. Of the studies used in 16 final meta-analysis, only five were found to have no bias, four using urine BPA and one with serum BPA.

Discussion

In this meta-analysis, we observed that the exposure of BPA was associated with an increased risk of T2DM. Both urine and serum BPA levels were positively associated with the risk of T2DM. The results of this study showed pooled OR of 1.28 (95% CI 1.14–1.44).

Previous studies have identified that the association between urinary BPA levels and T2DM may be biologically feasible. For example, BPA, an estrogen agonist that acts as an endocrine hormone disruptor, has been shown to be involved in several mechanisms of diabetes development including glucose homeostasis, obesity, insulin resistance, beta-cell dysfunction, inflammation, and oxidative stress [30]. BPA binding to estrogen receptors (ER) at concentrations at the physiological range or below can disrupt the pancreatic islets of Langherans, which are an essential tissue responsible for glucose metabolism [31]. BPA binding to pancreatic islet cells can induce impaired insulin or glucagon secretion, leading to an insulin-resistant state. In animal studies, adult mice exposed to low-dose BPA displayed both hyperinsulinemia and insulin resistance that are associated with pancreatic beta-cell dysfunction [32]. BPA can also act on peripheral insulin-sensitive tissues like muscle, liver, and adipose tissue [31]. Several in-vivo studies reported that BPA exposed mice showed decreased levels of circulating adiponectin as well as dysregulation of insulin signaling in skeletal muscle and liver. The mice also showed increased levels of pro-inflammatory cytokines, such as interleukin-6 and tumor necrosis factors, which favor the development of insulin resistance [33]. Additionally, BPA has an obesogen effect resulting in the development of obesity and metabolic disorders. Sheep exposed to BPA during the prenatal period became overweight, experienced an increase in adipocyte mass, and in insulin resistance [34–36]. The induction by BPA of the insulin resistance that precedes T2DM is mainly seen when humans and animals are in a rapid growth phase. Some studies have shown that BPA exposure during pregnancy or childhood causes metabolic disorders in both humans and animals [37, 38]. However, further studies are needed to clarify the complete mechanisms of BPA exposure and T2DM risk.

Previous meta-analyses, have not implemented the dose-response analytic method used in this study to determine the relationship between BPA exposure and the risk of T2DM. A significant dose-response relationship was found between urinary BPA concentrations (mg/dL) and T2DM risk. In addition, subgroup analysis was performed according to the type of sample (urine or serum), and the type of study (cross-sectional, case-control and prospective

Table 1 Risk estimates and study information from abstracts of original studies on BPA concentration and type 2 diabetes mellitus

Reference	Country	Type of study	Used sample	Unit	Population (Case / Total)	Comparison categories	Adjusted OR	95% CI	Adjustment in model	Quality score
Lang et al. (2008) [9]	The United States	Cross-sectional	Urine	ng/mL	136 / 1455	BPA continuous	1.39	1.21–1.60	Age, sex, race/ethnicity, education, income, smoking, BMI, waist circumference and urinary creatinine concentrations,	17
Melzer et al. (2010) [10]	The United States	Cross-sectional	Urine	ng/mL	277 / 2947	BPA continuous	1.24	1.10–1.40	Age, sex, race/ethnicity, education, income, smoking, BMI, waist circumference, and urinary creatinine concentration.	18
Silver et al. (2011) [11]	The United States	Cross-sectional	Urine	ng/mL	540 / 4389	BPA continuous	1.08	1.02–1.16	Age, age^2, urinary creatinine as natural splines (restricted cubic splines) with 4 degrees of freedom (knots at 25th, 50th, and 75th percentiles), BMI, waist circumference, and smoking status.	17
Ning et al. (2011) [12]	The United States	Cross-sectional	Urine	ng/mL	1087 / 3423	BPA in quartiles Q1: ≤0.47, Q2: 0.48–0.81, Q3: 0.82–1.43, Q4: > 1.43	1.37	1.08–1.74	Age, sex, educational level, family history of diabetes, WC, systolic blood pressure, ln(TG level), ln(hsCRP level), ln(ALT level), estimated glomerular filtration rate, albumin level and total bilirubin level.	15
Shanker & Teppala (2011) [13]	The United States	Cross-sectional	Urine	ng/mL	467 / 3967	BPA in quartiles Q1: < 1.10, Q2: 1.10–2.10, Q3: 2.11–4.20, Q4: > 4.20	1.68	1.22–2.30	Age (years), gender, race-ethnicity (non-Hispanic whites, non-Hispanic blacks, Mexican-Americans, others), education categories (below high school, high school, above high school), smoking (never, former, current), alcohol intake (never, former, current), BMI (normal, overweight, obese), systolic and diastolic blood pressure (mm Hg), urinary creatinine (mg/dl), and total cholesterol (mg/dl).	16
Wang et al. (2011) [14]	China	Cross-sectional	Urine	ng/mL	1048 / 3390	BPA in quartiles Q1: ≤0.47, Q2: 0.48–0.81, Q3: 0.82–1.43, Q4: > 1.43	1.37	1.06–1.77	Age, sex, BMI, urinary creatinine concentration, smoking, alcohol drinking, education levels, systolic blood pressure, HDL-C, LDL-C, TC, TG, hs-CRP, fasting plasma glucose, fasting serum insulin, and serum ALT and GGT.	17
LaKind et al. (2012) [15]	The United States	Cross-sectional	Urine	ng/mL	4823	BPA continuous	0.995	0.982–1.007	Creatinine, age, gender, ethnicity, education, income, smoking, drinking, BMI, waist circumference, hypertension, total cholesterol and family history.	15
Kim & Park (2013) [16]	Korea	Cross-sectional	Urine	ng/mL	99 / 1210	BPA in quartiles Q1: < 1.36, Q2: 1.36–2.14, Q3: 2.15–3.32, Q4: > 3.32	1.71	0.89–3.26	Creatinine, age, sex, BMI, education, smoking, income and place of residence.	17

Table 1 Risk estimates and study information from abstracts of original studies on BPA concentration and type 2 diabetes mellitus (*Continued*)

Reference	Country	Type of study	Used sample	Unit	Population (Case / Total)	Comparison categories	Adjusted OR	95% CI	Adjustment in model	Quality score
Sabanayagam et al. (2013) [17]	The United States	Cross-sectional	Urine	ng/mL	1108 / 3516	BPA in tertiles Q1: < 1.3, Q2: 1.3–3.2, Q3: > 3.2	1.34	1.03–1.73	Age (years), gender (male, female), race-ethnicity (non-Hispanic whites, non-Hispanic blacks, Mexican Americans, others), education categories (below high school, high school, above high school), smoking (never, former, current), alcohol intake (never, former, current), body mass index (normal, overweight, obese), physical inactivity (absent, present), mean arterial blood pressure (mm of Hg), C-reactive protein and total cholesterol/HDL ratio	13
Casey & Neidell et al. (2013) [18]	The United States	Cross-sectional	Urine	ng/mL	487 / 4658	BPA continuous	1.065	0.973–1.166	Age, sex, urinary creatinine concentration, race/ethnicity, income, smoking, BMI, waist circumference, veteran/military status, citizenship status, marital status, household size, pregnancy status, language at subject interview, health insurance coverage, employment status in the prior week, consumption of bottled water in the past 24 h, consumption of alcohol, annual consumption of tuna fish, presence of emotional support in one's life, being on a diet, using a water treatment device, access to a routine source of health care, vaccinated for Hepatitis A or B, consumption of dietary supplements (vitamins or minerals), and inability to purchase balanced meals on a consistent basis.	16
Sun et al. (2014) [19]	The United States (NHS)	Case-control	Urine	µg/L	394 / 787	BPA in quartiles Q1: < 1.0, Q2: 1.0–1.5, Q3: 1.5–2.7, Q4: > 2.7	0.98	0.6–1.61	Age, ethnicity, fasting status, time of sample collection, menopausal status, use of hormone replacement therapy (NHSII), urinary creatinine levels, smoking, postmenopausal hormone use (NHS), oral contraceptive use (NHSII), physical activity, drinking, family history of diabetes, history of hypercholesterolemia or hypertension, Alternative Health Eating Index score, BMI	15
	The United States (NHS II)	Case-control	Urine	µg/L	577 / 1154	BPA in quartiles Q1: < 1.0, Q2: 1.0–1.5, Q3: 1.5–2.7, Q4: > 2.7	2.08	1.17–3.69		
Ahmadkhaniha et al. (2014) [20]	Iran	Case-control	Urine	µg/L	119 / 239	BPA in two groups based on the median (< 0.85 and ≥ 0.85 µg/L)	57.6	21.1–157.05	Age, sex, BMI, hypertension, serum triglyceride level, serum cholesterol level, serum creatinine (smoking and consumption of sugared drinks in plastic bottles or canned food in two past weeks were exclusion criteria)	15
Andra S.S. et al. (2015) [21]	The United States	Cross-sectional	Urine	ng/mL	20/ 131	BPA continuous	0.77	0.24–2.04	Age, sex, BMI, fasting status, smoking, alcohol use, physical activity and family history	18

Table 1 Risk estimates and study information from abstracts of original studies on BPA concentration and type 2 diabetes mellitus (*Continued*)

Reference	Country	Type of study	Used sample	Unit	Population (Case / Total)	Comparison categories	Adjusted OR	95% CI	Adjustment in model	Quality score
Aekplakorn W et al. (2015) [22]	The Thailand	Cross-sectional	Serum	ng/mL	23 / 2558	BPA in quartiles Q1: < 1.0, Q2: 1.0–2.0, Q3: 2.0–3.7, Q4: > 3.7	1.88	1.18–2.99	Age, sex, urinary creatinine, race, education, smoking, physical activity, dietary energy intake and survey wave	17
Bi Y. et al. (2016) [23]	China	prospective	Urine	ng/mL	241 / 2209	BPA in quartiles	0.78	0.53–1.16	Age, sex, family history of diabetes, BMI (for weighted GRS), and further for smoking status, systolic blood pressure, diastolic blood pressure, lg (total cholesterol), lg (triglycerides), fasting plasma glucose,and lg (urinary creatinine) for BPA.	16
Shu et al. (2018) [24]	China	Case-control	Serum	ng/mL	232 / 464	BPA in tertiles	0.93	0.41–2.13	Age, sex, BMI, exercise, current smoking, systolic blood pressure, diastolic blood pressure, fasting plasma glucose, 2-h plasma glucose in oral glucose tolerance test, total cholesterol, triglyceride, high-density lipoprotein cholesterol and low-density lipoprotein cholesterol .	15

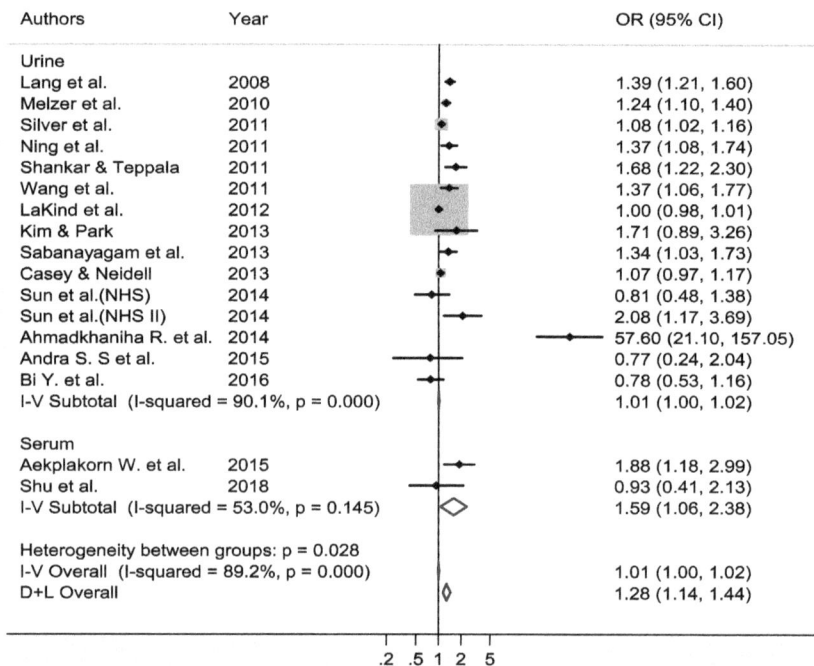

Fig. 2 Forest plot according to sample type

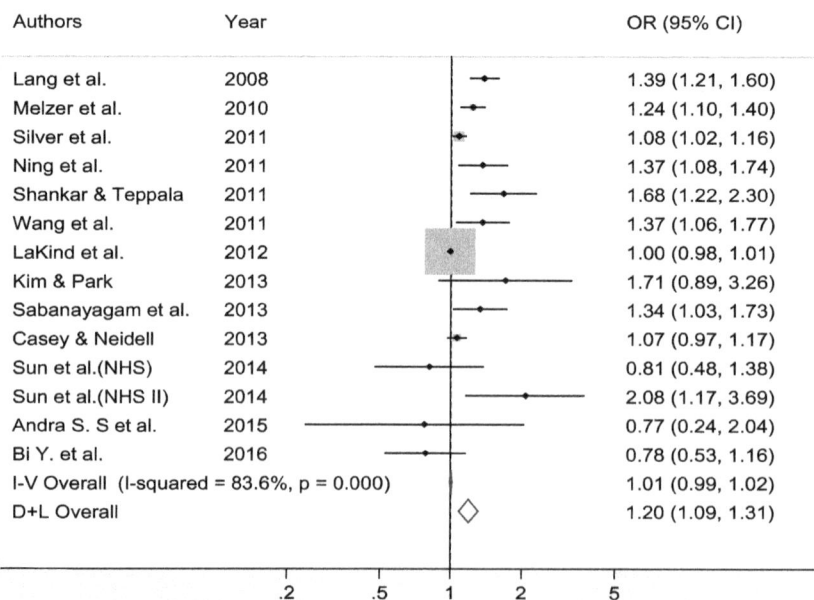

Fig. 3 Forest plot after exclusion of studies with serum BPA levels and high heterogeneity

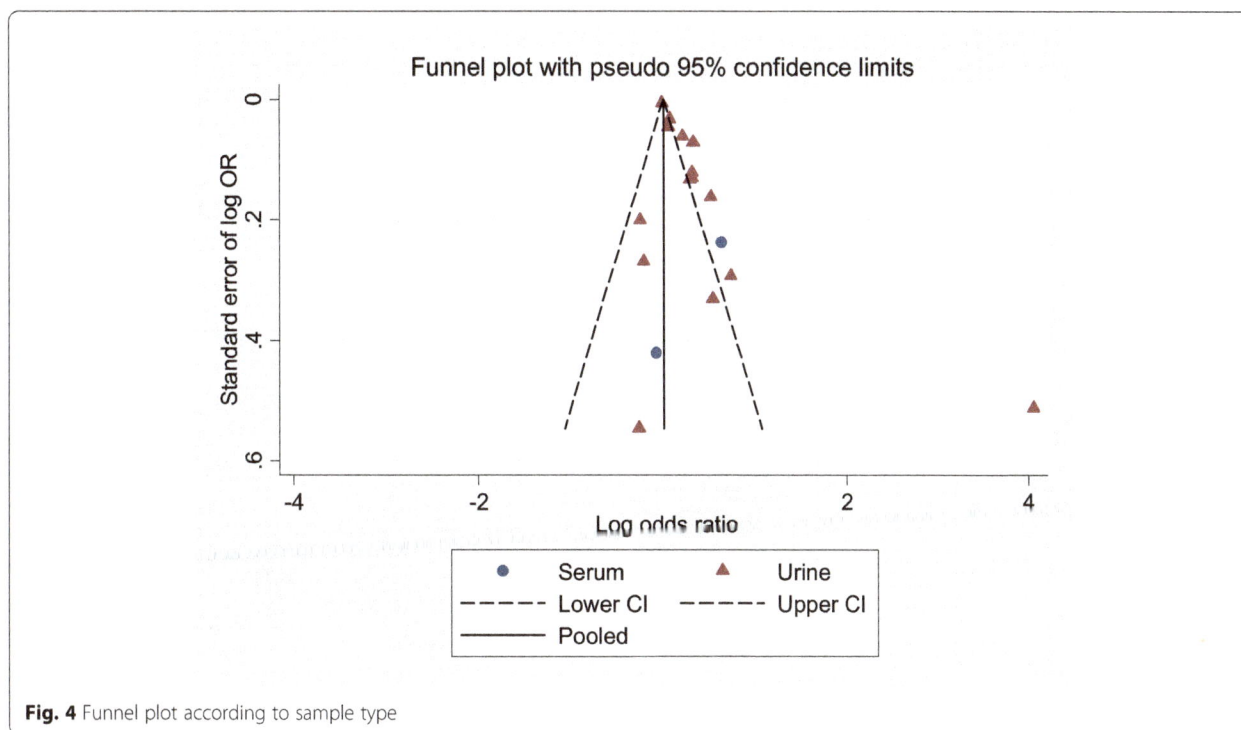

Fig. 4 Funnel plot according to sample type

study). Moreover, quality assessment methods were implemented to remove any irrelevant studies and to improve the validity of the meta-analysis. The current study considered only diabetes as a primary outcome variable as was the case with the final sixteen articles used for the meta-analysis. Despite the fact that diabetes mellitus is an important risk factor for cardiovascular disease, our study will focus specifically on T2DM, and as a result will be more focused and statistically significant than previous studies.

There were several limitations to the conduct and analysis in this study that must be considered. First, because of the limited number of cohort studies investigating the relationship between BPA exposure and T2DM risk that have been conducted, this meta-analysis included only thirteen cross-sectional, two case-control studies and one prospective studies. The inclusion of additional studies are required to validate and confirm these results. Second, this meta-analysis included fourteen studies which used spot urinary BPA concentrations and two study that used serum BPA concentrations as a surrogate marker of BPA exposure. It is unclear whether spot urinary BPA concentrations could accurately reflect the long term exposure level of BPA in individuals. Spot urinary BPA concentrations are the most commonly used method to assess BPA exposure levels because of it is short half-life and the convenience of the measurement method [11, 20]. Although some studies have demonstrated that spot urine samples can reasonably predict long-term exposures in adults [39, 40], the validity of

such results still needs to be proven. Some recent epidemiological studies used serum BPA concentrations to investigate the health effects of BPA [22, 40]. In these studies, the authors explained that serum BPA could be an appropriate surrogate for BPA exposure because serum BPA reflected the true levels of active BPA [22]. There is not sufficient information to determine the most suitable method for measuring BPA concentrations (e.g. spot urinary BPA concentrations, 24-h urinary BPA concentrations, serum BPA concentration) that accurately reflect the level of BPA exposure. Third, although linear relationships between BPA exposure and risk of T2DM were tested in this meta-analysis, several studies have suggested inverted U-shape or non-linear relationships [19, 21, 22]. To clarify this complex dose–response relationship, more detailed research is required. Fourth, a random effects model was implemented after performing statistical heterogeneity tests because of the significant effect that heterogeneity in inclusive studies could have on the meta-analystic results.

Conclusions

In conclusion, this meta-analysis demonstrated that BPA concentrations measured in urine or serum is positively associated with T2DM risk. Furthermore, prospective cohort studies, including carefully collected data about the dietary sources of BPA exposure and potential confounding, will help clarify the role of BPA in the pathogenesis of diabetes.

5s1624s i1te1seh

Abbreviations
BPA: Bisphenol A; CI: Confidence interval; EDC: Endocrine disrupting chemicals; OR: Odds ratio; T2DM : Type 2 diabetes mellitus

Acknowledgements
Not applicable

Funding
This research was funded by a grant (15162MFDS631) from the Ministry of Food and Drug Safety in 2015.

Authors' contributions
HS, LJE and JSH designed the study. HS collected the data and did the meta-analysis. HS, LJE contributed equally to the manuscript. CY discussed biological mechanism of in manuscript. HS, LJE and JSH contributed to study design and critically reviewed the paper. All authors read and approved the final manuscript.

Competing interests
The authors declare that they have no competing interests.

Author details
[1]Department of Epidemiology and Health Promotion, Institute for Health Promotion, Graduate School of Public Health, Yonsei University, 50-1 Yonsei-ro, Seodaemun-gu, Seoul 03722, Republic of Korea. [2]Department of Public Health, Graduate School, Yonsei University, Seoul, Republic of Korea.

References
1. Chamberlain JJ, Rhinehart AS, Shaefer CF Jr, Neuman A. Diagnosis and Management of Diabetes: synopsis of the 2016 American Diabetes Association standards of medical Care in Diabetes. Ann Intern Med. 2016; 164(8):542–52.
2. American Diabetes Association. Classification and diagnosis of diabetes. In: 2016 Standards of Medical Care in Diabetes. Diabetes Care. 2016;39:S13–22.
3. Ogurtsova K, da Rocha Fernandes JD, Huang Y, Linnenkamp U, Guariguata L, Cho NH, Cavan D, Shaw JE, Makaroff LE. IDF diabetes atlas: global estimates for the prevalence of diabetes for 2015 and 2040. Diabetes Res Clin Pract. 2017;128:40–50.
4. Arenholt-Bindslev D, Breinholt V, Preiss A, Schmalz G. Time-related bisphenol-a content and estrogenic activity in saliva samples collected in relation to placement of fissure sealants. Clin Oral Investig. 1999;3(3):120–5.
5. Sajiki J, Yonekubo J. Leaching of bisphenol a (BPA) to seawater from polycarbonate plastic and its degradation by reactive oxygen species. Chemosphere. 2003;51(1):55–62.
6. Calafat AM, Kuklenyik Z, Reidy JA, Caudill SP, Ekong J, Needham LL. Urinary concentrations of bisphenol a and 4-nonylphenol in a human reference population. Environ Health Perspect. 2005;113(4):391–5.
7. Stojanoska MM, Milosevic N, Milic N, Abenavoli L. The influence of phthalates and bisphenol a on the obesity development and glucose metabolism disorders. Endocrine. 2017;55(3):666–81.
8. Hu Y, Wen S, Yuan D, Peng L, Zeng R, Yang Z, Liu Q, Xu L, Kang D. The association between the environmental endocrine disruptor bisphenol a and polycystic ovary syndrome: a systematic review and meta-analysis. Gynecol Endocrinol. 2018;34(5):370–7.
9. Lang IA, Galloway TS, Scarlett A, Henley WE, Depledge M, Wallace RB, Melzer D. Association of urinary bisphenol a concentration with medical disorders and laboratory abnormalities in adults. JAMA. 2008;300(11):1303–10.
10. Melzer D, Rice NE, Lewis C, Henley WE, Galloway TS. Association of urinary bisphenol a concentration with heart disease: evidence from NHANES 2003/06. PLoS One. 2010;5:e8673.
11. Silver MK, O'Neill MS, Sowers MR, Park SK. Urinary bisphenol a and type-2 diabetes in US adults: data fromNHANES 2003-2008. PLoS One. 2011;6;e26868.
12. Ning G, et al. Relationship of urinary bisphenol a concentration to risk for prevalent type 2 diabetes in Chinese adults: a cross-sectional analysis. Ann Intern Med. 2011;155:368–74.
13. Shankar A, Teppala S. Relationship between urinary bisphenol a levels and diabetes mellitus. J Clin Endocrinol Metab. 2011;96(12):3822–6.
14. Wang T, Li M, Chen B, Xu M, Xu Y, Huang Y, Lu J, Chen Y, Wang W, Li X, Liu Y, Bi Y, Lai S, Ning G. Urinary bisphenol a (BPA) concentration associates with obesity and insulin resistance. J Clin Endocrinol Metab. 2012;97(2):E223–7.
15. LaKind JS, Goodman M, Naiman DQ. Use of NHANES data to link chemical exposures to chronic diseases: a cautionary tale. PLoS One. 2012;7(12): e51086.
16. Kim K, Park H. Association between urinary concentrations of bisphenol a and type 2 diabetes in Korean adults: a population-based cross-sectional study. Int J Hyg Environ Health. 2013;216(4):467–71.
17. Sabanayagam C, Teppala S, Shankar A. Relationship between urinary bisphenol a levelsand prediabetes among subjects free of diabetes. Acta Diabetol. 2013;50:625–31.
18. Casey MF. Disconcordance in statistical models of bisphenol a and chronic disease outcomes in NHANES 2003-08. PLoS One. 2013;8(11):e79944.
19. Sun Q, et al. Association of urinary concentrations of bisphenol a and phthalate metabolites with risk of type 2 diabetes: a prospective investigation in the nurses' health study (NHS) and NHSII cohorts. Environ Health Perspect. 2014;122:616–23.
20. Ahmadkhaniha R, Mansouri M, Yunesian M, Omidfar K, Jeddi MZ, Larijani B, Mesdaghinia A, Rastkari N. Association of urinary bisphenol a concentration with type-2 diabetes mellitus. J Environ Health Sci Eng. 2014;12(1):64.
21. Andra SS, Kalyvas H, Andrianou XD, Charisiadis P, Christophi CA, Makris KC. Preliminary evidence of the association between monochlorinated bisphenol a exposure and type II diabetes mellitus: a pilot study. J Environ Sci Health A Tox Hazard Subst Environ Eng. 2015;50(3):243–59.
22. Aekplakorn W, Chailurkit LO, Ongphiphadhanakul B. Association of serum bisphenol a with hypertension in thai population. Int J Hypertens. 2015;594189.
23. Bi Y, Wang W, Xu M, Wang T, Lu J, Xu Y, Dai M, Chen Y, Zhang D, Sun W, Ding L, Chen Y, Huang X, Lin L, Qi L, Lai S, Ning G. Diabetes genetic risk score modifies effect of bisphenol a exposure on deterioration in glucose metabolism. J Clin Endocrinol Metab. 2016;101(1):143–50.
24. Shu X, Tang S, Peng C, Gao R, Yang S, Luo T, Cheng Q, Wang Y, Wang Z, Zhen Q, Hu J, Li Q. Bisphenol a is not associated with a 5-year incidence of type 2 diabetes: a prospective nested case-control study. Acta Diabetol. 2018;55(4):369–75.
25. Dowans and Black. The feasibility of creating a checklist for the assessment of the methodological quality both of randomised and non-randomised studies of health care interventions . J Epidemiol Community Health. 1998; 52:377–384.
26. Borenstein M, Hedges LV, Higgins JPT, Rothstein HR. Introduction to Meta-Analysis. Wiley; 2009.
27. Begg CB, Mazumdar M. Operating characteristics of a rank correlation test for publication bias. Biometrics. 1994;50(4):1088–101.
28. Shim SR, Shin IS, Yoon BH, Bae JM. Dose-response meta-analysis using STATA software. J Health Info Stat. 2016;41(3):351–8.
29. Moher D, Liberati A, Tetzlaff J, Altman DG, The PRISMA. Preferred reporting items for systematic reviews and meta-analyses: the PRISMA statement. PLoS Med. 2009;6(7):e1000097.
30. Takeuchi T, Tsutsumi O, Ikezuki Y, et al. Positive relationship between androgen and the endocrine disruptor, bisphenol a, in normal women and women with ovarian dysfunction. Endocr J. 2004;21:165–9.
31. Alonso-Magdalena P, Morimoto S, Ripoll C, Fuentes E, Nadal A. The estrogenic effect of bisphenol a disrupts pancreatic beta-cell function in vivo and induces insulin resistance. Environ Health Perspect. 2006;114(1): 106–12.
32. Ariemma F, D'Esposito V, Liguoro D, Oriente F, Cabaro S, Liotti A, et al. Low-dose bisphenol-a impairs Adipogenesis and generates dysfunctional 3T3-L1 adipocytes. PLoS One. 2016;11(3):e0150762.
33. Moon MK, Jeong IK, Jung OT, Ahn HY, Kim HH, Park YJ, et al. Long-term oral exposure to bisphenol a induces glucose intolerance and insulin resistance. J Endocrinol. 2015;226:35–42.
34. Yadav A, Kataria MA, Saini V, Yadav A. Role of leptin and adiponectin in insulin resistance. Clin Chim Acta. 2013;417:80–4.
35. Trujillo ME, Scherer PE. Adiponectin–journey from an adipocyte secretory

protein to biomarker of the metabolic syndrome. J Intern Med. 2005;257: 167–75.

36. Veiga-Lopez A, Moeller J, Sreedharan R, Singer K, Lumeng CN, Ye W, et al. Developmental programming: interaction between prenatal BPA exposure and postnatal adiposity on metabolic variables in female sheep. Am J Physiol Endocrinol Metab. 2015;310:E238–47.

37. Menale C, Piccolo MT, Cirillo G, Calogero RA, Papparella A, Mita L, et al. Bisphenol A effects on gene expression in adipocytes from children: association with metabolic disorders. J Mol Endocrinol. 2015;54(3):289–303.

38. Chou WC, Chen JL, Lin CF, Chen YC, Shih FC, Chuang CY. Biomonitoring of bisphenol a concentrations in maternal and umbilical cord blood in regard to birth outcomes and adipokine expression:a birth cohort study in Taiwan. Environ Health A Glob Access Sci Source. 2011;10:94.

39. Mahalingaiah S, Meeker JD, Pearson KR, Calafat AM, Ye X, Petrozza J, Hauser R. Temporal variability and predictors of urinary bisphenol a concentrations in men and women. Environ Health Perspect. 2008;116(2):173–8.

40. Lin CY, Shen FY, Lian GW, Chien KL, Sung FC, Chen PC, Su TC. Association between levels of serum bisphenol a, a potentially harmful chemical in plastic containers, and carotid artery intima-media thickness in adolescents and young adults. Atherosclerosis. 2015;241(2):657–63.

26

Barriers and facilitators to taking on diabetes self-management tasks in pre-adolescent children with type 1 diabetes: a qualitative study

David Rankin[1]*[iD], Jeni Harden[1], Katharine Barnard[2], Louise Bath[3], Kathryn Noyes[3], John Stephen[4] and Julia Lawton[1]

Abstract

Background: When children with type 1 diabetes approach adolescence, they are encouraged to become more involved in diabetes self-management. This study explored the challenges pre-adolescent children encounter when self-managing diabetes and the factors which motivate and enable them to take on new diabetes-related tasks. A key objective was to inform the support offered to pre-adolescent children.

Methods: In-depth interviews using age-appropriate questioning with 24 children (aged 9–12 years) with type 1 diabetes. Data were analysed using an inductive, thematic approach.

Results: Children reported several barriers to taking on self-management tasks. As well as seeking respite from managing diabetes, children described relying on their parents to: perform the complex maths involved in working out carbohydrate content in food; calculate insulin doses if they did not use a bolus advisor; and administer injections or insert a cannula in hard-to-reach locations. Children described being motivated to take on diabetes tasks in order to: minimise the pain experienced when others administered injections; alleviate the burden on their parents; and participate independently in activities with their peers. Several also discussed being motivated to take on diabetes-management responsibilities when they started secondary school. Children described being enabled to take on new responsibilities by using strategies which limited the need to perform complex maths. These included using labels on food packaging to determine carbohydrate contents, or choosing foods with carbohydrate values they could remember. Many children discussed using bolus advisors with pre-programmed ratios and entering carbohydrate on food labels or values provided by their parents to calculate insulin doses. Several also described using mobile phones to seek advice about carbohydrate contents in food.

Conclusions: Our findings highlight several barriers which deter children from taking on diabetes self-management tasks, motivators which encourage them to take on new responsibilities, and strategies and technologies which enable them to become more autonomous. To limit the need to perform complex maths, children may benefit from using bolus advisors provided they receive regular review from healthcare professionals to determine and adjust pre-programmed insulin-to-carbohydrate ratios. Education and support should be age-specific to reflect children's changing involvement in self-managing diabetes.

Keywords: Type 1 diabetes, Children, Pre-adolescents, Self-management, Qualitative research

* Correspondence: a.d.rankin@ed.ac.uk
[1]The Usher Institute of Population Health Sciences and Informatics, University of Edinburgh, Edinburgh EH8 9AG, UK
Full list of author information is available at the end of the article

Background

Type 1 diabetes (T1D) is one of the most prevalent chronic diseases among children [1], and its incidence is rising globally by 2–3% per year [2]. Ensuring children are involved in diabetes-related care from an early age is considered essential to promoting optimal glycaemic control and minimising risk of long-term complications [3–5]. However, the daily demands of managing T1D are complex and difficult, including the requirement to undergo procedures such as frequent daily blood glucose monitoring, injecting (around 4 times daily) or inserting insulin pump infusion sets (at least every 2–3 days); regulating food intake and counting carbohydrate; calculating insulin doses; and recognising and taking action to prevent or treat hypoglycaemia and hyperglycaemia [6]. For these reasons, diabetes management is considered too difficult for young children to do independently and parental involvement and supervision remain critical throughout childhood. As children move towards adolescence, they are encouraged to gradually assume more responsibility for diabetes-related tasks [7], ideally working in partnership with their parents [8], in order to establish their own self-management practices [9].

Limited research has explored factors and considerations which prompt pre-adolescent children to take on more diabetes-related responsibilities and how they might be best supported to do so. When qualitative research has been undertaken with children, studies have tended to include participants up to 18 years [10–13], or report a mix of children's and parents' views together [12, 14], which makes extrapolation of the findings to pre-adolescents more challenging. Previous qualitative research has also tended to focus on specific aspects of managing diabetes in childhood, including: knowledge of the role of insulin and risks of high/low blood glucose [11, 15]; accounts of sharing care with adults [11, 14–16]; emotional responses to living with diabetes [10–12, 17–19]; knowledge of self-care [11, 13, 15]; and, views about managing diabetes at school [20–22] and attending paediatric diabetes clinics [23–25].

To supplement and enhance this research, we conducted interviews with children aged 9–12 years with T1D. Our aim was to understand and explore the challenges children in this age group encounter self-managing diabetes and the factors and considerations which motivate and enable them to take on new self-management tasks. A key objective was to identify ways in which pre-adolescent children can be better supported to take on responsibility for self-managing diabetes. The decision to focus on children aged 9–12 years was made because pre-adolescence is a critical stage of transition between young childhood where children are dependent on their parents and the teenage years where they become increasingly independent and autonomous [14, 26].

Methods

Study design

We used in-depth interviews and age-appropriate questioning, which incorporated optional play-based tasks, to elicit children's views. This design enabled each interview to be tailored to take into account differing ages and capabilities [27] and afforded the flexibility needed for children to discuss issues they perceived as salient, including those unanticipated at the study's outset [28]. Data collection and analysis took place concurrently, enabling issues identified in early interviews to inform areas explored in later ones in line with an inductive approach.

Recruitment and sample

Recruitment was undertaken in four Scottish paediatric diabetes centres located in diverse rural and urban catchment areas. After obtaining parents' permission, health professionals approached children during routine clinical consultations using an opt-in procedure. Purposive sampling was used to ensure there was diversity in terms of children's demographic and disease characteristics, and that approximately equal numbers of children using multiple daily injection (MDI) or pump regimens were recruited in line with usage by this age group across Scotland. To be eligible for the study, children needed to have been diagnosed at least 6 months to allow them to have had time to make emotional, physical and psychological adjustments to having T1D. Each participant, and their parents/carers, completed written, age-appropriate consent forms. Recruitment continued until data saturation was reached.

Data collection

Interviews were conducted DR who had received professional training on ways to involve young children in research and the use of age-appropriate methods. Interviews were informed by a topic guide developed in light of literature reviews and revised in light of emerging findings. During their interviews, children were offered opportunities to use participatory activities, including drawing and game-playing tasks, to prompt discussion [29, 30]. Relevant areas explored during the interviews are shown in Table 1. Face-to-face interviews took place between July 2016 and February 2017 with one third of children choosing to have a parent/carer present. Interviews averaged 45 min, were digitally recorded and transcribed in full.

Data analysis

Interviews were analysed by DR and JL using a thematic approach informed by the method of constant comparison. Both researchers read all participants' interviews in full before comparing them to identify issues and experiences which cut across different accounts [31]. Each researcher undertook their initial data analyses independently and

Table 1 Relevant areas explored in interview topic guides

• Children's views, and experiences of, being involved in managing diabetes.

• What do children recall about when and how they began to take on diabetes-related responsibilities; what were these tasks; and, why did they decide to become more involved?

• Children's perceptions of, and views about, the roles of significant others (e.g. parents, carers, family members, teachers, friends' parents) in helping them to manage diabetes.

• What are children's views about taking on new responsibilities for managing diabetes; what tasks do they envisage undertaking; and, what are their reasons for wanting to have more involvement?

wrote separate reports before meeting to discuss their interpretations and reach agreement on recurrent themes. A coding framework was then developed which captured key themes and contextual information needed to aid data interpretation. NVivo, a qualitative software package (QSR International, Doncaster, Australia), was used to facilitate data coding and retrieval and coded datasets were subjected to further in-depth analyses to identify sub-themes and illustrative quotations. Participants are referred to using unique identifiers throughout the paper.

Ethical approval was provided by the South East Scotland Research Ethics Committee 01, NHS Lothian (16-SS-0084).

Results

The sample comprised 24 children (see Table 2). In keeping with findings of other studies [32–34], children's involvement in diabetes related tasks, and the amount of support they received from their parents, was informed by their developmental maturity and individual needs. When invited to discuss their role and involvement in self-management, children highlighted various factors and

Table 2 Demographic characteristics of interview participants

Characteristic	N	%	Mean ± SD & range
Children (n = 24)			
Female	11	45.8	
Age – all children			10.3 ± 0.9, range 9–12
Female age at time of interview (Years)			10.4 ± 1.1, range 9–12
Male age at time of interview (Years)			10.2 ± 0.8, range 9–11
Female age at diagnosis (Years)			5.0 ± 3.0, range 1–10
Male age at diagnosis (Years)			6.7 ± 2.1, range 3–10
Diabetes duration – all children (Years since diagnosis)			4.3 ± 2.4, range 1–10
Regimen (at time of interview)			
Basal-Bolus	11	45.8	
CSII (Insulin pump)	13	54.2	

considerations which had influenced their decisions to assume new responsibilities. All but one participant chose to take part in a conventional interview, hence our findings focus exclusively on quotations elicited during face-to-face conversations. Below, we begin by exploring the factors and considerations which hindered children from taking on new responsibilities, followed by the motivators and tipping points informing their decisions to become more involved, before concluding with factors which helped them transition to having a more independent role in managing their diabetes.

Barriers to children taking on new self-management responsibilities

Over reliance on parents

Children reported how their parents undertook a range of diabetes management tasks on their behalf, including some which they described being competent to do themselves; in 015's case, to allow her respite from managing diabetes when at home, or in 014's, to allow her to have time to play:

"sometimes I'm too lazy to do it. It means when I'm on the couch and my mum and dad tell me to do my finger [blood glucose check], then I'll say, 'no, you just do it'. It's like mostly at night." (015, aged 10).

"at school I check myself and bolus. Em, but here [at home] I can't be bothered bolusing [administering insulin] (laughter). So my mum or dad does it. And they do my [blood glucose] checks here too because I just want to play." (014, aged 10).

Children of all ages also highlighted occasions when their parents undertook diabetes management tasks which they were normally capable of doing by themselves in order to protect them from harm. This included 005 who reported how her parents chose to administer insulin at times of day when they deemed she might be "too tired" to do so safely:

"I don't do the morning ones cause I'm too tired and I might make a mistake. So mum does my injections in the morning and dad does some of them in the evening... I kind of do about maybe 50% of my injections." (005, aged 11).

Lacking mathematical skills: Bewilderment when counting carbohydrate and calculating insulin doses

Virtually all children described experiencing difficulties with diabetes management tasks which required them to perform complex maths. This included determining the carbohydrate contents of meals and snacks which, as 008 noted, left them reliant on adult caregivers:

"there are some things that I just don't know at all about. And I tend to just do what other people tell me because I always have a fear that I'm doing something wrong. So I do tend to let other people take control." (008, aged 11).

A similar view was expressed by 012 who described knowing the carbohydrate value of specific items but being dependent on his father to work out carbohydrate in most foods, especially meals made from individual ingredients:

"I know one or two things, like the things that are my favourite number [but] my dad always does the calculating. And I'm always sitting there. I'm just like- I'm waiting for him to tell me them. I'm there like, 'What's the carbs? What's the carbs?'" (012, aged 9).

As many children also indicated, being unable to count carbohydrates meant they were sometimes unable to take part in activities with peers such as sleep-overs, going on school trips, or eating at friends' houses because, as 004 explained:

"[other] parents don't know what to do like if I'm having, or going to like somebody's for a barbecue, or something to eat, because they don't know how to weigh it" (004, aged 10).

Difficulties calculating insulin doses without access to a bolus advisor

Further challenges were reported by individuals who described struggling to apply ratios and perform the maths needed to determine their insulin doses because, as 001 (aged 10) explained: "a lot of the diabetes stuff is like times it by four, then divide it by two and when it comes to division or fractions or decimals, I'm just not very good". As 011, like others, discussed, this inability to perform complex maths, both to count carbohydrates and calculate insulin doses, meant he was dependent on his parents to undertake these tasks:

"she's [mother] really good at maths [and] she works out, like I think you work out everything about the jags [injections], and then I normally just turn it up to how many units, cause I hear her talk, like adding everything in her head, like she's talking to herself. I'm like: wow (laughter) I don't know what I'd do to learn that but it won't be anytime soon." (011, aged 10).

Accessing difficult to reach injection sites or locations to insert a cannula

Children also described having to rely on their parents to insert cannulas or administer injections when they were unable to reach certain parts of their bodies. This included several children using MDI regimens who had been advised to inject long-acting insulin into their buttocks to avoid over-using other sites which were used for meal-time injections. Similarly, several children who used pumps described depending on their parents to help insert a new cannula in difficult to reach locations:

"because I do it round on my bum, so they [parents] need to hold the cannula down and I can press the button for it, for the needle to go in. And then they take it out." (016, age 11).

Motivations and tipping points to taking on self-management responsibilities
To minimise the pain experienced when injections were administered by others

Many children also reported motivations and tipping points which made them decide, or acknowledge that, it was an appropriate time to take on new self-management responsibilities. For example, several children who used MDI regimens, including 006, described choosing to administer their own injections because having other people perform this task was a source of discomfort:

"I don't like somebody pinching my skin and then doing my injections. So I like doing that to myself because I don't feel very comfortable with people doing that. So my nurse in my school, she used to do that, and I needed to do it, cause I never felt very comfortable." (006, aged 10).

A similar motivation was reported by 024, who described taking on responsibility for administering his own long-acting injections soon after being diagnosed when he was nine:

"my dad stopped doing my night time insulin for me, because literally it was as sore as sore can be. ... it's usually that he put it in too quickly, that it makes like a really bad pain. So then I managed to do it by myself."

Alleviating parental burdens

Children also described taking on more self-management responsibilities to alleviate the burden on, and stress experienced by, their parents. This included 012 who described how, at age 9, he had decided to perform his own blood glucose checks and administer bolus doses of insulin using injections because:

"[I'm] in school now, and it was like my mum and dad were getting really bothered having to come in every day. I decided like, well they're getting annoyed at it, so I might as well just go ahead."

In other cases, children, including 013, described taking on new responsibilities if they noticed that their parents were struggling; for example, after beginning a new job or because of the pressures involved in caring for other dependents: "obviously she [mother] has to get dinner ready and all that, and see to everybody else. So it was just easier for her if like I knew how to do it [administer a bolus]" (013, aged 12). Similarly, 017 discussed wanting to learn how to change his pump infusion set in order to alleviate some of the demands his diabetes management placed on his mother when she was preparing other siblings for school:

"I'd like to kind of know how to put in my cannula by myself to stop my mum getting stressed and all annoyed in the mornings because before school she tries not to be late. And she needs to change my cannula and stuff like that, get everybody dressed." (017, aged 9).

Becoming more autonomous

As well as wanting to reduce demands on their parents, children described taking on self-management tasks so they could participate in activities with their peers. Several children, for example, discussed having learned how to calculate carbohydrates or change pump infusion sets so they could attend sleepovers at friends' houses or spend nights away on school trips/camps or, in 004's case, to be allowed to go and play at a friend's house:

"It's only when I kind, like got to eight or nine that I started doing it [blood glucose checks] myself. We made a deal that if you [father] did my injections then I would do my bloods, so I needed to do it because if I was at my friend's house, my dad wouldn't be able to come and do it every time." (004, aged 10).

Tipping points: Starting secondary school

Several older aged children (~ 11–12 years) also discussed how they would need to take on more self-management tasks when they transitioned to secondary school in order to adapt to having less dedicated support available from adults:

"when I go to high [secondary] school, well I guess I'll just have to be able to carb count by myself and do everything like that, because it's much more different,

cause you see we get a menu back for primary school. You get a menu and you pick... So you know what you're having. So when you go to the academy [secondary school], you don't know what's on that day. So you go in and then you have to go line up at whatever queue you want for whatever you want." (009, aged 11).

As well as recognising the need to become involved in counting carbohydrates, some children who used MDI regimens described how their forthcoming transition to secondary school had prompted them to consider using new locations on their bodies to administer injections because, as 022 described, he did not want to "miss out" on time spent with friends if he were to continue to remove clothing in order to inject:

"[I'll] probably learn how to do jags in more places, cause I can only do it in my arm myself ... if you're doing it in your arm you've got to take everything off. But with your belly you could slip, lift it up and do it under a table without going into another room." (022, aged 10).

Enablers to children taking on self-management responsibilities
Strategies to minimise needing to perform complex maths to count carbohydrates

As our findings have illustrated, some diabetes management tasks, such as counting carbohydrate contents in meals and determining insulin doses, were too difficult for children in this age group to do independently even if they were motivated to do so. To overcome these difficulties, some children described adopting strategies to limit the need to perform complex maths by choosing to eat snacks or meals with carbohydrate values they could remember:

"If I'm having cereal in the morning and I have to work it out myself, I just say, 'Mum, since I'm working it out today, can I please have toast?' Or can you help me with the sub-division?" (001, aged 10).

In addition, children who used a pump which incorporated a bolus advisor, or those who used MDI regimens and had access to a combined bolus advisor and blood glucose monitor, described how using these devices helped them to calculate their own insulin doses because they did not have to perform complex maths using ratios: "I don't have to do any working out and stuff, well you need to work out how many carbs, but the pump puts in the ratio for you" (003, aged 11). Some, including 008, also noted how, by using a bolus advisor, they did not need to take into account whether a correction dose was needed: "the pump does most of the work such as the correction, we don't have to figure out how much insulin to put through for that. It just does it" (008, aged 11).

As several children further pointed out, by using labels from packets to calculate carbohydrates in meals/snacks, and having access to a bolus advisor, they were able to assume responsibility for calculating insulin doses in instances where they did not want their parents to be involved:

"there's like carbs on the food that I eat, like on the packet. So I just look at that and then I put that into my [blood glucose] monitor, and then I keep adding all of that up. And then, say 40 grammes add to 15, that would be like 55. Then I put that into my monitor and that would be possibly 6.5 or 6 units." (006, aged 11).

While children struggled to count carbohydrates in meals made from multiple ingredients, several of those who used bolus advisors described how they were able to calculate their own insulin doses because their parents provided them with the total value of carbohydrate in their meals. For example, 018 (aged 11) described how for meals eaten at home, her mother "would tell me the grammes and my [blood glucose/bolus advisor] machine tells me how many units I've to get." Similarly, children discussed the benefits of parents providing them with a note containing the carbohydrate values of individual food items or the total count in their school lunch:

"my mum has like – she's got it on a bit of paper. ... And she sticks it on to my, well like my play piece [lunch box]. And then that's how I know my carbs at school" (020, aged 9).

Mobile phones

In related accounts, children reported how mobile phone technology enabled them to self-manage diabetes without their parents being present. Specifically, children who used bolus advisors discussed using phones to contact their parents remotely when they needed advice about carbohydrate contents in order to calculate their own insulin dose: "if I'm away with my friends to say the cinema and like I don't know the carbs of something, I'll just text her [mother] or phone her and see if she knows" (010, aged 11). Similarly, others described using the camera on their phone to seek advice from parents about carbohydrate contents:

"I have to take my phone everywhere, so I can take a picture, send it to her, and then she estimates how much [insulin] I put through for it. ... I'm not too sure about when it comes to the technical level of figuring everything out" (008, aged 11).

Discussion

This is one of the first qualitative studies to explore pre-adolescent children's experiences of, and views about, taking on T1D self-management tasks. In keeping with findings from a study involving parents [14], children in our study highlighted various motivations and tipping points which prompted them to take on more diabetes-related responsibilities. These included: wanting to gain more autonomy and spend time away from parents, wishing to alleviate the burden diabetes management placed on parents, a desire to minimise discomfort arising from administering injections, and needing to make preparations to begin secondary school. However, our findings also illustrate several novel issues and challenges which children in this age group may encounter, principally those relating to difficulties experienced performing the complex maths needed to count carbohydrates and calculate insulin doses. Furthermore, children described how bolus advisor technology enabled them to assume more independent responsibilities for managing diabetes by limiting the need to perform complex maths and how mobile phones allowed them to seek advice about the carbohydrate content of meals when remote from parents.

A key finding in our study is that pre-adolescent children found it extremely difficult to perform the complex maths required to self-manage their diabetes. As others have shown, people with T1D require numeracy skills equivalent to a General Certificate of Secondary Education (GCSE) grade A-C in order to perform the complex maths involved in managing diabetes, including counting carbohydrates, taking into account physical activity, and using insulin-to-carbohydrate ratios [35]. While we might therefore expect pre-adolescent children to be numerically challenged because they have yet to receive comprehensive mathematical teaching in secondary school, the numerical complexities of diabetes management are not confined to pre-adolescents. Indeed, in line with our participants' accounts, other studies have shown how adolescents and adults with T1D also encounter similar challenges [35–38], with poor numeracy skills being associated with lower levels of perceived self-efficacy and less participation in diabetes self-management behaviours [35, 36].

Reflecting findings from studies involving adults and parents of children with T1D diabetes [39, 40], our study has shown how having access to a bolus advisor allowed children to take on tasks which they hitherto found too challenging; specifically, by enabling them to calculate their own insulin doses without needing to use complex maths involving ratios. While a bolus advisor may be a useful and empowering tool for pre-adolescent children, physiological changes during childhood mean that a child's insulin requirements can change very frequently [41], which requires corresponding adjustments to be made to pre-set carbohydrate-to-insulin ratios in bolus advisors. As our findings have shown, children are dependent on others to determine and pre-programme ratios into bolus advisors. While pre-adolescent children would not be expected to adjust pre-set ratios on their own, for bolus advisors to remain a useful and clinically appropriate tool, regular review by health care professionals should be undertaken to help ensure whether the correct ratio and basal rate settings are always being used.

We have also highlighted how children benefited from having access to a mobile phone with a camera because this enabled them to seek advice from their parents remotely about carbohydrates in meals eaten away from home. This use of mobile phone technology, however, inevitably resulted in a continued level of dependency on parents to supply information about carbohydrates. Hence, our findings suggest that children (and adults) with T1D might benefit from ongoing research to develop mobile phone applications capable of identifying in real-time the carbohydrate contents in meals [42].

Children also described how parents undertook diabetes management tasks on their behalf in order to provide them with respite and enable them to have a normal childhood. While these findings are reported in other studies involving children [19, 43], studies involving parents of children with T1D have also demonstrated that parents choose to undertake diabetes-related tasks such as administering injections, to alleviate the burden of self-management [16] and help preserve their child's childhood [44].

Finally, our findings draw attention to how children's involvement and motivations to self-manage diabetes can change as they move towards adolescence. Specifically, pre-adolescent children in our study described actively seeking ways to become more involved in managing diabetes so they could fit in with and spend time with their friends and because they anticipated that less support would be available when they transitioned to secondary school. However, studies involving adolescents with T1D have demonstrated that the same motivations, particularly a desire to fit in with peers, can result in individuals in this older age group compromising their treatment regimens, including skipping blood glucose checks or administering insulin to avoid interrupting social activities [10, 43, 45, 46]. When taken together, findings from our own and adolescent studies indicate that a uniform approach to diabetes education is unlikely to address the needs of children of differing ages. Hence, we would recommend that education and support programmes should be age-specific and take into account children's changing involvement in diabetes-related tasks.

A key strength of our study is our use of an open-ended exploratory design using age-appropriate questions, as this has enabled us to identify a number of potentially important issues which have not yet been recognised or reported in the literature. An additional strength is related to the timing of our study as this enabled us to highlight and explore how new technologies, such as bolus advisors, can enable pre-adolescent children to assume more diabetes-related responsibilities. A potential limitation is that we had a mostly White, ethnically homogenous sample, which potentially limits the generalisability of the findings. Our sample size also limits exploration of how individual factors such as diabetes duration, age at diagnosis and pubertal status might affect pre-adolescent children's self-management decisions and future researchers might consider using quantitative methods to investigate these areas more fully. While the timing of our study enabled us to explore children's use of technology such as bolus advisors, technological advances will result in further changes to how children are involved in self-managing diabetes. Hence, we recommend that future studies exploring the development of self-management roles should include children from more ethnically diverse groups and those who use newly emerging technologies, such as such as continuous glucose monitoring and/or closed loop systems [47], and flash glucose monitoring [48].

Conclusions

This is one of the first qualitative studies to explore in depth factors and considerations which affect pre-adolescent children's decisions to take on responsibilities for self-managing T1D. Our findings identify several factors which may hinder children from taking on self-management tasks, motivators and tipping points which influence whether they take on new responsibilities, and how new technologies can help them to become more independent. To address the numerical challenges involved in managing diabetes, children may benefit from using bolus advisors which limit the need to perform complex maths, alongside regular review from health care professionals to adjust and re-programme insulin-to-carbohydrate ratios. Children (and parents) may also benefit from education and support which is age-specific to reflect their changing involvement in diabetes-related tasks.

Abbreviations
T1D: Type 1 diabetes

Acknowledgements
The authors would like to thank the children who generously contributed their time and views to this study. We would also like to thank the staff at each of the four research sites who gave generously of their time to help recruit children to the study. We are also very grateful to Rebecca Black for providing guidance about the methodology used in the study.

Funding
This work was undertaken as part of a post-doctoral fellowship awarded to DR by the Chief Scientist Office of the Scottish Government Health and Social Care Directorates (PDF/14/01). The views expressed here are those of the authors and not necessarily those of the funder.

Authors' contributions

DR designed the study, collected data, performed data analysis and interpretation and drafted the manuscript. JL performed data analysis and interpretation, contributed to the discussion, and reviewed and edited the manuscript. JH, KB, LB, KN and JS contributed to the discussion, and reviewed and edited the manuscript. All authors read and approved the final manuscript.

Competing interests

The authors declare that they have no competing interests.

Author details

[1]The Usher Institute of Population Health Sciences and Informatics, University of Edinburgh, Edinburgh EH8 9AG, UK. [2]BHR Ltd, 42 Kilmiston Drive, Portchester, Fareham, Hants, PO16 8EG and Faculty of Health & Social Science, Bournemouth University, Royal London House, Bournemouth BH1 3LT, UK. [3]Royal Hospital for Sick Children, Sciennes Road, Edinburgh EH9 1LF, UK. [4]Child Health Department, Borders General Hospital, Melrose TD6 9BS, UK.

References

1. Pettitt DJ, Talton J, Dabelea D, Divers J, Imperatore G, Lawrence JM, et al. Prevalence of diabetes in US youth in 2009: the SEARCH for diabetes in youth study. Diabetes Care. 2014;37:402–8.
2. Patterson CC, Dahlquist GG, Gyürüs E, Green A, Soltész G, Group ES. Incidence trends for childhood type 1 diabetes in Europe during 1989–2003 and predicted new cases 2005–20: a multicentre prospective registration study. Lancet. 2009;373:2027–33.
3. Dovey-Pearce G, Hurrell R, May C, Walker C, Doherty Y. Young adults' (16–25 years) suggestions for providing developmentally appropriate diabetes services: a qualitative study. Health Soc Care Community. 2005;13:409–19.
4. Lowes L. Managing type 1 diabetes in childhood and adolescence. Nurs Stand. 2008;22:50–6.
5. Streisand R, Monaghan M. Young children with type 1 diabetes: challenges, research, and future directions. Curr Diab Rep. 2014;14:1–9.
6. American Diabetes Association. 12. Children and adolescents: standards of medical care in diabetes—2018. Diabetes Care. 2018;41:S126–36.
7. Anderson B, Vangsness L, Connell A, Butler D, Goebel-Fabbri A, Laffel L. Family conflict, adherence, and glycaemic control in youth with short duration type 1 diabetes. Diabetic Med. 2002;19:635–42.
8. Schilling LS, Grey M, Knafl KA. The concept of self-management of type 1 diabetes in children and adolescents: an evolutionary concept analysis. J Adv Nurs. 2002;37:87–99.
9. Davis CL, Delamater AM, Shaw KH, La Greca AM, Eidson MS, Perez-Rodriguez JE, et al. Parenting styles, regimen adherence, and glycemic control in 4-to 10-year-old children with diabetes. J Pediatr Psychol. 2001;26:123–9.
10. Freeborn D, Dyches T, Roper SO, Mandleco B. Identifying challenges of living with type 1 diabetes: child and youth perspectives. J Clin Nurs. 2013; 22:1890–8.
11. Koller D, Khan N, Barrett S. Pediatric perspectives on diabetes self-care: a process of achieving acceptance. Qual Health Res. 2015;25:264–75.
12. Marshall M, Carter B, Rose K, Brotherton A. Living with type 1 diabetes: perceptions of children and their parents. J Clin Nurs. 2009;18:1703–10.
13. Roper SO, Call A, Leishman J, Cole Ratcliffe G, Mandleco BL, Dyches TT, et al. Type 1 diabetes: children and adolescents' knowledge and questions. J Adv Nurs. 2009;65:1705–14.
14. Newbould J, Smith F, Francis S-A. I'm fine doing it on my own': partnerships between young people and their parents in the management of medication for asthma and diabetes. J Child Health Care. 2008;12:116–28.
15. Alderson P, Sutcliffe K, Curtis K. Children as partners with adults in their medical care. Arch Dis Child. 2006;91:300–3.
16. Sutcliffe KAP, Curtis K. Children as partners in their diabetes care: an exploratory research study. London: social science research unit, University of London; 2004.
17. Miller S. Hearing from children who have diabetes. J Child Health Care. 1999;3:5–12.
18. Sparapani Vde C, Jacob E, Nascimento LC. What is it like to be a child with type 1 diabetes mellitus? Pediatr Nurs. 2015;41:17–22.
19. Tyler K. Levers and barriers to patient-centred care with school-age children living with long-term illness in multi-cultural settings: Type 1 diabetes as a case study [Ph.D.]. London: The City University; 2009.
20. Amillategui B, Mora E, Calle JR, Giralt P. Special needs of children with type 1 diabetes at primary school: perceptions from parents, children, and teachers. Pediatr Diabetes. 2009;10:67–73.
21. Nabors L, Lehmkuhl H, Christos N, Andreone TL. Children with diabetes: perceptions of supports for self-Management at School. J Sch Health. 2003; 73:216–21.
22. Newbould J, Francis SA, Smith F. Young people's experiences of managing asthma and diabetes at school. Arch Dis Child. 2007;92:1077–81.
23. Curtis-Tyler K. Facilitating children's contributions in clinic? Findings from an in-depth qualitative study with children with type 1 diabetes. Diabetic Med. 2012;29:1303–10.
24. Dedding C, Reis R, Wolf B, Hardon A. Revealing the hidden agency of children in a clinical setting. Health Expect. 2015;18:2121–8.
25. Lowes L, Eddy D, Channon S, McNamara R, Robling M, Gregory JW, et al. The experience of living with type 1 diabetes and attending clinic from the perception of children, adolescents and carers: analysis of qualitative data from the DEPICTED study. J Pediatr Nurs. 2015;30:54–62.
26. Pradel FG, Hartzema AG, Bush PJ. Asthma self-management: the perspective of children. Patient Educ Couns. 2001;45:199–209.
27. Gabb J. Researching intimacy in families. London: Palgrave Macmillan; 2008.
28. Britten N. Qualitative research: qualitative interviews in medical research. Br Med J. 1995;311:251–3.
29. O'Kane C. The development of participatory techniques: facilitating children's views about decisions which affect them. In: Christensen P, James A, editors. Research with children: perspectives and practices. London: Routledge; 2008.
30. Punch S. Research with children: the same or different from research with adults? Childhood. 2002;9:321–41.
31. Strauss A, Corbin JM. Basics of qualitative research: grounded theory procedures and techniques. London: Sage Publications; 1990.
32. Curtis-Tyler K. Levers and barriers to patient-centred care with children: findings from a synthesis of studies of the experiences of children living with type 1 diabetes or asthma. Child Care Health Dev. 2011;37:540–50.
33. Kelo M, Martikainen M, Eriksson E. Self-care of school-age children with diabetes: an integrative review. J Adv Nurs. 2011;67:2096–108.
34. Rankin D, Harden J, Jepson R, Lawton J. Children's experiences of managing type 1 diabetes in everyday life: a thematic synthesis of qualitative studies. Diabetic Med. 2017;34:1050–60.
35. Marden S, Thomas P, Sheppard Z, Knott J, Lueddeke J, Kerr D. Poor numeracy skills are associated with glycaemic control in type 1 diabetes. Diabetic Med. 2012;29:662–9.
36. Cavanaugh K, Huizinga MM, Wallston KA, Gebretsadik T, Shintani A, Davis D, et al. Association of numeracy and diabetes control. Ann Intern Med. 2008; 148:737–46.
37. Chaney D, Coates V, Shevlin M. Running a complex educational intervention for adolescents with type 1 diabetes–lessons learnt. J Diabetes Nurs. 2010; 14:370–9.
38. Lawton J, Rankin D, Cooke D, Elliott J, Amiel S, Heller S, et al. Patients' experiences of adjusting insulin doses when implementing flexible intensive insulin therapy: a longitudinal, qualitative investigation. Diabetes Res Clin Pract. 2012;98:236–42.
39. Lawton J, Kirkham J, Rankin D, Barnard K, Cooper C, Taylor C, et al. Perceptions and experiences of using automated bolus advisors amongst people with type 1 diabetes: a longitudinal qualitative investigation. Diabetes Res Clin Pract. 2014;106:443–50.
40. Rankin D, Harden J, Noyes K, Waugh N, Barnard K, Lawton J. Parents' experiences of managing their child's diabetes using an insulin pump: a qualitative study. Diabetic Med. 2015;32:627–34.
41. Kushion W, Salisbury PJ, Seitz KW, Wilson BE. Issues in the care of infants and toddlers with insulin-dependent diabetes mellitus. Diabetes Educ. 1991;17:107–10.
42. Hartz J, Yingling L, Powell-Wiley TM. Use of Mobile health Technology in the Prevention and Management of diabetes mellitus. Curr Cardiol Rep. 2016;18:130.
43. Herrman JW. Children's and young adolescents' voices: perceptions of

the costs and rewards of diabetes and its treatment. J Pediatr Nurs. 2006;21:211–21.

44. Lawton J, Waugh N, Barnard K, Noyes K, Harden J, Stephen J, et al. Challenges of optimizing glycaemic control in children with type 1 diabetes: a qualitative study of parents' experiences and views. Diabetic Med. 2015;32:1063–70.

45. Lambert V, Keogh D. Striving to live a normal life: a review of children and young people's experience of feeling different when living with a long term condition. J Pediatr Nurs. 2015;30:63–77.

46. Spencer J, Cooper H, Milton B. The lived experiences of young people (13–16 years) with type 1 diabetes mellitus and their parents–a qualitative phenomenological study. Diabetic Med. 2013;30:e17–24.

47. Hovorka R, Allen JM, Elleri D, Chassin LJ, Harris J, Xing D, et al. Manual closed-loop insulin delivery in children and adolescents with type 1 diabetes: a phase 2 randomised crossover trial. Lancet. 2010;375:743–51.

48. Bailey T, Bode BW, Christiansen MP, Klaff LJ, Alva S. The performance and usability of a factory-calibrated flash glucose monitoring system. Diabetes Technol Ther. 2015;17:787–94.

27

Vitamin D status in healthy black African adults at a tertiary hospital in Nairobi, Kenya: a cross sectional study

Elizabeth Kagotho[1]*(iD), Geoffrey Omuse[1], Nancy Okinda[1] and Peter Ojwang[2]

Abstract

Background· Vitamin D has been known since the twentieth Century for its benefits in bone health. Recent observational studies have demonstrated its benefits in infectious diseases such as tuberculosis and non-communicable diseases such as diabetes mellitus, cardiovascular diseases and cancer. This has led to a dramatic increase in testing among adults.

The cut-offs for vitamin D deficiency have been debated for decades and the current cut off is derived from a Caucasian population. Studies done among black African adults in Africa are few with vitamin D deficiency ranging from 5 to 91%. A few cut- offs have correlated vitamin D deficiency to physiological markers such as parathyroid hormone (PTH), calcium and phosphate with varying results.

Methods: This was a cross sectional study carried out among blood donors at Aga Khan University hospital, Nairobi (AKUHN) from March to May 2015. Vitamin D (25(OH)D) levels were assayed and correlated with PTH, calcium and phosphate.

Results: A total of 253 individuals were included in the final analysis. The proportion of study participants who had a 25(OH) D level of < 20 ng/ml thus classified as vitamin D deficient was 17.4% (95% C.I 12.73–22.07). The 25(OH) D level that coincided with a significant increase in PTH was 30 ng/ml.

Males were less likely to be vitamin D deficient (O.R 0.48 (C.I 0.233–0.993) p 0.04). Sunshine exposure for ≥3 h per day reduced the odds of being Vitamin D deficient though this was not statistically significant after multivariate regression analysis.

Conclusions: We found a much lower prevalence of Vitamin D deficiency compared to many similar studies carried out in sub-Saharan Africa possibly due to the recruitment of healthy individuals and the proximity of Nairobi to the equator which allows for considerable exposure to sunshine. Vitamin D levels below 30 ng/mL was associated with a significant rise in PTH levels, suggesting that this cut off could be appropriate for defining Vitamin D deficiency in the population served by our laboratory.

Keywords: Vitamin D deficiency, Cut-offs, Kenya, Africa

* Correspondence: elizabeth.kagotho@gmail.com
[1]Department of Pathology, Aga Khan University Hospital Nairobi, P.O. Box 30270-00100, Nairobi, Kenya
Full list of author information is available at the end of the article

Background

Vitamin D is a prohormone, which is widely known for its role in bone health [1]. Observational studies in the last decade have implicated its role in reducing the risk of non-communicable diseases such as cancers, auto-immune diseases, cardiovascular diseases, disorders of glucose metabolism, neurodegenerative diseases and communicable diseases [2–4].

Due to the increasing evidence of the importance of vitamin D in relation to various health outcomes, many clinical laboratories in the USA have seen requests for vitamin D testing increase by up to 100% [5]. We have observed similar increments in the requests for vitamin D determination at the Aga Khan University Hospital, Nairobi laboratory.

Africa is a heterogeneous continent that straddles the equator and has northern and southern temperate zones. Most countries in the continent enjoy sunshine all year round due to their proximity to the equator [6]. Data on vitamin D levels among healthy Africans is scant with vitamin D deficiency ranging from 5 to 91% and mean vitamin D levels ranging from 4.4–46.1 ng/ml [7–10].

These studies however used different cut offs to define vitamin D deficiency making direct comparisons on its prevalence difficult. Majority did not correlate Vitamin D levels to surrogate markers of physiological deficiency such as calcium, phosphate and PTH and had insufficient sample sizes.

Other factors that influence the production of vitamin D3 by the skin include the melanin content of the skin, use of sunscreens, time of day, season, air pollution, cloud cover, age and the extent of clothing covering the body [11, 12]. Thus due to high melanin content (skin type V-VI) among Africans, vitamin D production is not as efficient as in light skinned individuals (skin type I-IV) [13]. However most African countries enjoy sunshine throughout the year. The use of sunscreens reduces the absorption of UVB radiation. Sun protection factor (SPF 30) reduces vitamin D3 synthesis by more than 95%. Increasing age reduces the amount of 7-dehydrocholesterol in the skin leading to less production of vitamin D3 [12]. Season, latitude and time of day affects the amount of solar UVB photons reaching the earth thus affecting vitamin D3 production by the skin [11].

We therefore sought to determine the vitamin D status of Kenyan blood donors of African origin and explore the possible risk factors for vitamin D deficiency. We also determined whether vitamin D deficiency as determined using published cut offs translated into a functional deficiency by assaying PTH, total calcium and inorganic phosphate.

Methods

Study design and site

This was a cross sectional study involving blood donors that was conducted at the AKUH,N Kenya blood donor unit from March to May 2015. AKUH,N is a private referral hospital that caters for the residents of Nairobi, Kenya and the greater East African region and receives 400–500 blood donors per month. Nairobi is located at latitude $1^018'S$ and experiences sunshine throughout the year due to its proximity to the equator.

Study participants

Blood donors of African origin between the ages of 18–65 years who met the criteria of blood donation as per the hospital policies were eligible to join the study. It was assumed that those who met the strict criteria for qualifying as a blood donor were healthy. Consecutive sampling was used until the desired sample size was achieved. Blood donors with a positive HIV, hepatitis B, hepatitis C, malaria or syphilis result were excluded from the final analysis.

Data collection

Upon obtaining an informed written consent, the study participants filled a questionnaire. Its purpose was to collect information regarding sun exposure, which was expressed in terms of the number of hours spent outside, dietary intake of vitamin D rich foods such as oily fish and dietary intake of calcium and phosphate rich foods. This was in addition to the blood donor screening questionnaire that checks whether one is fit to qualify as a blood donor based on appropriate age, weight, haemoglobin level, exposure to infectious diseases and medication intake.

Sample collection and processing

Blood samples were collected in EDTA tubes for PTH and 25(OH) D and serum clot activator tubes for total calcium, inorganic phosphate and albumin. Centrifugation was done immediately at 4000 rpm for 5 min. Plasma and serum was then aliquoted into 2 ml plastic tubes and stored at -20 °C and analysed in batches of 50.

Sample analysis

All samples were analysed on the ROCHE COBAS ® platform e601 for PTH, 25(OH) D and e501 for total calcium, inorganic phosphate and albumin. Analysis of 25 (OH) D was done using an electrochemiluminescent competitive immunoassay assay and reported in nanograms per milliliter (ng/ml). PTH was analysed using an electrochemiluminescent sandwich immunoassay and reported in picograms/milliliter (pg/ml). Serum calcium and phosphate levels were measured photometrically using the o-cresolphthalein complexone and molybdate methods respectively and reported in mmol/l. Serum albumin was analysed using a calorimetric assay and reported in in g/l.

Daily quality controls were within acceptable ranges. All analytes had been registered under the Randox International Quality Assessment Scheme (RIQAS) with acceptable running means standard deviation index of − 0.21,-0.80, -0.44,-0.30,0.03 for 25 (OH) D, PTH, Calcium, phosphate and albumin respectively.

Vitamin D levels were categorized as sufficient (> 30 ng/ml), insufficient (21-29 ng/ml) and deficient (< 20 ng/ml) based on the IOM classification that has been widely adopted globally. The reference ranges for PTH were 15-65 pg/ml, total calcium 2.1–2.66 mmol/l, inorganic phosphate 0.84–1.45 mmol/l. Corrected calcium was calculated for all study participants who had a low albumin level and this was used in the final analysis.

Statistical analysis

Data was analysed using IBM® SPSS® Statistics V22.0. The prevalence of vitamin D deficiency was expressed as a percentage with 95% confidence intervals (CI). Continuous variables i.e. 25(OH)D, PTH, phosphate and calcium were presented in form of medians and inter quartile ranges.

A scatter plot was used to determine the relationship between vitamin D and PTH and a quadratic equation was used to arrive at the level of vitamin D beyond which a decline resulted in an increase in PTH levels. This was determined using the point of inflection on the graph.

Man Whitney U test was used to compare medians or mean ranks of calcium and phosphate levels between the vitamin D deficient (25(OH)D levels of < 20 ng/ml) and non-deficient group (25(OH)D levels of ≥20 ng/ml). Binary logistic regression and multivariate regression analysis was used to calculate crude and adjusted odds ratios for risk factors of vitamin D deficiency. These risk factors included sunshine exposure in hours, gender and dietary intake of oily fish. Age was not adjusted for, since there was no statistically significant difference between the vitamin D deficient and non-deficient group. A p value < 0.05 was considered statistically significant.

Results

A total of 258 participants were recruited into the study of whom 5 were excluded from the final analysis due to a positive screen for HIV, Hepatitis B or C virus.

The median (IQR) age of the study participants was 33.07(40) years. Overall 62 (24.5%) of the study participants were female.

Table 1 shows the baseline demographic and biochemical variables of the study participants.

Vitamin D status

Study participants who were classified as vitamin D deficient (levels < 20 ng/ml) was 17.4% (95% C.I 12.73–22.07). Those classified as vitamin D insufficient were 42.6% (95% C.I 36.51–48.69) while 40% (95% C.I 33.96–46.04) were classified as vitamin D sufficient. Figure 1 shows the distribution of vitamin D levels.

Males were less likely to be vitamin D deficient (O.R 0.481(C.I 0.233–0.933) $p = 0.04$). Sunshine exposure for > 3 h significantly reduced the odds of one been vitamin D deficient however this was not statistically significant after multivariate regression analysis. The use of sunscreens and dietary intake of oily fish did not significantly increase or reduce the odds of one been vitamin D deficient respectively though the numbers in these categories were very small as shown in Table 2.

There was an inverse relationship between vitamin D levels and PTH and the vitamin D level that coincided with a significant increase in PTH was 30 ng/ml as shown in Fig. 2.

There was no statistically significant difference in calcium and phosphate levels between the vitamin D deficient and non- deficient individuals.

Discussion

The prevalence of vitamin D deficiency was 17.4% (95% C.I 12.73–22.07). This study population was representative of a healthy black African population in Kenya and despite being vitamin D deficient they did not have any related symptomatology. Furthermore, there was no statistically significant difference in calcium and phosphate levels between the vitamin D deficient non-deficient individuals. This puts into question whether levels below 20 ng/mL should trigger a medical intervention in the absence of related symptomatology.

The prevalence we found in our study is in stark contrast to a study done by Luxwolda et al. in Tanzania on the Hadzabe's and Maasai's who had a mean vitamin D of 46.1 ng/ml with none of the participants being vitamin D Deficient [8]. The difference in vitamin D levels might have been due to the fact that Maasai's and Hadzabe's are pastoralists, hunters and gatherers and spend most of their time outdoors with minimal clothing.

The US National Nutrition and Health survey (NHANES) III reported that at least 53–76% of African Americans were vitamin D deficient during winter [14] and Powe et al. reported a mean vitamin D level of 15 ± 0.2 ng/ml among 1181 black Americans [15]. The reasons cited for this level of deficiency included dark skin colour thus resulting in inefficient vitamin D production by the skin and lack of regular vitamin D supplementation.

We found that females were more likely to be vitamin D deficient. Possible explanations for this observation include increased subcutaneous adiposity and higher Body mass index (BMI) among females resulting in increased 25(OH) D storage in adipose tissue thus not readily available for conversion to calcitriol [16]. Subcutaneous adiposity and BMI were however not taken for the study participants.

Studies have been done correlating vitamin D to physiological markers of vitamin D deficiency such as PTH,

Table 1 Descriptive characteristics of the study participants

	Male (n = 191)		Female (n = 62)		Total (n = 253)		Male vs female
	Median(IQR)	Min-Max	Median (IQR)	Min-Max	Median (IQR)	Min-Max	p- value
Age (years)	33 (40)	19–59	31 (30)	21–51	33.07 (40)	19–59	0.304
Vitamin D (ng/ml)	28.24 (44.47)	8.89–53.36	25.08 (34.12)	8.57–42.71	27.80 (44.79)	8.57–53.36	0.002
PTH (pg/ml)	36.46 (72.69)	10.38–83.07	36.71 (83.38)	16.72–100.1	36.7 (89.72)	10.38–100.1	0.534
Calcium (mmol/l)	2.42 (1.50)	1.23–2.73	2.38 (0.72)	2.05–2.77	2.41 (1.54)	1.23–2.77	0.168
Phosphate (mmol/l)	1.17 (3.32)	0.66–3.98	1.17 (2.58)	0.82–3.40	1.13 (3.32)	0.66–3.98	0.360

IQR interquartile range

calcium and phosphate. These studies have reported that PTH is inversely associated with vitamin D and begins to plateau at a vitamin D level between 16 and 40 ng/ml [17–19]. This is the lowest vitamin D level beyond which PTH starts rising. Whether these values would be suitable cut-offs still remains controversial. The US Institute of Medicine 2011 guidelines quoted that one of the reasons behind the current recommendation of the cut off 20 ng/ml to define deficiency was the lowest vitamin D level at which PTH started rising [17]. From our study, the derived vitamin D cut-off based on the point of inflection i.e. the vitamin D level when PTH starts rising is 30 ng/ml. This was similar to a cross-sectional study done by Nusrat et al. in Kenya, unpublished data who looked at vitamin D levels and PTH in exclusively 97 breast fed infants and came up with a cut-off of 30 ng/ml. If a cut off of 30 ng/ml was adopted then 60.1% (95% C.I. 54.07–66.13%) of the study population would have been vitamin D deficient.

This raises the question whether there are other factors such as bioavailable vitamin D and vitamin D binding protein that should be considered when interpreting 25(OH) D levels since this was essentially a healthy population. This was reported in a study by Powe et al. where Black Americans compared to whites had low Vitamin D levels (15.6 ± 0.2 ng/ml vs. 25.8 ± 0.4 ng/ml, $P < 0.001$) and vitamin D binding protein (168 ± 3 µg/ml vs. 337 ± 5 µg/ml, $P < 0.001$) but similar concentrations of bioavailable Vitamin D 2.9 ± 0.1 ng/ml vs 3.1 ± 0.1 ng/ml, $P = 0.71$. Genetic polymorphisms partially explained the differences in Vitamin D binding protein in the two populations [15].

Sunshine exposure for ≥3 h was associated with a decreased likelihood of being vitamin D deficient as compared to < 1 h. This was however not statistically significant using

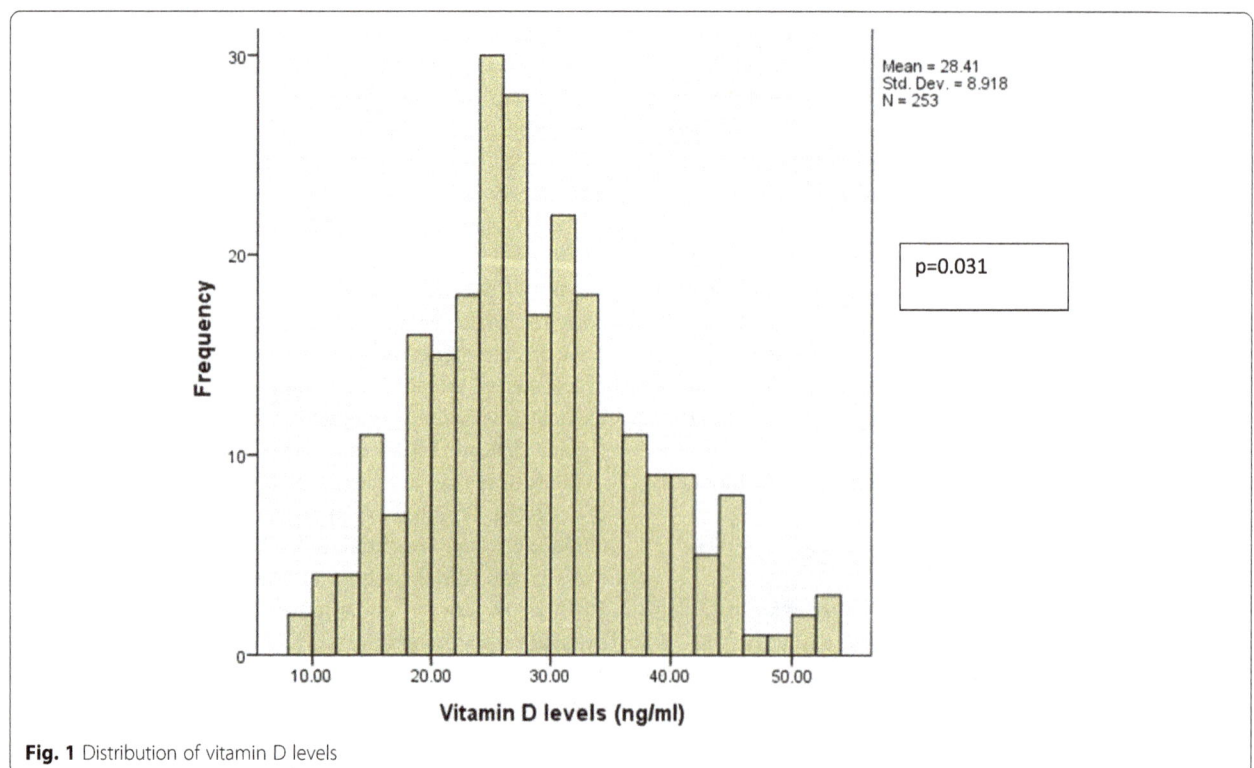

Fig. 1 Distribution of vitamin D levels

Table 2 Comparison of risk factors for Vitamin D deficiency

	Deficient	Non-deficient	P value	Crude O.R (C.I)	P value	Adjusted O.R. (C.I)
Gender: N (%)						
Female[a]	17 (27.4%)	45 (72.6%)				
Male	27 (14.1%)	164 (85.9%)	0.03	0.463 (0.212–0.784)	0.04	0.481 (0.233–0.933)
Sunshine exposure: N (%)						
≤ 1 h daily[a]	66 (76.7%)	20 (23.3%)				
1–3 h daily	57 (81.4%)	13 (18.6%)	0.48	0.753 (0.344–0.1647)	0.13	0.893 (0.0.658–4.912)
> 3 h daily	86 (88.7%)	11 (11.3%)	0.03	0.422 (0.189–0.942)	0.08	0.623 (0.487–3.889)
Oily fish intake: N (%)						
None[a]	30 (19.9%)	121 (80.1%)				
≥ once a week	14 (13.7%)	88 (86.3%)	0.20	0.642 (0.231–1.281)		
Sunscreen use: N (%)						
None[a]	42 (17.6%)	197 (82.4%)				
Yes	2 (14.3%)	12 (85.7%)	0.75	0.782 (0.169–3.623)		

[a]Reference group, *O.R* Odds ratio, *C.I* Confidence interval

multiple logistic regression. More than 95% of vitamin D 3 is from the sun [20]. Nairobi lies at latitude 1018'S thus enjoying sunshine all year round. Increased skin pigmentation reduces the production of vitamin D 3 on the skin. Since most Africans are skin type V and VI longer sunshine exposure would be required to make vitamin D 3.

Sunscreen use increases the risk of vitamin D deficiency, with sunscreens with an SPF of 30 and above reducing vitamin D production by upto 95% [20]. From this study 14 out of the 253 study participants reported the use of sunscreen or sunscreen containing lotions and there was no statistically significant difference in vitamin D levels between those who did and didn't use sunscreen. This study was however not sufficiently powered to test for this association.

Limitations

This study was not sufficiently powered to show significant differences for the different risk factors and as such, most of the analysis was exploratory. The absence of statistically significant differences could be due to the small sample size, which increases the risk of a type II error.

Sun exposure, use of sunscreens and dietary intake of vitamin D and calcium rich foods data collected for this study was self-reported thus liable to a reporting bias.

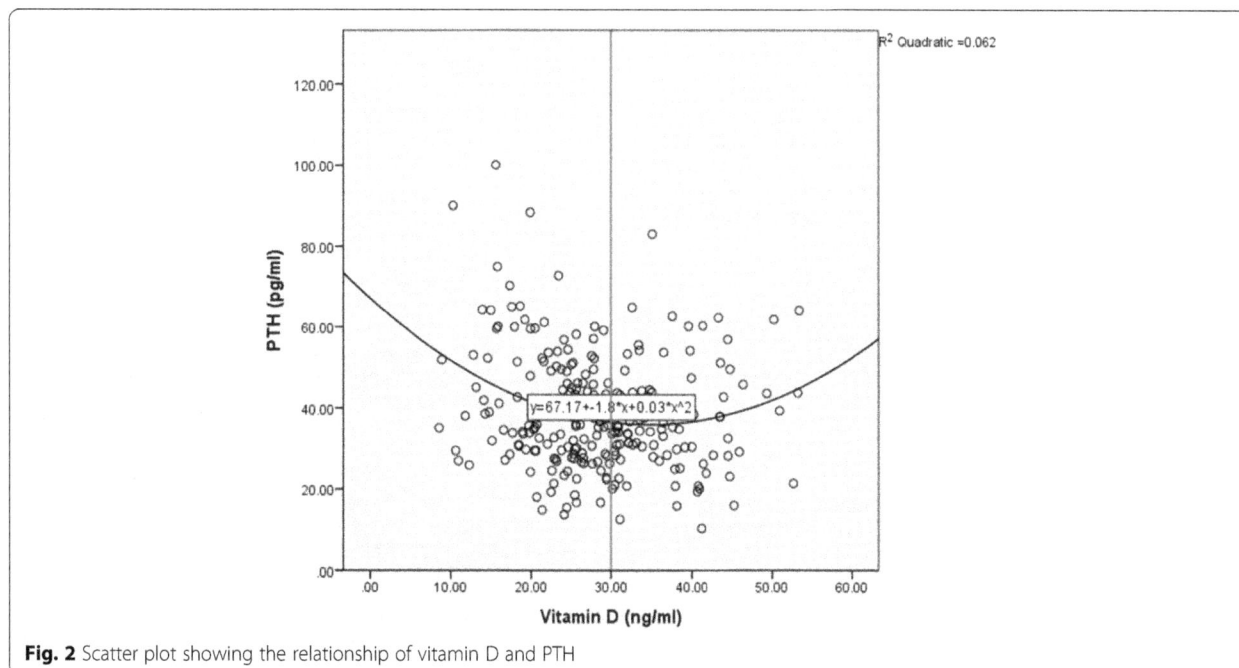

Fig. 2 Scatter plot showing the relationship of vitamin D and PTH

Skin type for the study participants was also not determined. Potentially, variation in skin types could influence the impact of some risk factors on Vitamin D levels.

Factors that can affect vitamin D levels such as Vitamin D supplementation, Body Mass Index (BMI) and subcutaneous adiposity were not taken.

Conclusion

This study highlights that one in every six healthy Kenyan adults of African origin donating blood at AKUHN is vitamin D deficient using the cut-off of 20 ng/ml. These adults had no signs and symptoms of deficiency and biochemically appeared not to have any significant abnormality. Clinicians need to be aware of the level of deficiency in the healthy population so that they can take this into account when interpreting Vitamin D results in patients. Whether such individuals should have vitamin D supplementation to boost their levels above 30 ng/mL is a question that still needs to be answered. Vitamin D testing should also be restricted to patients at risk as per the Endocrine society 2011 guidelines. This includes patients with osteoporosis, chronic kidney disease, pregnant and lactating mothers, hyperparathyroidism and malabsorption syndromes.

Studies being carried out linking vitamin D to various health outcomes also need to bear in mind the baseline level of deficiency in the healthy Kenyan population.

Suitable 25 (OH) D cut-offs need to be established in the African population and these need to be predictive of specific well defined outcomes. Since total vitamin D and not the active form is what is routinely assayed, studies correlating 25(OH)D levels, vitamin D binding protein and physiological markers of vitamin D deficiency among Africans need to be done.

Abbreviations

25(OH)D: 25 hydroxyvitamin D; AKUHN: Aga Khan University Hospital Nairobi; BMI: Body Mass Index; EDTA: Ethylenediaminetetraacetic acid; IOM: Institute of medicine; NHANES: National Health and Nutrition Examination Survey; PTH: Parathyroid hormone; RIQAS: Randox International Quality Assessment Scheme; SPF: Sun protection factor; UVB: Ultraviolet Radiation B; VDBP: Vitamin D binding protein

Acknowledgements

Esther Cuma and Luke Kilonzo, Aga Khan University Hospital Nairobi, assisted in participant recruitment, sample collection and processing.

Funding

Part of this study was funded by an Aga Khan University Research Council seed grant for master's students and the reagents were provided by Roche diagnostics.

Authors' contribution

EK designed the study, collected data, performed statistical analysis and wrote the manuscript. GO, NO and PJ designed the study, assisted with statistical analysis and critiqued the manuscript. All authors read and approved the final manuscript.

Competing interests

The author(s) declare they have no competing interests.

Author details

[1]Department of Pathology, Aga Khan University Hospital Nairobi, P.O. Box 30270-00100, Nairobi, Kenya. [2]Department of Pathology, Maseno University, P.O. Box Private Bag, Maseno, Kenya.

References

1. Holick MF. Vitamin D: A millenium perspective. J Cell Biochem. 2003;88(2): 296–307.
2. Autier P, Boniol M, Pizot C, Mullie P. Vitamin D status and ill health: a systematic review. Lancet Diabetes Endocrinol. 2014;2(1):76–89.
3. Chu MP, Alagiakrishnan K, Sadowski C. The cure of ageing: vitamin D--magic or myth? Postgrad Med J. 2010;86(1020):608–16.
4. Theodoratou E, Tzoulaki I, Zgaga L, Ioannidis JPA. Vitamin D and multiple health outcomes: umbrella review of systematic reviews and meta-analyses of observational studies and randomised trials. BMJ. 2014;348(4):g2035.
5. Krasowski MD. Pathology consultation on vitamin D testing. Am J Clin Pathol. 2011 Oct;136(4):507–14.
6. Brooks RA. Africa. Cambr Intell 1999;
7. Feleke Y, Abdulkadir J, Mshana R, Mekbib T, Brunvand L, Berg JP, et al. Low levels of serum calcidiol in an African population compared to a north European population. Eur J Endocrinol. 1999;21(4):358–60.
8. Luxwolda MF, Kuipers RS, Kema IP, Dijck-brouwer DAJ, Muskiet FAJ. Traditionally living populations in East Africa have a mean serum 25-hydroxyvitamin D concentration of 115 nmol/l. Br J Nutr. 2012;108(9):1557–61.
9. Prentice A, Schoenmakers I, Jones KS, Jarjou LM a, Goldberg GR. Vitamin D deficiency and its health consequences in Africa. Clin Rev Bone Miner Metab. 2009;7(1):94–106.
10. Arabi A, El Rassi R, El-Hajj Fuleihan G. Hypovitaminosis D in developing countries-prevalence, risk factors and outcomes. Nat Rev Endocrinol. 2010;6(10):550–61.
11. Alshahrani FM, Almalki MH, Aljohani N, Alzahrani A, Alsaleh Y, Holick MF, Vitamin D. Light side and best time of sunshine in Riyadh, Saudi Arabia. Dermatoendocrinol. 2013;5(1):177–80.
12. Holick MF. Vitamin D deficiency. N Engl J Med. 2007;357(3):266–81.
13. Fitzpatrick TB. The validity and practicality of sun reactive skin types 1 through VI. JAMA dermatology. 1988;124(6):869–71.
14. Mayer J, Harris SS. Symposium : optimizing vitamin D intake for populations with special Needs : barriers to effective food fortification and supplementation barriers to optimizing vitamin D 3 intake for the elderly 1. J Nutr. 2006;25(4):1123–5.
15. Powe CE, Evans MK, Wenger J, Zonderman AB, Berg AH, Nalls M, et al. Vitamin D-binding protein and vitamin D status of black Americans and white Americans. N Engl J Med. 2013;369(21):1991–2000.
16. Hannemann A, Thuesen BH, Friedrich N, Völzke H, Steveling A, Ittermann T, et al. Adiposity measures and vitamin D concentrations in Northeast Germany and Denmark. Nutr Metab (Lond). 2015;12(1):24–33.
17. Holick MF, Binkley NC, Bischoff-Ferrari HA, Gordon CM, Hanley DA, Heaney RP, et al. Evaluation, treatment, and prevention of vitamin D deficiency: an endocrine society clinical practice guideline. J Clin Endocrinol Metab. 2011;96(7):1911–30.
18. Chapuy MC, Preziosi P, Maamer M, Arnaud S, Galan P, Hercberg S, et al. Prevalence of vitamin D insufficiency in an adult normal population. OsteoporosInt. 1997;7(5):439–43.
19. Aspray TJ, Yan L, Prentice A. Parathyroid hormone and rates of bone formation are raised in perimenopausal rural Gambian women. Bone. 2005;36:710–20.
20. Holick MF. Sunlight and vitamin D for bone health and prevention of autoimmune diseases , cancers , and cardiovascular disease. Am J Clin Nutr. 2004;80(suppl):1678–88.

28

Usefulness of core needle biopsy for the diagnosis of thyroid Burkitt's lymphoma: a case report and review of the literature

Stella Bernardi[1,2]* (iD), Andrea Michelli[1], Deborah Bonazza[1,3], Veronica Calabrò[2], Fabrizio Zanconati[1,3], Gabriele Pozzato[1,4] and Bruno Fabris[1,2]

Abstract

Background: Thyroid lymphomas are an exceptional finding in patients with thyroid nodules. Burkitt's lymphoma is one of the rarest and most aggressive forms of thyroid lymphomas, and its prognosis depends on the earliness of medical treatment. Given the rarity of this disease, making a prompt diagnosis can be challenging. For instance, fine-needle aspiration (FNA) cytology, which is the first-line diagnostic test that is performed in patients with thyroid nodules, is often not diagnostic in cases of thyroid lymphomas, with subsequent delay of the start of therapy.

Case presentation: Here we report the case of a 52-year-old woman presenting with a rapidly enlarging thyroid mass. Thyroid ultrasonography demonstrated a solid hypoechoic nodule. FNA cytology was only suggestive of a lymphoproliferative disorder and did not provide a definitive diagnosis. It is core needle biopsy (CNB) that helped us to overcome the limitations of routine FNA cytology, showing the presence of thyroid Burkitt's lymphoma. Subsequent staging demonstrated bone marrow involvement. The early start of an intensive multi-agent chemotherapy resulted in complete disease remission. At 60 months after the diagnosis, the patient is alive and has not had any recurrence.

Conclusions: Clinicians should be aware that thyroid Burkitt's lymphoma is an aggressive disease that needs to be treated with multi-agent chemotherapy as soon as possible. To diagnose it promptly, they should consider to order/perform a CNB in any patient with a rapidly enlarging thyroid mass that is suspicious for lymphoma.

Keywords: Thyroid, Burkitt's lymphoma, Thyroid lymphomas, Core needle biopsy, Case report

Background

Thyroid nodules are an extremely common occurrence. It is estimated that up to 67% of the population has a thyroid nodule that could be detected by ultrasonography [1]. Thyroid cancer occurs in 7–15% of cases depending on risk factors such as age, sex, family history, and radiation exposure [2]. Thyroid lymphoma accounts for less than 5% of all thyroid cancers. Nevertheless, clinicians should know how to manage this extremely rare

occurrence, as the prognosis of the most aggressive subtypes depends on the earliness of the diagnosis and the subsequent start of multiagent chemotherapy regimens.

Routine medical work-up of patients with thyroid nodules is based on the evidence that fine-needle aspiration (FNA), preferably performed under ultrasonographic guidance and with rapid on-site evaluation by a cytopathologist [3], is the most sensitive and cost-effective method to assess their nature and/or the need for surgery [2, 4–6]. By contrast, FNA has a low accuracy for the diagnosis of thyroid lymphomas [7, 8], often leading to diagnostic surgery. It has been argued that in cases suspicious of thyroid lymphomas, core needle biopsy (CNB) could help to reduce diagnostic surgery [7] and, most importantly, to obtain earlier the diagnosis

* Correspondence: stella.bernardi@asuits.sanita.fvg.it; shiningstella@gmail.com
[1]Department of Medical Surgical and Health Sciences, Università degli Studi di Trieste, Cattinara Teaching Hospital, Strada di Fiume 447, 34149 Trieste, Italy
[2]Endocrinology Unit - Azienda Sanitaria Universitaria Integrata Trieste, Cattinara Teaching Hospital, Strada di Fiume 447, 34149 Trieste, Italy
Full list of author information is available at the end of the article

necessary to start life-saving treatment with multiagent chemotherapy.

Here we report the case of a woman with Burkitt's lymphoma of the thyroid gland, where CNB helped us to overcome the limitations of routine FNA cytology and to prescribe the right medical treatment. We also performed a review of the literature and a search in Pubmed of other clinical cases of adult patients affected by Burkitt's lymphoma of the thyroid gland. For this purpose, we used the combined terms "Burkitt", "thyroid", and "case", and we selected only English written articles [9–24], while we excluded a few reports in other languages, such as Spanish [25–28], French [29, 30], and Japanese [31, 32].

Case presentation

A 52-year-old woman presented to our Endocrinology Unit with a growing thyroid mass, which had enlarged so rapidly she had become unable to wear her motorcycle helmet in the weeks prior to her visit. She suffered from Hashimoto's thyroiditis for which she was taking levothyroxine. There was no history of neck irradiation or family history of thyroid cancer. On examination, there was a large, firm thyroid nodule on the right side of the neck, without palpable cervical lymphadenopathy. TSH was 4.79 μU/mL with FT3 and FT4 within the reference range. Otherwise, there was only a mild thrombocytopenia. Thyroid ultrasonography showed a solid hypoechoic nodule in the right lobe of the gland, with significant internal vascularity and absence of calcifications (Figure 1). FNA cytology with rapid on-site evaluation of the material adequacy showed that there were only atypical lymphoid cells with no thyrocytes and the specimens were considered suggestive of a lymphoproliferative disorder but insufficient to make a diagnosis, such that a CNB was scheduled for the following day.

After checking the blood coagulation profile, the patient underwent a CNB, which allowed histological/morphological tissue analysis. This showed that normal thyrocytes were virtually all replaced by homogeneous medium-sized lymphocytes with scanty blue cytoplasm, round nuclei, coarse chromatin, and multiple small nucleoli. There were frequent mitotic figures and scattered macrophages ingesting apoptotic cells, giving to the tissue section the so-called 'starry sky' appearance (Fig. 1). Overall, these features were consistent with the presence of a thyroid Burkitt's lymphoma, and further investigations were ordered to confirm the diagnosis and evaluate the disease extent. A CT of chest and abdomen showed the 44x43x87 mm thyroid nodule with left tracheal deviation (Figure 1) without other visible masses or lymph nodes. Bone marrow biopsy showed almost 100% lymphoid infiltration, consisting of a population of intermediate-sized

blast-like cells, with prominent nucleoli, which were replacing all normal cells. These cells expressed CD10, CD20, and were negative for Bcl2, CD34, and TdT. Altogether these results led us to the final diagnosis of stage IV Burkitt's lymphoma [33].

The patient was admitted to our hospital's Haematology Unit and was successfully treated with 3 cycles of Hyper-CVAD chemotherapy (cyclophosphamide, vincristine, doxorubicin and dexamethasone) completed in five months. The thyroid mass disappeared (Fig. 1) and the platelets returned to baseline levels. At 60 months after diagnosis the patient is alive, and remains disease-free at regular follow-up.

Discussion

Burkitt's lymphoma is one of the rarest [34] and also most aggressive subtypes of thyroid lymphomas [11]. It is considered the fastest growing human tumor, with a cell doubling time of 24–48 h [33]. It arises from B cells, where a chromosomal translocation, more frequently t(8;14)(q24;q32) and less frequently either t(2;8)(p12;q24) or t(8;22)(q24;q11), leads to the deregulated expression of the oncogene C-Myc, which promotes cell cycle progression [35]. As a result, this lymphoma is characterized by the presence of monomorphic medium-sized B cells with a very high proliferation rate and increased apoptosis. To the best of our knowledge, 23 cases of thyroid Burkitt's lymphoma have been described in the English medical literature [9–24] (Table 1). The majority of them (13 out of 23) were cases of Burkitt's lymphoma with disseminated disease (stage III/IV). Among them, at least 5 patients (22%) died within the first 2 years of follow-up [11, 21, 22, 24] (Table 1). These were cases of age greater than 60 years, advanced disease, or disease onset complicated by cavernous sinus thrombosis (Table 1). Consistent with this, advanced age, poor performance status, advanced stage, and central nervous system or bone marrow involvement are considered the most relevant prognostic factors of a poor outcome in Burkitt's lymphoma [35]. Therefore, starting chemotherapy as soon as possible is key for a complete response.

Unfortunately, given the rarity of this disease, making a prompt diagnosis can be challenging. The first aspect that should raise the suspicion of a thyroid lymphoma should be the presence of a rapidly growing goiter or nodule. It is estimated that 70% of patients with aggressive thyroid lymphomas complain of a rapidly expanding cervical mass that causes obstructive symptoms, such as dyspnea and dysphagia [8, 36]. In line with this figure, these symptoms were reported by 65% (15 out of 23) of patients with thyroid Burkitt's lymphoma (Table 1). However, these symptoms are not specific and they might also be due to other conditions, such as anaplastic carcinoma or Riedel's thyroiditis. Moreover, sometimes,

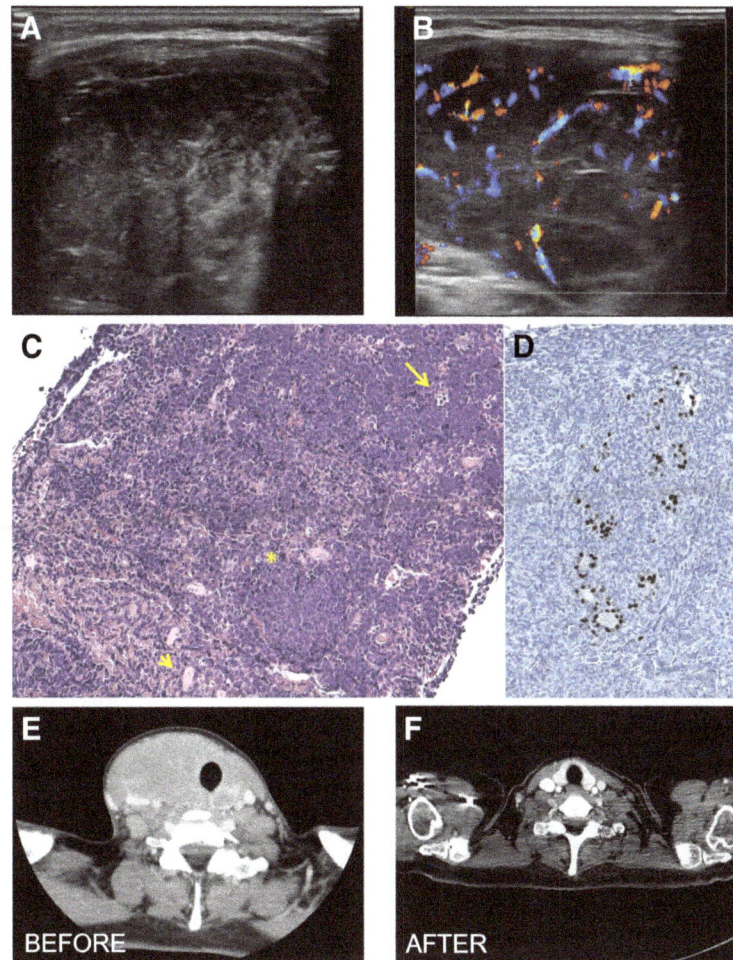

Fig. 1 Endocrine imaging of a patient with Burkitt's lymphoma. Thyroid US showed a solid hypoechoic mass (**a**) with significant internal vascularity (**b**) and no calcifications. Core needle biopsy showed homogeneous medium-sized B cells infiltrating the thyroid (**c**, arrowhead), mitotic figures (**c**, asterisk), and scattered macrophages ingesting apoptotic cells (**c**, arrow), giving a "starry sky" appearance. The extent of thyroid infiltration can be appreciated on (**d**) where follicular cells are only those positively stained for TTF1 (thyroid transcription factor 1). The CT scan performed before treatment showed a 44x43x87 mm thyroid nodule (**e**), which disappeared at the CT scan performed one year after treatment completion (**f**)

the thyroid mass due to a lymphoma can be an incidental occurrence in patients with fever, malaise, weight loss, or hypothyroidism due to Hashimoto's thyroiditis, as reported by [9, 16, 20]. Otherwise, there have been also a few reports of exceptional presentations such as a pathological fracture due to a secondary lytic lesion [13], and the onset of diplopia and headache due to a bilateral cavernous sinus thrombosis [24].

According to current guidelines [2, 6], ultrasonography is the first exam that should be performed in patients with a goiter or a thyroid nodule, and it should be generally followed by FNA cytology, whenever a solid thyroid nodule greater than 1-2 cm is detected. However, in case of a thyroid lymphoma, these procedures are often non-diagnostic. For instance, the ultrasound features of thyroid lymphomas, which include very low echogenicity, enhanced posterior echoes, increased vascularity, and lack of internal calcifications, are all aspecific [36]. In addition, as shown by the rapid on-site evaluation of our specimens, FNA cytology is often suggestive but insufficient to make a diagnosis of thyroid lymphoma. Apart from not providing adequate material, other pitfalls of FNA include the cytological similarities with thyroiditis and the high rate at which both pathologies occur simultaneously in the same gland, as 60–90% of lymphomas arise on a background of thyroiditis [36]. For these reasons, it has been argued that patients with suspected thyroid lymphomas require CNB or excision for diagnosis [8].

Tissue biopsies can provide the material necessary to assess tissue morphology and to perform a panel of immunostains, which should be the first aspects to evaluate when a Burkitt's lymphoma is suspected [37]. In

Table 1 Reported cases of thyroid Burkitt's lymphomas

Authors (ref)	Age (y) Sex	Sites of involvement	Stage	Symptoms (S) Diagnosis (D)	Follow-up (mo)	Outcome
Thieblemont [9]	46 M	Thyroid, cervical and mediastinal nodes, bone marrow, stomach	IV	S: asymptomatic D: CNB	NA	NA
Iqbal [10]	6 M	Thyroid, right atrium, right ventricle, pericardium, abdominal masses, CNS	IV	S: thyroid enlargement, anorexia, weight loss, shortness of breath D: biopsy of suprarenal mass	NA	Alive, CR
Ruggiero [11]	40 F	Thyroid, other sites	IV	S: obstructive symptoms D: FNA + CNB	Died after 3 months	
Kalinyak [12]	53 M	Thyroid, bone marrow	IV	S: obstructive symptoms D: FNA + bone marrow	27	Alive, CR
Camera [13]	56 M	Thyroid, mediastinum, kidneys, right femur	IV	S: pathological fracture D: FNA + open surgery	NA	Reduction of all lesions
Kandil [14]	60 F	Thyroid and cervical nodes	I	S: obstructive symptoms D: FNA + incisional biopsy	NA	Succesfully treated after 1 cycle of CT
Yildiz [15]	31 M	Thyroid, cervical and jugulodigastric nodes	I	S: obstructive symptoms D: open surgery	6	Alive, CR
Bongiovanni [16]	72 F	Thyroid, cervical nodes, liver and skeletal lesions	IV	S: fever D: FNA + CNB	NA	NA
Mweempwa [17]	58 F	Thyroid	I	S: obstructive symptoms D: FNA + CNB	4	Alive, CR
Albert [18]	16 M	Thyroid	I	S: obstructive symptoms D: open surgery	NA	Alive, CR
Zhang [19]	8 M	Thyroid	I	S: obstructive symptoms D: open surgery	48	Alive, CR
Cooper [20]	14 M	Thyroid, lung, kidney and pancreas	IV	S: malaise, lethargy, weight loss D: FNA + OWB	36	Alive, CR
Alloui [21]	70 M	Thyroid	I	S: obstructive symptoms D: CNB	Patient died of septic shock after 17 days	
Quesada [22]	24 NA	Thyroid, cervical, aortcaval, preaortic, and paraortic nodes	III	S: obstructive symptoms 5/7 D: FNA 5/7 + either CNB 4/7, or open surgery 3/7	41	Alive, CR
	28 NA	Thyroid and cervical nodes	I		361	Alive, CR
	47 NA	Thyroid, cervical nodes, CNS	IV		25	Alive, CR
	45 NA	Thyroid	I		12	Alive, PD
	41 NA	Thyroid, cervical, pretracheal and retrocrural nodes, mediastinum, bone marrow	IV		113	Alive, CR
	49 NA	Thyroid, cervical and iliac nodes	III		Died after 12 months	
	19 NA	Thyroid, cervical, jugulodigastric nodes, lumbar vertebrae	IV		Dieta after 23 months	
Akshintala [23]	21 F	Thyroid and cervical nodes	I	S: obstructive symptoms D: CNB + incisional biopsy	NA	Alive, CR
Moghaddasi [24]	47 F	Thyroid and cervical nodes	I	S: diplopia D: incisional biopsy	Died after 30 days	
Claudi [45]	56 F	Thyroid, liver	IV	S: obstructive symptoms D: open surgery	NA	NA

CNB is for core needle biopsy; CNS is for central nervous system; CR is for complete remission; FNA is for fine needle aspiration; NA is for not applicable; PD is for persistent disease; OWB is for open wedge biospy

particular, typical morphological features of this lymphoma include the presence of homogeneous medium-sized lymphocytes with round nuclei, coarse chromatin and multiple small nucleoli, surrounded by a scanty blue cytoplasm with frequent small vacuoles and indistinct edges [38]. Another typical feature is the "starry sky" pattern [16], which is due to the presence of macrophages containing apoptotic tumor cells on a background of proliferating B cells. Then, to reach a final diagnosis of Burkitt's lymphoma, immunohistochemical stainings should provide evidence that lymphomatous cells express CD19, CD20, CD10, and CD79a and no CD3, CD5, Bcl2, and

TdT [37, 38]. Additional diagnostic criteria for Burkitt's lymphoma include Ki67 positivity/proliferation index > 90%, light chain restriction, nuclear c-myc positivity at immunocytochemistry, and t(8;14)(q24;q32) by fluorescence in situ hybridization [38], as reported by [9, 11, 16, 17, 21–23] (Table 1).

Core needle biopsy (CNB) is an exam that is not routinely performed in the work-up of patients with thyroid nodules. This is ascribed to higher cost, technical requirements, and concerns about potential complications as compared to FNA [39]. In addition, also CNB can fail to diagnose follicular carcinomas [40], whose presence is diagnosed based on vascular invasion and/or capsular breakthrough [39]. Consistent with these issues, the AACE/ACE/AME guidelines suggest considering the use of CNB only in solid nodules with persistently inadequate cytology [6], and the ATA guidelines do not even recommend its use [2]. Nevertheless, our case reminds that CNB should not be dismissed as it can become extremely useful in cases of thyroid lymphomas, where it allows to obtain a specimen that is adequate for histological/morphological tissue analysis, as well as for other key diagnostic tests. This is supported also by our literature review showing that CNB (but no FNA) was able to provide the final diagnosis without additional exams [9, 11, 16, 17, 21–23] (Table 1). In particular, in the 23 reports of Burkitt's lymphoma, FNA cytology was performed in 12 patients (52%) and was able to provide the diagnosis without core needle or open surgical biopsy only in one case [12] (Table 1). Overall, in the reported cases of thyroid Burkitt's lymphoma, diagnosis was provided by core needle biospy (43%; 10 cases out of 23), open surgery (35%; 8 cases out of 23), incisional/open wedge biopsy (17%; 4 cases out of 23), rarely by FNA (1 case out of 23) [12] or biopsy of other sites of involvement, such as a renal mass (1 cases out of 23) [10] (Table 1).

In line with the concept that CNB should be the advised modality for thyroid lymphoma diagnosis, Sharma and colleagues have recently shown that CNB diagnostic sensitivity for detecting thyroid lymphomas is 93% [41]. This is in line with the results of Ha and colleagues, who found that CNB sensitivity for thyroid lymphoma was 94.7% with a positive predictive value of 100%, such that CNB was able to significantly reduce the rate of diagnostic surgery from 37.9 to 5.3%, as compared to FNA [7]. Interestingly, in a work comparing CNB to open surgical biopsy in patients with lymphoadenopathies, CNB turned out to have greater sensitivity for detecting malignancy, and it was also faster, cheaper and safer than the conventional surgical approach [42].

Having said that, current treatment of Burkitt's lymphoma in adults is based on the delivery of short-duration, dose-intensive, multi-agent chemotherapy with minimization of treatment delays, and maintenance of serum drug concentrations over at least 48 to 72 h [35]. Some protocols, like the French LMB, the German BFM, and the CODOX-M/IVAC [43], have been adapted from pediatric regimens. Others, such the Hyper-CVAD regimen [44], which is the one we used, have been evaluated primarily in adults, but incorporate the principles found to be effective in pediatric populations [35]. Overall, with these regimens, 65 to 100% of patients achieve a complete response and 47 to 86% of patients maintain these remissions at least 1 year after treatment completion [35].

Conclusions

This case describes a patient with thyroid Burkitt's lymphoma, which is a rare and highly aggressive thyroid malignancy that requires a prompt diagnosis in order to start as soon as possible life-saving multi-agent chemotherapy. In particular, our case highlights the usefulness of CNB for the diagnosis of thyroid lymphomas and reminds clinicians to order/perform it in any patient with a rapidly enlarging thyroid mass that is suspicious for lymphoma.

Abbreviations
AACE/ACE/AME: American association of clinical endocrinologists/Association of clinical endocrinologists/Associazione medici endocrinologi; ATA: American thyroid association; BFM: Berlin-Frankfurt-Münster; CNB: core needle biopsy; CODOX-M/IVAC: cyclophosphamide, vincristine, doxorubicin, high-dose methotrexate/ifosfamide, etoposide, and high-dose cytarabine; CVAD: cyclophosphamide, vincristine, doxorubicin, and dexamethasone; FNA: fine needle biopsy; FT3: free triiodothyronine; FT4: free thyroxine; LMB: lymphoma malignancy B; TSH: thyroid stimulating hormone

Acknowledgments
Not applicable.

Funding
No funding was received for this study.

Authors' contributions
SB, BF examined the patient and contributed to manuscript conception, preparation, and editing. AM contributed to manuscript preparation and editing. DB and FZ performed the tissue sections readings, and contributed to image preparation and manuscript editing. VC examined the patient and contributed to manuscript editing. GP examined the patient and contributed to manuscript preparation and editing. All authors read and approved the final manuscript.

Competing interests
The authors declare that they have no competing interests.

Author details

[1]Department of Medical Surgical and Health Sciences, Università degli Studi di Trieste, Cattinara Teaching Hospital, Strada di Fiume 447, 34149 Trieste, Italy. [2]Endocrinology Unit - Azienda Sanitaria Universitaria Integrata Trieste, Cattinara Teaching Hospital, Strada di Fiume 447, 34149 Trieste, Italy. [3]Pathology Unit - Azienda Sanitaria Universitaria Integrata Trieste, Cattinara Teaching Hospital, Strada di Fiume 447, 34149 Trieste, Italy. [4]Haematology Unit - Azienda Sanitaria Universitaria Integrata Trieste, Cattinara Teaching Hospital, Strada di Fiume 447, 34149 Trieste, Italy.

References

1. Tan GH, Gharib H. Thyroid incidentalomas: management approaches to nonpalpable nodules discovered incidentally on thyroid imaging. Ann Intern Med. 1997;126(3):226–31.
2. Haugen BR, Alexander EK, Bible KC, Doherty GM, Mandel SJ, Nikiforov YE, Pacini F, Randolph GW, Sawka AM, Schlumberger M, et al. 2015 American Thyroid Association management guidelines for adult patients with thyroid nodules and differentiated thyroid Cancer the American Thyroid Association guidelines task force on thyroid nodules and differentiated thyroid Cancer. Thyroid. 2016;26(1):1–133.
3. Witt BL, Schmidt RL. Rapid onsite evaluation improves the adequacy of fine-needle aspiration for thyroid lesions: a systematic review and meta-analysis. Thyroid. 2013;23(4):428–35.
4. Burman KD, Wartofsky L. CLINICAL PRACTICE. *Thyroid Nodules N Engl J Med.* 2015;373(24):2347–56.
5. Frates MC, Benson CB, Charboneau JW, Cibas ES, Clark OH, Coleman BG, Cronan JJ, Doubilet PM, Evans DB, Goellner JR, et al. Management of thyroid nodules detected at US: Society of Radiologists in ultrasound consensus conference statement. Radiology. 2005;237(3):794–800.
6. Gharib H, Papini E, Garber JR, Duick DS, Harrell RM, Hegedus L, Paschke R, Valcavi R, Vitti P. No AAATFT: American Association of Clinical Endocrinologists, American College of Endocrinology, and Associazione Medici Endocrinologi medical guidelines for clinical Practice for the diagnosis and Management of Thyroid Nodules-2016 update. Endocr Pract. 2016;22:1–60.
7. Ha EJ, Baek JH, Lee JH, Kim JK, Song DE, Kim WB, Hong SJ. Core needle biopsy could reduce diagnostic surgery in patients with anaplastic thyroid cancer or thyroid lymphoma. Eur Radiol. 2016;26(4):1031–6.
8. Graff-Baker A, Sosa JA, Roman SA. Primary thyroid lymphoma: a review of recent developments in diagnosis and histology-driven treatment. Curr Opin Oncol. 2010;22(1):17–22.
9. Thieblemont C, Mayer A, Dumontet C, Barbier Y, Callet-Bauchu E, Felman P, Berger F, Ducottet X, Martin C, Salles G, et al. Primary thyroid lymphoma is a heterogeneous disease. J Clin Endocrinol Metab. 2002;87(1):105–11.
10. Iqbal Y, Al-Sudairy R, Abdullah MF, Al-Omari A, Crankson S. Non-Hodgkin lymphoma manifesting as thyroid nodules and cardiac involvement. J Pediatr Hematol Oncol. 2003;25(12):987–8.
11. Ruggiero FP, Frauenhoffer E, Stack BC Jr. Thyroid lymphoma: a single institution's experience. Otolaryngol Head Neck Surg. 2005;133(6):888–96.
12. Kalinyak JE, Kong CS, McDougall IR. Burkitt's lymphoma presenting as a rapidly growing thyroid mass. Thyroid. 2006;16(10):1053–7.
13. Camera A, Magri F, Fonte R, Villani L, Della Porta MG, Fregoni V, Manna LL, Chiovato L. Burkitt-like lymphoma infiltrating a hyperfunctioning thyroid adenoma and presenting as a hot nodule. Thyroid. 2010;20(9):1033–6.
14. Kandil E, Safah H, Noureldine S, Abdel Khalek M, Waddadar J, Goswami M, Friedlander P. Burkitt-like lymphoma arising in the thyroid gland. Am J Med Sci. 2012;343(1):103–5.
15. Yildiz I, Sen F, Toz B, Kilic L, Agan M, Basaran M. Primary Burkitt's lymphoma presenting as a rapidly growing thyroid mass. Case Rep Oncol. 2012;5(2):388–93.
16. Bongiovanni M, Mazzucchelli L, Martin V, Crippa S, Bolli M, Suriano S, Giovanella L. Images in endocrine pathology: a starry-sky in the thyroid. Endocr Pathol. 2012;23(1):79–81.
17. Mweempwa A, Prasad J, Islam S. A rare neoplasm of the thyroid gland. N Z Med J. 2013;126(1369):75–8.
18. Albert S. Primary Burkitt lymphoma of the thyroid. Ear Nose Throat J. 2013;92(12):E1–2.
19. Zhang L, Gao L, Liu G, Wang L, Xu C, Li L, Tian Y, Feng H, Guo Z. Primary Burkitt's lymphoma of the thyroid without Epstein-Barr virus infection: a case report and literature review. Oncol Lett. 2014;7(5):1519–24.
20. Cooper K, Gangadharan A, Arora RS, Shukla R, Pizer B. Burkitt lymphoma of thyroid gland in an adolescent. Case Rep Pediatr. 2014;2014:187467.
21. Allaoui M, Benchafai I, Mahtat el M, Regragui S, Boudhas A, Azzakhmam M, Boukhechba M, Al Bouzidi A, Oukabli M. Primary Burkitt lymphoma of the thyroid gland: case report of an exceptional type of thyroid neoplasm and review of the literature. BMC Clin Pathol. 2016;16:6.
22. Quesada AE, Liu H, Miranda RN, Golardi N, Billah S, Medeiros LJ, Jaso JM. Burkitt lymphoma presenting as a mass in the thyroid gland: a clinicopathologic study of 7 cases and review of the literature. Hum Pathol. 2016;56:101–8.
23. Akshintala D, Paturi BT, Liu J, Emani VK. A rare diagnosis of a thyroid mass. Am J Med. 2016;129(9):e191–2.
24. Moghaddasi M, Nabovvati M, Razmeh S. Bilateral cavernous sinus thrombosis as first manifestation of primary Burkitt lymphoma of the thyroid gland. Neurol Int. 2017;9(2):7133.
25. Garcia Calzado MC, Ruiz Buendia A, Lopez Aranda JF, Martin Villacanas JA: [Burkitt's lymphoma with onset in the thyroid gland. A case report]. *Med Clin (Barc)* 1997, 108(14):556–557.
26. Hernandez JA, Reth P, Ballestar E. primary thyroid lymphoma with bone marrow and central nervous system infiltration at presentation. Med Clin (Barc). 2001;116(9):357–8.
27. Duran HJ, Diaz-Morfa M, Garcia-Parrenoa J, Bellon JM. Burkitt's lymphoma affecting only the thyroid. Med Clin (Barc). 2008;131(1):38–9.
28. Pereyra Zenklusen A, Burgesser MV. thyroid Burkitt lymphoma. Rev Fac Cien Med Univ Nac Cordoba. 2011;68(2):70–1.
29. Bouges S, Daures JP, Hebrard M. incidence of acute leukemias, lymphomas and thyroid cancers in children under 15 years, living around the Marcoule nuclear site from 1985 to 1995. Rev Epidemiol Sante Publique. 1999;47(3):205–17.
30. Mongalgi MA, Chakroun D, el Bez M, Boussen H, Debabbi A. thyroid goiter revealing Burkitt's lymphoma. Arch Fr Pediatr. 1992;49(6):594–5.
31. Matsuo T, Murase K, Wago M, Matsuo S, Ikeda T, Yamaguchi T. acute B-cell lymphoblastic leukemia with Burkitt's lyphoma cells--a case report. Gan No Rinsho. 1983;29(9):1035–9.
32. Fujii H, Maekawa T, Kamezaki H, Ohno H, Nishida K, Urata Y. Burkitt's lymphoma with an initial symptom of thyroid tumor during pregnancy. Rinsho Ketsueki. 1986;27(10):1957–63.
33. Molyneux EM, Rochford R, Griffin B, Newton R, Jackson G, Menon G, Harrison CJ, Israels T, Bailey S. Burkitt's lymphoma. Lancet. 2012;379(9822):1234–44.
34. Graff-Baker A, Roman SA, Thomas DC, Udelsman R, Sosa JA. Prognosis of primary thyroid lymphoma: demographic, clinical, and pathologic predictors of survival in 1,408 cases. Surgery. 2009;146(6):1105–15.
35. Blum KA, Lozanski G, Byrd JC. Adult Burkitt leukemia and lymphoma. Blood. 2004;104(10):3009–20.
36. Stein SA, Wartofsky L. Primary thyroid lymphoma: a clinical review. J Clin Endocrinol Metab. 2013;98(8):3131–8.
37. Naresh KN, Ibrahim HA, Lazzi S, Rince P, Onorati M, Ambrosio MR, Bilhou-Nabera C, Amen F, Reid A, Mawanda M, et al. Diagnosis of Burkitt lymphoma using an algorithmic approach--applicable in both resource-poor and resource-rich countries. Br J Haematol. 2011;154(6):770–6.
38. Zeppa P, Cozzolino I. Non-Hodgkin lymphoma. Monogr Clin Cytol. 2018;23:34–51.
39. Paja M, del Cura JL, Zabala R, Corta I, Lizarraga A, Oleaga A, Exposito A, Gutierrez MT, Ugalde A, Lopez JI. Ultrasound-guided core-needle biopsy in thyroid nodules. A study of 676 consecutive cases with surgical correlation. Eur Radiol. 2016;26(1):1–8.
40. Yoon JH, Kim EK, Kwak JY, Moon HJ. Effectiveness and limitations of core needle biopsy in the diagnosis of thyroid nodules: review of current literature. J Pathol Transl Med. 2015;49(3):230–5.
41. Sharma A, Jasim S, Reading CC, Ristow KM, Villasboas Bisneto JC, Habermann TM, Fatourechi V, Stan M. Clinical presentation and diagnostic challenges of thyroid lymphoma: a cohort study. Thyroid. 2016;26(8):1061–7.
42. Pugliese N, Di Perna M, Cozzolino I, Ciancia G, Pettinato G, Zeppa P, Varone V, Masone S, Cerchione C, Della Pepa R, et al. Randomized comparison of power Doppler ultrasonography-guided core-needle biopsy with open surgical biopsy for the characterization of lymphadenopathies in patients with suspected lymphoma. Ann Hematol. 2017;96(4):627–37.
43. Oosten LEM, Chamuleau MED, Thielen FW, de Wreede LC, Siemes C, Doorduijn JK, Smeekes OS, Kersten MJ, Hardi L, Baars JW, et al. Treatment of sporadic Burkitt lymphoma in adults, a retrospective comparison of four treatment regimens. Ann Hematol. 2018;97(2):255–66.

Permissions

The contributors of this book come from diverse backgrounds, making this book a truly international effort. This book will bring forth new frontiers with its revolutionizing research information and detailed analysis of the nascent developments around the world.

We would like to thank all the contributing authors for lending their expertise to make the book truly unique. They have played a crucial role in the development of this book. Without their invaluable contributions this book wouldn't have been possible. They have made vital efforts to compile up to date information on the varied aspects of this subject to make this book a valuable addition to the collection of many professionals and students.

This book was conceptualized with the vision of imparting up-to-date information and advanced data in this field. To ensure the same, a matchless editorial board was set up. Every individual on the board went through rigorous rounds of assessment to prove their worth. After which they invested a large part of their time researching and compiling the most relevant data for our readers.

The editorial board has been involved in producing this book since its inception. They have spent rigorous hours researching and exploring the diverse topics which have resulted in the successful publishing of this book. They have passed on their knowledge of decades through this book. To expedite this challenging task, the publisher supported the team at every step. A small team of assistant editors was also appointed to further simplify the editing procedure and attain best results for the readers.

Apart from the editorial board, the designing team has also invested a significant amount of their time in understanding the subject and creating the most relevant covers. They scrutinized every image to scout for the most suitable representation of the subject and create an appropriate cover for the book.

The publishing team has been an ardent support to the editorial, designing and production team. Their endless efforts to recruit the best for this project, has resulted in the accomplishment of this book. They are a veteran in the field of academics and their pool of knowledge is as vast as their experience in printing. Their expertise and guidance has proved useful at every step. Their uncompromising quality standards have made this book an exceptional effort. Their encouragement from time to time has been an inspiration for everyone.

The publisher and the editorial board hope that this book will prove to be a valuable piece of knowledge for researchers, students, practitioners and scholars across the globe.

List of Contributors

Zhihua Zuo and Yibing Lu
Department of Endocrinology, The Second Affiliated Hospital of Nanjing Medical University, 125 Jiangjiayuan Road, Nanjing 211166, China

Bin Song
Department of Endocrinology, The Second Affiliated Hospital of Nanjing Medical University, 125 Jiangjiayuan Road, Nanjing 211166, China
Department of Endocrinology, Clinical Medical College, Yangzhou University, 98 Nantong West Road, Yangzhou 225001, China

Juan Tan
Department of Gerontology, Huai'an First People's Hospital, Nanjing Medical University, 6 Beijing West Road, Huai'an 223300, China

Jianjin Guo
Department of Endocrinology, Second Hospital of Shanxi Medical University, 382 Wuyi Road, Taiyuan 030001, China

Weiping Teng
Department of Endocrinology and Metabolism, The First Hospital of China Medical University, 155 Nanjing Road, Shenyang 110001, China

Chao Liu
Endocrine and Diabetes Center, Affiliated Hospital of Integrated Traditional Chinese and Western Medicine, Nanjing University of Chinese Medicine, 8 Huadian East Road, Nanjing 210028, China

Leonardo de Andrade Mesquita, Luciana Pavan Antoniolli and Giordano Fabricio Cittolin-Santos
Faculdade de Medicina da Universidade Federal do Rio Grande do Sul, Ramiro Barcelos, 2400, Porto Alegre 90035-003, Brazil

Fernando Gerchman
Faculdade de Medicina da Universidade Federal do Rio Grande do Sul, Ramiro Barcelos, 2400, Porto Alegre 90035-003, Brazil
Serviço de Endocrinologia do Hospital de Clínicas de Porto Alegre, Ramiro Barcelos, 2350, Porto Alegre 90035-903, Brazil

Yuan-yuan Wang, Hui-min Ying, Hui-li Li and Fang Tian
Department of Endocrinology, Xixi Hospital of Hangzhou, Hangzhou, Hangzhou 315000, Zhejiang Province, China

Shuang-fei Hu, Long Chen and Zhen-feng Zhou
Department of Anesthesiology, Zhejiang Provincial People's Hospital (People's Hospital of Hangzhou Medicine College), Hangzhou 315000, China

Chun-Lin Liu
Graduate Institute of Medicine, College of Medicine, Kaohsiung Medical University, No. 100, Shih-Chuan 1st Road, Kaohsiung 80708, Taiwan
Calo Psychiatric Center, No.12-200, Jinhua Rd., Xinpi Township, Pingtung County 925, Taiwan

Ching-Kuan Liu
Graduate Institute of Medicine, College of Medicine, Kaohsiung Medical University, No. 100, Shih-Chuan 1st Road, Kaohsiung 80708, Taiwan
Department of Neurology, Kaohsiung Medical University Hospital, Kaohsiung Medical University, No. 100, Shih-Chuan 1st Road, Kaohsiung 80708, Taiwan

Shang-Jyh Hwang
Graduate Institute of Medicine, College of Medicine, Kaohsiung Medical University, No. 100, Shih-Chuan 1st Road, Kaohsiung 80708, Taiwan
Department of Renal Care, College of Medicine, Kaohsiung Medical University, No. 100, Shih-Chuan 1st Road, Kaohsiung 80708, Taiwan
Division of Nephrology, Department of Internal Medicine, Kaohsiung Medical University Hospital, Kaohsiung Medical University, No. 100, Shih-Chuan 1st Road, Kaohsiung 80708, Taiwan
Institute of Population Health Sciences, National Health Research Institutes, No. 35 Keyan Road, Zhunan, Miaoli 35053, Taiwan

Ming-Tsang Wu
Graduate Institute of Medicine, College of Medicine, Kaohsiung Medical University, No. 100, Shih-Chuan 1st Road, Kaohsiung 80708, Taiwan
Research Center for Environmental Medicine, Kaohsiung Medical University, No. 100, Shih-Chuan 1st Road, Kaohsiung 80708, Taiwan
Department of Public Health, Kaohsiung Medical University, No. 100, Shih-Chuan 1st Road, Kaohsiung 80708, Taiwan
Graduate Institute of Clinical Medicine, Kaohsiung Medical University, No. 100, Shih-Chuan 1st Road, Kaohsiung 80708, Taiwan

Ming-Yen Lin
Department of Renal Care, College of Medicine, Kaohsiung Medical University, No. 100, Shih-Chuan 1st Road, Kaohsiung 80708, Taiwan

Division of Nephrology, Department of Internal Medicine, Kaohsiung Medical University Hospital, Kaohsiung Medical University, No. 100, Shih-Chuan 1st Road, Kaohsiung 80708, Taiwan

Huei-Lan Lee
Division of Nephrology, Department of Internal Medicine, Kaohsiung Medical University Hospital, Kaohsiung Medical University, No. 100, Shih-Chuan 1st Road, Kaohsiung 80708, Taiwan

Mei Lyn Tan, Jo-Anne Manski-Nankervis, Sharmala Thuraisingam and John Furler
Department of General Practice, University of Melbourne, Level 1, 200 Berkeley St, Carlton, VIC 3010, Australia

Alicia Jenkins
NHMRC Clinical Trials Centre, University of Sydney, Levels 4-6 Medical Foundation Building, 92-94 Parramatta Rd, Camperdown, NSW 2050, Australia

David O'Neal
Department of Medicine, St Vincent's Hospital, The University of Melbourne, Level 4, Clinical Sciences Building, 29 Regent St, Fitzroy, VIC 3065, Australia

Jianran Sun, Cancan Hui, Tongjia Xia, Min Xu, Datong Deng and Youmin Wang
Department of Endocrinology, Institute of Endocrinology and Metabolism, The First Affiliated Hospital of Anhui Medical University, 218 Jixi Road, Hefei 230022, Anhui, China

Faming Pan
Department of Epidemiology and Biostatistics, School of Public Health, Anhui Medical University, 81Meishan Road, Hefei 230032, Anhui, China

Risa Ozaki, Ronald C. W. Ma, Alice P. S. Kong, Francis C. C. Chow and Juliana C. N. Chan
Department of Medicine and Therapeutics, The Chinese University of Hong Kong, Shatin, Hong Kong
Li Ka Shing Institute of Health Science, The Chinese University of Hong Kong, Prince of Wales Hospital, Shatin, Hong Kong

Andrea O. Y. Luk
Department of Medicine and Therapeutics, The Chinese University of Hong Kong, Shatin, Hong Kong
Li Ka Shing Institute of Health Science, The Chinese University of Hong Kong, Prince of Wales Hospital, Shatin, Hong Kong
Diabetes and Endocrine Research Centre, The Prince of Wales Hospital, Shatin, New Territories, Hong Kong

Benny C. Y. Zee and Marc Chong
School of Public Health and Primary Care, The Chinese University of Hong Kong, Prince of wales Hospital, Shatin, Hong Kong

Carl W. Rausch
Boston Therapeutics Inc., 354 Merrimack Street #4, Lawrence, MA 01843, USA

Michael H. M. Chan
Department of Chemical Pathology, The Chinese University of Hong Kong, Prince of Wales Hospital, Shatin, Hong Kong

Huiying Shi, Chaoqun Han, Ding Zhen and Rong Lin
Department of Gastroenterology, Union Hospital, Tongji Medical College, Huazhong University of Science and Technology, Wuhan 430022, China

Qin Zhang
Department of Pathology, Union Hospital, Tongji Medical College, Huazhong University of Science and Technology, Wuhan 430022, China

Ziyan Zhang and Jianlin Zhang
Department of Biochemistry and Molecular Biology, Shanxi Medical University, Taiyuan, No.56, Xinjian South Road, Taiyuan, Shanxi 030001, People's Republic of China

Lingxia Zhao and Xuemei Fan
Department of Biochemistry and Molecular Biology, Shanxi Medical University, Taiyuan, No.56, Xinjian South Road, Taiyuan, Shanxi 030001, People's Republic of China
Department of Endocrinology Medicine, Dayi Hospital Affiliated to Shanxi Medical University, Taiyuan, Shanxi 030032, People's Republic of China

Guoping Zheng
Department of Biochemistry and Molecular Biology, Shanxi Medical University, Taiyuan, No.56, Xinjian South Road, Taiyuan, Shanxi 030001, People's Republic of China
Centre for Transplantation and Renal Research, University of Sydney at Westmead Millennium Institute, Sydney, NSW 2145, Australia

Guangxia Xi
Department of Endocrinology Medicine, Dayi Hospital Affiliated to Shanxi Medical University, Taiyuan, Shanxi 030032, People's Republic of China

Lin Zuo
Department of Physiology, Shanxi Medical University, Taiyuan, Shanxi 030001, People's Republic of China

Qiang Guo
Department of Medical Statistics, School of Public Health of Shanxi Medical University, Taiyuan, Shanxi 030001, People's Republic of China

Xiaole Su
Renal Division, Shanxi Medical University Second Hospital, Shanxi Kidney Disease Institute, Taiyuan, Shanxi 030001, People's Republic of China

S. P. Vibha, Muralidhar M. Kulkarni and A. B. Kirthinath Ballala
Department of Community Medicine, Kasturba Medical College, Manipal Academy of Higher Education, Manipal, Karnataka 576104, India

Asha Kamath
Department of Statistics, Prasanna School of Public Health, Manipal Academy of Higher Education, Manipal, Karnataka 576104, India

G. Arun Maiya
Department of Physiotherapy, School of Allied Health Sciences, Manipal Academy of Higher Education, Manipal, Karnataka 576104, India

Sharon D. Yeatts, Renee' H. Martin, Anbesaw Selassie and Marvella E. Ford
Department of Public Health Sciences, Medical University of South Carolina, Charleston, SC, USA

Colleen Bauza
Department of Public Health Sciences, Medical University of South Carolina, Charleston, SC, USA
Department of Health Informatics, Johns Hopkins All Children's Hospital, 601 5th Street South, Suite 707, St. Petersburg, FL 33701, USA

Keith Borg
Department of Emergency Medicine, Medical University of South Carolina, Charleston, SC, USA

Gayenell Magwood
Department of Nursing, Medical University of South Carolina, Charleston, SC, USA

Miso Jang
Department of Family Medicine and Center for Cancer Prevention and Detection, Hospital, National Cancer Center, 323, Ilsan-ro, Ilsandong, Goyang-si, Gyeonggi-do 10408, Republic of Korea

Hyunkyung Kim
Department of Family Medicine, DDH Hospital, 60, Hi park 2-ro, Ilsanseo-gu, Goyang-si, Gyeonggi-do 10234, Republic of Korea

Shorry Lea
Center for Health Promotion, Cheil General Hospital, 17, Seoae-ro 1-gil, Jung-gu, Seoul 04619, Republic of Korea

Sohee Oh
Department of Biostatistics, SMG-SNU Boramae Medical Center, 20, Boramae-ro 5-gil, Dongjak-gu, Seoul 07061, Republic of Korea

Jong Seung Kim and Bumjo Oh
Department of Family Medicine, SMG-SNU Boramae Medical Center, 20, Boramae-ro 5-gil, Dongjak-gu, Seoul 07061, Republic of Korea

Hua-Pin Chang
Department of Nursing, Asia University, Taichung, Taiwan
Department of Nursing, Asia University Hospital, Taichung, Taiwan

Shun-Fa Yang
Institute of Medicine, Chung Shan Medical University, Taichung, Taiwan
Department of Medical Research, Chung Shan Medical University Hospital, Taichung, Taiwan

Shu-Li Wang
National Institute of Environmental Health Sciences, Zhuman, Taiwan
The Department of Public Health, China Medical University, Taichung, Taiwan

Pen-Hua Su
Department of Pediatrics, Chung Shan Medical University Hospital, Taichung, Taiwan
School of Medicine, Chung Shan Medical University, Number 110, Section 1, Chien-Kou North Road, Taichung 402, Taiwan

Natalie Terens
Trenton Health Team, Trenton, New Jersey, USA

Simona Vecchi, Anna Maria Bargagli, Nera Agabiti, Zuzana Mitrova, Laura Amato and Marina Davoli
Department of Epidemiology, Lazio Region- ASL Rome1, Rome, Italy

Francesca Sassi, Ilaria Buondonno, Chiara Luppi, Elena Spertino, Emanuela Stratta, Marco Di Stefano, Marco Ravazzoli, Giovanni Carlo Isaia and Patrizia D'Amelio
Department of Medical Science, Gerontology and Bone Metabolic Diseases, University of Torino, Corso Bramante 88/90, 10126 Torino, Italy

Marina Trento, Pietro Passera and Massimo Porta
Department of Medical Science, Internal Medicine, University of Torino, Torino, Italy

Gianluca Isaia
Geriatric Division, University of Turin, San Luigi Gonzaga Hospital, Orbassano, Turin, Italy

Koichi Yabiku
Division of Endocrinology, Diabetes and Metabolism, Hematology, Rheumatology (Second Department of Internal Medicine), Graduate School of Medicine, University of the Ryukyus, 207 Uehara, Nishihara, Okinawa 903-0215, Japan

Keiko Nakamoto
GenomIdea Incorporated, Okinawa, Japan

Akihiro Tokushige
Clinical Pharmacology and Therapeutics University of the Ryukyus School of Medicine, Okinawa, Japan

Mohammed J. Alramadan, Afsana Afroz and Baki Billah
Department of Epidemiology and Preventive Medicine, School of Public Health and Preventive Medicine, Monash University, Melbourne, Australia

Dianna J. Magliano
Department of Epidemiology and Preventive Medicine, School of Public Health and Preventive Medicine, Monash University, Melbourne, Australia
Baker Heart and Diabetes Institute, Melbourne, VIC, Australia

Turky H. Almigbal and Mohammed Ali Batais
College of Medicine, King Saud University, Riyadh, Saudi Arabia

Hesham J. Alramadhan
College of Medicine, King Faisal University, Al-Ahsa, Saudi Arabia

Waad Faozi Mahfoud
Ibn Sina National College, Jeddah, Saudi Arabia

Adel Mehmas Alragas
Medical City - King Saud University, Riyadh, Saudi Arabia

Romildo Luiz Monteiro Andrade
University Hospital Cassiano Antônio de Moraes (HUCAM) of the Federal, University of Espírito Santo (UFES), Vitória-ES, Brazil
Post-Graduate Program in Epidemiology, Federal University of Pelotas (UFPel), Pelotas-RS, Brazil
Vitória, Brazil

Denise P. Gigante, Isabel Oliveira de Oliveira and Bernardo Lessa Horta
Post-Graduate Program in Epidemiology, Federal University of Pelotas (UFPel), Pelotas-RS, Brazil

Elena Chertok Shacham, Hila Kfir and Avraham Ishay
Endocrinology Unit, Haemek Medical Center, Rabin Ave 21, Afula, Israel, 18134 Afula, Israel

Naama Schwartz
Statistics Department, Haemek Medical Center, Afula, Israel

Miguel Ángel Gómez-Sámano, Lucía Palacios-Báez, Daniel Cuevas-Ramos and Francisco Javier Gomez-Perez
Department of Endocrinology and Metabolism, Instituto Nacional de Ciencias Medicas y Nutricion Salvador Zubiran, Vasco de Quiroga #15, Sección XVI Tlalpan, 14000 Mexico City, Mexico

Jorge Enrique Baquerizo-Burgos, Melissa Fabiola Coronel Coronel and Buileng Daniela Wong-Campoverde
Universidad Catolica de Santiago de Guayaquil, Av. Carlos Julio Arosemena Km. 1½ vía Daule, Guayaquil, Ecuador

Fernando Villanueva-Martinez
Department of Internal Medicine, Hospital San Angel Inn, Av Chapultepec 489, Juárez, 06600 Mexico City, Mexico

Diego Molina-Botello
Universidad Anahuac Mexico Sur, Av. de las Torres No. 131, Alvaro Obregon, Olivar de los padres, 01780 Mexico City, Mexico

Jose Alonso Avila-Rojo
Universidad Autonoma de Baja California, Campus Mexicali, Av. Alvaro Obregon y Julian Carrillo S/N, Colonia Nueva, 21100 Mexicali, B.C, Mexico

Alejandro Zentella-Dehesa
Department of Biochemistry, Instituto Nacional de Ciencias Medicas y Nutricion Salvador Zubiran, Vasco de Quiroga #15, Sección XVI Tlalpan, 14000 Mexico City, Mexico

Álvaro Aguayo-González
Department of Hematology, Instituto Nacional de Ciencias Medicas y Nutricion Salvador Zubiran, Vasco de Quiroga #15, Sección XVI Tlalpan, 14000 Mexico City, Mexico

Alfonso Gulias-Herrero
Department of Internal Medicine, Instituto Nacional de Ciencias Medicas y Nutricion Salvador Zubiran, Vasco de Quiroga #15, Sección XVI Tlalpan, 14000 Mexico City, Mexico

Xiu Zhao, Zhe Su, Xia Liu, LiWang and Lili Pan
Department of Endocrinology, Shenzhen Children's Hospital, 7019# Yitian Road, Futian District, Shenzhen 518038, Guangdong Province, China

Jianming Song
Pathology Department, Shenzhen Children's Hospital, Shenzhen 518038, China

Yungen Gan
Radiology Department, Shenzhen Children's Hospital, Shenzhen 518038, China

Pengqiang Wen
Pediatrics Research Institute, Shenzhen Children's Hospital, Shenzhen 518038, China

Shoulin Li
Department of Urology, Shenzhen Children's Hospital, Shenzhen 518038, China

Jing Li, Liming Wang, Fen Chen, Dongxia Xia and Lingling Miao
Department of Endocrinology, The Affiliated Hospital of Medical School of Ningbo University, Zhejiang, China

Anjali Gopalan
Division of Research, Kaiser Permanente Northern California, 2000 Broadway, Oakland, CA 94612, USA
Michael J. Crescenz VA Medical Center, 3900 Woodland Ave, Philadelphia, PA 19104, USA

Marilyn M. Schapira
Michael J. Crescenz VA Medical Center, 3900 Woodland Ave, Philadelphia, PA 19104, USA
Division of General Internal Medicine, The Perelman School of Medicine at the University of Pennsylvania, 3400 Civic Center Blvd, Philadelphia, PA 19104, USA

Katherine Kellom
Policy Lab, The Children's Hospital of Philadelphia, 3401 Civic Center Blvd, Philadelphia, PA 19104, USA

Kevin McDonough
Division of General Internal Medicine, The Perelman School of Medicine at the University of Pennsylvania, 3400 Civic Center Blvd, Philadelphia, PA 19104, USA

Kuang-Hsing Chiang
Division of Cardiology and Cardiovascular Research Center, Department of Internal Medicine, Taipei Medical University Hospital, Taipei, Taiwan
Graduate Institute of Biomedical Electronics and Bioinformatics, National Taiwan University, Taipei, Taiwan

Po-Hsun Huang
Division of Cardiology, Department of Internal Medicine, Taipei Veterans General Hospital, Taipei, Taiwan
Cardiovascular Research Center, National Yang-Ming University, Taipei, Taiwan
Institute of Clinical Medicine, National Yang-Ming University, Taipei, Taiwan

Jaw-Wen Chen
Division of Cardiology, Department of Internal Medicine, Taipei Veterans General Hospital, Taipei, Taiwan
Department of Medical Research and Education, Taipei Veterans General Hospital, Taipei, Taiwan
Cardiovascular Research Center, National Yang-Ming University, Taipei, Taiwan
Institute of Pharmacology, National Yang-Ming University, Taipei, Taiwan

Shao-Sung Huang and Hsin-Bang Leu
Division of Cardiology, Department of Internal Medicine, Taipei Veterans General Hospital, Taipei, Taiwan
Cardiovascular Research Center, National Yang-Ming University, Taipei, Taiwan
Healthcare and Service Center, Taipei Veterans General Hospital, Taipei, Taiwan
Institute of Clinical Medicine, National Yang-Ming University, Taipei, Taiwan

Shing-Jong Lin
Division of Cardiology, Department of Internal Medicine, Taipei Veterans General Hospital, Taipei, Taiwan
Department of Medical Research and Education, Taipei Veterans General Hospital, Taipei, Taiwan
Cardiovascular Research Center, National Yang-Ming University, Taipei, Taiwan
Institute of Clinical Medicine, National Yang-Ming University, Taipei, Taiwan
Department of Internal Medicine, School of Medicine, College of Medicine, Taipei Medical University, Taipei, Taiwan

Semi Hwang, Jung-eun Lim and Sun Ha Jee
Department of Epidemiology and Health Promotion, Institute for Health Promotion, Graduate School of Public Health, Yonsei University, 50-1 Yonsei-ro, Seodaemun-gu, Seoul 03722, Republic of Korea

Yoonjeong Choi
Department of Public Health, Graduate School, Yonsei University, Seoul, Republic of Korea.

David Rankin, Jeni Harden and Julia Lawton
The Usher Institute of Population Health Sciences and Informatics, University of Edinburgh, Edinburgh EH8 9AG, UK

Katharine Barnard
BHR Ltd, 42 Kilmiston Drive, Portchester, Fareham, Hants, PO16 8EG and Faculty of Health and Social Science, Bournemouth University, Royal London House, Bournemouth BH1 3LT, UK

Louise Bath and Kathryn Noyes
Royal Hospital for Sick Children, Sciennes Road, Edinburgh EH9 1LF, UK

John Stephen
Child Health Department, Borders General Hospital, Melrose TD6 9BS, UK

Elizabeth Kagotho, Geoffrey Omuse and Nancy Okinda
Department of Pathology, Aga Khan University Hospital Nairobi, Nairobi, Kenya

Peter Ojwang
Department of Pathology, Maseno University, Private Bag, Maseno, Kenya

Andrea Michelli
Department of Medical Surgical and Health Sciences, Università degli Studi di Trieste, Cattinara Teaching Hospital, Strada di Fiume 447, 34149 Trieste, Italy

Stella Bernardi and Bruno Fabris
Department of Medical Surgical and Health Sciences, Università degli Studi di Trieste, Cattinara Teaching Hospital, Strada di Fiume 447, 34149 Trieste, Italy Endocrinology Unit - Azienda Sanitaria Universitaria Integrata Trieste, Cattinara Teaching Hospital, Strada di Fiume 447, 34149 Trieste, Italy

Deborah Bonazza and Fabrizio Zanconati
Department of Medical Surgical and Health Sciences, Università degli Studi di Trieste, Cattinara Teaching Hospital, Strada di Fiume 447, 34149 Trieste, Italy Pathology Unit - Azienda Sanitaria Universitaria Integrata Trieste, Cattinara Teaching Hospital, Strada di Fiume 447, 34149 Trieste, Italy

Gabriele Pozzato
Department of Medical Surgical and Health Sciences, Università degli Studi di Trieste, Cattinara Teaching Hospital, Strada di Fiume 447, 34149 Trieste, Italy Haematology Unit - Azienda Sanitaria Universitaria Integrata Trieste, Cattinara Teaching Hospital, Strada di Fiume 447, 34149 Trieste, Italy

Veronica Calabrò
Endocrinology Unit - Azienda Sanitaria Universitaria Integrata Trieste, Cattinara Teaching Hospital, Strada di Fiume 447, 34149 Trieste, Italy

Index